Approved Abbreviations for Medications

Abbreviation	Meaning	Abbreviation	Meaning
$\bar{a}$	before	Write out	milliunit
ac	before meals	ml or mL	milliliter
ad lib	as desired; freely	NG, NGT	nasogastric
ADE	adverse drug event	NKA	no known allergies
AM, am	in the morning; before noon	NKDA	no known drug allergies
amp	ampule	NPO	nothing by mouth
aq	water	NS	normal saline
bid	twice a day	oz	ounce
BSA	body surface area	OTC	over the counter
C	Celsius	$\bar{p}$	after
$\bar{c}$	with	pc	after meals
cap or caps	capsule	PCA	patient-controlled analgesia
CD*	controlled dose	per	through, by (route)
comp	compound	per	each (math term)
CR*	controlled release	PO, po	by mouth
dil.	dilute	PM, pm	afternoon; evening
DS	double strength	prn	as needed; when necessary
elix	elixir	q	each, every
ext	external; extract	q2h, q4h, etc.	every 2 hours, every 4 hours, etc.
F	Fahrenheit	qs	as much as needed; quantity sufficient
fl. or fld	fluid	rep.	repeat
g	gram	Rx	give, treatment, prescription
gt, gtt	drop, drops	$\bar{s}$	without
h, hr	hour	SL, subl	sublingual (under the tongue)
ID	intradermal(ly)	sol. or soln.	solution
IM	intramuscular(ly)	SR*	sustained release
inj	injection	stat	immediately, at once
IV	intravenous(ly)	subcut	subcutaneous(ly)
IVPB	intravenous piggyback	supp	suppository
kg	kilogram	susp.	suspension
KVO	keep vein open	Syr	syrup
L	liter	tab	tablet
LA*	long acting	tbs., tbsp, or T	tablespoon
lb	pound	tid	three times a day
liq.	liquid	tinct	tincture
m	meter	TKO	to keep open
m^2	square meter	tsp	teaspoon
mcg	microgram	ung	ointment
mEq	milliequivalent	vag	vaginal
mg	milligram	XR*	extended release

CLINICAL ALERT!

*The manufacturer acronyms that follow medication names have caused confusion and errors. CD, CR, DR, E-R, LA, SA, SR, TR, XL, XR, XT all refer to various timed-release forms of the drug. They cannot be used interchangeably. Some need to be taken more than once a day; some tablets can be cut, others cannot. Double check the order and the acronym with a current drug reference and the patient medication history to protect the patient from a medication type or dose error.

Do NOT confuse DS—double strength—with other acronyms. DS pertains *only* to strength, not timing of release.

The Joint Commission's Official "Do Not Use" List

Official "Do Not Use" List[1]

Do Not Use	Potential Problem	Use Instead
U (unit)	Mistaken for "0" (zero), the number "4" (four) or "cc"	Write "unit"
IU (International Unit)	Mistaken for IV (intravenous) or the number 10 (ten)	Write "International Unit"
Q.D., QD, q.d., qd (daily) Q.O.D., QOD, q.o.d, qod (every other day)	Mistaken for each other Period after the Q mistaken for "I" and the "O" mistaken for "I"	Write "daily" Write "every other day"
Trailing zero (X.0 mg)* Lack of leading zero (.X mg)	Decimal point is missed	Write X mg Write 0.X mg
MS MSO_4 and $MgSO_4$	Can mean morphine sulfate or magnesium sulfate Confused for one another	Write "morphine sulfate" Write "magnesium sulfate"

[1] Applies to all orders and all medication-related documentation that is handwritten (including free-text computer entry) or on pre-printed forms.

***Exception:** A "trailing zero" may be used only where required to demonstrate the level of precision of the value being reported, such as for laboratory results, imaging studies that report size of lesions, or catheter/tube sizes. It may not be used in medication orders or other medication-related documentation.

Additional Abbreviations, Acronyms and Symbols

(For possible future inclusion in the Official "Do Not Use" List)

Do Not Use	Potential Problem	Use Instead
> (greater than) < (less than)	Misinterpreted as the number "7" (seven) or the letter "L" Confused for one another	Write "greater than" Write "less than"
Abbreviations for drug names	Misinterpreted due to similar abbreviations for multiple drugs	Write drug names in full
Apothecary units	Unfamiliar to many practitioners Confused with metric units	Use metric units
@	Mistaken for the number "2" (two)	Write "at"
cc	Mistaken for U (units) when poorly written	Write "mL" or "ml" or "milliliters" ("mL" is preferred)
µg	Mistaken for mg (milligrams) resulting in one thousand-fold overdose	Write "mcg" or "micrograms"

Institute for Safe Medication Practices (ISMP) List of Error-Prone Abbreviations, Symbols, and Dose Designations			
Abbreviation	**Write**	**Abbreviation**	**Write**
AD, AS, or AU	right ear, left ear, or each ear	X 3d	for 3 days
OD, OS, or OU	right eye, left eye, or each eye	SC, SQ, or sub q	subcut or subcutaneous(ly)
BT	bedtime	ss	one half or 1/2; spell out sliding scale
cc	mL for milliliters	SSI	sliding scale (insulin)
HS	half-strength	μg	mcg
hs	bedtime	< >	less than more than
qhs	nightly	+	and
qn	nightly	@	at
q1d	daily		

Please note: This is a partial list. For a more complete list, refer to www.ISMP.org.

11TH EDITION

BROWN AND MULHOLLAND'S

Drug Calculations

RATIO AND PROPORTION PROBLEMS FOR CLINICAL PRACTICE

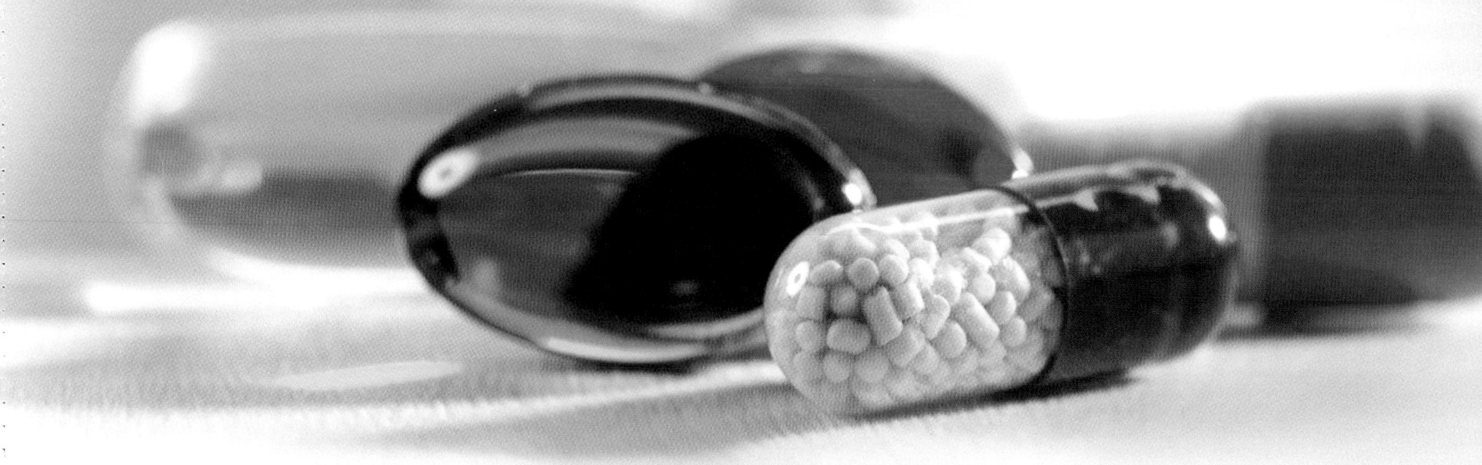

ANN TRITAK, EdD, RN

AACN-Wharton Executive Fellow
Former Professor and Associate Dean
Department of Graduate Nursing
Director DNP Program (Retired) School of Nursing, Felician University
Lodi, New Jersey
Curriculum and Accreditation Consultant
EdD, Rutgers, The State University of New Jersey
New Brunswick, New Jersey
MA, Nursing Education, New York University
New York, New York
BSN, William Paterson College
Wayne, New Jersey

MARGARET A. FARRELL DAINGERFIELD, EdD, RN, CNE

Professor and Associate Dean
Department of Graduate Nursing
School of Nursing, Felician University
Lodi, New Jersey
EdD, Rutgers, The State University of New Jersey
New Brunswick, New Jersey
MA, Nursing Education, New York University
New York, New York
BSN, Seton Hall University
South Orange, New Jersey

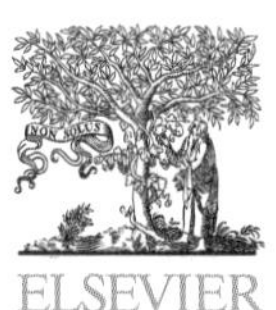

ELSEVIER

3251 Riverport Lane
St. Louis, Missouri 63043

BROWN AND MULHOLLAND'S DRUG CALCULATIONS: RATIO AND PROPORTION PROBLEMS FOR CLINICAL PRACTICE, ELEVENTH EDITION
ISBN: 978-0-323-55129-8

Previous editions copyrighted 2016, 2012, 2008, 2000, 1996, 1992, 1988, 1984, 1979.

Library of Congress Control Number: 2019942175

Senior Content Strategist: Yvonne Alexopoulos
Content Development Manager: Lisa Newton
Senior Content Development Specialist: Danielle M. Frazier
Publishing Services Manager: Julie Eddy
Senior Project Manager: Tracey Schriefer
Design Direction: Renee Duenow

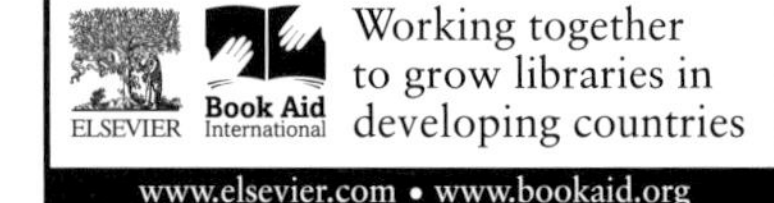

Printed in China

Last digit is the print number: 9 8 7 6 5 4 3 2 1

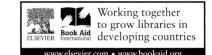

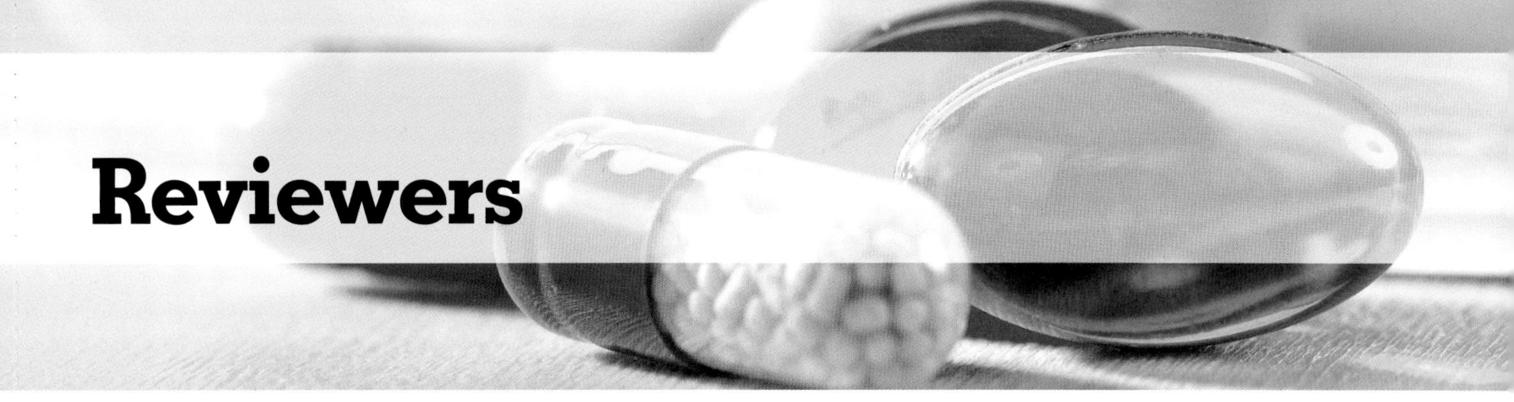

Reviewers

Lou Ann Boose, MSN, RN
Senior Professor of Nursing
Health and Public Service Department
HACC- Central Pennsylvania's Community College
Harrisburg, Pennsylvania

Becky Farmer, MSRS, RT(R)(M)
Associate Professor
Allied Health
Northwestern State University
Shreveport, Louisiana

Jessica Gonzales, ARNP
Advanced Registered Nurse Practitioner
Private Practice
Redmond, Washington

Janice Elaine Pinheiro, BSN, MSN, RNC-OB, MSN
Senior Clinical Instructor, Staff RN, Level III, Captain USAF (inactive)
Department of Baccalaureate and Graduate Nursing, Obstetrics
Eastern Kentucky University, Baptist Health Lexington
Richmond, Kentucky
Lexington, Kentucky

Paula Denise Silver, BS Biology, PharmD
Medical Instructor
Medical Assisting, Dental Assisting, LPN, RN, BSN
ECPI University: School of Health Science
Newport News, Virginia

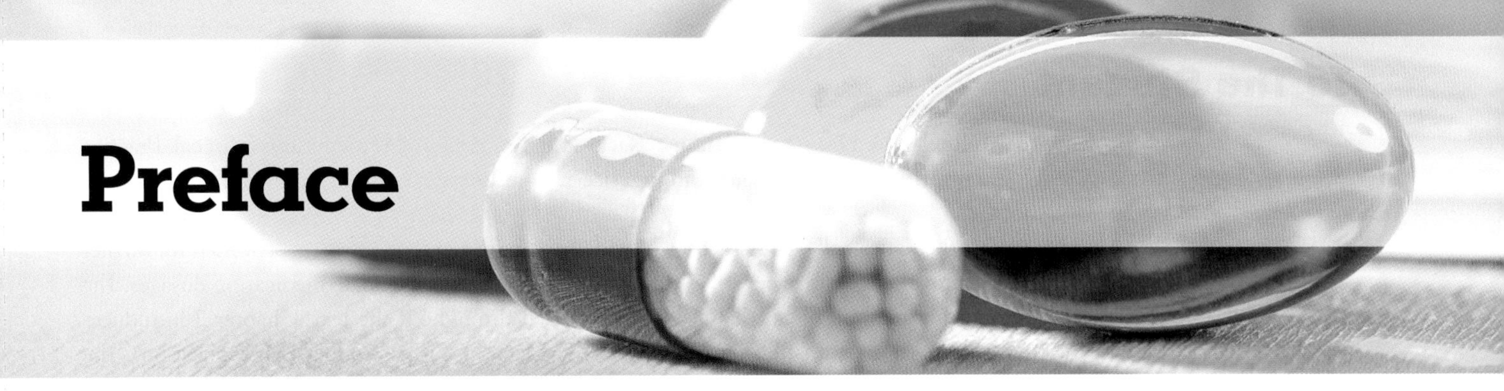

Preface

To The Instructor

Drug Calculations was originally designed in the late 1970s as a basic practical resource for nursing students and faculty in classrooms and clinical areas. Additional content was added over the years to be current with the increased roles and responsibilities of the nurse and to be useful for refresher courses, nurses practicing in specialty areas, distance-learning nursing students, and nursing students who must master the material independently.

The current text has been updated to reflect feedback from reviewers, colleagues, and students, and student needs related to current trends in nursing education and practice that will result in safe practice and best patient outcomes.

Continuing in This Edition

Ratio and proportion calculations are presented in the second chapter following a math review so that the student has the method reinforced throughout the rest of the text for maximum competence. As with earlier editions, the text presents one calculation method—ratio and proportion—to maximize the teaching and learning time for reinforcement, practice, and mastery within the brief time the student has to devote to this critical subject.

The material is sequential with logical steps and ample practice problems to facilitate mastery of the concepts.

The quizzes and tests are brief and can be completed in one sitting. Answers are worked out.

Each medication problem has a frequently encountered diagnosis attached to make the problem more realistic and help the student assimilate clinical relevance.

A high-alert red flag is attached to the Institute for Safe Medication Practices (ISMP)–identified medication labels to call attention to these medications.

The sample hand-off communication report in Appendix D has highlighted medication-related inclusions.

The Joint Commission (TJC) and ISMP abbreviations and QSEN patient safety recommendations are emphasized.

Clinical relevance and patient safety measures are included for the benefit of students who are studying independently as well as those in the classroom.

New to This Edition

- Chapter objectives are logically organized and reflect the progression of chapter content.
- Vocabulary definitions are updated to reflect current practice.
- The fraction cross product multiplication setup of ratio and proportion calculations and the colon setup show color coded means and extremes examples to ensure correct factor placement.
- Medication administration "rights" are expanded to include pre-administration assessment, reason and post administration evaluation.
- Examples of cultural responsiveness in the administration of medications are included.
- Chapters address the 2017 Hospital National Patient Safety Goals of Identifying Patients Correctly, Use Medications Safely, and Prevent Infection.

To The Student

Brown and Mulholland's Drug Calculations: Ratio and Proportion Problems for Clinical Practice provides all the information, explanation and practice you need to competently and confidently calculate drug dosages.

A General Mathematics Self-Assessment is provided as a refresher to identify areas needed for further study. Chapter 1 provides a basic review of all the arithmetic needed to calculate medication dosages. The Ratio and Proportion method of calculating dosages is used throughout the text. Chapter 2 introduces two Ratio and Proportion setups: Using colons and the Fraction Cross-Product (Multiplication). The "means" and" extremes" have been color coded to assist you in setting up and solving the dosage calculation or problem using either of the R and P methods. You may use whichever R and P method you prefer. Be sure that you have complete mastery of Chapter 1 and 2 before proceeding with the rest of the text.

Each chapter has a series of quizzes with a Multiple-Choice and Final test at the end of each chapter. Each of the quizzes and tests can be completed in one sitting. Answers with proofs are worked out in the Answer Key at the end of each chapter.

Clinical Alerts in red will point out potential errors that can occur in the clinical setting. Clinical Relevance information is provided to help you connect math to the safe application in the clinical setting. A high-alert medication icon flag is a visual reminder of high-risk drugs identified by the Institute for Safe Medication Practices (ISMP).

Samples of look-alike medications (ISMP) that have caused medication errors are included. Pay close attention to all of the icons and textbox notes. They relate to actual safe and unsafe practice. Tall Man letters distinguish differences between similar names.

Critical Thinking Exercises at the end of each chapter help you understand how medication errors occur and how they might have been prevented. Discuss the exercises with other nursing students to elicit various ways to avoid medication errors.

Multiple-Choice and Comprehensive Finals test your knowledge on all of the chapters studied. Spend extra review time in the text on any questions that you cannot answer correctly.

NEW! Elsevier's Interactive Drug Calculation Application, Version 1

This interactive drug calculations application provides hands on, interactive practice for the user to master drug calculations. Users can select the mode (Study, Exam, or Comprehensive Exam) and then the category for study and exam modes. There are eight categories that cover the main drug calculation topics. Users are also able to select the number of problems they want to complete and their preferred drug calculation method. A calculator is available for easy access within any mode, and the application also provides history of the work done by the user.

Refer to *Elsevier's Interactive Drug Calculation Application, Version 1* for additional practice problems and content information.

Acknowledgments

Acknowledgments

We extend our thanks to all the reviewers, editors, production, and marketing teams who contributed to this edition. We included as many of their recommendations as permitted by space, content, and text design.

Ann Tritak is deeply grateful to her family and former students who have taught her so much and encouraged her to keep learning and sharing her love of nursing with others. A special thank you to "Peggy" Daingerfield who agreed to work with her on this important publication. She is a great colleague, educator, and friend.

Margaret A. Farrell Daingerfield is eternally grateful for the love of her husband, Richard, who is always proud of any accomplishment, great or small; is thankful for her parents, Peggy and Joseph Farrell, who supported her vision to become a nurse educator; and is proud of her children and grandchildren as they strive to realize their dreams.

Ann Tritak
Margaret A. Farrell Daingerfield

Contents

General Mathematics Self-Assessment, 1

1 General Mathematics, 5

2 Ratio and Proportion, 41

3 Safe Medication Administration, 57

4 Medication Measurements and Oral Dose Calculations, 101

5 Injectable Medication Calculations, 147

6 Reconstitution of Medications From Powders and Crystals: Oral and Intramuscular, 181

7 Basic Intravenous Therapy Calculations, 231

8 Advanced Intravenous Calculations, 275

9 Insulin Administration and Type 2 Diabetes Medications, 307

10 Parenteral Nutrition, 355

11 Anticoagulants, 381

12 Pediatric Dosages, 417

Multiple-Choice Final, 451

Comprehensive Final, 461

Appendices

A ISMP List of High-Alert Medications in Acute Care Settings, 477

B ISMP's List of Error-Prone Abbreviations, Symbols, and Dose Designations, 479

C Sample Medication Administration Errors With Potential Clinical Outcomes, 481

D 5-Minute Sample Verbal Communication From Nurses to Subsequent Caregivers, 483

Index, 485

General Mathematics Self-Assessment

The accurate calculation of medication dosages, a skill that is central to patient safety, builds on a knowledge of fundamental mathematics. Competency and skill in using the basic principles of arithmetic are essential for safe medication administration. To progress in the *Drug Calculations* text, students must know how to solve problems using addition, subtraction, multiplication, division, fractions, decimals, and percentages. Use the problems provided in the following self-assessment to gauge current knowledge. Answers are on page 4. Chapter 1, General Mathematics, provides a refresher for each type of problem in the self-assessment. Consult a text for general mathematics as needed.

Fractions

Change to whole or mixed numbers.

1. $\frac{9}{2}$ **2.** $\frac{26}{5}$

Change to improper fractions.

3. $8\frac{1}{3}$ **4.** $5\frac{2}{5}$

Find the lowest common denominator.

5. $\frac{4}{11}$ and $\frac{1}{8}$ **6.** $\frac{2}{5}$ and $\frac{5}{9}$

Add.

7. $\frac{1}{5}$, $\frac{1}{6}$, and $\frac{2}{3}$ **8.** $1\frac{1}{2} + 3\frac{1}{8} + 2\frac{1}{6}$

Subtract.

9. $\frac{5}{7} - \frac{1}{3}$ **10.** $8\frac{1}{4} - 3\frac{3}{8}$

Multiply and reduce to lowest terms.

11. $\frac{1}{6} \times \frac{1}{3}$ **12.** $\frac{2}{8} \times 1\frac{1}{3}$

Divide and reduce to lowest terms.

13. $\frac{1}{3} \div \frac{2}{5}$ **14.** $1\frac{1}{8} \div 2\frac{1}{2}$

Reduce to lowest terms (numbers).

15. $\frac{4}{120}$

16. $\frac{3}{7}$

Decimals

Write as decimals.

17. Twelve hundredths

18. Three and sixteen thousandths

Add.

19. 3.04 + 1.864

20. 25.7 + 3.008

Subtract.

21. 3 − 0.04

22. 0.96 − 0.1359

Multiply.

23. 0.05 × 2

24. 3 × 0.4

Divide and carry to the third decimal place.

25. 500 ÷ 15

26. 20.6 ÷ 0.21

Change to decimals and carry to the third decimal place.

27. $\frac{24}{44}$

28. $9\frac{1}{8}$

Percentages

Find the percentages.

29. 25% of 300

30. 1% of 50

Change the decimals to fractions and reduce to lowest terms.

31. 0.005

32. 0.05

Change the fractions to a decimal and a percentage.

33. $\frac{3}{4}$

34. $\frac{1}{8}$

Rounding

Round the decimals (35–39) in the chart below.

	Decimal	Nearest Whole Number	Nearest Hundredth	Nearest Tenth
35.	0.8734			
36.	0.842			
37.	0.553			
38.	0.689			
39.	2.75			

Answer the questions.

40. What is 25% of 2? Ans: fraction ______ Ans: decimal ______

41. What is $\frac{1}{4}$ of 2? Ans: fraction ______ Ans: decimal ______

42. What is 75% of 2? Ans: fraction ______ Ans: decimal ______

43. Divide 0.5 by 0.25:

44. Divide 0.2 by 0.1:

45. Divide $\frac{1}{100}$ by $\frac{1}{200}$:

Answer Key

General Mathematics Self-Assessment (page 1)

1. $4\frac{1}{2}$ **2.** $5\frac{1}{5}$ **3.** $\frac{25}{3}$ **4.** $\frac{27}{5}$

5. 88 **6.** 45 **7.** $1\frac{1}{30}$ **8.** $6\frac{19}{24}$

9. $\frac{8}{21}$ **10.** $4\frac{7}{8}$ **11.** $\frac{1}{18}$ **12.** $\frac{1}{3}$

13. $\frac{5}{6}$ **14.** $\frac{9}{20}$ **15.** $\frac{1}{30}$ **16.** $\frac{3}{7}$

17. 0.12 **18.** 3.016 **19.** 4.904 **20.** 28.708

21. 2.96 **22.** 0.8241 **23.** 0.1 **24.** 1.2

25. 33.333 **26.** 98.095 **27.** 0.545 **28.** 9.125

29. 75 **30.** 0.5 **31.** $\frac{5}{1000} = \frac{1}{200}$ **32.** $\frac{5}{100} = \frac{1}{20}$

33. 0.75 75% **34.** 0.125 $12\frac{1}{2}\%$

	Decimal	Nearest Whole Number	Nearest Hundredth	Nearest Tenth
35.	0.8734	1	0.87	0.9
36.	0.842	1	0.84	0.8
37.	0.553	1	0.55	0.6
38.	0.689	1	0.69	0.7
39.	2.75	3	2.75	2.8

40. $\frac{1}{2}$ (0.5) **41.** $\frac{1}{2}$ (0.5) **42.** $1\frac{1}{2}$ (1.5) **43.** 2

44. 2 **45.** 2

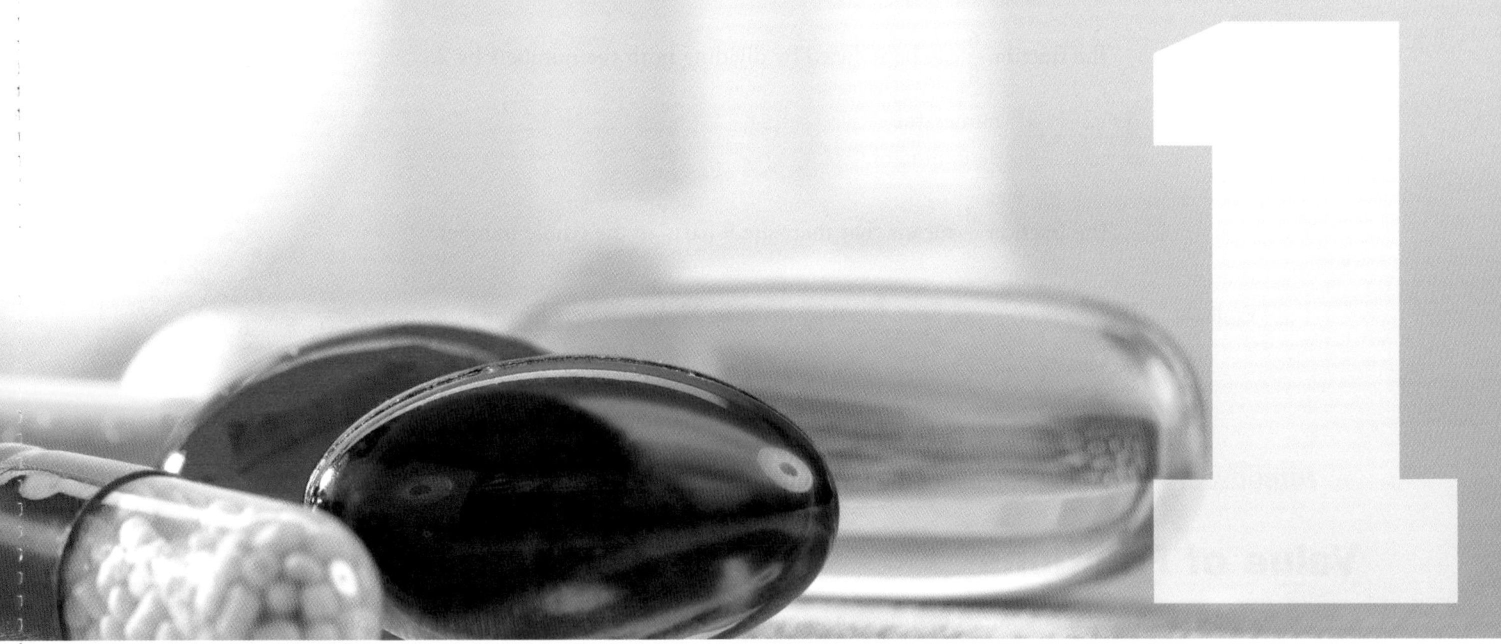

General Mathematics

Objectives

- Define the term *fraction*, including parts of a fraction.
- Reduce fractions to lowest terms.
- Understand the value of fractions.
- Convert improper fractions and mixed numbers.
- Create equivalent fractions and compare values.
- Add, subtract, multiply, and divide fractions and mixed numbers.
- Compare decimal values.
- Round decimals.
- Add, subtract, multiply, and divide decimals.
- Convert decimals, fractions, and percentages.

Introduction

The Quality and Safety Education for Nurses (QSEN) project centers on the knowledge, skills, and attitudes necessary for nurses to provide safe, high-quality, evidence-based, patient-centered care as part of the interprofessional team (http://qsen.org). Proficiency in general mathematical calculations is an essential step towards safe medication administration, one means of ensuring quality patient outcomes.

This chapter provides a thorough and easy-to-follow review of the arithmetic needed for accurate medication dose calculations. Many examples, practice problems, and answers related to fractions, decimals, rounding, and percentages are offered. Your ability to avoid medication errors and solve medication dose-related problems starts with competence in basic arithmetic. If you need further review, refer to a basic mathematics text. Mastery of these concepts is essential before you proceed to the following chapters and medication-related calculations.

Fractions

A fraction is part of a whole number. The fraction $\frac{6}{8}$ means that there are 8 parts to the whole number (bottom number, or denominator), but you want to measure only 6 of those parts (top number, or numerator).

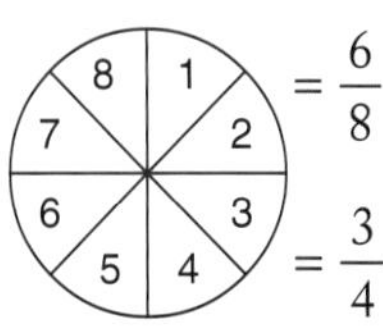

The fraction $\frac{6}{8}$ can be reduced by dividing both the numbers by 2.

$\frac{6 \div 2}{8 \div 2} = \frac{3}{4}$ numerator / denominator

The fraction $\frac{3}{9}$ means that there are 9 parts to the whole number.

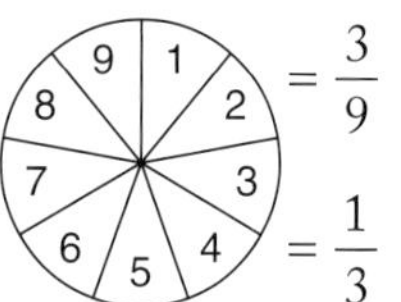

$= \frac{3}{9}$

$= \frac{1}{3}$

Example The fraction $\frac{3}{9}$ can be reduced by dividing both numbers by the same number.

$\frac{3 \div 3 = 1}{9 \div 3 = 3}$ numerator / denominator

remember **The whole number of the fraction is always the denominator.**

Value of Fractions

RULE **The denominator determines the number of parts into which the whole number is divided. The smaller the denominator of a fraction, the greater the fraction's value if the numerators are the same.**

Example Which would you rather have, $\frac{1}{6}$ or $\frac{1}{9}$ of your favorite candy bar? $\frac{1}{6}$ is greater than $\frac{1}{9}$. It represents a larger part of the whole unit.

$\frac{1}{6}$	$\frac{1}{6}$	$\frac{1}{6}$	$\frac{1}{6}$	$\frac{1}{6}$	$\frac{1}{6}$

= 6 parts   Each $\frac{1}{6}$ part is **larger** than the $\frac{1}{9}$ part.

$\frac{1}{9}$	$\frac{1}{9}$	$\frac{1}{9}$	$\frac{1}{9}$	$\frac{1}{9}$	$\frac{1}{9}$	$\frac{1}{9}$	$\frac{1}{9}$	$\frac{1}{9}$

= 9 parts   Each $\frac{1}{9}$ part is **smaller** than the $\frac{1}{6}$ part.

Answers on page 32

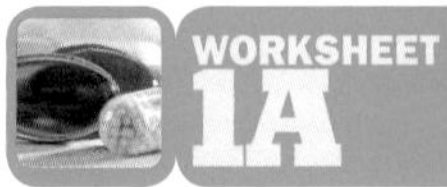

WORKSHEET 1A Value of Fractions

Answer the following questions by circling the correct answer.

1. Would you rather own $\frac{1}{10}$ or $\frac{1}{20}$ of a lottery ticket?

2. Would you rather have 2 out of 7 or 2 out of 14 days off?

3. If you had a choice of a bonus of $\frac{1}{20}$ or $\frac{1}{30}$ of your annual salary, which would you prefer?

4. Which would be the *greater* incidence of a disease, 1 out of approximately every 100,000 people $\left(\frac{1}{100,000}\right)$ or 1 out of approximately 250,000 people $\left(\frac{1}{250,000}\right)$?

5. If a tablet was ordered for a patient at grain $\frac{1}{4}$ and you had tablets labeled grain $\frac{1}{8}$, would you need to give *more* or *less* than what is on hand?

6. Which is **greater?** $\frac{1}{5}$ or $\frac{1}{8}$

7. Which is **smaller?** $\frac{1}{100}$ or $\frac{1}{150}$

8. Which is **greater?** $\frac{1}{250}$ or $\frac{1}{300}$

9. Which is **smaller?** $\frac{1}{7}$ or $\frac{1}{9}$

10. Which is **smaller?** $\frac{1}{50}$ or $\frac{1}{200}$

Changing Improper Fractions to Whole or Mixed Numbers

An improper fraction has a numerator that is larger than the denominator, as in $\frac{8}{4}$.

Steps for Changing Improper Fractions to Whole or Mixed Numbers

1. When the top number (numerator) is larger than the bottom number (denominator), divide the bottom number (denominator) into the top number (numerator).
2. Write the remainder as a fraction and reduce to lowest terms.

Examples

$\frac{8}{4} = 8 \div 4 = 2$ *This is a whole number.*

$\frac{16}{6} = 16 \div 6 = 2\frac{4}{6} = 2\frac{2}{3}$ This is a *mixed number* because it has a whole number plus a fraction.

Answers on page 32

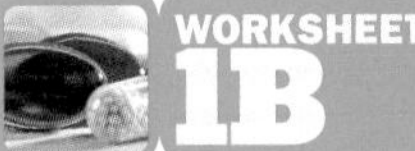

WORKSHEET 1B Changing Improper Fractions to Whole or Mixed Numbers

Change the following to whole numbers or mixed fractions and reduce to lowest terms.

1. $\frac{6}{6} =$

2. $\frac{10}{2} =$

3. $\frac{13}{4} =$

4. $\frac{14}{9} =$

5. $\frac{34}{6} =$

6. $\frac{100}{20} =$

7. $\frac{9}{4} =$

8. $\frac{120}{64} =$

9. $\frac{18}{3} =$

10. $\frac{41}{6} =$

Changing Mixed Numbers to Improper Fractions

Steps for Changing Mixed Numbers to Improper Fractions

1. Multiply the whole number by the denominator of the fraction.
2. Add this to the numerator of the fraction.
3. Write the sum as the numerator of the fraction; the denominator of the fraction remains the same.

Examples

$2\frac{3}{8} = \frac{8 \times 2 + 3}{8} = \frac{19}{8}$ $\frac{\text{Numerator}}{\text{Denominator}}$

$4\frac{2}{5} = \frac{5 \times 4 + 2}{5} = \frac{22}{5}$ $\frac{\text{Numerator}}{\text{Denominator}}$

Answers on page 32

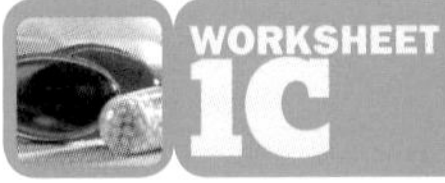

WORKSHEET 1C Changing Mixed Numbers to Improper Fractions

Change the following to improper fractions.

1. $3\frac{1}{2} =$ **2.** $1\frac{1}{6} =$ **3.** $4\frac{1}{8} =$

4. $3\frac{7}{12} =$ **5.** $13\frac{3}{5} =$ **6.** $16\frac{1}{3} =$

7. $3\frac{5}{6} =$ **8.** $2\frac{5}{8} =$ **9.** $10\frac{3}{6} =$

10. $125\frac{2}{3} =$

Finding a Common Denominator for Two or More Fractions

To add and subtract fractions, the denominators must be the *same.*

Example Fractions with same denominators

$$\frac{5}{16} - \frac{2}{16} \quad \text{or} \quad \frac{3}{8} + \frac{1}{8} \quad \text{or} \quad \frac{3}{4} + \frac{1}{4}$$

These fractions can be added and subtracted. Each set's value is also easier to compare because of the common denominators.

Example Different denominators in fractions with the same value as the fractions in example A:

$$\frac{5}{16} - \frac{1}{8} \quad \text{or} \quad \frac{3}{8} + \frac{2}{16} \quad \text{or} \quad \frac{3}{4} + \frac{2}{8}$$

These fractions cannot be added or subtracted until they are converted to *equivalent* fractions with a *common* denominator. The relative value of each set is harder to compare until they are converted to equivalent fractions. A *common* denominator is a number that can be divided evenly by *all* the denominators in the problem. It is easier to add or subtract fractions if the lowest common denominator is used.

Steps for Finding a Common Denominator for Two or More Fractions

1. Examine the largest denominator in the group to determine whether the other denominators will divide *evenly* into it.
2. If any of the denominators will not divide evenly into the largest denominator, begin multiplying the largest denominator by 2. If the other denominators cannot be divided by 2 evenly, then proceed to multiply the denominator by 3, 4, 5, 6, and so on until all denominators can be divided into the number equally. This becomes the common denominator.

Example $\frac{5}{16}$ and $\frac{1}{8}$: the largest denominator, 16, can be divided by 8 without a remainder. Therefore 16 is the common denominator.

Example $\frac{2}{8}$ and $\frac{3}{4}$ and $\frac{1}{2}$: the largest denominator, 8, can be divided by 4 and by 2 without a remainder. Therefore 8 is the common denominator.

Example $\frac{1}{7}, \frac{1}{6}$, and $\frac{1}{3}$
3 and 6 will *not* divide evenly into 7.

Multiples of 7: 14, 21, 28, 35, and 42.
42 is the lowest number that can be divided evenly by 6 and 3. Therefore **42** is a common denominator, the lowest common denominator.

Changing Fractions to Equivalent Fractions

RULE **To maintain equivalence, the numerator and the denominator must be divided (or multiplied) by the *same* number.**

Whatever you do to the denominator (multiply or divide by a number), you must do the *same* to the numerator so that the value does not change.

Steps for Changing Fractions to Equivalent Fractions

1. Find the common denominator—in this case 24.
2. Multiply each *numerator* by the *same* number used to obtain the common denominator for that fraction.

Example $\frac{3}{8}$ and $\frac{2}{3}$ and $\frac{1}{4}$: 3 will *not* divide evenly into 8.

The largest denominator in the group is **8**.
$8 \times 2 = 16$ 3 will *not* divide evenly into 16.
$8 \times 3 = 24$ Both 3 and 4 will divide evenly into **24**.
$8 \times 4 = 32$ 3 will *not* divide evenly into 32.
$8 \times 5 = 40$ 3 will *not* divide evenly into 40.
$8 \times 6 = 48$ Both 3 and 4 will divide evenly into **48**.

Therefore 24 and 48 are common denominators for $\frac{3}{8}$ and $\frac{2}{3}$ and $\frac{1}{4}$, but 24 is the *lowest* common denominator for the three numbers.

Examples

Proving Fractions Are Equivalent by Using the Cross Fraction Product Method

$\frac{3}{8} = \frac{?}{24}$ (×3) $3 \times 3 = 9$ Therefore $\frac{3}{8} = \frac{9}{24}$ = $3 \times 24 = 72$, $9 \times 8 = 72$

$\frac{2}{3} = \frac{?}{24}$ (×8) $2 \times 8 = 16$ Therefore $\frac{2}{3} = \frac{16}{24}$ = $2 \times 24 = 48$, $3 \times 16 = 48$

$\frac{1}{4} = \frac{?}{24}$ (×6) $1 \times 6 = 6$ Therefore $\frac{1}{4} = \frac{6}{24}$ = $1 \times 24 = 24$, $4 \times 6 = 24$

Reducing Fractions to Lowest Terms

A fraction is in lowest terms when the numerator and denominator cannot be divided by any other number except one.

RULE **To reduce a fraction to *lowest* terms, *divide* the numerator and denominator by the *largest* same whole number that will divide evenly into both. When there are no whole numbers that can be used except one, the fraction is in lowest terms.**

The fraction $\frac{6}{8}$ is not in lowest terms because it can be reduced by dividing both the numerator and the denominator by 2, a common denominator. $\frac{3}{4}$ is expressed in lowest terms.

Example $\frac{6 \div 2}{8 \div 2} = \frac{3}{4}$ Note that both 6 and 8 are divided by 2.

Example $\frac{10 \div 5}{15 \div 5} = \frac{2}{3}$ Note that both 10 and 15 are divided by 5.

Example $\frac{4 \div 4}{24 \div 4} = \frac{1}{6}$ Note that both 4 and 24 are divided by 4.

$\frac{3}{4}$ and $\frac{2}{3}$ and $\frac{1}{6}$ cannot be further reduced. No other number than one will divide evenly into both the numerator and denominator. They are now in their simplest or *lowest* terms.

Changing to Equivalent Fractions Using Higher Terms

RULE **To change a fraction to *higher* terms and maintain equivalence, *multiply* both the numerator and the denominator by the *same* number.**

Example $\frac{6 \times 2}{8 \times 2} = \frac{12}{16}$ $\frac{6}{8} = \frac{12}{16}$

The value has not changed because the multiplier 2 is used for both the numerator and the denominator, and $\frac{2}{2} = 1$.

Multiplying or dividing numbers by one does *not* change the value. Equivalence is maintained.

Addition of Fractions and Mixed Numbers

RULE **If fractions have the same denominator, add the numerators, and place the result over the denominator and reduce.**

Example

$$\frac{1}{5} + \frac{2}{5} = \frac{3}{5}$$

$$\frac{2}{6} + \frac{1}{6} = \frac{3}{6} = \frac{1}{2}$$

RULE **If fractions have different denominators, convert each fraction to an equivalent fraction using the lowest common denominator and then add the numerators. Then convert the fraction to a mixed number if greater than 1.**

Example

$$\begin{array}{rl} \frac{3}{5} = & \frac{9}{15} \\ +\frac{2}{3} = & +\frac{10}{15} \\ \hline & \frac{19}{15} = 19 \div 15 = 1\frac{4}{15} \end{array}$$

$$\frac{3(\times 3)}{5(\times 3)} = \frac{9}{15}$$
$$\frac{2(\times 5)}{3(\times 5)} = \frac{10}{15}$$

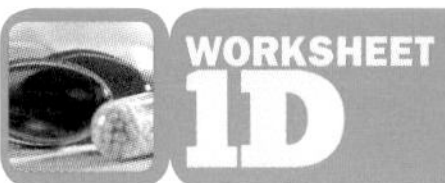

To add mixed numbers, first add the fractions by converting to a common denominator and then add this to the sum of the whole numbers.

Example

$$\begin{array}{rl} 9\frac{5}{8} = & 9\frac{15}{24} \\ +6\frac{1}{6} = & +6\frac{4}{24} \\ \hline & 15\frac{19}{24} \end{array}$$

$$\frac{5(\times 3)}{8(\times 3)} = \frac{15}{24}$$
$$\frac{1(\times 4)}{6(\times 4)} = \frac{4}{24}$$

Answers on page 32

WORKSHEET 1D Addition of Fractions and Mixed Numbers

Add the following fractions and mixed numbers, using the common denominator, and reduce to lowest terms.

1. $\frac{2}{5} + \frac{2}{5}$

2. $\frac{4}{5} + \frac{2}{3}$

3. $6\frac{1}{6} + 9\frac{5}{8}$

4. $2\frac{1}{4} + 3\frac{1}{8}$

5. $1\frac{3}{4} + 9\frac{9}{10}$

6. $\frac{1}{8}$, $\frac{1}{4}$, $+\frac{3}{9}$

7. $\frac{7}{9}$, $\frac{4}{5}$, $+\frac{9}{10}$

8. $3\frac{1}{4} + 9\frac{3}{4}$

9. $8\frac{2}{5}$, $14\frac{7}{10}$, $+9\frac{9}{10}$

10. $2\frac{1}{3} + 4\frac{1}{6}$

Subtraction of Fractions and Mixed Numbers

RULE **If fractions have the same denominator, find the difference between the numerators and write it over the common denominator. Reduce the fraction if necessary.**

Example

$$\begin{array}{r} \frac{27}{32} \\ -\frac{18}{32} \\ \hline \frac{9}{32} \end{array}$$

The difference between the numerators (27 minus 18) equals 9. The denominator is 32.

RULE **If fractions have different denominators, find the lowest common denominator and proceed as above.**

Example

$$\begin{array}{rcr} \frac{7}{8} & = & \frac{21}{24} \\ -\frac{2}{3} & = & \frac{16}{24} \\ \hline & & \frac{5}{24} \end{array}$$

The difference between the numerators (21 minus 16) equals 5. The lowest common denominator is 24.

RULE **To subtract mixed numbers, first subtract the fractions and then find the difference in the whole numbers. If the lower fraction is larger than the upper fraction, you cannot subtract it.** ***You must borrow from the whole number before subtracting the fraction.***

Example

$$\begin{array}{r} 21\frac{7}{16} \\ -7\frac{12}{16} \\ \hline \end{array}$$

You cannot subtract 12 from 7 because 12 is larger than 7. Therefore you must borrow a whole number (1) from the 21, make a fraction out of $1\left(\frac{16}{16}\right)$, and add the 7.

$$\frac{16}{16} + \frac{7}{16} = \frac{23}{16}$$

Because you added a whole number to the fraction, you must take a whole number away from 21 and make it 20. The problem is now set up as follows:

$$\begin{array}{r} 21\frac{7}{16} = 20\frac{16}{16} + \frac{7}{16} = 20\frac{23}{16} \\ -7\frac{12}{16} \\ \hline 13\frac{11}{16} \end{array}$$

RULE **Reduce your answer to lowest terms.**

Answers on page 33

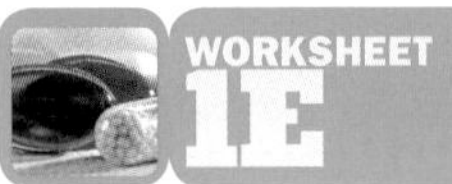

WORKSHEET 1E Subtraction of Fractions and Mixed Numbers

Subtract fractions and mixed numbers, and reduce the answers to lowest terms.

1. $\frac{2}{3} - \frac{1}{2}$

2. $\frac{27}{32} - \frac{18}{32}$

3. $10\frac{2}{5} - 6\frac{1}{4}$

4. $7\frac{16}{24} - 3\frac{1}{8}$

5. $6\frac{3}{10} - 2\frac{1}{5}$

6. $\frac{7}{8} - \frac{1}{3}$

7. $3\frac{5}{8} - 1\frac{3}{8}$

8. $5\frac{3}{7} - 1\frac{6}{7}$

9. $7 - 1\frac{3}{4}$

10. $2\frac{7}{8} - \frac{3}{4}$

Multiplication of Fractions and Mixed Numbers

Steps for Multiplication of Fractions and Mixed Numbers

1. Change the mixed number to an improper fraction if necessary.
2. Cancel, if possible, by dividing the numerators and denominators by the largest common divisor contained in each.
3. Multiply the remaining numerators to find a result, or product.
4. Multiply the denominators to find a result, or product.
5. Reduce the answer to lowest terms.

Example

$$\frac{4}{5} \times \frac{15}{16} = \frac{\overset{1}{\cancel{4}}}{\underset{1}{\cancel{5}}} \times \frac{\overset{3}{\cancel{15}}}{\underset{4}{\cancel{16}}} = \frac{3}{4}$$

$$4\frac{1}{2} \times 2\frac{1}{4} = \frac{9}{2} \times \frac{9}{4} = \frac{81}{8} = 10\frac{1}{8}$$

$$6 \times \frac{3}{8} = \frac{6}{1} \times \frac{3}{8} = \frac{\overset{3}{\cancel{6}}}{1} \times \frac{3}{\underset{4}{\cancel{8}}} = \frac{9}{4} = 2\frac{1}{4}$$

Answers on page 33

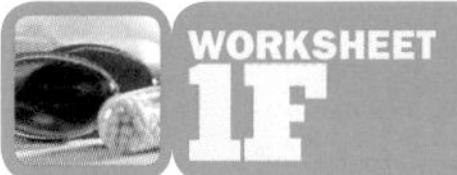

WORKSHEET 1F Multiplication of Fractions and Mixed Numbers

Multiply the following fractions and mixed numbers, and reduce the answers to lowest terms.

1. $\frac{1}{5} \times \frac{2}{4} =$ **2.** $\frac{1}{5} \times \frac{1}{6} =$ **3.** $\frac{3}{5} \times \frac{5}{8} =$

4. $4 \times 3\frac{1}{3} =$ **5.** $\frac{2}{4} \times 2\frac{1}{6} =$ **6.** $5\frac{1}{2} \times 3\frac{1}{8} =$

7. $1\frac{3}{4} \times 3\frac{1}{7} =$ **8.** $\frac{5}{6} \times 1\frac{9}{16} =$ **9.** $\frac{5}{100} \times 900 =$

10. $2\frac{1}{10} \times 4\frac{1}{3} =$

Division of Fractions and Mixed Numbers

Steps for Division of Fractions and Mixed Numbers

1. Change mixed numbers to improper fractions if necessary.
2. Invert the number after the ÷ (division) sign.
3. Follow the steps for multiplication, and reduce any fractions.

Examples

$$\frac{1}{2} \div \frac{1}{3} = \frac{1}{2} \times \frac{3}{1} = \frac{3}{2} = 1\frac{1}{2}$$

$$8\frac{3}{4} \div 15 = \frac{\overset{7}{\cancel{35}}}{4} \times \frac{1}{\underset{3}{\cancel{15}}} = \frac{7}{12}\,*$$

---

*Reducing fractions to $\left(\frac{7}{4} \times \frac{1}{3}\right)$ makes the math easier and reduces errors.

Answers on page 34

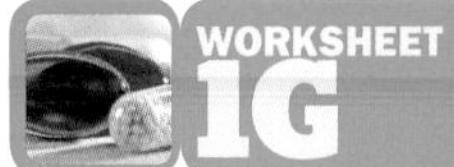

WORKSHEET 1G Division of Fractions and Mixed Numbers

Divide the following fractions and mixed numbers, and reduce the answers to lowest terms.

1. $\frac{1}{5} \div \frac{1}{8} =$ **2.** $\frac{1}{3} \div \frac{1}{2} =$ **3.** $\frac{3}{4} \div \frac{1}{8} =$

4. $\frac{1}{16} \div \frac{1}{4} =$ **5.** $8\frac{3}{4} \div 15 =$ **6.** $\frac{3}{4} \div 6 =$

7. $2 \div \frac{1}{5} =$ **8.** $3\frac{3}{8} \div 4\frac{1}{2} =$ **9.** $\frac{3}{5} \div \frac{3}{8} =$

10. $4 \div 2\frac{1}{8} =$

Value of Decimals

A decimal fraction is a fraction whose denominator (bottom number) is 10, 100, 1000, 10,000, and so on. It differs from a common fraction in that the denominator is *not* written but is expressed by the proper placement of the decimal point.

Observe the scale below. All whole numbers are to the left of the decimal point; all decimal fractions are to the right.

RULE **All whole numbers are to the left of the decimal; all decimal fractions are to the right of the decimal point.**

To read a decimal fraction, read the number to the right of the decimal and use the name that applies to "place value" of the *last* figure other than zero. Decimal fractions read with a *ths* on the end.

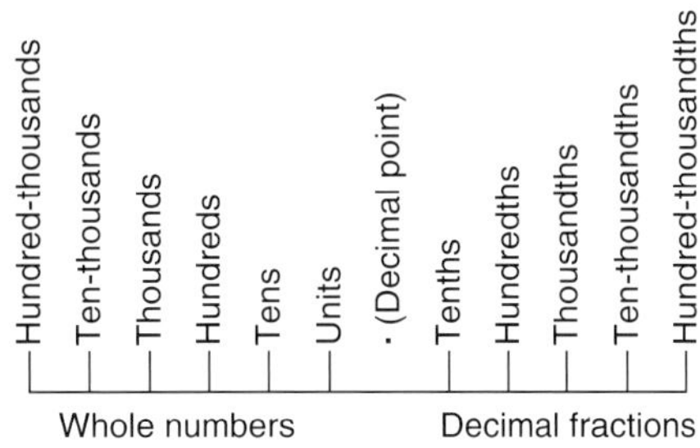

Examples
0.2 = Two Ten*ths*
0.25 = Twenty-five hundred*ths*
0.257 = Two hundred fifty-seven thousand*ths*
0.2057 = Two thousand fifty-seven ten-thousand*ths*
0.20057 = Twenty thousand fifty-seven hundred-thousand*ths*

RULE **For a whole number and a fraction, read the decimal point as an and. Read the whole number first and then read the decimal point as an and.**

Example 327.006 = Three hundred twenty-seven *and* six thousand*ths*

Comparison of Decimals

To determine which decimal is larger or smaller, compare the decimals from left to right, starting with the tenths place value, then the hundredths if needed, and so on.

Examples

0.4 and 0.5	5 is greater than 4, and 0.5 is greater than 0.4.
0.123 and 0.234	2 is greater than 1 in the tenths place, so 0.234 is greater than 0.123.
0.189 and 0.194	Both have 1 in the tenths column, but comparing the hundredths column reveals that the 9 is greater than 8. Therefore 0.194 is greater than 0.189.
0.34 and 0.269	Avoid distraction because of the length of the numbers. Compare the tenths place value first: 3 is greater than 2. Therefore 0.34 is greater than 0.269.

Rounding Decimals

Steps for Rounding Decimals

1. Calculate *one* decimal place beyond the desired place.
2. If the final digit is **4** or less, make no adjustment. If the final digit is **5** or more, *increase* the prior digit by one number.
3. Drop the final digit.

tenths

Examples

- Round 2.7 to the nearest whole number. Examine the tenths column.
- Because 7 is greater than 5, the answer is 3 and 0.7 is dropped.

tenths hundredths

- Round 2.55 to the nearest tenth.
  Examine the second decimal place (hundredths column).
  Because the hundredths column is 5, the 2.5 is rounded up to 2.6 and the final 0.05 (hundredths) is dropped.
- Round 3.762 to the nearest hundredth.
  Examine the third decimal place (thousandths column).
  Because 2 is less than 5, no adjustment will be made in the hundredths column and the 2 is dropped. 3.76 is the answer.

	Nearest Whole Number	Nearest Tenth	Nearest Hundredth
3.689	4	3.7	3.69
204.534	205	204.5	204.53
7.87	8	7.9	7.87
3.366	3	3.4	3.37
0.845*	1	0.8	0.85

*To reduce reading errors, develop the habit of placing a zero (0) in front of the decimal when a whole number is absent.

CLINICAL ALERT!

Do ***not*** round dosages of oral medication or injections to the nearest whole number because this could result in an overdose. Syringes are calibrated in tenths and hundredths of a milliliter; therefore rounding to a whole number could result in an overdose. For instructions on how to round medication doses, refer to Chapter 4.

Answers on page 34

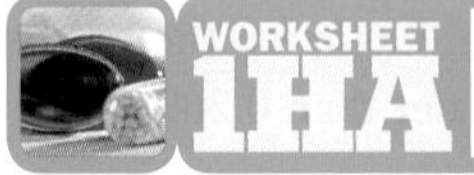

WORKSHEET 1HA Rounding Decimals

Round the decimal to the nearest whole number, the nearest tenth, and the nearest hundredth.

	Nearest Whole Number	Nearest Tenth	Nearest Hundredth
1. 93.489	______	______	______
2. 25.43	______	______	______

	Nearest Whole Number	Nearest Tenth	Nearest Hundredth
3. 38.2	______	______	______
4. 57.8888	______	______	______
5. 0.0092	______	______	______
6. 3.144	______	______	______
7. 8.999	______	______	______
8. 77.788	______	______	______
9. 12.959	______	______	______
10. 5.7703	______	______	______

Answers on page 34

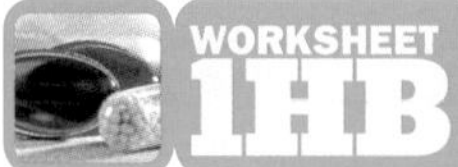

WORKSHEET 1HB Value of Decimals

Read the following decimals and write them out in words.

1. 0.06 ______________________

2. 0.096 ______________________

3. 0.005 ______________________

4. 100.01 ______________________

5. 0.9 ______________________

Write the following as decimals.

6. Thirty-four hundredths

7. Four thousandths ________

8. Two and seventeen thousandths ________

9. Nine and two ten-thousandths ________

10. Thirty-four and one tenth ________

CLINICAL ALERT!

Make it your habit to always insert a zero (0) in front of a decimal fraction when a whole number is absent. This draws attention to the decimal and avoids two potentially critical errors: missing the decimal or mistaking it for a number "1."

Answers on page 34

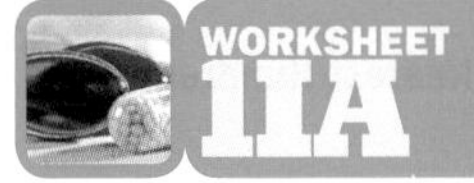

WORKSHEET 1IA Rounding Decimals

Round to tenths 0.0

1. 0.297 ______________
2. 4.435 ______________
3. 2.754 ______________
4. 0.845 ______________
5. 6.766 ______________

Round to hundredths 0.00

6. 0.297 ______________
7. 4.435 ______________
8. 2.754 ______________
9. 0.845 ______________
10. 6.766 ______________

Round to thousandths 0.000

11. 8.9374 ______________
12. 5.6256 ______________
13. 10.8976 ______________
14. 4.6255 ______________
15. 3.7386 ______________

Round to ten-thousandths 0.0000

16. 8.93749 ______________
17. 5.62568 ______________
18. 10.89763 ______________
19. 4.62557 ______________
20. 3.73869 ______________

Answers on page 35

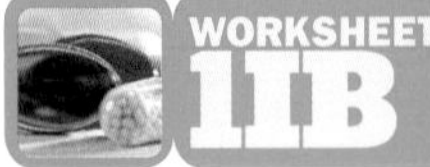

WORKSHEET 1IB Rounding Decimals

One of the keys to avoiding decimal errors when calculating medication doses is to know at a glance whether the amount you will give is *more* or *less* than the amount provided. Refer to page 16 for a review.

Which is *smaller?* Circle the correct answer.

1. 0.2 or 0.3
2. 0.5 or 0.25
3. 0.125 or 0.25
4. 2.309 or 2.07
5. 1.465 or 1.29

Which is *larger?* Circle the correct answer.

6. 0.9 or 0.1
7. 0.07 or 0.7
8. 0.58 or 0.09
9. 0.25 or 0.05
10. 0.001 or 0.1

Addition of Decimals

Steps for Adding Decimals

1. Write decimals in a column, keeping the decimal points under each other (A).
2. Add as in whole numbers, from right to left.
3. Place the decimal point in the answer directly under the decimal points in the numbers to be added.
4. Insert zeros as placeholders if desired within the problem after the last number (B).

Examples

A	B	C
0.8	1.64	2.42
+ 0.5	+ 2.10	+ 1.08
1.3	3.74	3.5~~0~~

remember **Line up the decimal points.**
Remove trailing zeros from the final answer (C).

Answers on page 35

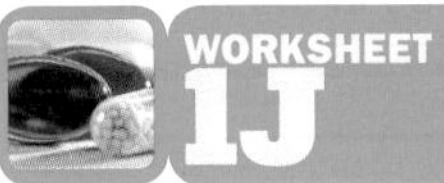

WORKSHEET 1J

Addition of Decimals

Add the following decimals.

1. 0.4 + 0.7 =

2. 5.03 + 2.999 =

3. 2.27 + 0.07 + 4 =

4. 15.6 + 0.19 + 500 =

5. 210.79 + 2 + 68.41 =

Subtraction of Decimals

Steps for Subtracting Decimals

1. Write decimals in a column, keeping the decimal points under each other.
2. Subtract as in whole numbers, from right to left.
3. Place the decimal point in the answer directly under the decimal points in the numbers to be subtracted (zeros can be added *after* the decimal point without changing the value).

Examples

0.604	0.500
− 0.524	− 0.123
0.08~~0~~	0.377

remember **Line up the decimal points.**
Remove trailing zeros from the final answer.

Answers on page 35

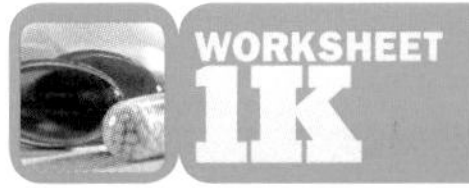

WORKSHEET 1K | Subtraction of Decimals

Subtract the following decimals.

1. 2.5 − 1.25 =

2. 0.5 − 0.25 =

3. 0.45 − 0.367 =

4. 108.56 − 5.4 =

5. 1.25 − 0.75 =

Multiplication of Decimals

Steps for Multiplying Decimals

1. Multiply as with whole numbers.
2. Count the total number of decimal places in the multiplier and in the number to be multiplied.
3. Start from the right and count off the same number of places in the answer.
4. If the answer does not have enough places, supply as many zeros as needed, counting from right to left as illustrated on the following page. Eliminate trailing zeros in the answer.

Example $2.5 \times 0.0002 =$

2.5	(1 decimal place)
× 0.0002	(4 decimal places)
0.00050̸	(5 decimal places from right to left in the answer before the trailing zero is deleted)

Answers on page 35

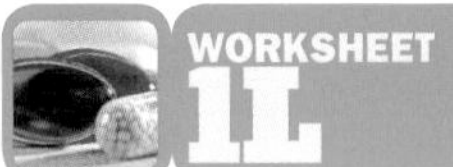

WORKSHEET 1L | Multiplication of Decimals

Multiply the following decimals.

1. 100 × 0.5 =

2. 0.25 × 2 =

3. 3.14 × 0.072 =

4. 2.14 × 0.03 =

5. 58.7 × 70.1 =

Division of Decimals

Examine the divisor—the number you are dividing by. Is it a *whole* number or a *decimal?*

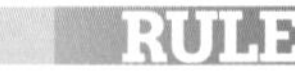

RULE **If the divisor is a *whole* number, the dividend decimal place is unchanged. Immediately place the decimal point prominently on the answer line directly *above* the decimal point in the dividend. Use zeros in the answer to hold places until you can divide. Prove your answer.**

Example 1.20 ÷ 15

```
              0.08  ← Answer
Divisor → 15)1.20  ← Dividend
              1 20
```

PROOF (Divisor × answer = dividend)

```
  0.08
×   15
  1.20̸
```

Example 3.15 ÷ 7

```
   0.45
7)3.15
  2 8
  ---
    35
    35
    --
```

PROOF
```
  0.45
×    7
  ----
  3.15
```

RULE If the divisor has a *decimal*, you must make it a whole number by moving the decimal point to the right. Move the decimal point in the dividend the same number of places to the right and immediately place the decimal point directly above on the answer line. Then divide as with whole numbers. Prove your answer.

Example 10 ÷ 4.4

```
         2.27
4.4)10.0 00
     8 8
     -----
     1 2 0
       8 8
       ----
       3 20
       3 08
       ----
         12  Remainder
```

PROOF
```
   2.27  (2 decimal places)
 × 4.4   (1 decimal place)
   ----
    908
   908
   ----
   9988
 +   12  Remainder
 ------
 10.000  Move decimal 3 places.
```

Example 30 ÷ 5.2

```
          5.7
5.2)30.0 0
    26 0
    -----
     4 0 0
     3 6 4
     -----
       3 6  Remainder
```

PROOF
```
   5.2  (1 decimal place)
 × 5.7  (1 decimal place)
  ----
  36 4
 260
 -----
 296 4
 + 3 6  Remainder
 -----
 30.00  Move decimal 2 places
```

Note that, as with whole division, a remainder is not just added to the answer in decimal division. Additional division will allow the remainder to be converted to a decimal fraction.

Example 2.6 ÷ 4

```
   0.6              0.65
4)2.6             4)2.60
  2 4               2 4
  ---               ---
    2 Remainder      20
                     20
                     --
```

remember Keep all the decimal points dark for accuracy.

Answers on page 36

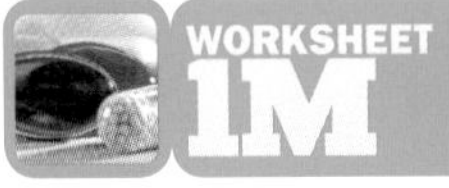

WORKSHEET 1M Division of Decimals

In the following problems, the divisor is a whole number. Place the decimal point on the answer line as illustrated in red in #1. Do NOT do the math in these problems.

1. 60)1.35

2. 20)15.6

3. 19)10.14

4. 7)60.5

5. 25)35.9

In the following problems, the divisor has a decimal. Make the divisor a whole number, move the decimal place an equal number of places in the dividend, and place the decimal point on the answer line as illustrated in red in #6. Calculate the answer to the *nearest tenth*. Add zeros to the dividend as necessary.

6. $0.25\overline{)0.50}$

7. $0.1\overline{)0.5}$

8. $4.8\overline{)2.04}$

9. $0.5\overline{)0.25}$

10. $0.12\overline{)0.44}$

Answers on page 36

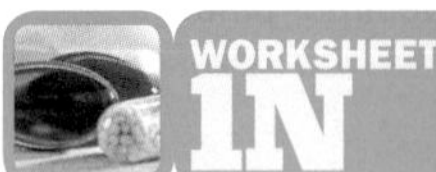

WORKSHEET 1N More Division of Decimals

Divide the following and carry to the *third* decimal place if necessary. Prove the answers.

1. 200 ÷ 6 =

2. 15.06 ÷ 6 =

3. 79.4 ÷ 0.87 =

4. 158.4 ÷ 48 =

5. 670.8 ÷ 0.78 =

Changing Decimals to Fractions

RULE **The numbers to the *right* of the decimal can be written as a fraction because they are only part of the whole number.**

remember **The first number past the decimal to the *right* is ten*ths,* the second is hundred*ths,* the third is thousand*ths,* the fourth is ten-thousand*ths,* and so on.**

So if your problem has 3 numbers to the *right* of the decimal, just remove the decimal and put the number over 1000.

Example 0.376 has 3 numbers to the *right* of the decimal. To make a fraction out of 0.376 and also get rid of the decimal, place it over 1000.

0.376 written as a fraction is $\frac{376}{1000}$.

Example It's easy to remember: 3 numbers on top and 3 zeros on the bottom.

0.95 written as a fraction is $\frac{95}{100}$.

The idea is the same as above: 2 numbers on top and 2 zeros on the bottom. The fraction $\frac{90}{100}$ can be reduced to $\frac{9}{10}$ by dividing the numerator and the denominator by 10.

Answers on page 37

WORKSHEET 10 Changing Decimals to Fractions

Change the following decimals to fractions, and reduce to lowest terms.

1. 0.8 =
2. 0.4 =
3. 0.25 =
4. 1.32 =
5. 4.08 =
6. 0.5 =
7. 0.75 =
8. 0.2 =
9. 0.65 =
10. 0.7 =

Changing Common Fractions to Decimals

RULE **To change a common fraction to a decimal, divide the numerator by the denominator and place the decimal point in the proper position on the answer line.**

Examples

$$\frac{2}{5} = 5\overline{)2.0} = 0.4 \qquad \begin{array}{r} 0.4 \\ 5\overline{)2.0} \\ \underline{2\,0} \end{array}$$

$$\frac{1}{8} = 8\overline{)1.000} \qquad \begin{array}{r} 0.125 \\ 8\overline{)1.000} \\ \underline{8} \\ 20 \\ \underline{16} \\ 40 \\ \underline{40} \end{array}$$

Answers on page 37

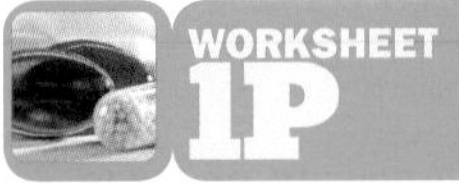

WORKSHEET 1P Changing Common Fractions to Decimals

Carry out the following division problems to the *third* decimal place as needed.

1. $\frac{1}{5} =$
2. $\frac{2}{3} =$
3. $\frac{1}{2} =$
4. $\frac{1}{12} =$
5. $\frac{6}{8} =$

Percentages, Decimals, and Fractions

The term "percent" and its symbol (%) mean parts per hundred. A percent number is a fraction whose numerator is already known and whose denominator is always understood to be 100. 25% means 25 parts per hundred.

Changing a Percentage to a Decimal

RULE To change a percentage to a decimal, divide the percentage by 100, moving the decimal point two places to the *left*. Remove the percent sign. (Remember that an implied decimal point immediately follows a whole number.)

Examples $5\% \div 100 = 0.05$ (5% has an implied decimal point after the 5)

$0.5\% = 0.005$

$10\% = 0.1$ (10% has an implied decimal point after the 10)

Changing a Percentage to a Fraction

RULE To change the percentage to a fraction, *first* change the percentage to a decimal by dividing the percentage by 100, moving the decimal point two places to the *left*. Write the decimal as a fraction.

Example $5\% (\div 100) = 0.05 = \frac{5}{100}$

The fraction can then be further reduced to $\frac{1}{20}$

$0.1\% = 0.001 = \frac{1}{1000}$

$10\% = 0.1 = \frac{10}{100} = \frac{1}{10}$

Converting a Decimal to a Percentage

RULE To change a decimal to a percentage, multiply the decimal by 100 by moving the decimal point 2 places to the *right*. Then add the percent sign.

Examples $0.1 (\times 100) = 10\%$

$0.01 = 1\%$

$0.5 = 50\%$

Answers on page 37

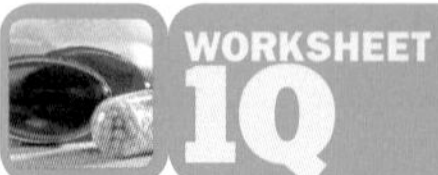

WORKSHEET 1Q

Percentages, Decimals, and Fractions

Fill in the following blanks with the appropriate equivalents.

	Fraction	Decimal	Percentage
1.	$\frac{1}{2}$		
2.			50%
3.		0.05	
4.	$\frac{1}{12}$		
5.	$\frac{3}{1000}$		
6.		0.10	
7.			250%

8.		0.35	
9.	$\frac{4}{5}$		
10.			75%

Steps for Finding the Percentage

1. Change the percentage to a decimal or common fraction.
2. *Multiply* the number by this decimal.

Examples $50\% \text{ of } 120 = 0.5 \times 120 = 60 \text{ or } \frac{1}{2} \times 120 = 60$

$10\% \text{ of } 120 = 0.1 \times 120 = 12 \text{ or } \frac{1}{10} \times 120 = 12$

Answers on page 37

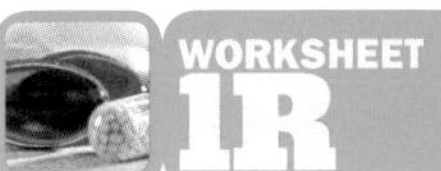

WORKSHEET 1R Finding the Percentage

Solve the following problems.

1. 2% of 1500 =
2. 114% of 240 =
3. 28% of 50 =
4. 9% of 200 =
5. $\frac{1}{2}$% of 9328 =
6. $\frac{1}{3}$% of 930 =
7. 120% of 400 =
8. 5% of 105.80 =
9. 10% of 520 =
10. 3% of 40.80 =

Answers on page 38

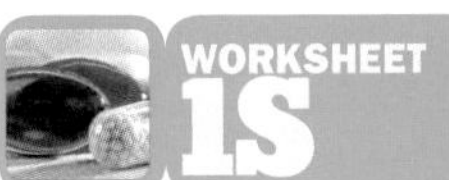

WORKSHEET 1S Using Fractions to Percentages to Make Solutions

In the hospital, you might be asked to prepare a baby formula diluted to 50% ($\frac{1}{2}$) strength from a full-strength formula. If the baby was to receive 120 mL (4 oz) at each feeding, the nurse would multiply 0.5 (or $\frac{1}{2}$) × 120 for a result of 60 mL. 60 mL of full strength formula would be measured and 60 mL of water added (120 mL − 60) for the total 120 mL to make a 50%-strength formula.

For 10% strength, the nurse would multiply 0.1 × 120 for a result of 12 mL full-strength formula. The nurse would measure 12 mL of full-strength formula and add 108 mL of water (120 mL total − 12 mL formula = 108 mL) for the total of 120 mL of 10%-strength formula.

Another way to do the math would be by ratio and proportion. This method will be introduced in Chapter 2. It is simpler to convert percentages, decimals, and fractions using basic arithmetic.

10 mL : 100 mL = x mL : 120 mL

$100x = 10 \times 120$

x = 12 mL of full-strength formula

120 − 12 = 108 mL of water to be added

Multiply the two inside numbers (the means). Then multiply the two outside numbers (the extremes). Divide the x number 100 into the product of 10 × 120 = 1200. The answer is the amount of formula needed.

Make 150 mL of a 50% Betadine solution using normal saline (NS). 50% can be written as 50 : 100 or 1 : 2. The Betadine solution is the active solution and the NS is the solvent.

1 mL : 2 mL = x mL : 150 mL.

Multiply the two inside numbers (means) and then the 2 outside numbers (extremes). Always divide the x number into the number on the right to get the answer. The resulting answer is the amount of solvent (Betadine) needed to make a 50% solution. The formula is called a ratio and proportion:

1 mL : 2 mL = x mL : 150 mL

Example

$2x = 1 \times 150 = 150$

$2x = 150$

$x = 75$ mL Betadine + 75 mL of NS = 150 mL of a 50% solution.

Make the following solutions using Betadine solution as the active ingredient and NS as the diluent.

1. Make 450 mL yielding a $\frac{2}{3}$ strength solution.
2. Make 6 oz of a $\frac{1}{3}$ strength solution.
3. Make a $\frac{1}{4}$ strength solution for a total of 500 mL.
4. Make 800 mL yielding a $\frac{3}{4}$ strength solution.
5. Make a $\frac{2}{5}$ ratio solution for a total of 120 mL.

Answers on page 38

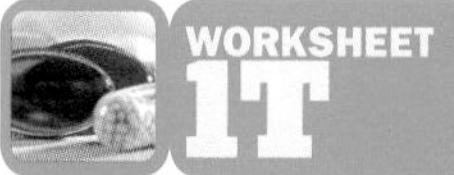

WORKSHEET 1T Multiple-Choice Practice

Solve the following problems and select the correct answer. Estimate the correct answer before working the problem.

1. $\frac{30}{9}$ can be converted to which whole and mixed number?

a. $3\frac{3}{9} = 3\frac{1}{3}$

b. $2\frac{1}{30}$

c. $2\frac{1}{8}$

d. $4\frac{2}{9}$

2. Select the *fraction* equivalent for $3\frac{5}{6}$.

a. $\frac{15}{6}$

b. $\frac{23}{6}$

c. $4\frac{1}{6}$

d. $\frac{8}{6}$

3. $\frac{7}{8}$ and $\frac{3}{5}$ have which lowest common denominator?

a. 8

b. 10

c. 13

d. 40

4. $5\frac{1}{8} + 1\frac{1}{4} + 4\frac{1}{2} =$

a. $10\frac{7}{8}$
b. $9\frac{1}{6}$
c. $12\frac{1}{2}$
d. $10\frac{3}{4}$

5. $6\frac{3}{4} - 5\frac{1}{3} =$

a. $\frac{1}{2}$
b. $1\frac{1}{2}$
c. $1\frac{5}{12}$
d. $1\frac{5}{8}$

6. $\frac{5}{6} \times \frac{2}{8} =$

a. $\frac{1}{12}$
b. $\frac{5}{24}$
c. $\frac{7}{14}$
d. $\frac{10}{44}$

7. Divide the following fraction and reduce to the lowest term: $\frac{1}{6} \div \frac{1}{3}$

a. $\frac{2}{12}$
b. $\frac{1}{2}$
c. $\frac{1}{6}$
d. $\frac{1}{3}$

8. Divide the following fraction and reduce to the lowest term: $\frac{5}{6} \div \frac{1}{3}$

a. $\frac{1}{6}$
b. $\frac{5}{18}$
c. $1\frac{1}{6}$
d. $2\frac{1}{2}$

9. Two and eighteen thousandths can be written in decimal form as:
a. 2.0018
b. 2.018
c. 2.18
d. 2.118

10. 0.41 − 0.2538 =
a. 0.1562
b. 0.2503
c. 0.4138
d. 0.6638

11. 5 × 0.9 =
a. 0.45
b. 4.5
c. 5.09
d. 45

12. 79.4 ÷ 0.87 =
a. 12.024
b. 21.084
c. 80.276
d. 91.264

13. Change $\frac{1}{6}$ to a decimal and round the answer to the nearest *hundredth.*

a. 0.02
b. 0.0625
c. 0.167
d. 0.17

14. 20% of 450 =

a. 90
b. 135
c. 150
d. 185

15. $6\frac{1}{4}$% of 9328 =

a. 0.56
b. 540
c. 583
d. 5596

16. Change 0.285 to a fraction.

a. $\frac{285}{1000}$
b. $\frac{28}{100}$
c. $\frac{285}{100}$
d. $\frac{29}{1000}$

17. Change $\frac{2}{5}$ to a decimal to the nearest *tenth.*

a. 0.4
b. 0.25
c. 0.04
d. 0.025

18. Change $\frac{1}{8}$ to a decimal to the nearest *hundredth.*

a. 0.13
b. 0.12
c. 0.17
d. 0.125

19. Round 58.09 to the nearest *tenth.*

a. 58
b. 58.07
c. 58.1
d. 58.7

20. Change 4% to a decimal.

a. 0.4
b. 0.04
c. 0.25
d. 0.2

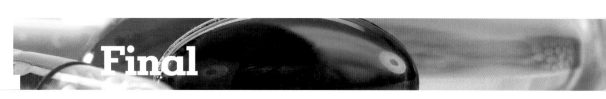

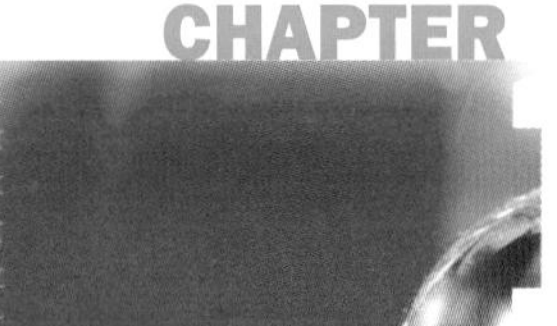

CHAPTER 1 Final

Change to whole or mixed numbers.

1. $\frac{25}{4}$ **2.** $\frac{48}{6}$

Change to an improper fraction.

3. $10\frac{1}{5}$ **4.** $3\frac{5}{6}$

Find the lowest common denominator in the following pairs of fractions.

5. $\frac{17}{20}$ and $\frac{4}{5}$ **6.** $\frac{7}{8}$ and $\frac{3}{5}$

Add the following.

7. $\frac{2}{18} + \frac{1}{4} + \frac{2}{9}$ **8.** $5\frac{1}{8} + 1\frac{1}{4} + 4\frac{1}{2}$

Subtract the following.

9. $\frac{7}{8} - \frac{2}{3}$ **10.** $6\frac{2}{4} - 5\frac{1}{2}$

Multiply the following.

11. $\frac{5}{6} \times \frac{2}{8}$ **12.** $\frac{1}{5} \times \frac{1}{6}$

Divide the following.

13. $\frac{3}{4} \div \frac{1}{8}$ **14.** $3\frac{3}{8} \div 4\frac{1}{2}$

Reduce the following fractions to lowest terms (numbers).

15. $\frac{2}{500}$ **16.** $\frac{9}{27}$

Write the following as decimals.

17. Five hundredths **18.** Two and seventeen thousandths

Add the following.

19. 5.01 + 2.999 **20.** 36.87 + 8.26 + 15.84

Subtract the following.

21. $4 - 0.176$

22. $0.53 - 0.2538$

Multiply the following.

23. 0.0005×0.02

24. 5×0.7

Divide the following and carry to the third decimal place.

25. $158.4 \div 48$

26. $79.4 \div 0.87$

Change the following to decimals.

27. $\frac{57}{48}$

28. $8\frac{1}{16}$

Find the following percentages.

29. 24% of 52

30. $6\frac{1}{4}$% of 9328

Change the following decimals to fractions.

31. 0.4

32. 0.285

Fill in the following blanks with the appropriate equivalents.

	Fraction	Decimal to Nearest Tenth	Decimal to Nearest Hundredth	Percentage
33.	$\frac{1}{3}$			
34.				5%
35.	$\frac{2}{5}$			
36.				22%
37.	$\frac{1}{8}$			
38.				10%
39.	$\frac{1}{12}$			
40.				$\frac{1}{2}$%
41.	$\frac{5}{16}$			
42.				15%
43.	$\frac{1}{4}$			
44.				12%
45.	$\frac{1}{100}$			
46.				80%
47.	$\frac{1}{200}$			
48.				33%
49.	$\frac{1}{250}$			
50.				75%

Answer Key

1 General Mathematics

WORKSHEET **1A** (page 6)

1. $\frac{1}{10}$
2. $\frac{2}{7}$
3. $\frac{1}{20}$
4. $\frac{1}{100,000}$
5. More
6. $\frac{1}{5}$
7. $\frac{1}{150}$
8. $\frac{1}{250}$
9. $\frac{1}{9}$
10. $\frac{1}{200}$

WORKSHEET **1B** (page 7)

1. 1
2. 5
3. $3\frac{1}{4}$
4. $1\frac{5}{9}$
5. $5\frac{2}{3}$
6. 5
7. $2\frac{1}{4}$
8. $1\frac{7}{8}$
9. 6
10. $6\frac{5}{6}$

WORKSHEET **1C** (page 8)

1. $\frac{7}{2}$
2. $\frac{7}{6}$
3. $\frac{33}{8}$
4. $\frac{43}{12}$
5. $\frac{68}{5}$
6. $\frac{49}{3}$
7. $\frac{23}{6}$
8. $\frac{21}{8}$
9. $\frac{63}{6}$
10. $\frac{377}{3}$

WORKSHEET **1D** (page 11)

1. $\frac{2}{5} + \frac{2}{5} = \frac{4}{5}$
2. $\frac{4}{5} = \frac{12}{15}$; $+\frac{2}{3} = \frac{10}{15}$; $\frac{22}{15} = 1\frac{7}{15}$
3. $6\frac{1}{6} = 6\frac{4}{24}$; $+9\frac{5}{8} = 9\frac{15}{24}$; $15\frac{19}{24}$
4. $2\frac{1}{4} = 2\frac{2}{8}$; $+3\frac{1}{8} = 3\frac{1}{8}$; $5\frac{3}{8}$
5. $1\frac{3}{4} = 1\frac{30}{40}$; $+9\frac{9}{10} = 9\frac{36}{40}$; $10\frac{66}{40} = 11\frac{13}{20}$
6. $\frac{1}{8} = \frac{9}{72}$; $\frac{1}{4} = \frac{18}{72}$; $+\frac{3}{9} = \frac{24}{72}$; $\frac{51}{72}$
7. $\frac{7}{9} = \frac{70}{90}$; $\frac{4}{5} = \frac{72}{90}$; $+\frac{9}{10} = \frac{81}{90}$; $\frac{223}{90} = 2\frac{43}{90}$
8. $3\frac{1}{4}$; $+9\frac{3}{4}$; $12\frac{4}{4} = 13$

9.
$$\begin{array}{rcl} 8\frac{2}{5} & = & 8\frac{4}{10} \\ 14\frac{7}{10} & = & 14\frac{7}{10} \\ +9\frac{9}{10} & = & 9\frac{9}{10} \\ \hline & & 31\frac{20}{10} = 33 \end{array}$$

10.
$$\begin{array}{rcl} 2\frac{1}{3} & = & 2\frac{2}{6} \\ +4\frac{1}{6} & = & 4\frac{1}{6} \\ \hline & & 6\frac{3}{6} = 6\frac{1}{2} \end{array}$$

WORKSHEET **1E** (page 13)

1.
$$\begin{array}{rcl} \frac{2}{3} & = & \frac{4}{6} \\ -\frac{1}{2} & = & \frac{3}{6} \\ \hline & & \frac{1}{6} \end{array}$$

2.
$$\begin{array}{r} \frac{27}{32} \\ -\frac{18}{32} \\ \hline \frac{9}{32} \end{array}$$

3.
$$\begin{array}{rcl} 10\frac{2}{5} & = & 10\frac{8}{20} \\ -6\frac{1}{4} & = & 6\frac{5}{20} \\ \hline & & 4\frac{3}{20} \end{array}$$

4.
$$\begin{array}{rcl} 7\frac{16}{24} & = & 7\frac{16}{24} \\ -3\frac{1}{8} & = & 3\frac{3}{24} \\ \hline & & 4\frac{13}{24} \end{array}$$

(Must borrow from the whole number.)

5.
$$\begin{array}{rcl} 6\frac{3}{10} & = & 6\frac{3}{10} \\ -2\frac{1}{5} & = & 2\frac{2}{10} \\ \hline & & 4\frac{1}{10} \end{array}$$

6.
$$\begin{array}{rcl} \frac{7}{8} & = & \frac{21}{24} \\ -\frac{1}{3} & = & \frac{8}{24} \\ \hline & & \frac{13}{24} \end{array}$$

7.
$$\begin{array}{r} 3\frac{5}{8} \\ -1\frac{3}{8} \\ \hline 2\frac{2}{8} = 2\frac{1}{4} \end{array}$$

8.
$$\begin{array}{rcl} 5\frac{3}{7} & = & 4\frac{10}{7} \\ -1\frac{6}{7} & = & 1\frac{6}{7} \\ \hline & & 3\frac{4}{7} \end{array}$$

(Must borrow from the whole number.)

9.
$$\begin{array}{rcl} 7 & = & 6\frac{4}{4} \\ -1\frac{3}{4} & = & 1\frac{3}{4} \\ \hline & & 5\frac{1}{4} \end{array}$$

10.
$$\begin{array}{rcl} 2\frac{7}{8} & = & 2\frac{7}{8} \\ -\frac{3}{4} & = & \frac{6}{8} \\ \hline & & 2\frac{1}{8} \end{array}$$

(Must borrow from the whole number.)

WORKSHEET **1F** (page 14)

1. $\frac{1}{5} \times \frac{2}{4} = \frac{2}{20} = \frac{1}{10}$

2. $\frac{1}{5} \times \frac{1}{6} = \frac{1}{30}$

3. $\frac{3}{5} \times \frac{5}{8} = \frac{15}{40} = \frac{3}{8}$

4. $4 \times 3\frac{1}{3} = 4 \times \frac{10}{3} = \frac{40}{3} = 13\frac{1}{3}$

5. $\frac{2}{4} \times 2\frac{1}{6} = \frac{\overset{1}{\cancel{2}}}{4} \times \frac{13}{\underset{3}{\cancel{6}}} = \frac{13}{12} = 1\frac{1}{12}$

6. $5\frac{1}{2} \times 3\frac{1}{8} = \frac{11}{2} \times \frac{25}{8} = \frac{275}{16} = 275 \div 16 = 17\frac{3}{16}$

7. $1\frac{3}{4} \times 3\frac{1}{7} = \frac{\overset{1}{\cancel{7}}}{4} \times \frac{22}{\underset{1}{\cancel{7}}} = \frac{22}{4} = 22 \div 4 = 5\frac{1}{2}$

8. $\frac{5}{6} \times 1\frac{9}{16} = \frac{5}{6} \times \frac{25}{16} = \frac{125}{96} = 125 \div 96 = 1\frac{29}{96}$

9. $\frac{5}{100} \times 900 = \frac{5}{\underset{1}{\cancel{100}}} \times \frac{\overset{9}{\cancel{900}}}{1} = 45$

10. $2\frac{1}{10} \times 4\frac{1}{3} = \frac{\overset{7}{\cancel{21}}}{10} \times \frac{13}{\underset{1}{\cancel{3}}} = \frac{91}{10} = 9\frac{1}{10}$

WORKSHEET 1G (page 14)

1. $\frac{1}{5} \div \frac{1}{8} = \frac{1}{5} \times \frac{8}{1} = \frac{8}{5} = 1\frac{3}{5}$

2. $\frac{1}{3} \div \frac{1}{2} = \frac{1}{3} \times \frac{2}{1} = \frac{2}{3}$

3. $\frac{3}{4} \div \frac{1}{8} = \frac{3}{\cancel{4}_{1}} \times \frac{\cancel{8}^{2}}{1} = 6$

4. $\frac{1}{16} \div \frac{1}{4} = \frac{1}{\cancel{16}_{4}} \times \frac{\cancel{4}^{1}}{1} = \frac{1}{4}$

5. $8\frac{3}{4} \div 15 = \frac{\cancel{35}^{7}}{4} \times \frac{1}{\cancel{15}_{3}} = \frac{7}{12}$

6. $\frac{3}{4} \div 6 = \frac{\cancel{3}^{1}}{4} \times \frac{1}{\cancel{6}_{2}} = \frac{1}{8}$

7. $2 \div \frac{1}{5} = \frac{2}{1} \times \frac{5}{1} = 10$

8. $3\frac{3}{8} \div 4\frac{1}{2} = \frac{27}{8} \div \frac{9}{2} = \frac{\cancel{27}^{3}}{\cancel{8}_{4}} \times \frac{\cancel{2}^{1}}{\cancel{9}_{1}} = \frac{3}{4}$

9. $\frac{3}{5} \div \frac{3}{8} = \frac{\cancel{3}^{1}}{5} \times \frac{8}{\cancel{3}_{1}} = \frac{8}{5} = 1\frac{3}{5}$

10. $4 \div 2\frac{1}{8} = \frac{4}{1} \times \frac{8}{17} = \frac{32}{17} = 1\frac{15}{17}$

WORKSHEET 1HA (page 16)

	Nearest Whole Number	Nearest Tenth	Nearest Hundredth
1. 93.489	93	93.5	93.49
2. 25.43	25	25.4	25.43
3. 38.2	38	38.2	38.20
4. 57.8888	58	57.9	57.89
5. 0.0092	0	0	0.01
6. 3.144	3	3.1	3.14
7. 8.999	9	9.0	9.00
8. 77.788	78	77.8	77.79
9. 12.959	13	13.0	12.96
10. 5.7703	6	5.8	5.77

WORKSHEET 1HB (page 17)

1. Six hundredths
2. Ninety-six thousandths
3. Five thousandths
4. One hundred and one hundredth
5. Nine tenths
6. 0.34
7. 0.004
8. 2.017
9. 9.0002
10. 34.1

WORKSHEET 1IA (page 18)

Round to tenths

1. 0.3
2. 4.4
3. 2.8
4. 0.8
5. 6.8

Round to hundredths

6. 0.30
7. 4.44
8. 2.75
9. 0.85
10. 6.77

Round to thousandths

11. 8.937
12. 5.626
13. 10.898
14. 4.626
15. 3.739

Round to ten-thousandths

16. 8.9375
17. 5.6257
18. 10.8976
19. 4.6256
20. 3.7387

WORKSHEET 1IB (page 18)

Smaller:

1. 0.2
2. 0.25
3. 0.125
4. 2.07
5. 1.29

Larger:

6. 0.9
7. 0.7
8. 0.58
9. 0.25
10. 0.1

WORKSHEET 1J (page 19)

```
     0.4
   + 0.7
   -----
1.   1.1
```

```
     5.030
   + 2.999
   -------
2.   8.029
```

```
     2.27
     0.07
   + 4.00
   ------
3.   6.34
```

```
      15.60
       0.19
   + 500.00
   --------
4.   515.79
```

```
     210.79
       2.00
   +  68.41
   --------
5.   281.20*
```

WORKSHEET 1K (page 20)

```
     2.50
   - 1.25
   ------
1.   1.25
```

```
     0.50
   - 0.25
   ------
2.   0.25
```

```
     0.450
   - 0.367
   -------
3.   0.083
```

```
     108.56
   -   5.40
   --------
4.   103.16
```

```
     1.25
   - 0.75
   ------
5.   0.50*
```

WORKSHEET 1L (page 20)

```
    100
   × 0.5
   -----
1. 50.0
```

Count 1 decimal place in from the right.

```
   0.25
   ×  2
   ----
2. 0.50
```

Count 2 decimal places in from the right.

```
       3.14
   × 0.072
   -------
3. 0.22608
```

You do not have to multiply zeros. Count 5 decimal places in from the right, adding zeros where needed.

```
     2.14
   × 0.03
   ------
4. 0.0642
```

Count 4 decimal places in from the right, adding zeros as needed.

```
      58.7
    × 70.1
    ------
      58.7
    41090
   -------
5. 4114.87
```

*Trailing zeros must be removed from answers.

WORKSHEET 1M (page 21)

1. 60)1.35

2. 20)15.6

3. 19)10.14

4. 7)60.5

5. 25)35.9

6.
```
         2.
0.25)0.50
      50
      ——
       0
```
ANSWER: 2

7.
```
        5.
0.1 )0.5
```
ANSWER: 5

8.
```
       0.425
4.8 )2.0400
     1 9 2
     ——————
       120
       –96
       ———
        240
        240
        ———
          0
```
ANSWER: 0.4

9.
```
        0.5
0.5 )0.2 5
        2 5
        ———
```
ANSWER: 0.5

10.
```
         3.66
0.12)0.44 00
      36
      ————
       8 0
       7 2
       ———
        80
        72
        ——
         8
```
ANSWER: 3.7

WORKSHEET 1N (page 22)

1.
```
   3 3.333
6)200.0 000
  180
  ———
   20 0
   18 0
   ————
    2 0 0
    1 8 0
    —————
     2 00
     1 80
     ————
      200
      180
      ———
```
PROOF
```
   33.333
×      60
—————————
 1999.980
```

2.
```
   2.51
6)15.06
  12
  ——
   3 0
   3 0
   ———
    06
     6
    ——
```
PROOF
```
  2.51
×    6
——————
 15.06
```

3.
```
        91.264
0.87)79.40 000
      78 30
      —————
       1 10
         87
       ————
         23 0
         17 4
         ————
          5 60
          5 22
          ————
            380
            348
            ———
```
PROOF
```
  91.264
×     87
————————
 638 848
7301 12
————————
7939.968
```

4.
```
     3.3
48)158.4
   144
   —————
    14 4
    14 4
    ————
```
PROOF
```
   48
× 3.3
—————
 14 4
144
—————
158.4
```

5.
```
        860.
0.78)670.80
      624
      ———
       46 8
       46 8
       ————
```
PROOF
```
  860
  ×78
 ————
 6880
6020
—————
67080
```

WORKSHEET 1O (page 23)

1. $\frac{8}{10} = \frac{4}{5}$
2. $\frac{4}{10} = \frac{2}{5}$
3. $\frac{25}{100} = \frac{1}{4}$
4. $1\frac{32}{100} = 1\frac{8}{25}$
5. $4\frac{8}{100} = 4\frac{2}{25}$
6. $\frac{5}{10} = \frac{1}{2}$
7. $\frac{75}{100} = \frac{3}{4}$
8. $\frac{2}{10} = \frac{1}{5}$
9. $\frac{65}{100} = \frac{13}{20}$
10. $\frac{7}{10}$

WORKSHEET 1P (page 23)

1. $$\begin{array}{r} 0.2 \\ 5\overline{)1.0} \\ \underline{1\ 0} \end{array}$$

2. $$\begin{array}{r} 0.666 \\ 3\overline{)2.000} \\ \underline{1\ 8} \\ 20 \\ \underline{18} \\ 20 \\ \underline{18} \end{array}$$

3. $$\begin{array}{r} 0.5 \\ 2\overline{)1.0} \\ \underline{1\ 0} \end{array}$$

4. $$\begin{array}{r} 0.083 \\ 12\overline{)1.000} \\ \underline{96} \\ 40 \\ \underline{36} \end{array}$$

5. $$\begin{array}{r} 0.75 \\ 8\overline{)6.00} \\ \underline{5\ 6} \\ 40 \\ \underline{40} \end{array}$$

WORKSHEET 1Q (page 24)

1. Decimal: 0.5
   Percentage: 50%
2. Fraction: $\frac{1}{2}$
   Decimal: 0.5
3. Fraction: $\frac{5}{100} = \frac{1}{20}$
   Percentage: 5%
4. Decimal: 0.083
   Percentage: 8.33%
5. Decimal: 0.003
   Percentage: 0.3%
6. Fraction: $\frac{1}{10}$
   Percentage: 10%
7. Fraction: $\frac{250}{100} = \frac{5}{2}$
   Decimal: 2.5
8. Fraction: $\frac{7}{20}$
   Percentage: 35%
9. Decimal: 0.8
   Percentage: 80%
10. Fraction: $\frac{75}{100} = \frac{3}{4}$
    Decimal: 0.75

WORKSHEET 1R (page 25)

1. $$\begin{array}{r} 1500 \\ \underline{\times 0.02} \\ 30.0\cancel{0}^{*} \end{array}$$

2. $$\begin{array}{r} 240 \\ \underline{\times 1.14} \\ 960 \\ 240 \\ \underline{240} \\ 273.6\cancel{0}^{*} \end{array}$$

3. $$\begin{array}{r} 50 \\ \underline{\times 0.28} \\ 400 \\ \underline{100} \\ 14.0\cancel{0}^{*} \end{array}$$

4. $$\begin{array}{r} 200 \\ \underline{\times 0.09} \\ 18.0\cancel{0}^{*} \end{array}$$

5. $$\frac{\frac{1}{2}}{100} = \frac{1}{2} \div \frac{100}{1} = \frac{1}{2} \times \frac{1}{100} = \frac{1}{200} = \begin{array}{r} 0.005 \\ 200\overline{)1.000} \end{array} \qquad \begin{array}{r} 9328 \\ \underline{\times 0.005} \\ 46.64\cancel{0}^{*} \end{array}$$

6. $$\frac{\frac{1}{3}}{100} = \frac{1}{3} \div \frac{100}{1} = \frac{1}{3} \times \frac{1}{100} = \frac{1}{300} = \begin{array}{r} 0.003 \\ 300\overline{)1.000} \\ \underline{900} \\ 100 \end{array} \qquad \begin{array}{r} 930 \\ \underline{\times 0.003} \\ 2.79\cancel{0}^{*} \end{array}$$

7.
$$\begin{array}{r} 400 \\ \times 1.20 \\ \hline 8000 \\ 400 \\ \hline 480.\not{0}\not{0}^* \end{array}$$

8.
$$\begin{array}{r} 105.80 \\ \times 0.05 \\ \hline 5.29\not{0}\not{0}^* \end{array}$$

9.
$$\begin{array}{r} 520 \\ \times 0.10 \\ \hline 52.\not{0}\not{0}^* \end{array}$$

10.
$$\begin{array}{r} 40.80 \\ \times 0.03 \\ \hline 1.224\not{0}^* \end{array}$$

WORKSHEET 1S (page 25)

1. $2 : 3 = x : 450$
$3x = 2 \times 450 = 900$
$x = 300$ mL of Betadine + 150 mL NS = $\frac{2}{3}$ strength solution

2. $1 : 3 = x : 6$
$3x = 6$
$x = 2$ oz of Betadine + 4 oz of NS = 6 oz of $\frac{1}{3}$ strength solution

3. $1 : 4 = x : 500$
$4x = 500$
$x = 125$ mL Betadine + 375 mL NS = 500 mL $\frac{1}{4}$ strength solution

4. $3 : 4 = x : 800$
$4x = 3 \times 800 = 2400$
$x = 600$ mL Betadine + 200 mL NS = 800 mL $\frac{3}{4}$ strength solution

5. $2 : 5 = x : 120$
$5x = 2 \times 120 = 240$
$x = 48$ mL Betadine + 72 mL NS = 120 mL $\frac{2}{5}$ strength solution

WORKSHEET 1T (page 26)

1. a The other responses can be eliminated quickly because only **a** offers 3 as the whole number.

2. b	**3.** d	**4.** a	**5.** c
6. b	**7.** b	**8.** d	**9.** b
10. a	**11.** b	**12.** d	**13.** d
14. a	**15.** c	**16.** a	**17.** a
18. a	**19.** c	**20.** b	

CHAPTER 1 FINAL: GENERAL MATHEMATICS (page 29)

1. $6\frac{1}{4}$	**2.** 8	**3.** $\frac{51}{5}$	**4.** $\frac{23}{6}$
5. 20	**6.** 40	**7.** $\frac{21}{36}$	**8.** $10\frac{7}{8}$
9. $\frac{5}{24}$	**10.** 1	**11.** $\frac{10}{48} = \frac{5}{24}$	**12.** $\frac{1}{30}$
13. $\frac{24}{4} = 6$	**14.** $\frac{3}{4}$	**15.** $\frac{1}{250}$	**16.** $\frac{1}{3}$

*When calculating medication dosages, trailing zeros must be removed from answers.

17. 0.05 **18.** 2.017 **19.** 8.009 **20.** 60.97

21. 3.824 **22.** 0.2762 **23.** 0.00001~~0~~* **24.** 3.5

25. 3.3* **26.** 91.264 **27.** 1.1875 **28.** 8.0625

29. 12.48 **30.** 583 **31.** $\frac{2}{5}$ **32.** $\frac{57}{200}$

	Fraction	Decimal to Nearest Tenth	Decimal to Nearest Hundredth	Percentage
33.	$\frac{1}{3}$	0.3	0.33	33%
34.	$\frac{5}{100} = \left(\frac{1}{20}\right)$	0.1	0.05	5%
35.	$\frac{2}{5}$	0.4	0.40	40%
36.	$\frac{22}{100} = \left(\frac{11}{50}\right)$	0.2	0.22	22%
37.	$\frac{1}{8}$	0.1	0.13	12.5%
38.	$\frac{10}{100} = \left(\frac{1}{10}\right)$	0.1	0.10	10%
39.	$\frac{1}{12}$	0.1	0.08	8%
40.	$\frac{1}{200}$	0.0	0.01	$\frac{1}{2}$%
41.	$\frac{5}{16}$	0.3	0.31	31%
42.	$\frac{15}{100} = \left(\frac{3}{20}\right)$	0.2	0.15	15%
43.	$\frac{1}{4}$	0.3	0.25	25%
44.	$\frac{12}{100} = \left(\frac{3}{25}\right)$	0.1	0.12	12%
45.	$\frac{1}{100}$	0.0	0.01	1%
46.	$\frac{80}{100} = \left(\frac{4}{5}\right)$	0.8	0.80	80%
47.	$\frac{1}{200}$	0.0	0.01	$\frac{1}{2}$%
48.	$\frac{33}{100}$	0.3	0.33	33%
49.	$\frac{1}{250}$	0.0	0.00	$\frac{2}{5}$%
50.	$\frac{75}{100} = \left(\frac{3}{4}\right)$	0.8	0.75	75%

*When calculating medication dosages, trailing zeros must be removed from answers.

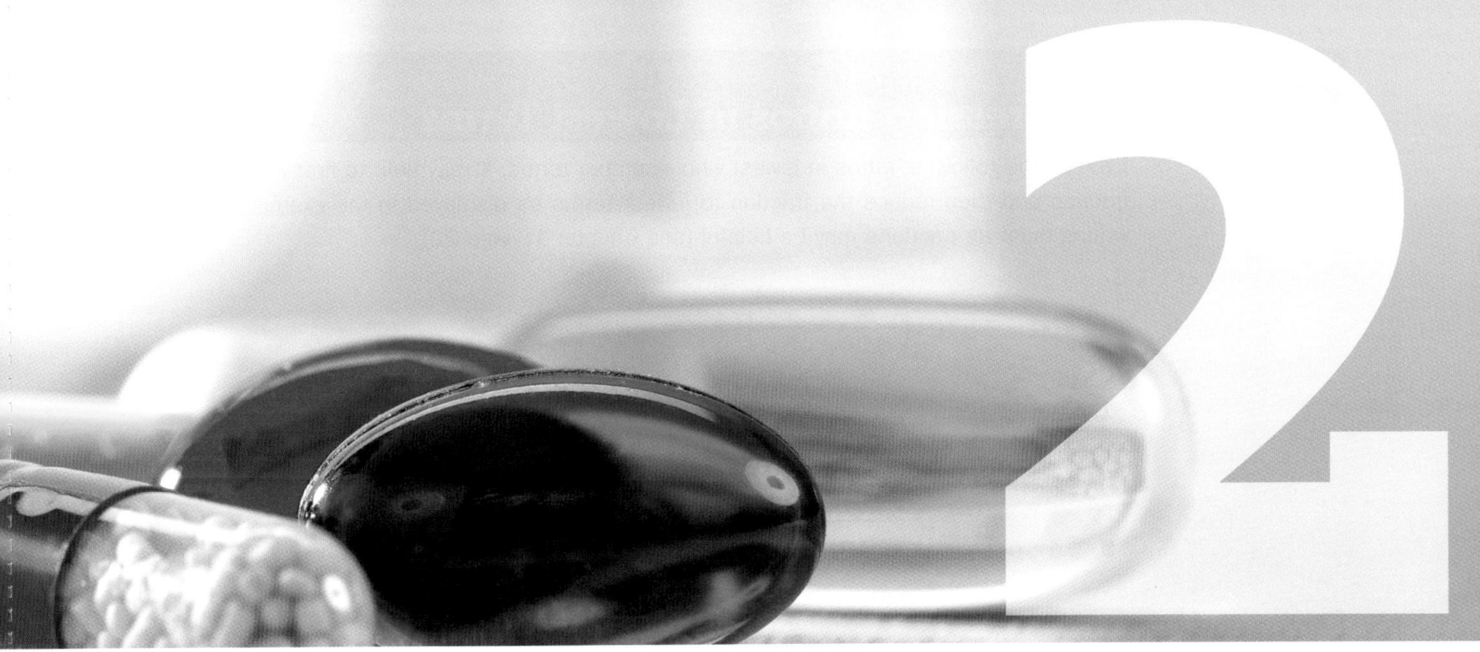

Ratio and Proportion

Objectives

- Understand the relationship between accurate ratio and proportion calculations and safe medication administration.
- Define ratio and proportion.
- Identify the differences between ratio and proportion.
- Solve proportion problems for a missing quantity (the value of *x*).
- Set up one-step ratio and proportion problems from a word problem.
- Estimate, solve, and prove answers.

Introduction

Ratio and proportion is a precise, provable method for solving medication dose problems. Estimating and then correctly setting up, solving, and proving problems from given information, using the ratio and proportion method, is one of several safe medication practices essential for accurate medication administration.

Ratio

A ratio is a comparison of two quantities. Two ways to express a ratio are with a colon (:), as in 2 : 3, or as a fraction $\left(\frac{2}{3}\right)$. *A colon is read as the word "to" or "is to."*

Examples *one to three* $\left(1 : 3 \text{ or } \frac{1}{3}\right)$ *three to five* $\left(3 : 5 \text{ or } \frac{3}{5}\right)$

2 scoops coffee to 1 cup water $\left(\text{two to one, } 2 : 1, \text{ or } \frac{2}{1}\right)$

Ratios, like fractions, can be expressed in lowest terms to simplify problem recognition and the arithmetic.

Examples 2 : 8 reduced to 1 : 4 50 : 100 reduced to 1 : 2

Answers on page 51

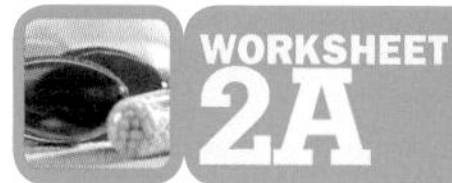

WORKSHEET 2A Expressing Ratios in Lowest Terms

Express the following ratios in lowest whole-number terms. It may help to first write the ratio as a fraction and then reduce the fraction to lowest terms as displayed in the example. Reading and writing them as fractions may be helpful (see Chapter 1, page 22).

Example 70 : 100 = 7 : 10 $\left(\frac{70}{100} = \frac{7}{10}\right)$

1. 2 : 4 **2.** 250 : 125 **3.** 2 : 5 **4.** 0.5 : 1

5. 2 : 3 **6.** 0.5 : 0.25 **7.** 100 : 10 **8.** 0.1 : 1

9. 0.1 : 0.2 **10.** 0.2 : 0.05

Proportion

A proportion is a statement that shows the relationship between *two equal* ratios. We calculate proportions when we alter quantities on hand but want to maintain the same ratio. You may use a colon or fraction setup. In order to maintain the SAME ratio, we must be careful to keep the QUANTITIES and the NUMBERS in the correct order or sequence. If we were to switch them, we would no longer have the same ratio and our answer would be incorrect. We can use a colon or a fraction to set up the ratio, but the quantities and numbers must be in the correct order.

Let's look at an example that we can set up with the use of a colon and the fraction to determine how many pizzas we should order for movie night.

Examples

Using Colons

1 pizza : 3 guests = 3 pizzas : 9 guests

(1 : 3 = 3 : 9)

Using Fractions

$$\frac{1 \text{ pizza}}{3 \text{ guests}} = \frac{3 \text{ pizzas}}{9 \text{ guests}}$$

$$\left(\frac{1}{3} = \frac{3}{9}\right)$$

In this example, you want to paint a room that is 400 square feet (sq. ft) and the paint comes in quarts (qt). How many quarts would you need to paint the room? The ratio proportion problem can be solved using either a colon or fraction setup.

1 qt paint : 100 sq. ft = 4 qt paint : 400 sq. ft

(1 : 100 = 4 : 400)

$$\frac{1 \text{ qt paint}}{100 \text{ sq. ft}} = \frac{4 \text{ qt paint}}{400 \text{ sq. ft}}$$

$$\left(\frac{1}{100} = \frac{4}{400}\right)$$

Steps to Prove a Proportion Is Correct

Example

Using Colons 1 : 5 = 5 : 25

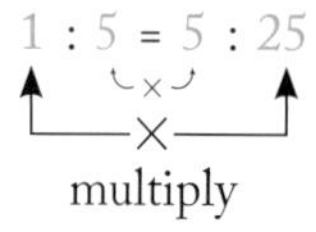

Using Fractions
Cross product

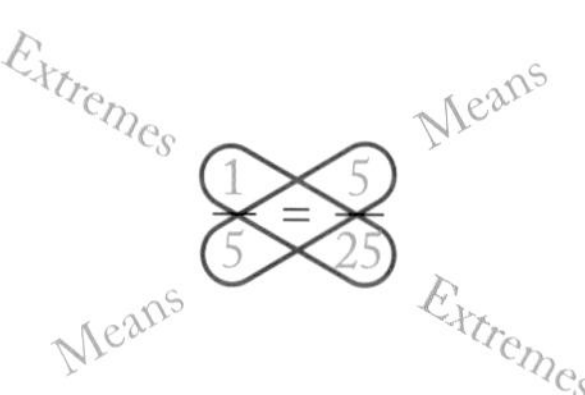

1. Multiply the *means* (two middle numbers) 5 × 5 = 25.
2. Multiply the *extremes* (two end numbers) 1 × 25 = 25.
3. Compare the two products. If the ratios are equal, the products of the means and extremes will be equal. The proportion will be correct.

Example 3 : 5 = 6 : 10

multiply

3 6
=
5 10

Multiply the means: 5 × 6 = 30.
Multiply the extremes: 3 × 10 = 30.

Solving Proportion Problems When One of the Numbers Is *Unknown*, or *x*

Example $2 : 8 = x : 24$

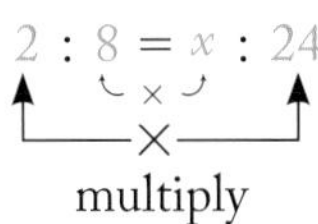

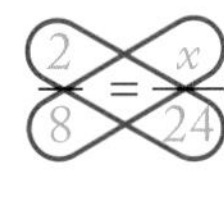

Multiply the means.

$8 \times x = 8x$

Multiply the extremes.

$2 \times 24 = 48$

Move the x product to the **left** side of the equation. It will look like this:

$8x = 48$

Now you must get x to stand alone.

RULE **To solve for the value of *x*, *divide* both sides of the equation by the number *next* to *x*. Those numbers will cancel each other. The result will be that *x* will stand alone.**

What you do to one side of the equation, you must do to the other to keep the sides equal.

Example

$$\frac{\not{8}}{\not{8}}x = \frac{48}{8}$$

$x = 6$

Example KNOW WANT TO KNOW

$2 : 3 = 6 : x$

multiply

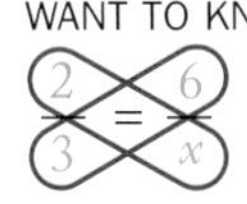

$2x = 3 \times 6$

$2x = 18$ Keep the x product on the left side of the equation.

$\frac{\not{2}x}{\not{2}} = \frac{18}{2}$ Divide both sides of the equation by the number next to x.

$x = 9$

$2 : 3 = 6 : 9$

Example KNOW WANT TO KNOW

$10 : 5 = x : 3$

10 x
=
5 3

$5x = 30$

$\frac{\not{5}x}{\not{5}} = \frac{30}{5}$

$x = 6$

$10 : 5 = 6 : 3$

RULE **To check your answer and prove the proportion is correct, substitute the answer for *x* in the original problem. Multiply the means and extremes. The products must be equal.**

Steps 1. *Substitute the answer (6) for x.*
2. *Multiply the means. Multiply the extremes.* The products must be equal.

KNOW

$2 : 8 = x : 24$

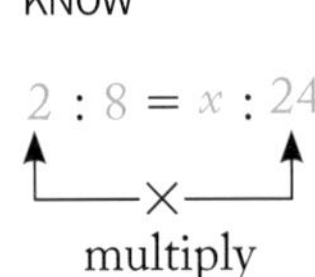

WANT TO KNOW

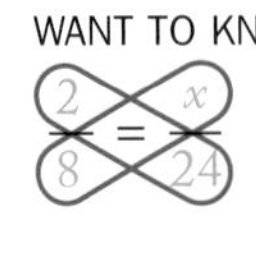

$2 : 8 = 6 : 24$

Proof $8 \times 6 = 48$ product of means $= 2 \times 24 = 48$ product of extremes

The ratios are equal. The proportion is correct.

Answers on page 51

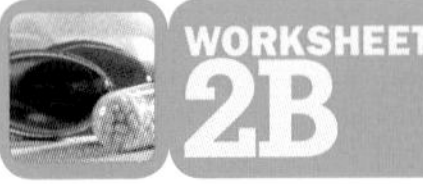

WORKSHEET 2B Solving Proportion Practice Problems for the Value of *x*

Use the colon or fraction cross-multiplication process to arrive at the products. First, multiply the means and extremes, then move the x product to the left side of the equation, solve for the unknown quantity (x), and prove the answer.

1. $5 : 100 = 9 : x \quad \left(\frac{5}{100} = \frac{9}{x}\right)$

2. $9 : 27 = 300 : x \quad \left(\frac{9}{27} = \frac{300}{x}\right)$

3. $1 : 8 = \frac{1}{2} : x \quad \left(\frac{1}{8} = \frac{\frac{1}{2}}{x}\right)$

4. $4 : 120 = x : 600 \quad \left(\frac{4}{120} = \frac{x}{600}\right)$

5. $0.7 : 70 = x : 1000 \quad \left(\frac{0.7}{70} = \frac{x}{1000}\right)$

Answers on page 52

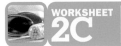

WORKSHEET 2C Solving Proportion Practice Problems for the Value of *x*

Use the colon or fraction cross-multiplication process to arrive at the products. First estimate, then solve, for the unknown quantity (x) and prove the answer.

1. $15 : 30 = x : 12$

2. $5 : 10 = 15 : x$

3. $6 : 12 = 0.25 : x$

4. $7.5 : 12 = x : 28$

5. $0.4 : 12 = 10 : x$

Setting Up Ratios and Proportions from Given Information

1. Read the problem and identify the unknown wanted quantity (*x*). This is expressed as *x*.
2. Estimate the size of the *x* (wanted) quantity. Remember, this is the quantity you are looking for or trying to calculate.
3. Always enter the ratio of what you already *KNOW* or already *have* on the *LEFT* side of the equal sign.
4. On the *RIGHT* side of the equal sign, write or enter the *x* or unknown quantity ratio—what you want to know.
5. Now you are ready to solve for *x*. Make sure that you prove the proportion to demonstrate that you correctly set up and solved for the unknown quantity.
6. Finally, check your estimate with the answer you calculated for *x*.

Remember, each of the two ratios must be set up in the *same sequence for the answer to be correct.*

Apples : Pears = Apple : *x* Pears   Sugar : Tea = Sugar : Tea

Example

Let's try putting the above steps into action by working through the following example. You are making coffee for a group meeting. The label says 2 scoops per cup. You will need 20 cups. How many scoops will you use?

Estimate The *x* unknown is how many scoops of coffee you need. Because the label says to use 2 scoops for 1 cup, you know you will need many more than 2 scoops to make 20 cups. (Remember, make the estimate *before* the setup and math.) Now follow the steps in the box above to set up the ratio and proportion from the information supplied.

Correct Setup

KNOW   WANT TO KNOW

2 scoops : 1 coffee = *x* scoops : 20 coffees

$$\left(\frac{2}{1} = \frac{x}{20}\right)$$

$x = 20 \times 2$

$x = 40$ scoops.

$2 : 1 = 40 : 20$ Estimate is correct. 40 is many more than 2

PROOF $1 \times 40 = 40$
$2 \times 20 = 40$

Example of Incorrect Setup

$2 : 20 = x : 2$

$20x - 4$

$$\frac{\cancel{20}}{\cancel{20}}x = \frac{\cancel{4}}{\cancel{20}}$$

$x = \frac{1}{5}$ cup

remember

The math can be correct and the proportion can be correct, but if the setup is wrong, the answer to the problem will be wrong.

This is an example of a proof that appears to be set up correctly. The answer doesn't make sense. The problem is looking for the number of scoops and this has provided the number of cups.

$20 \times \frac{1}{5} = 4$

$2 \times 2 = 4$

remember **Placements, labels, estimates, and proofs are important to reduce errors. Estimates provide a rough guide to the approximate size of the answer. Estimates *are not* a substitute for proofs. They may protect from major math errors if the setup is correct. Recheck the setup, numbers, and placements if the estimate and/or the proof is incorrect.**

Example You wish to make a floral bouquet of 6 daffodils for every 4 roses. How many daffodils will you use for 30 roses?

Estimate: x daffodils will be many more than 6 daffodils.

KNOW WANT TO KNOW

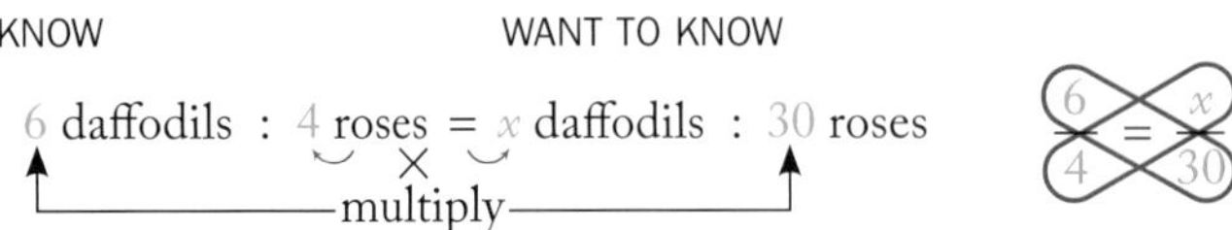

$4x = 6 \times 30$

$\frac{\not{4}}{\not{4}}x = \frac{180}{4}$

$x = 45$ daffodils

My estimate is correct. 6 : 4 = 45 : 30

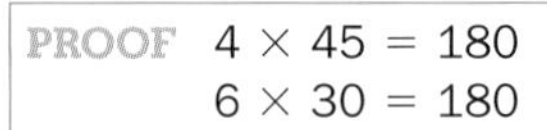

PROOF $4 \times 45 = 180$
$6 \times 30 = 180$

The product of the means = the product of the extremes.

Example Make a necklace that has 19 blue beads for every yellow bead. How many blue beads are needed if you have 8 yellow beads?

Estimate: x blue beads will be many more than 19 blue beads (8 times more).

KNOW WANT TO KNOW

19 blue beads : 1 yellow bead = x blue beads : 8 yellow beads

multiply

$x = 19 \times 8$

$x = 152$ blue beads needed

My estimate is correct.

PROOF $19 \times 8 = 152$
$1 \times 152 = 152$

Answers on page 52

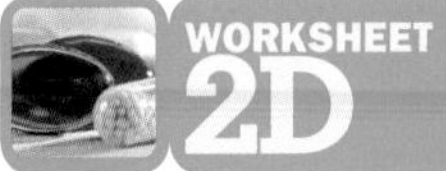

WORKSHEET 2D Setting Up and Solving Ratios and Proportions

Set up a proportion for each of the following problems. Estimate the value of x, label, and prove your answers. Use the colon or fraction cross-product method.

1. You have to make a fruit basket with 6 bananas for every 9 apples. How many bananas will there be for 72 apples?

2. You are making coffee, and 7 scoops make 8 cups. How many scoops make 40 cups?

3. You have a recipe for cocoa: 4 scoops make 6 cups of cocoa. You want to make 18 cups for a party. How many scoops of cocoa are needed? Set up a proportion.

4. Ordered: 2 tablets each day. The patient will be taking the medication for 21 days. How many tablets will the patient need for discharge?

5. You wish to plant 8 bushes for every 2 trees in your yard. How many bushes will there be if there are 36 trees?

6. Ordered: 2 cups of green tea every day. How many days would it take to consume 24 cups of green tea?

7. It takes 4 cups of flour to make 3 loaves of bread. How many loaves of bread can be made from 24 cups of flour?

8. Your recipe for punch calls for 3 cups of soda for every $\frac{1}{2}$ cup of fruit juice. How many cups of soda will be needed for 2 cups of fruit juice?

9. You need 4 tablespoons of sugar for every glass of lemonade you prepare. How many tablespoons of sugar will be needed for 6 glasses of lemonade?

10. Ordered: 4 capsules every day. How many capsules would be needed for 14 days?

Answers on page 54

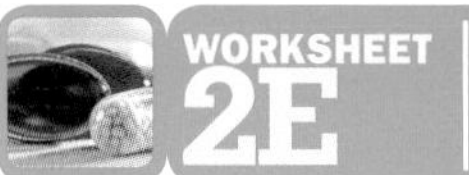

WORKSHEET 2E Ratio and Proportion Practice

Use ratio and proportion to set up and solve the following problems, estimate, label, and prove your answers. Use the colon or fraction cross-product method.

1. The office needs 4000 envelopes. The boxes on hand contain 200 envelopes per box. How many boxes will you send to the office?

2. The order is for 300 operating room gowns. The packages on hand contain 10 gowns per package. How many packages will you send?

3. If one computer is allocated for every 18 students, how many computers will be needed for an enrollment of 1260 students?

4. Your doctor tells you to drink 3 glasses of water and eat 2 apples every day. How many apples will you have eaten when you have drunk 24 glasses of water?

5. If all the teachers were to receive 6 pens for every 8 pencils, how many pens would you give them if the teachers have 72 pencils?

6. The nurse is assigned 6 patients per shift. How many nurses will be needed for 36 patients?

7. If baby formula calls for 4 tablespoons of powdered formula for every 8 ounces of water, how many tablespoons of powdered formula would be needed for 56 ounces of water?

8. The hospital requires 2 nurses for every unit for each 12-hour shift. How many nurses are needed for each unit for 72 hours?

9. If a patient takes 3 aspirin tablets per day, how many aspirin tablets will the patient need for a 2-week vacation?

10. If a multidose liquid medication contains 100 mL and the patient takes 5 mL (1 teaspoon) per day, how many days will the medication last?

Answers on page 55

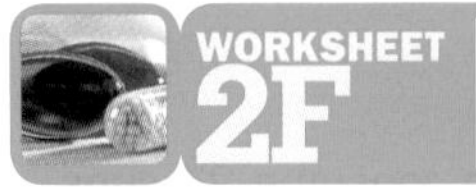

WORKSHEET 2F Multiple-Choice Practice

Use ratio and proportion to solve the following problems. Label, estimate, and prove your answers.

1. If you need 10 diapers a day, how many days will a package of 50 diapers last?

a. 5 days **c.** 15 days
b. 10 days **d.** 20 days

2. Ordered: 120 insulin syringes. They are delivered in units of 10 per package. How many packages will you receive?

a. 10 packages **c.** 15 packages
b. 12 packages **d.** 20 packages

3. You have to take 4 teaspoons of medicine every day. The bottle contains 80 teaspoons. How many days will the bottle last?

a. 2 days **c.** 10 days
b. 5 days **d.** 20 days

4. Ordered: 3 capsules per day. How many capsules will the patient need for 21 days?

a. 12 capsules **c.** 31 capsules
b. 20 capsules **d.** 63 capsules

5. You have a vial holding 30 mL of liquid. If the average dose given is 5 mL, how many doses are available?

a. 5 doses **c.** 8 doses
b. 6 doses **d.** 10 doses

6. The hospital has allotted 120 days of inservice for 15 departments. How many days of inservice can each department use?

a. 4 days **c.** 12 days
b. 8 days **d.** 15 days

7. The hospital staffs every 8 patients with one RN. How many RNs will be needed when the census is 240?

a. 30 RNs **c.** 90 RNs
b. 60 RNs **d.** 120 RNs

8. The directions state that for every $\frac{1}{2}$ cup portion of baby cereal you will need 4 ounces of milk. How many ounces of milk will you need to prepare 20 portions?

a. 20 ounces **c.** 80 ounces
b. 40 ounces **d.** 100 ounces

9. If you receive $15 an hour in overtime pay, how many hours would you need to work overtime to receive $450 in overtime earnings?

a. 3 hours **c.** 30 hours
b. 15 hours **d.** 45 hours

10. If a patient is to receive 3 liters of an intravenous fluid every 8 hours, how many liters would be needed for 72 hours?

a. 9 liters **c.** 27 liters
b. 18 liters **d.** 36 liters

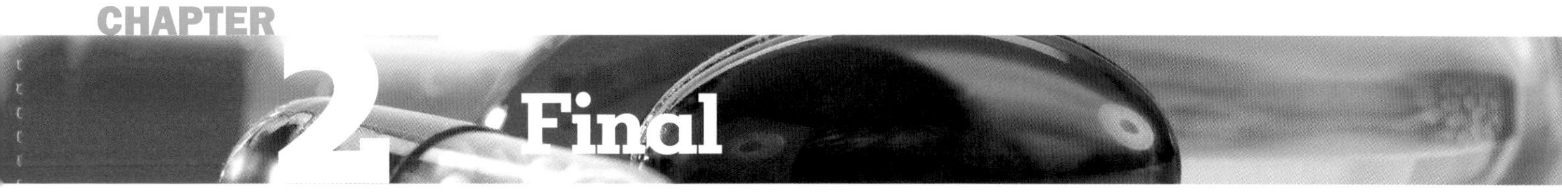

CHAPTER 2 Final

Solve each problem using ratio and proportion. Label, estimate, and prove your answers.

1. The hospital assigns 5 nursing supervisors per shift. How many supervisors are needed for 3 shifts?

2. Each nurse is assigned 6 patients. How many nurses are needed for 150 patients in a hospital?

3. The hospital laundry provides 4 sheets per bed per day. How many sheets are needed per day for a 200-bed hospital?

4. The average number of discharges is 32 patients per day. How many patients are discharged each week?

5. A nurse earns $20 an hour in extra pay for overtime hours. How much extra pay will the nurse earn for 24 hours of overtime in a pay period?

6. A CNA is hired for every 12 beds in the hospital. How many CNAs would be hired for a 360-bed hospital?

7. There is 1 administrator for every 50 beds. How many administrators would be needed for a 200-bed hospital?

8. The hospital spends $750 a day for portable oxygen canister rentals. How much will a 4-week supply of canisters cost?

9. Approximately 1 resident and 2 interns are assigned for every 20 patients. How many interns are needed for 210 patients?

10. Some studies show that approximately 1 of every 6 medications given involves an error. Approximately how many medication errors would occur for every 240 medications given?

11. If a patient has to take 1 antiinflammatory tablet every 6 hours, how many tablets will he or she need for 3 days?

12. If a staff member is allotted 1.5 PTO (personal time off) days per month, how many PTO days will be accumulated in 6 months?

13. Ordered: 2 tablets, 3 times daily. How many days will a bottle of 60 tablets last? Hint: You need to enter total tablets per day in the equation.

14. The patient is to drink 4 ounces of water every $\frac{1}{2}$ hour. How much water should the patient have consumed in 8 hours?

15. The budget permits 48 inservice days per year. There are 12 units. How many inservice days could each unit receive for a year?

16. A multidose vial contains 20 mL. If each dose is 2.5 mL, how many doses are in the vial?

17. If the average adult weight is 150 pounds and the elevator can hold 1800 pounds, how many people, on average, can the elevator safely carry at one time?

18. If each orientation for an RN costs approximately $3000, how many RNs can the hospital plan to hire with an annual orientation budget of $96,000?

19. If a guest speaker is paid a $50 honorarium, how many guest speakers can be invited if the budget is $600?

20. If a patient needs a 30-day supply of tablets and takes 2 tablets four times a day, how many tablets will the patient need at discharge?

Answer Key

2 Ratio and Proportion

WORKSHEET **2A** (page 42)

1. $2:4 = 1:2 \quad \left(\frac{2}{4} = \frac{1}{2}\right)$

2. $250:125 = 2:1 \quad \left(\frac{250}{125} = \frac{2}{1}\right)$

3. $2:5 = 2:5 \quad \left(\frac{2}{5} = \frac{2}{5}\right)$

4. $0.5:1 = 1:2 \quad \left(\frac{0.5}{1} = \frac{1}{2}\right)$

5. $2:3 = 2:3 \quad \left(\frac{2}{3} = \frac{2}{3}\right)$

6. $0.5:0.25 = 2:1 \quad \left(\frac{0.5}{0.25} = \frac{2}{1}\right)$

7. $100:10 = 10:1 \quad \left(\frac{100}{10} = \frac{10}{1}\right)$

8. $0.1:1 = 1:10 \quad \left(\frac{0.1}{1} = \frac{1}{10}\right)$

9. $0.1:0.2 = 1:2 \quad \left(\frac{0.1}{0.2} = \frac{1}{2}\right)$

10. $0.2:0.05 = 4:1 \quad \left(\frac{0.2}{0.05} = \frac{4}{1}\right)$

WORKSHEET **2B** (page 44)

1. $5:100 = 9:x$

$5x = 9 \times 100$

$5x = 900$

$\frac{\cancel{5}}{\cancel{5}}x = \frac{900}{5} = 900 \div 5$

$x = 180$

PROOF

$180 \times 5 = 900$

$9 \times 100 = 900$

2. $9:27 = 300:x$

$9x = 27 \times 300 = 8100$

$\frac{\cancel{9}}{\cancel{9}}x = \frac{8100}{9} = 8100 \div 9$

$x = 900$

PROOF

$27 \times 300 = 8100$

$9 \times 900 = 8100$

3. $1:8 = \frac{1}{2}:x$

$x = \frac{8}{1} \times \frac{1}{2}$

$x = \frac{8}{2}$

$x = 4$

PROOF

$4 \times 1 = 4$

$\frac{1}{2} \times 8 = 4$

4. $4:120 = x:600$

$120x = 4 \times 600 = 2400$

$\frac{\cancel{120}}{\cancel{120}}x = \frac{240\cancel{0}}{12\cancel{0}} = 240 \div 12$

$x - 20$

PROOF

$600 \times 4 = 2400$

$20 \times 120 = 2400$

5. $0.7:70 = x:1000$

$70x = 0.7 \times 1000 = 700$

$\frac{\cancel{70}}{\cancel{70}}x = \frac{70\cancel{0}}{7\cancel{0}} = 70 \div 7$

$x = 10$

PROOF

$70 \times 10 = 700$

$0.7 \times 1000 = 700$

WORKSHEET **2C** (page 44)

1. $15 : 30 = x : 12$

$30x = 15 \times 12$

$30x = 180$

$\frac{\not{30}}{\not{30}}x = \frac{180}{30} = 180 \div 30$

$x = 6$

PROOF

$30 \times 6 = 180$

$15 \times 12 = 180$

2. $5 : 10 = 15 : x$

$\frac{\not{5}x}{\not{5}} = \frac{150}{5}$

$x = 30$

PROOF

$10 \times 15 = 150$

$5 \times 30 = 150$

3. $6 : 12 = 0.25 : x$

$6x = 12 \times 0.25 = 3$

$\frac{\not{6}}{\not{6}}x = \frac{3}{6} = 3 \div 6$

$x = 0.5$

PROOF

$12 \times 0.25 = 3$

$6 \times 0.5 = 3$

4. $7.5 : 12 = x : 28$

$12x = 7.5 \times 28 = 210$

$\frac{\not{12}}{\not{12}}x = \frac{210}{12} = 210 \div 12$

$x = 17.5$

PROOF

$7.5 \times 28 = 210$

$12 \times 17.5 = 210$

5. $0.4 : 12 = 10 : x$

$0.4x = 10 \times 12 = 120$

$\frac{\not{0.4}}{\not{0.4}}x = \frac{120}{0.4} = 120 \div 0.4$

$x = 300$

PROOF

$10 \times 12 = 120$

$300 \times 0.4 = 120$

WORKSHEET **2D** (page 46)

1. KNOW WANT TO KNOW

Bananas : Apples = x Bananas : Apples

$6 : 9 = x : 72$

$9x = 6 \times 72 = 432$

$\frac{\not{9}}{\not{9}}x = \frac{432}{9}$

$x = 48$ bananas

PROOF

$6 : 9 = 48 : 72$

$9 \times 48 = 432$

$6 \times 72 = 432$

2. KNOW WANT TO KNOW

Scoops : Cups = x Scoops : Cups

$7 : 8 = x : 40$

$8x = 40 \times 7 = 280$

$\frac{\not{8}}{\not{8}}x = \frac{280}{8}$

$x = 35$ scoops

PROOF

$7 : 8 = 35 : 40$

$8 \times 35 = 280$

$7 \times 40 = 280$

remember **Scoops : Cups = Scoops : Cups**
Apples : Bananas = Apples : Bananas
Miles : Gallons = Miles : Gallons

3. KNOW WANT TO KNOW

Scoops : Cups = x Scoops : Cups

$4 : 6 = x : 18$

$6x = 72$

$\frac{\not{6}}{\not{6}}x = \frac{72}{6}$

$x = 12$ scoops of cocoa

PROOF

$4 : 6 = 12 : 18$

$6 \times 12 = 72$

$4 \times 18 = 72$

4. KNOW WANT TO KNOW

2 tablets : 1 day = x tablets : 21 days

$x = 2 \times 21$

$x = 42$ tablets

PROOF

$2 : 1 = 42 : 21$

$2 \times 21 = 42$

$1 \times 42 = 42$

5. KNOW WANT TO KNOW

Bushes : Trees = x Bushes : Trees

$8 : 2 = x : 36$

$2x = 8 \times 36 = 288$

$\frac{\not{2}}{\not{2}}x = \frac{288}{2}$

$x = 144$ bushes

PROOF

$8 : 2 = 144 : 36$

$8 \times 36 = 288$

$2 \times 144 = 288$

6. KNOW WANT TO KNOW

Cups : Day = Cups : x Days

$2 : 1 = 24 : x$

$2x = 24$

$\frac{\not{2}}{\not{2}}x = \frac{24}{2}$

$x = 12$ days

PROOF

$2 : 1 = 24 : 12$

$1 \times 24 = 24$

$2 \times 12 = 24$

7. KNOW WANT TO KNOW

Cups : Loaves = Cups : x Loaves

$4 : 3 = 24 : x$

$4x = 24 \times 3 = 72$

$\frac{\not{4}}{\not{4}}x = \frac{72}{4}$

$x = 18$ loaves

PROOF

$4 : 3 = 24 : 18$

$4 \times 18 = 72$

$3 \times 24 = 72$

8. KNOW WANT TO KNOW

3 soda : $\frac{1}{2}$ fruit juice = x soda : 2 fruit juice

$\frac{1}{2}x = 3 \times 2$

$\frac{\not{1}/\not{2}}{\not{1}/\not{2}}x = \frac{6}{\frac{1}{2}} = 6 \div \frac{1}{2} = 6 \times \frac{2}{1}$

$x = 12$ cups soda

PROOF

$3 : \frac{1}{2} = 12 : 2$

$3 \times 2 = 6$

$\frac{1}{2} \times 12 = 6$

9. KNOW WANT TO KNOW

4 Tbsp sugar : 1 glass = x Tbsp sugar : 6 glasses

$x = 6 \times 4$

$x = 24$ Tbsp sugar

PROOF

$4 : 1 = 24 : 6$

$4 \times 6 = 24$

$1 \times 24 = 24$

10. KNOW WANT TO KNOW

4 capsules : 1 day = x capsules : 14 days

$x = 4 \times 14$

$x = 56$ capsules

PROOF

$4 : 1 = 56 : 14$

$4 \times 14 = 56$

$1 \times 56 = 56$

WORKSHEET 2E (page 47)

1. KNOW WANT TO KNOW

200 envelopes : 1 box = 4000 envelopes : x boxes

$200x = 4000$

$$\frac{\cancel{200}}{\cancel{200}}x = \frac{400\cancel{0}}{20\cancel{0}}$$

$x = 20$ boxes

PROOF

$200 \times 20 = 4000$

$1 \times 4000 = 4000$

2. KNOW WANT TO KNOW

10 gowns : 1 package = 300 gowns : x packages

$10x = 300$

$$\frac{\cancel{10}}{\cancel{10}}x = \frac{30\cancel{0}}{1\cancel{0}}$$

$x = 30$ packages of gowns

PROOF

$10 \times 30 = 300$

$1 \times 300 = 300$

3. KNOW WANT TO KNOW

1 computer : 18 students =
x computers : 1260 students

$18x = 1260$

$$\frac{\cancel{18}}{\cancel{18}}x = \frac{1260}{18}$$

$x = 70$ computers

PROOF

$1 \times 1260 = 1260$

$18 \times 70 = 1260$

4. KNOW WANT TO KNOW

3 glasses : 2 apples = 24 glasses : x apples

$3x = 48$

$$\frac{\cancel{3}}{\cancel{3}}x = \frac{48}{3}$$

$x = 16$ apples

PROOF

$3 \times 16 = 48$

$2 \times 24 = 48$

5. KNOW WANT TO KNOW

6 pens : 8 pencils = x pens : 72 pencils

$8x = 432$

$$\frac{\cancel{8}}{\cancel{8}}x = \frac{432}{8}$$

$x = 54$ pens

PROOF

$6 \times 72 = 432$

$8 \times 54 = 432$

6. KNOW WANT TO KNOW

1 nurse : 6 patients = x nurses : 36 patients

$6x = 36$

$$\frac{\cancel{6}}{\cancel{6}}x = \frac{36}{6}$$

$x = 6$ nurses

PROOF

$1 \times 36 = 36$

$6 \times 6 = 36$

7. KNOW WANT TO KNOW

4 Tbsp : 8 oz water = x Tbsp : 56 oz water

$8x = 4 \times 56 = 224$

$$\frac{\cancel{8}}{\cancel{8}}x = \frac{224}{8}$$

$x = 28$ Tbsp formula

PROOF

$4 \times 56 = 224$

$8 \times 28 = 224$

8. KNOW WANT TO KNOW

2 nurses : 12 hr = x nurses : 72 hr

$12x = 144$

$$\frac{\cancel{12}}{\cancel{12}}x = \frac{144}{12}$$

$x = 12$ nurses needed

PROOF

$12 \times 12 = 144$

$2 \times 72 = 144$

9. KNOW WANT TO KNOW

3 aspirin : 1 day = x aspirin : 14 days

$x = 3 \times 14$

$x = 42$ aspirin tablets

PROOF

$3 \times 14 = 42$

$1 \times 42 = 42$

10. KNOW WANT TO KNOW

5 mL : 1 day = 100 mL : x days

$$\frac{\cancel{5}}{\cancel{5}}x = \frac{100}{5}$$

$x = 20$ days

PROOF

$5 \times 20 = 100$

$1 \times 100 = 100$

WORKSHEET 2F (page 48)

1. a. KNOW WANT TO KNOW

10 diapers : 1 day = 50 diapers : x days

$\frac{10}{10}x = \frac{50}{10}$

$x = 5$ days

PROOF

$10 \times 5 = 50$

$1 \times 50 = 50$

2. b. KNOW WANT TO KNOW

10 syringes : 1 package = 120 syringes : x packages

$\frac{10}{10}x = \frac{120}{10}$

$x = 12$ packages

PROOF

$10 \times 12 = 120$

$1 \times 120 = 120$

3. d. KNOW WANT TO KNOW

4 tsp : 1 day = 80 tsp : x days

$\frac{4}{4}x = \frac{80}{4}$

$x = 20$ days

PROOF

$4 \times 20 = 80$

$1 \times 80 = 80$

4. d. KNOW WANT TO KNOW

3 capsules : 1 day = x capsules : 21 days

$x = 3 \times 21$

$x = 63$ capsules

PROOF

$3 \times 21 = 63$

$1 \times 63 = 63$

5. b. KNOW WANT TO KNOW

5 mL : 1 dose = 30 mL : x doses

$\frac{5}{5}x = \frac{30}{5}$

$x = 6$ doses

PROOF

$5 \times 6 = 30$

$1 \times 30 = 30$

6. b. KNOW WANT TO KNOW

120 days : 15 depts = x days : 1 dept

$\frac{15}{15}x = \frac{120}{15}$

$x = 8$ days

PROOF

$120 \times 1 = 120$

$15 \times 8 = 120$

7. a. KNOW WANT TO KNOW

8 patients : 1 RN = 240 patients : x RNs

$\frac{8}{8}x = \frac{240}{8}$

$x = 30$ RNs

PROOF

$8 \times 30 = 240$

$1 \times 240 = 240$

8. c. KNOW WANT TO KNOW

4 oz : 1 portion = x oz : 20 portions

$x = 4 \times 20$

$x = 80$ oz

PROOF

$4 \times 20 = 80$

$1 \times 80 = 80$

9. c. KNOW WANT TO KNOW

$15 : 1 hr = $450 : x hr

$\frac{15}{15}x = \frac{450}{15}$

$x = 30$ hr

PROOF

$15 \times 30 = 450$

$1 \times 450 = 450$

10. c. KNOW WANT TO KNOW

3 liters : 8 h = x liters : 72 h

$8x = 3 \times 72$

$\frac{8}{8}x = \frac{216}{8}$

$x = 27$ liters

PROOF

$3 \times 72 = 216$

$8 \times 27 = 216$

CHAPTER 2 FINAL: RATIO AND PROPORTION (page 49)

1. 15 supervisors
2. 25 nurses
3. 800 sheets
4. 224 patient discharges
5. $480
6. 30 CNAs
7. 4 administrators
8. $21,000 for 4 weeks
9. 21 interns
10. approximately 40 medication errors
11. 12 tablets
12. 9 PTO (personal time off) days
13. 10 days
14. 64 oz
15. 4 inservice days
16. 8 doses
17. 12 people
18. 32 RNs
19. 12 guest speakers
20. 240 tablets

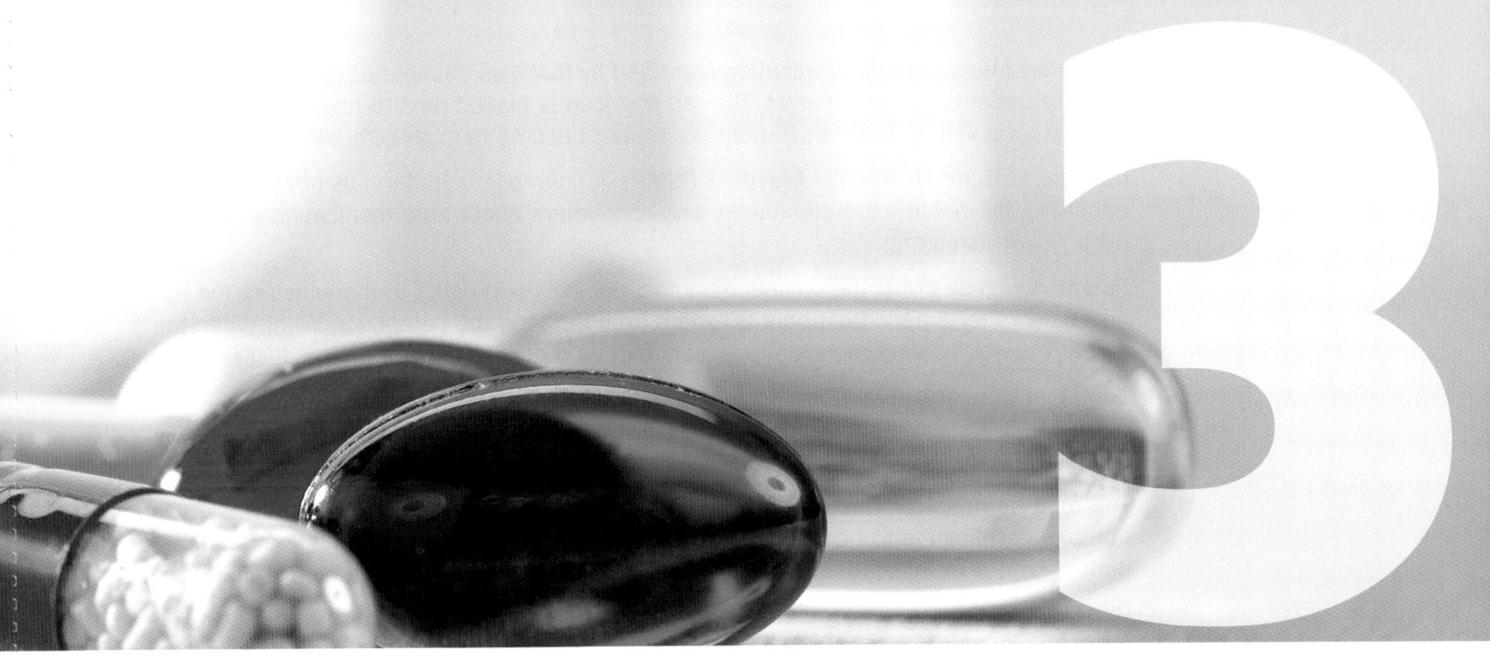

Safe Medication Administration

Objectives

- State all medication-related patient rights.
- Use The Joint Commission (TJC)– and Institute for Safe Medication Practices (ISMP)–approved abbreviations.
- Distinguish forms of oral medications.
- Name the two major divisions of routes of medication administration.
- Interpret medication labels, prescriber orders, and medication administration records.
- Convert 12-hour clock time to 24-hour clock time (military time).
- Identify abbreviations and prescriber orders that require clarification.
- State recommended patient-safety practices related to medication administration.
- State the need for medication-related incident reports.
- Analyze medication errors using critical thinking.

Introduction

Safe medication administration involves more than accurate dose measurement and calculations. Before calculation, the nurse must be able to interpret a variety of medication-related documents. Interpretation requires knowledge of medical terminology and abbreviations, as well as familiarity with drug label information and current drug references. Attention to detail and observance of patient medication-related rights are key elements of patient safety.

Vocabulary

Adverse Drug Event (ADE): A medication-related occurrence that causes harm to a patient.

Drug Concentration (strength): The ratio of medication amount to a specific amount of liquid or solid (e.g., the amount of drug, such as 50 milligrams) per tablet or metric-calibrated teaspoon, or the amount of drug in the total quantity or weight supplied (e.g., 1 gram per 500-milliliter container).

Food and Drug Administration (FDA): The federal agency responsible for ensuring the safety, efficacy, and security of drugs, biological products such as vaccines, medical devices, and more. FDA approves medications for specific uses and sale in the United States.

Generic Drug: Drug product that is comparable to a brand-name drug product in dosage form, strength, route of administration, quality and performance characteristics, and intended use.

High-Alert Medication: 🚩 Medication identified by ISMP as capable of causing significant harm to patients if used in error. The red flag icon is placed next to high-alert medications in the text as a visual reminder to help the reader become familiar with some of these drugs.

Institute for Safe Medication Practices (ISMP): A nonprofit, voluntary agency dedicated to educating the health care community and consumers about safe medication practices (http://www.ismp.org).

Patent: A license giving the original manufacturer exclusive rights to manufacture the approved new product for a period of about 20 years from the time the patent was filed. When the patent expires, other companies may manufacture a generic copy of the product (e.g., drug).

Sentinel Event: The Joint Commission definition is an unexpected occurrence involving death or serious physical or psychological injury or the risk thereof. Serious injury specifically includes the loss of limb or function.

The Joint Commission (TJC): A national nonprofit, independent agency that provides accreditation and certification to health care organizations, with an emphasis on high standards and patient safety, including medication administration safety (http://www.jointcommission.org).

Unit-Dose Packaging: Non-reusable packaged and labeled single serving of drug dose ordered for the patient; usually used in health care institutions. May contain more than one unit of the drug, depending on the order (e.g., 2 tablets per serving). Keeps the medication free from contaminants, is opened just before using, and reduces the need for measurement and calculations, thus reducing the chance of dosage errors.

Usual Dose: The average dose ordered for the desired therapeutic effect for the target population (e.g., usual dose for children age 5 to 12 years: 1 teaspoon at bedtime for itching). Seen on manufacturers' prepared labels.

Patient Rights

There are many patient rights related to safe medication administration. As you read through a summary of major rights, think about the implications should one or more of these rights be violated.

Right Patient

The patient for whom the medication is ordered must be the patient who receives the medication. Because of the number of wrong patient errors, this issue is addressed in the first goal of The Joint Commission (TJC) Patient Safety Council: Improve the accuracy of patient identification. (https://www.jointcommission.org/assets/1/6/NPSG_Chapter_HAP_Jan2018.pdf). A minimum of two separate written patient identifiers must be used. Identifiers may include the patient's name, an assigned identification number (which may be on the patient's wristband), telephone number, or other person-specific identifiers. Room number and bed number may not be used.

Right Drug

The nurse must be able to interpret drug orders and drug labels and to match the supplied drug exactly to the order. It must be the right drug for the right patient. Any portion of the process that is unclear or unfamiliar needs to be clarified promptly with a current drug reference, the prescriber, or the pharmacist before administering the medication (http://www.ismp.org/tools/confuseddrugnames.pdf). Medication orders must be checked against patient allergies to ensure no allergies to the medication exist.

Right Dose

The nurse needs to know that it is the ordered dose and the dose will be safe for the intended patient. The nurse should be aware of the patient's medical history and current conditions that may influence dosage. Certain factors such as age or height/weight may also affect dosage. Knowledge of measurement systems, abbreviations, dose calculation, and preparation technique is essential. A reliable current drug reference and/or pharmacist or prescriber must be consulted if there are questions. Attention to detail, decimals, and zeros is also vital to prevent errors.

Right Time

If administration of a medication is delayed, omitted, or given too early, there can be serious consequences. Some drugs must be given at specific, timed intervals to maintain stable blood levels for effectiveness. The Joint Commission and clinical agencies have policies and guidelines pertaining to prioritization of medication administration when several are to be given at about the same time. Certain medications and certain patient conditions take priority (http://www.ismp.org/tools/guidelines/acutecare/tasm.pdf).

CLINICAL ALERT!

It is very important to ask for help if the workload is too heavy to safely prepare or administer medications on time.

Right Route

The nurse must prepare the medication for the prescribed and safe drug route for the individual patient. Consult the prescriber if a medication order does not contain a route. Abbreviations are often used to designate the route. Many medications are available in solid and liquid forms for oral, intramuscular, and/or intravenous administration. The label must match the ordered route. If the patient refuses or is unable to tolerate the route ordered, the nurse must document the reason and include an assessment of the mental status of the patient. The prescriber must be reached promptly for a change in the order.

Right Reason

Medication orders may provide a specific reason for administration. For example, a medication such as acetaminophen ordered to reduce the pain of a headache should not be administered to reduce a fever.

Right Assessment

The nurse should understand the actions of the medication and should perform a pre-administration assessment of the patient. This may include vital signs, pain level, mental status, or recent laboratory results, for example.

Right Documentation

Accurate and timely reporting and documentation in the patient medication record, as well as other records, is essential for patient safety. Documentation varies among agencies and is best learned during on-site orientation. Most agencies use some form of electronic documentation. "If it wasn't documented, it wasn't done" is an old adage that still holds true. Lack of prompt recording of medications given or omitted can lead to serious errors.

CLINICAL ALERT!

Documents are confidential. They cannot be photocopied and cannot be altered. Agencies have guidelines for entering amended information.

Right Evaluation

Following medication administration, assess the patient to evaluate the response to the medication, including effectiveness and adverse side effects. Document the post-administration assessment.

Right to Refuse

The American Hospital Association Patient Care Partnership (2003) (https://www.aha.org/system/files/2018-01/aha-patient-care-partnership.pdf) identifies a patient's right to consent to or refuse treatment. Nurses need to keep patients informed of all medications to be administered, including the name, reason for administration, action, purpose, and potential adverse or unintended effects. Should a patient refuse a medication, the provider should be notified and the refusal documented according to the agency's policies and procedures.

CLINICAL ALERT!

It is illegal for the nurse to change a medication order. The prescriber must be contacted for a new order if any part of an order—the drug, the dose, the route, or the frequency—needs to be changed.

Medication Errors

Estimated rates of medication errors range from 2% to well over 10% when underreporting and wrong time of administration are considered. Many national organizations are working with manufacturers and health care agencies to reduce the error rate. Medication errors by the prescriber, the pharmacist, and the nurse may and do occur at any stage in the process:

- Prescription errors: drug type, dose, route, frequency, use of unapproved abbreviations, directions for use; if handwritten—legibility.
- Pharmacy errors: drug order misinterpretation or contraindication, transcribing and transferal, computer data entry, drug selection, preparation, labeling (including directions for use).
- Nurse errors: wrong patient, drug order misinterpretation or contraindication, drug selection, time, dose calculation and preparation, route, administration technique, and inappropriate follow-up evaluation.

CLINICAL ALERT!

The nurse who prepares and administers the medication offers the last step in administration safeguards to the patient.

CLINICAL ALERT!

Agency policies and needed corrective actions must be carried out promptly by the person who encounters an error *even* if the patient shows no sign of ill effects.

The following are a few of the many web sites that provide updates and articles about medication errors: their causes and prevention.

http://www.fda.gov/drugs/drugsafety/medicationerrors
http://www.ismp.org
http://www.medscape.com
http://www.pharmacist.com

Abbreviations

The trend has been to reduce the number of approved abbreviations used in medical records and to decrease handwritten orders and records because of medication errors due to misinterpretation. Nevertheless, there are still many approved abbreviations to be learned to interpret patient medical records, including prescriber orders, medication administration records, drug literature, and drug labels. The nurse must also avoid writing abbreviations that are on TJC's "Do Not Use" list (Table 3.1) and ISMP's List of Error-Prone Abbreviations, Symbols, and Dose Designations" (Figure 3.1). You will have to double check and review the approved abbreviations frequently. Use the worksheets provided to reinforce your memory.

Table 3.1 The Joint Commission's Official "Do Not Use" List*

Do Not Use	Potential Problem	Use Instead
U, u (unit)	Mistaken for "0" (zero), the number "4" (four), or "cc"	Write "unit"
IU (International Unit)	Mistaken for "IV" (intravenous) or the number "10" (ten)	Write "International Unit"
Q.D., QD, q.d., qd (daily)	Mistaken for each other	Write "daily"
Q.O.D., QOD, q.o.d., qod (every other day)	Period after the Q mistaken for "I" and the "O" mistaken for "I"	Write "every other day"
Trailing zero (X.0 mg)†	Decimal point is missed	Write X mg
Lack of leading zero (.X mg)		Write 0.X mg
MS	Can mean morphine sulfate or magnesium sulfate	Write "morphine sulfate"
MSO_4 and $MgSO_4$	Confused for one another	Write "magnesium sulfate"

From The Joint Commission: Official "Do Not Use" List, June 9, 2017. Retrieved from www.jointcommission.org/facts_about_do_not_use_list/.

*Applies to all orders and all medication-related documentation that is handwritten (including free-text computer entry) or on preprinted forms.

†Exception: A "trailing zero" may be used only where required to demonstrate the level of precision of the value being reported, such as for laboratory results, imaging studies that report size of lesions, or catheter/tube sizes. It may not be used in medication orders or other medication-related documentation.

Institute for Safe Medication Practices

ISMP's List of *Error-Prone Abbreviations, Symbols,* and *Dose Designations*

The abbreviations, symbols, and dose designations found in this table have been reported to ISMP through the ISMP National Medication Errors Reporting Program (ISMP MERP) as being frequently misinterpreted and involved in harmful medication errors. They should **NEVER** be used when communicating medical information. This includes internal communications, telephone/verbal prescriptions, computer-generated labels, labels for drug storage bins, medication administration records, as well as pharmacy and prescriber computer order entry screens.

Abbreviations	Intended Meaning	Misinterpretation	Correction
µg	Microgram	Mistaken as "mg"	Use "mcg"
AD, AS, AU	Right ear, left ear, each ear	Mistaken as OD, OS, OU (right eye, left eye, each eye)	Use "right ear," "left ear," or "each ear"
OD, OS, OU	Right eye, left eye, each eye	Mistaken as AD, AS, AU (right ear, left ear, each ear)	Use "right eye," "left eye," or "each eye"
BT	Bedtime	Mistaken as "BID" (twice daily)	Use "bedtime"
cc	Cubic centimeters	Mistaken as "u" (units)	Use "mL"
D/C	Discharge or discontinue	Premature discontinuation of medications if D/C (intended to mean "discharge") has been misinterpreted as "discontinued" when followed by a list of discharge medications	Use "discharge" and "discontinue"
IJ	Injection	Mistaken as "IV" or "intrajugular"	Use "injection"
IN	Intranasal	Mistaken as "IM" or "IV"	Use "intranasal" or "NAS"
HS **hs**	Half-strength At bedtime, hours of sleep	Mistaken as bedtime Mistaken as half-strength	Use "half-strength" or "bedtime"
IU**	International unit	Mistaken as IV (intravenous) or 10 (ten)	Use "units"
o.d. or OD	Once daily	Mistaken as "right eye" (OD-oculus dexter), leading to oral liquid medications administered in the eye	Use "daily"
OJ	Orange juice	Mistaken as OD or OS (right or left eye); drugs meant to be diluted in orange juice may be given in the eye	Use "orange juice"
Per os	By mouth, orally	The "os" can be mistaken as "left eye" (OS-oculus sinister)	Use "PO," "by mouth," or "orally"
q.d. or QD**	Every day	Mistaken as q.i.d., especially if the period after the "q" or the tail of the "q" is misunderstood as an "i"	Use "daily"
qhs	Nightly at bedtime	Mistaken as "qhr" or every hour	Use "nightly"
qn	Nightly or at bedtime	Mistaken as "qh" (every hour)	Use "nightly" or "at bedtime"
q.o.d. or QOD**	Every other day	Mistaken as "q.d." (daily) or "q.i.d. (four times daily) if the "o" is poorly written	Use "every other day"
q1d	Daily	Mistaken as q.i.d. (four times daily)	Use "daily"
q6PM, etc.	Every evening at 6 PM	Mistaken as every 6 hours	Use "daily at 6 PM" or "6 PM daily"
SC, SQ, sub q	Subcutaneous	SC mistaken as SL (sublingual); SQ mistaken as "5 every;" the "q" in "sub q" has been mistaken as "every" (e.g., a heparin dose ordered "sub q 2 hours before surgery" misunderstood as every 2 hours before surgery)	Use "subcut" or "subcutaneously"
ss	Sliding scale (insulin) or ½ (apothecary)	Mistaken as "55"	Spell out "sliding scale;" use "one-half" or "½"
SSRI **SSI**	Sliding scale regular insulin Sliding scale insulin	Mistaken as selective-serotonin reuptake inhibitor Mistaken as Strong Solution of Iodine (Lugol's)	Spell out "sliding scale (insulin)"
i/d	One daily	Mistaken as "tid"	Use "1 daily"
TIW or tiw	3 times a week	Mistaken as "3 times a day" or "twice in a week"	Use "3 times weekly"
U or u**	Unit	Mistaken as the number 0 or 4, causing a 10-fold overdose or greater (e.g., 4U seen as "40" or 4u seen as "44"); mistaken as "cc" so dose given in volume instead of units (e.g., 4u seen as 4cc)	Use "unit"
UD	As directed ("ut dictum")	Mistaken as unit dose (e.g., diltiazem 125 mg IV infusion "UD" misinterpreted as meaning to give the entire infusion as a unit [bolus] dose)	Use "as directed"
Dose Designations and Other Information	**Intended Meaning**	**Misinterpretation**	**Correction**
Trailing zero after decimal point (e.g., 1.0 mg)**	1 mg	Mistaken as 10 mg if the decimal point is not seen	Do not use trailing zeros for doses expressed in whole numbers
"Naked" decimal point (e.g., .5 mg)**	0.5 mg	Mistaken as 5 mg if the decimal point is not seen	Use zero before a decimal point when the dose is less than a whole unit
Abbreviations such as mg. or mL. with a period following the abbreviation	mg mL	The period is unnecessary and could be mistaken as the number 1 if written poorly	Use mg, mL, etc. without a terminal period

FIGURE 3.1 ISMP's List of Error-Prone Abbreviations, Symbols, and Dose Designations. (© ISMP, 2015. Reprinted with permission.)

Continued

ISMP's List of *Error-Prone Abbreviations, Symbols,* and *Dose Designations* (continued)

Dose Designations and Other Information	Intended Meaning	Misinterpretation	Correction
Drug name and dose run together (especially problematic for drug names that end in "l" such as Inderal40 mg; Tegretol300 mg)	Inderal 40 mg Tegretol 300 mg	Mistaken as Inderal 140 mg Mistaken as Tegretol 1300 mg	Place adequate space between the drug name, dose, and unit of measure
Numerical dose and unit of measure run together (e.g., 10mg, 100mL)	10 mg 100 mL	The "m" is sometimes mistaken as a zero or two zeros, risking a 10- to 100-fold overdose	Place adequate space between the dose and unit of measure
Large doses without properly placed commas (e.g., 100000 units; 1000000 units)	100,000 units 1,000,000 units	100000 has been mistaken as 10,000 or 1,000,000; 1000000 has been mistaken as 100,000	Use commas for dosing units at or above 1,000, or use words such as 100 "thousand" or 1 "million" to improve readability
Drug Name Abbreviations	**Intended Meaning**	**Misinterpretation**	**Correction**
To avoid confusion, do not abbreviate drug names when communicating medical information. Examples of drug name abbreviations involved in medication errors include:			
APAP	acetaminophen	Not recognized as acetaminophen	Use complete drug name
ARA A	vidarabine	Mistaken as cytarabine (ARA C)	Use complete drug name
AZT	zidovudine (Retrovir)	Mistaken as azathioprine or aztreonam	Use complete drug name
CPZ	Compazine (prochlorperazine)	Mistaken as chlorpromazine	Use complete drug name
DPT	Demerol-Phenergan-Thorazine	Mistaken as diphtheria-pertussis-tetanus (vaccine)	Use complete drug name
DTO	Diluted tincture of opium, or deodorized tincture of opium (Paregoric)	Mistaken as tincture of opium	Use complete drug name
HCl	hydrochloric acid or hydrochloride	Mistaken as potassium chloride (The "H" is misinterpreted as "K")	Use complete drug name unless expressed as a salt of a drug
HCT	hydrocortisone	Mistaken as hydrochlorothiazide	Use complete drug name
HCTZ	hydrochlorothiazide	Mistaken as hydrocortisone (seen as HCT250 mg)	Use complete drug name
MgSO4**	magnesium sulfate	Mistaken as morphine sulfate	Use complete drug name
MS, MSO4**	morphine sulfate	Mistaken as magnesium sulfate	Use complete drug name
MTX	methotrexate	Mistaken as mitoxantrone	Use complete drug name
PCA	procainamide	Mistaken as patient controlled analgesia	Use complete drug name
PTU	propylthiouracil	Mistaken as mercaptopurine	Use complete drug name
T3	Tylenol with codeine No. 3	Mistaken as liothyronine	Use complete drug name
TAC	triamcinolone	Mistaken as tetracaine, Adrenalin, cocaine	Use complete drug name
TNK	TNKase	Mistaken as "TPA"	Use complete drug name
ZnSO4	zinc sulfate	Mistaken as morphine sulfate	Use complete drug name
Stemmed Drug Names	**Intended Meaning**	**Misinterpretation**	**Correction**
"Nitro" drip	nitroglycerin infusion	Mistaken as sodium nitroprusside infusion	Use complete drug name
"Norflox"	norfloxacin	Mistaken as Norflex	Use complete drug name
"IV Vanc"	intravenous vancomycin	Mistaken as Invanz	Use complete drug name
Symbols	**Intended Meaning**	**Misinterpretation**	**Correction**
ʒ ♍	Dram Minim	Symbol for dram mistaken as "3" Symbol for minim mistaken as "mL"	Use the metric system
x3d	For three days	Mistaken as "3 doses"	Use "for three days"
> and <	Greater than and less than	Mistaken as opposite of intended; mistakenly use incorrect symbol; "< 10" mistaken as "40"	Use "greater than" or "less than"
/ (slash mark)	Separates two doses or indicates "per"	Mistaken as the number 1 (e.g., "25 units/10 units" misread as "25 units and 110" units)	Use "per" rather than a slash mark to separate doses
@	At	Mistaken as "2"	Use "at"
&	And	Mistaken as "2"	Use "and"
+	Plus or and	Mistaken as "4"	Use "and"
°	Hour	Mistaken as a zero (e.g., q2° seen as q 20)	Use "hr," "h," or "hour"
Φ or ⊘	zero, null sign	Mistaken as numerals 4, 6, 8, and 9	Use 0 or zero, or describe intent using whole words

**These abbreviations are included on The Joint Commission's "minimum list" of dangerous abbreviations, acronyms, and symbols that must be included on an organization's "Do Not Use" list, effective January 1, 2004. Visit www.jointcommission.org for more information about this Joint Commission requirement.

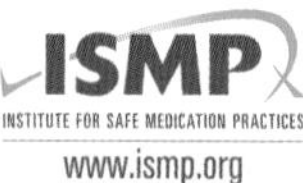

FIGURE 3.1, cont'd ISMP's List of Error-Prone Abbreviations, Symbols, and Dose Designations. (© ISMP, 2015. Reprinted with permission.)

The Joint Commission's Official "Do Not Use" List

The Joint Commission developed its first "do not use" list of abbreviations in 2004. The list was incorporated into the Information Management Standards in 2010. This list currently does not apply to preprogrammed health information technology systems such as electronic medical records or computerized physician order entry (CPOE) systems, although these systems may be brought into compliance in the future. It is advised that these dangerous abbreviations, acronyms, symbols, and dose designations should be eliminated from future development and upgrades to software used by health care providers.

Answers on page 94

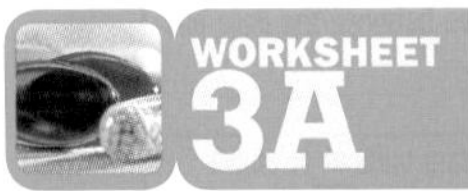

WORKSHEET 3A Abbreviations, Symbols, and Acronyms

Directions: For medication safety, it is important to be very familiar with The Joint Commission "Do Not Use" list (see Table 3.1) and the Institute for Safe Medication Practices (ISMP) Error-Prone Abbreviations list (see Figure 3.1). Answer the following questions:

TJC: "Do Not Use" List (p. 61)

1. What are three mistakes that can be made if the abbreviation "U" for units is misread?
2. How can periods and "0" be misread?
3. How can trailing zeros and lack of leading zeros result in a dose error?
4. Which documents must be in compliance with the TJC official "Do Not Use" list?
5. Which is the preferred abbreviation for milliliters? cc, ml, or mL? Why?

ISMP: Dose Designation and Symbols Sections (p. 63):

6. How can medication names ending in the letter "l" cause a major dose error?
7. Why should large doses in the thousands have commas?
8. How should a numerical dose and unit of measure such as "ten milligrams" be spaced to avoid 10- to 100-fold overdoses?
9. How can a slash mark be misread, and what word should be used instead of a slash?
10. How can x3d be misinterpreted, and how can it be avoided?

Medication Forms: Solids and Liquids

Medications can be provided in a variety of forms: solids, liquids, inhalants, skin patches, suppositories, and others. It is very important to distinguish the forms and to ascertain the precise form ordered by the prescriber and supplied for administration. The form affects the rate of absorption and distribution in the body. It also affects the route of administration.

Solid Oral Medications

- Plain tablets (Figure 3.2, *A*): compressed powdered drugs
- Scored tablets (Figure 3.2, *B*): tablets with a dividing line; the *only kind* of tablet that can be cut, if an ordered dose amount is for half a tablet
- Caplets: tablets small or large, oval-shaped like a capsule
- Enteric-coated tablets (Figure 3.2, *C*): tablets with coating to permit them to dissolve in the small intestine instead of the stomach, where it might cause gastric irritation
- Capsules (Figure 3.2, *D*): soluble case—usually gelatin—that holds liquid or dry particles of the drug; can be hard or soft (softgels), in one piece or two pieces

- Delayed release (DR) (Figure 3.2, *E*): extended release (ER), slow release (SR), controlled release (CR), long acting (LA), extra long acting (EL), controlled dose (CD)
- Double strength (DS, ES): extra-strength medications
- Powders and granules (Figure 3.2, *F*): loose or molded drug substance usually to be dissolved in liquid or nonessential food

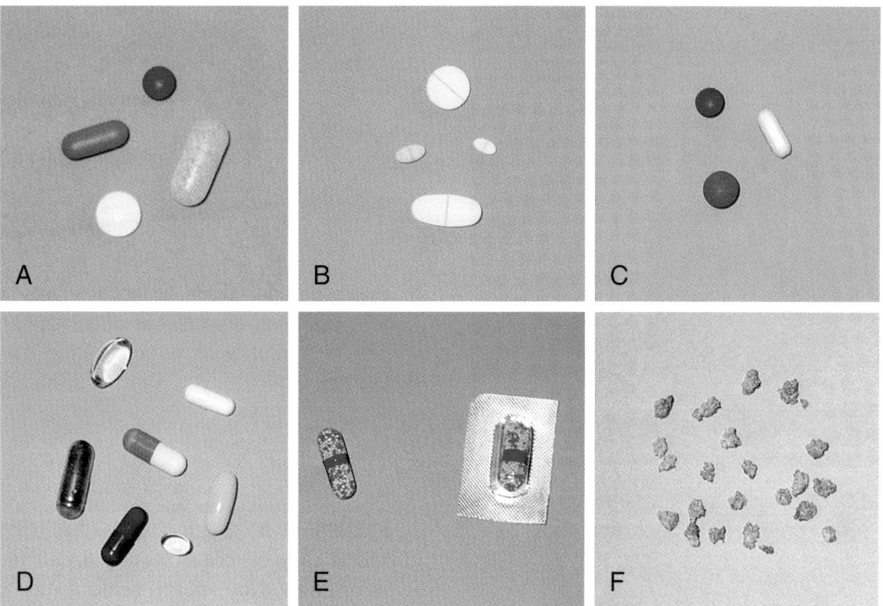

FIGURE 3.2 Various solid oral drug forms. **A,** Plain tablets. **B,** Scored tablets. **C,** Enteric-coated tablets. **D,** Capsules. **E,** Extended-release capsules. **F,** Granules. (Courtesy Amanda Politte, St. Louis, MO.)

CLINICAL ALERT!

Be aware that the names, abbreviations, and length of release time for these medications vary among tablets and capsules. They are not standardized among manufacturers.

CLINICAL ALERT!

Never crush or cut delayed-release gel or enteric-coated medications. Doing so will accelerate their release into the body's circulation and is a reportable medication error. Only cut scored tablets if needed (Figures 3.3 to 3.5).

CLINICAL ALERT!

Never crush or cut capsules. Occasionally a two-piece capsule may be opened and the contents placed in a nonessential food or liquid for a patient who cannot swallow capsules, but only if the prescriber permits.

Liquid Oral Medications

- Aqueous suspensions: solid particles suspended in liquid that must be well mixed before administration
- Elixirs: sweetened alcohol and water solutions
- Emulsions: fats or oils suspended in liquid by an emulsifier
- Extracts: syrups or derived forms of active drugs
- Fluid extracts: concentrated alcoholic liquid extracts of plants or vegetables
- Solutions: mixtures in which solids are fully dissolved (vs. aqueous suspensions)

The trend is to supply liquid oral medications in individual, calibrated unit-dose cups and calibrated plastic droppers and spoons to reduce calculation and measurement errors* (Figures 3.6 and 3.7).

Occasionally a liquid medication must be poured from a multidose bottle into a metric-calibrated cup. The dose must be measured on a level surface and at eye level.

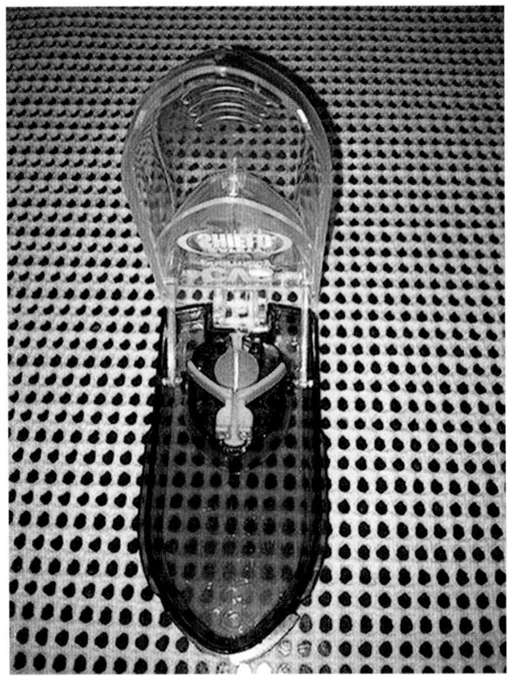

FIGURE 3.3 Pill splitter. Pill splitter only splits pills that are scored with an indented line.

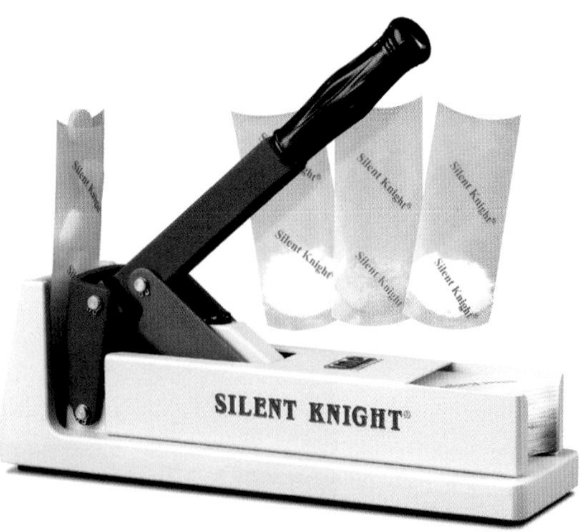

FIGURE 3.4 Silent Knight® Tablet Crushing System. A pill crusher that contains disposable pouches for each tablet to prevent cross-contamination with prior crushed medications. (Used with permission by Links Medical Products, Inc., Irvine, California.)

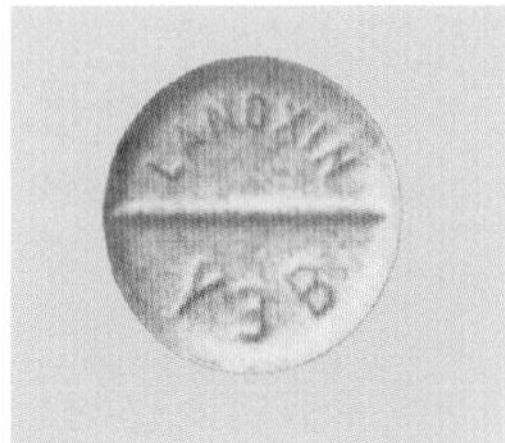

FIGURE 3.5 Scored tablet. A scored tablet may be cut in half if a half dose is ordered. Non-scored tablets may not be cut.

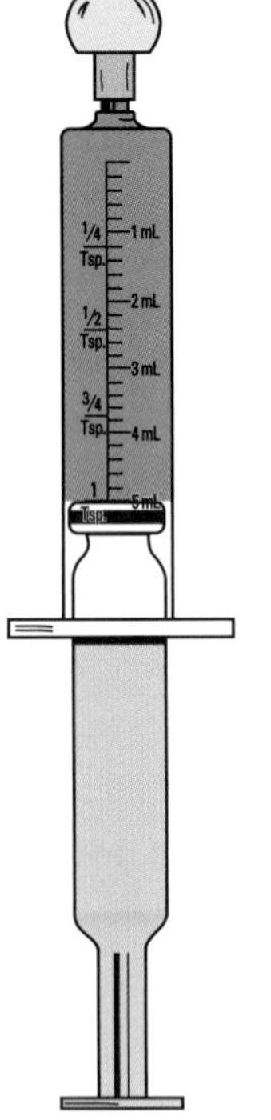

FIGURE 3.6 Prefilled oral syringe.

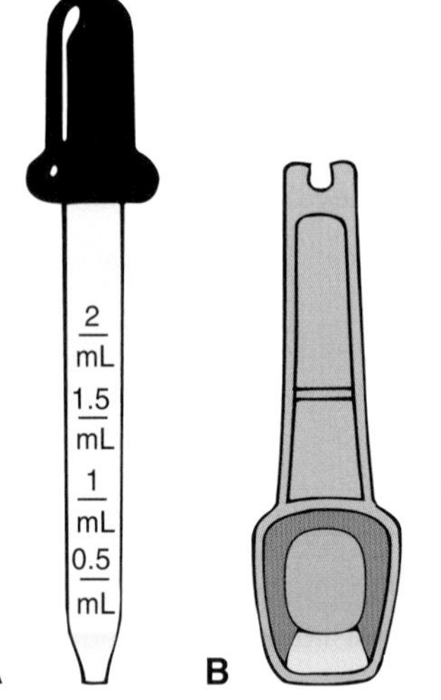

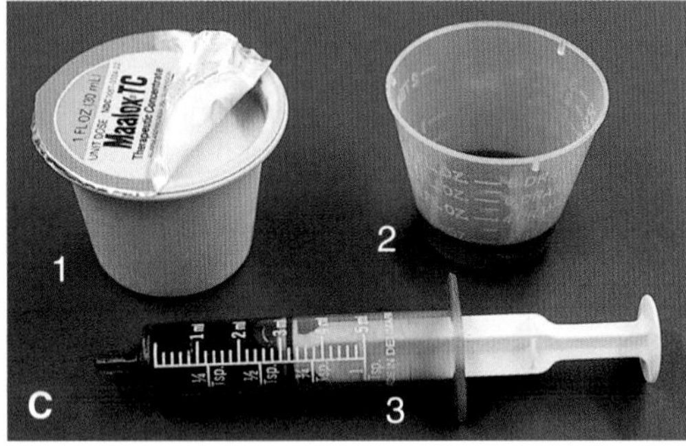

FIGURE 3.7 **A,** Medicine dropper. **B,** Measuring teaspoon. **C,** Liquid medication in *(1)* a single-unit-dose package, *(2)* liquid measured in medicine cup, and *(3)* oral liquid medicine in syringe. (**A** and **B** from Clayton BD, Willihnganz M: *Basic pharmacology for nurses,* ed. 17, St. Louis, 2017 Mosby. **C** from Perry AG, Potter PA, Ostendorf WR: *Clinical nursing skills and techniques,* ed. 8, St. Louis, 2014, Mosby.)

CLINICAL ALERT!

Teach patients not to substitute household utensils such as spoons and cups when measuring medications at home. The sizes vary considerably and, if used, will result in an underdose or overdose of the medication. The metric-calibrated equipment that is supplied with the medication must be used to obtain the exact dose ordered. Also teach patients to discard unused or excess medication rather than to save it or pour it back into the original container.

---

*Liquids are also supplied in injectable (also known as parenteral) forms, such as ampules, vials, and prefilled injectable syringes and other devices. These are discussed in Chapter 5 and later chapters.

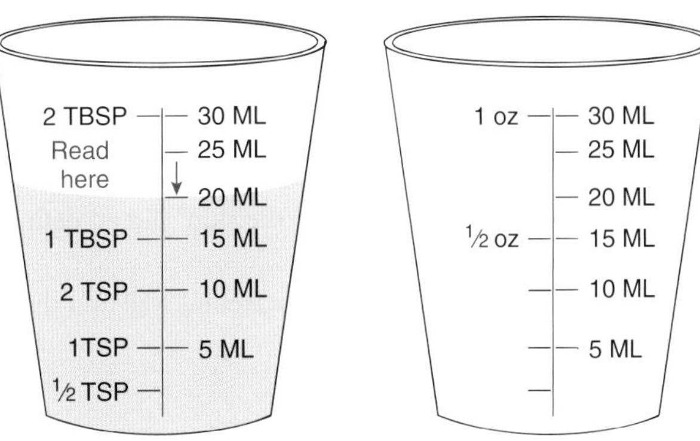

The "Read Here" arrow points to the meniscus, the center of the slightly concave liquid surface where liquid medications should be measured. The meniscus is best seen on a flat surface at eye level.

Answers on page 94

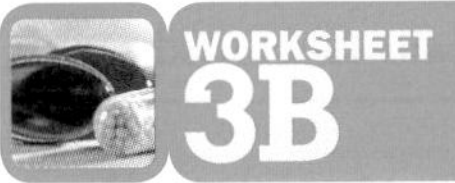

WORKSHEET 3B Abbreviations for Drug Forms

Study the abbreviations on the first page of the text. Then provide the abbreviations in the spaces provided.

Term	Recommended Abbreviation
capsule*	
tablet	
fluid	
solution	
suspension	
elixir	
teaspoon	
tablespoon	
liquid	
ounce	
double-strength	
extended release*	
long acting*	
sustained release*	
controlled release*	

*Do not crush these medications.

CLINICAL ALERT!

Study examples of abbreviations that have caused errors and should be written out (see Table 3.1 and Figure 3.1).

Routes of Medication Administration

There are two major divisions of routes:

1. **Parenteral** (injectables)
   - *Intradermal (ID):* between epidermis and dermis
   - *Intravenous (IV):* into vein
   - *Intramuscular (IM):* into muscle
   - *Subcutaneous (Subcut):* "under the skin" (literal definition); in practice, injected into fatty layer below the dermis
   - *Epidural:* into space between vertebral wall and dura mater (dural membrane that holds spinal fluid and nerve roots)
   - *Intrathecal:* into spinal fluid
2. **Nonparenteral** (all routes administered as a noninjectable)
   - *Oral (PO, po):* swallowed by mouth
   - *Sublingual (SL):* dissolved under the tongue directly into circulation, bypassing the gastrointestinal tract for faster absorption (e.g., nitroglycerin for cardiac-related pain)
   - *Buccal (bucc):* dissolved inside the cheek, absorbed directly into circulation, bypassing the gastrointestinal tract for faster absorption
   - *Topical (top):* applied to skin surface for local effects
   - *Transdermal (skin):* for systemic effects (e.g., transdermal patches deliver pain-relief medication, hormones)
   - *Other:* eyes, ears, lungs (respiratory) (inhalants), nose, nasogastric (NG) (nose to stomach), gastric (g) (stomach), intestine (enteral), rectum, vagina (vag)

CLINICAL RELEVANCE

Most nonparenteral medications are ordered for the oral (po) route. Most parenteral medications are ordered for the intravenous (IV), intramuscular (IM), or subcutaneous (Subcut) routes.

CLINICAL ALERT!

An error with medication routes may result in a serious adverse drug event (ADE). The patient and family must be taught the correct use and/or application of the drug and give return demonstrations during hospitalization and at the time of discharge. One session of teaching is often insufficient. Provide the patient with written follow-up instructions. Patients have been known to apply narcotic transdermal patches over old ones or on the wrong part of the body; to chew or swallow sublingual or buccal medications, or to use bare hands for topically applying a medication when hands should be gloved or an implement used for application to avoid an overdose or injury to the patient (or person applying the medication) and/or contamination of the product.

To reduce the chance of errors, have a family member present and use effective communication, including assessment of mental status and comprehension via feedback. Document all patient and family education.

CLINICAL ALERT!

The nurse may not legally change the route of medication administration. The provider must be contacted.

Answers on page 95

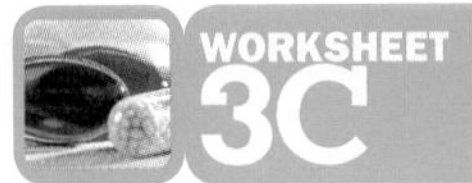

WORKSHEET 3C Abbreviations for Time and Route

Study the approved and recommended abbreviations on the first page of the text and their patterns of similarities and differences as well as The Joint Commission's "Do Not Use" list in Table 3.1 and the Institute for Safe Medication Practices List of Error-Prone Abbreviations, Symbols, and Dose Designations (see Figure 3.1). Then enter the approved or recommended abbreviation in the space provided.

Worksheet 3C: Abbreviations for Time and Route Table

Time	Abbreviation (if Applicable)	Time	Abbreviation (if Applicable)
before		after	
before meals		after meals	
daily	Write out daily	three times a day	
twice a day		every other day	Write out every other day
every day	Write out every day	every 6 hours	
every 4 hours		every 12 hours	
whenever necessary		as desired, freely	
immediately, at once		bedtime	Write out bedtime
with		without	
Route	**Abbreviation (if Applicable)**	**Route**	**Abbreviation (if Applicable)**
by mouth		nothing by mouth	
intravenous		intramuscular	
sublingual		subcutaneous	
intradermal		suppository*	
left eye	Write out left eye	right ear	Write out right ear
nasogastric		per gastrostomy tube	

*Orders for suppositories require further route identification per vagina, per rectum, or per urethra.

Measurement Abbreviations

Metric abbreviations for weight and volume are the most frequently seen abbreviations in medication orders. They will be used for calculations in future chapters. Metric abbreviations are the same for single and plural measurements. They are not pluralized. Two milligrams would be written *2 mg* not *2 mgs*.

Answers on page 95

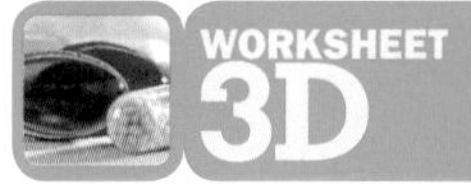

WORKSHEET 3D Abbreviations for Drug Measurements

Study the abbreviations on the first page of the text. Pay attention to uppercase and lowercase letters when learning the abbreviations. There are only a few instances when uppercase is employed. Then provide the approved abbreviations for the measurements.

Metric Measurement Term*	Abbreviation (if Applicable)
microgram(s)	
milligram(s)	
gram(s)	
kilogram(s)	
milliliter(s)	
milliequivalent(s)	
unit	Write out unit
international unit	Write out international unit
liter	
square meter	
Other Measurement Term	**Abbreviation (if Applicable)**
one half	Write out one half
teaspoon	
tablespoon	
pound	

*The metric abbreviations are the same for singular and plural measurements.

Medication Labels

Medication labels contain required critical information for patient safety. The label must be read carefully to ensure that the medication is precisely what the prescriber ordered.

Drug Names

Drugs may have three names:

1. The **brand name,** which begins with a capital letter, that distinguishes a manufacturer's product from similar products from other manufacturers
2. The **generic name** is the official name by which a drug is commonly available, unprotected by trademark; all drugs, including over-the-counter medications, must have the generic name on the label
3. A long **chemical name,** such as acetylsalicylic acid (the chemical name for aspirin); this name is rarely seen on labels.

Brand/Trade Name and Registration of Name

Companies that spend millions of dollars and years to be the first to develop an FDA-approved new drug can receive two important official protections from U.S. governmental agencies. The first is registration of the **brand name** (proprietary name) the company selects with the U.S. Food and Drug Administration; it is designated on the label with the **registration symbol** ® after the proprietary name. As long as the registration is maintained, *no other company can use that name.* The second protection is the **patent,** which gives exclusive manufacturing rights to the company for a specific amount of time.

Generic Drugs

Generic drugs are copies of the original drug product that are produced by companies after the original manufacturer's patent expires. The *only* differences permitted by the FDA between the original and the generic product are (1) inactive ingredients, (2) size, (3) color, and (4) shape. There are thousands of generic drugs with and without their own brand names on the market because many patents have expired in recent years. Generic drugs are considerably *less expensive* than the original product because the drug formula has already been invented, tested, and approved and is available.

Examine the following labels. They contain a surprisingly large amount of information in a small space. They *may* contain a trade/brand name, registered or unregistered. They *must* contain a generic (official name); national drug code (NDC) number; manufacturer name; drug concentration (unit dose) and form (tablet, capsule, liquid, suppository, etc.); bar code; total amount in container; route to be administered; expiration date; lot (batch) number; any special storage needs; warnings, if needed; and directions for use.

Additional information, such as the usual dose, may be included. The abbreviations for United States Pharmacopeia (USP) and National Formulary (NF) may appear next to the name, indicating that the product adheres to the national legal standards of identity, purity, quality, strength, labeling, and other specific requirements.

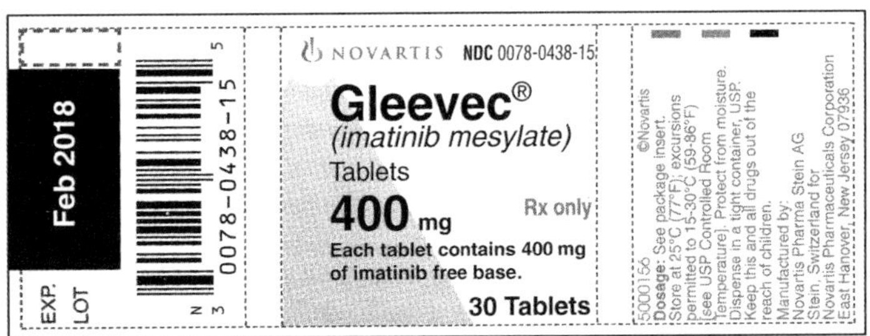

Note that the generic name is in lowercase. The main information on the label is contained in the bar code as well. This lot (batch) expired in 2018. The nurse cannot give an expired medication. "Rx only" means this is a prescription-only medication. The lot (batch) number and expiration date are added when the container is filled and are placed close to each other.

The FDA web site http://www.accessdata.fda.gov/scripts/cder/ndc/dsp_searchresult.cfm maintains all the information on drug labels and more. You can search the site for information on a drug by entering any one of five types of data from the label: proprietary name, application number, active ingredient, NDC number, and labeler. The web site will then show the current status of the drug. It will either state "no match" if the drug is not currently approved or has been withdrawn, or it will list the current manufacturers and all the forms and dosages available by each manufacturer. Additional important information about the medication will be shown.

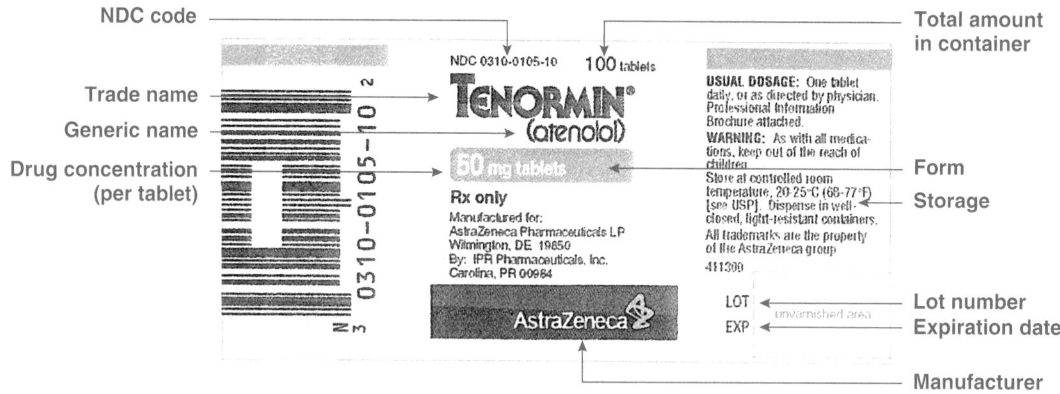

Registered trademark brand name: Tenormin, the exclusive brand name for this antihypertensive medication.

Generic official name: atenolol; all manufacturers must include the generic official name on all labels of the drug.

Drug dose: 50 mg.

Drug form (tablet, capsule, granules, suppository, inhaler, liquid, etc.): tablet.

Drug concentration (dose per weight or quantity): 50 mg per tablet.

Bar code: placed near the drug dose; contains the NDC code.

NDC code: national drug code contains label information.

Total amount in container: 100 tablets in this multidose container.

Lot (specific batch) and *expiration date:* lot and expiration date appear adjacent to each other on the label when the container was filled.

Storage directions: storage temperatures and conditions (some storage directions pertain to keeping a drug in a dark or light area).

Special warnings: "Keep out of reach of children."

Other information: usual dose.

Note: the implied oral route is not on this label. All new labels must specify the route.

There are about 128 generic copies of Tenormin. Many of the manufacturers have their own brand names, which can be very similar, such as Alol, Adelol, Atol, Atenol, to name a few. Always refer to the ISMP's List of Confused Drug Names to be sure you do not confuse look alike/sound alike medications. The list can be retrieved from https://www.ismp.org/sites/default/files/attachments/2017-11/confuseddrugnames%2802.2015%29.pdf

To calculate a dose, enter the drug concentration on the left side of the equation:

WHAT YOU HAVE

$$50 \text{ mg} : 1 \text{ tablet} = or \left(\frac{50 \text{ mg}}{1 \text{ tablet}} = \right)$$

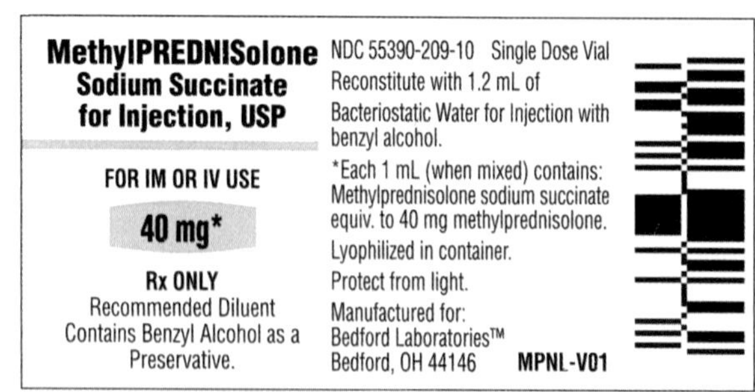

Note that the route for this drug is *injectable:* intramuscular (IM) or intravenous (IV). Also note the two types of print on the registered brand name—MethylPREDNISolone—an antiinflammatory drug used for allergies, arthritis, psoriasis, and other indications. The tall letters are called "tall man letters"

to draw attention to a drug name that is similar to one or more other drugs by emphasizing the main differences in the spelling. Other examples include medroxyPROGESTERone, a hormone used for female contraception, among other uses; and methylTESTOSTERone, a hormone used to treat testosterone deficiency, among other uses. Many drugs are "look alike, sound alike," which has led to serious medication errors (https://www.ismp.org/tools/confuseddrugnames.pdf). Obviously, confusion about these three names could lead to serious medical issues. Because of medication errors attributed to labels, the FDA, ISMP, and other organizations have been working with manufacturers to reduce errors by improving and standardizing label packaging, design, and content.

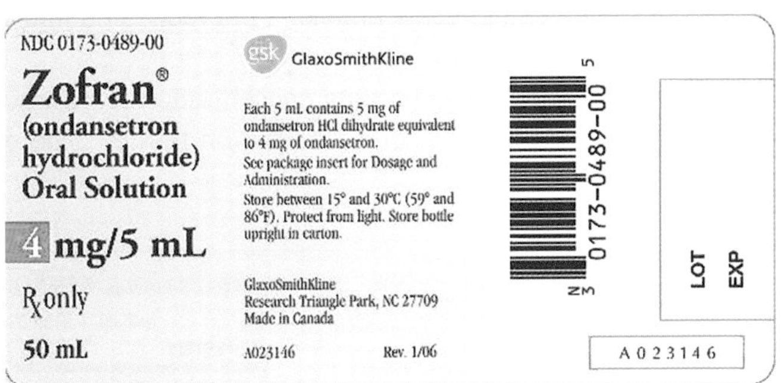

This form of Zofran (ondansetron) is a *liquid oral solution* in a multidose container. The usual order for medications is 1 or 2 servings of the supplied concentration, in this case 4 mg per 5 mL or 8 mg per 10 mL. The trend for patient safety is to increase the supply of unit-dose packaging. If this multidose container was mistaken for the unit-dose ordered, such an error would amount to a dose of 40 mg, 10 times the usual dose.

CLINICAL ALERT!

Distinguish unit-dose containers from multidose containers.
NOTE: Both of these labels indicate they are multidose containers.

Do not use a slash for "per." It can be mistaken for the number 1; for example, 4 mg/5 mL might be misinterpreted as 15 mL.

This oral-route liquid suspension is packaged in a unit-dose (usual single serving) container. Unit-dose containers are not reusable. Acetaminophen is a generic form of the original drug Tylenol. The patent for Tylenol expired in 2011, and over 600 generics containing acetaminophen—many with their own brand names—have been manufactured. This solution concentration is 160 mg per 5 mL and is indicated for pediatric use. The trend is to package more medications specifically in doses that are usually prescribed for children. This reduces the need for calculating a child's fractional portion of an adult dose, thereby reducing the chance of error.

Drug Facts (continued)

- use only enclosed dosing cup designed for use with this product. Do not use any other dosing device.
- if needed, repeat dose every 4 hours while symptoms last
- do not give more than 5 times in 24 hours
- do not give for more than 5 days unless directed by a doctor
- **this product does not contain directions or complete warnings for adult use**

Weight (lb)	Age (yr)	Dose (tsp or mL)
under 24	under 2 years	ask a doctor
24-35	2-3 years	1 tsp or 5 mL
36-47	4-5 years	1 1/2 tsp or 7.5 mL
48-59	6-8 years	2 tsp or 10 mL
60-71	9-10 years	2 1/2 tsp or 12.5 mL
72-95	11 years	3 tsp or 15 mL

Attention: use only enclosed dosing cup specifically designed for use with this product. Do not use any other dosing device.

Other information

- **each teaspoon contains:** sodium 3 mg
- store at 20°-25°C (68°-77°F)
- do not use if printed neckband is broken or missing

Inactive ingredients anhydrous citric acid, butylparaben, carboxymethylcellulose sodium, carrageenan, D&C red no. 33, FD&C blue no. 1, flavor, glycerin, high fructose corn syrup, hydroxyethyl cellulose, microcrystalline cellulose, propylene glycol, purified water, sodium benzoate, sorbitol solution

Questions? Call 1-800-910-6874

*This product is not manufactured or distributed by the Tylenol Company, owner of the registered trademark Tylenol®.

094 01 0137 ID209441
Distributed by Target Corporation
Minneapolis, MN 55403
© 2009 Target Brands, Inc.
All Rights Reserved Shop Target.com

NDC 11673-130-26

children's acetaminophen

oral suspension

80 mg per ½ teaspoon
(160 mg per 5 mL)
fever reducer/pain reliever

Compare to active ingredient in Children's Tylenol® Oral Suspension*

see new warnings information

alcohol free
ibuprofen free
aspirin free

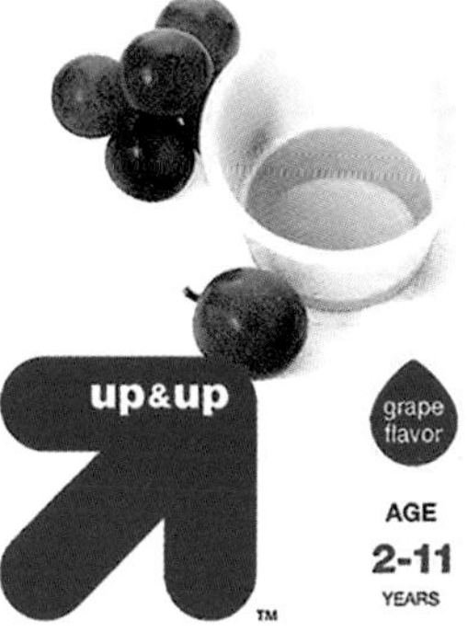

4 FL OZ (118 mL)

To calculate a dose, place the given concentration per unit on the left side of the equation:

$$160 \text{ mg} : 5 \text{ mL} = or \left(\frac{160 \text{ mg}}{5 \text{ mL}} = \right)$$

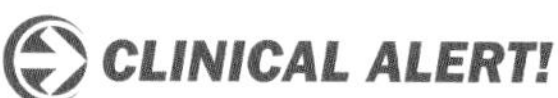

CLINICAL ALERT!

Do not confuse aspirin with acetaminophen products. The two often are prescribed for similar conditions. Injury or death can result. They are contained in many hundreds of products. Many have their own brand names.

Answers on page 96

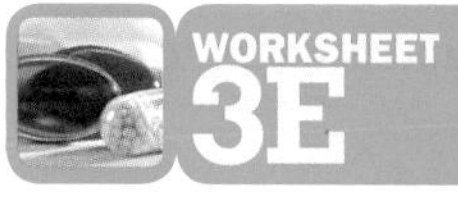

WORKSHEET 3E Interpreting Medication Labels

Examine the following labels and fill in the requested information.

What you have, the supplied drug concentration (e.g., 100 mg per tablet or 50 mg per 2 mL), is determined from the label and inserted on the left side of your ratio and proportion in colon or fraction form.

1.

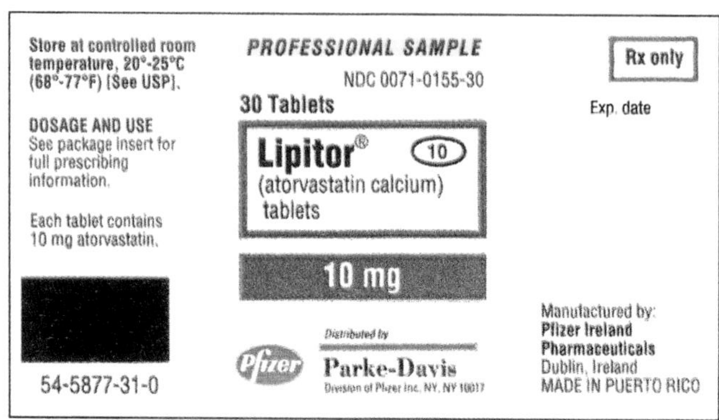

a. National Drug Code number
b. Proprietary (registered) brand name
c. Generic (official) name
d. Drug concentration
e. Ratio for "what you have" (dose concentration supplied per tablet, capsule, milliliter)

2.

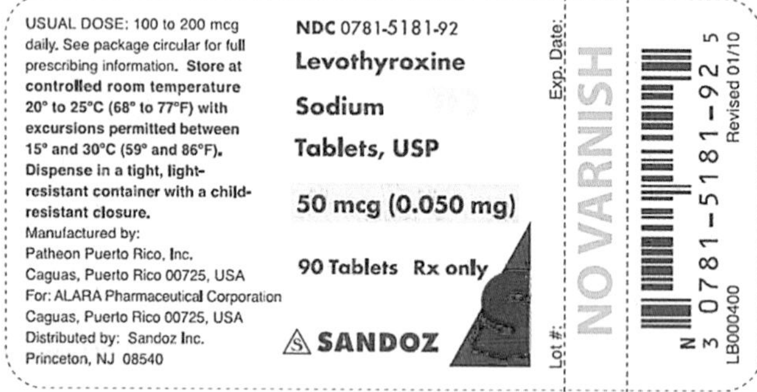

a. Generic name
b. Dose in micrograms (mcg) and equivalent dose in milligrams (mg)
c. Ratio for "what you have"

3.

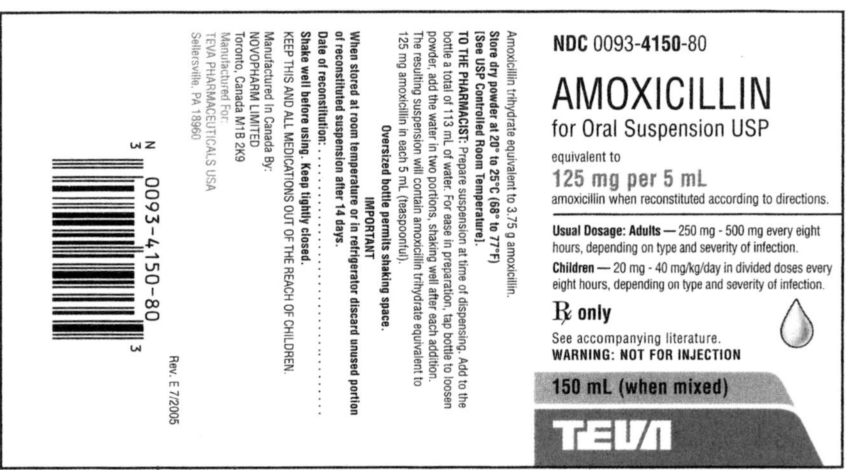

NDC 0093-4150-80
AMOXICILLIN
for Oral Suspension USP
equivalent to
125 mg per 5 mL
amoxicillin when reconstituted according to directions.
Usual Dosage: Adults — 250 mg - 500 mg every eight hours, depending on type and severity of infection.
Children — 20 mg - 40 mg/kg/day in divided doses every eight hours, depending on type and severity of infection.
℞ only
See accompanying literature.
WARNING: NOT FOR INJECTION
150 mL (when mixed)
TEVA

a. Drug form
b. Drug concentration
c. Usual dose for adults
d. Is this a single-dose or multidose container?
e. If multidose, how many times more is total dose in mL after reconstitution than the single dose in mL?
f. Ratio for "what you have"

4. a. Proprietary name for this compound drug
b. Generic names and dose for each drug
c. Form
d. Meaning of "DS"
e. Ratio for "what you have," if applicable

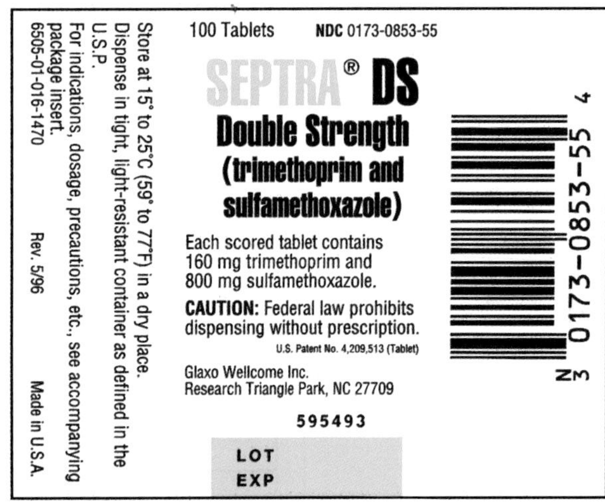

100 Tablets
NDC 0173-0853-55
SEPTRA® DS
Double Strength
(trimethoprim and sulfamethoxazole)
Each scored tablet contains 160 mg trimethoprim and 800 mg sulfamethoxazole.
CAUTION: Federal law prohibits dispensing without prescription.
U.S. Patent No. 4,209,513 (Tablet)
Glaxo Wellcome Inc.
Research Triangle Park, NC 27709
595493
LOT
EXP
Store at 15° to 25°C (59° to 77°F) in a dry place.
Dispense in tight, light-resistant container as defined in the U.S.P.
For indications, dosage, precautions, etc., see accompanying package insert.
6505-01-016-1470
Rev. 5/96
Made in U.S.A.
N 3 0173-0853-55 4

CLINICAL ALERT!

Compound drugs, such as Septra DS, are usually ordered by name and number of servings of the dose provided. The labels *always* provide the concentration of each drug. The medication *orders* for a compound drug seldom mention the drug concentrations for a compound drug *unless it is a scored tablet* that allows a half dose of the drug on hand.

Three Reasons to Double Check a DS Medication

1. The abbreviation DS reveals that there is also a weaker concentration, "regular strength," available. It alerts the nurse to double check the dose and whether the order is actually for DS or regular strength.
2. The most common order for an oral compound drug is one tablet or capsule. Recheck an order that exceeds a single dose of a compound drug.
3. When medication is provided in a scored tablet, the dose needs to be rechecked. Just because the tablet is scored does not necessarily mean that the order will call for half the dose on hand.

5.

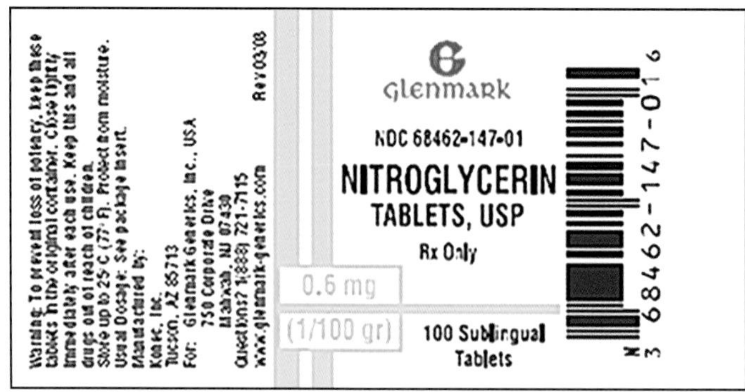

a. Generic name

b. Route on label and definition

c. Reason you would assess patient's mental status and experience with this medication before administering

d. Ratio for "what you have"

Medication Orders

Medication orders must be legible and complete. They may be handwritten, faxed, or entered into a computer (computerized physician order entry [CPOE]) by the provider or pharmacist (Figure 3.8). Handwritten orders are becoming less common because of misinterpretations resulting in medication errors.

GENERAL HOSPITAL

Patient: Greiga, Anna R. Female ID# C239479 DOB 01/03/60 Age: 58
Allergies: Morphine, Sulfa, Tree nuts
Primary Attending: Jenson, Olaf R. 14589-134
Date: 01/11/18

Medication Orders

Order ID	Order	
122766	Lanoxin (digoxin) tablet 0.25 mg PO AM daily Hold if pulse under 50.	
122767	Calcium 600 + D tablet PO bedtime	
122769	Lantus (insulin glargine) inj 10 units, Subcut, AM daily at same time	
122770	Crestor 10 mg tablet at bedtime (generic allowed)	
122771	Furosemide 20 mg IV push 2 mg per minute in AM after breakfast one time only	
	PRN ORDERS	
122772	Oxycodone tab 30 mg q6h PRN severe pain *	

Electronic Signature: Olaf R Jensen, MD Date/Time: 01/11/18

A separate signed prescription for controlled substance must accompany this form.

Electronic signature: Olaf R Jensen, MD Date/Time: 01/11/18 0930 Phone: (602 315 3930)

This is an example of electronically entered Prescriber Medication Order.
These orders will be transfered to a Medication Administration Record by Pharmacy with more details if necessary, such as the number of tablets based on what they will supply or a warning about a known side effect to watch for or a flag for controlled substance. The nurse should check for new orders periodically during the shift to see if any orders have been discontinued.

FIGURE 3.8 Sample medication orders.

All medication orders must contain the complete date and time, the name of the patient, the name of the medication, the dosage, the form (if supplied in more than one form), the route, the frequency (dosing) schedule, and the prescriber's signature. Additional directions may be needed for specific medications. Questions about an order need to be clarified with an instructor, pharmacist, and/or the prescriber.

CLINICAL RELEVANCE

Example of a call to a provider: "This is Mark Keene, RN, calling from General Hospital, 5 West, to clarify a medication order for morphine for your patient, Michael Carrana, in Room 600. The patient says that he has an allergy to morphine and gets low blood pressure and feels faint and nauseated."

In most agencies, the pharmacy provides the unit with a printed daily medication administration record (MAR or EMAR) based on the provider's orders. It often includes additional brief but important information for the nurse who administers the medication.

CLINICAL ALERT!

Consult TJC and your clinical agency's policies pertaining to verbal and telephone orders. There are specific requirements limiting verbal and telephone orders to reduce chances of error. This becomes more important each year as more sound-alike drugs appear on the market.

Answers on page 97

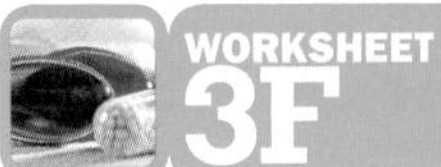

WORKSHEET 3F Identifying Incomplete Medication Orders

Read the physician orders that follow and in a few words state why the order would have to be clarified. Hint: Think of the patient rights list.

1. Cozaar 25 mg daily in AM

2. Aspirin 2 tablets q4h po prn headache

3. Ampicillin 500 mg q6h × 3 days

4. Morphine sulfate 5 mg IV for pain

5. Tylenol 2 teaspoons q6h for fever over 100° F

The 24-Hour Clock

The 24-hour clock is used in most hospitals and governmental and military agencies. It is computer compatible. It runs sequentially from 0001 h (1 minute after midnight) to 2400 h (midnight). Each hour is written in increments of 100: 1200, 1300, 1400, etc. No number is repeated. Use of the 12-hour clock can cause errors because the same number is used twice: once for AM once for PM hours. With an order such as "Give the medicine at 9 o'clock," it is unclear whether 9 AM or 9 PM is intended. Also 12 AM and 12 PM are often misinterpreted.

- Four digits indicate the hours and minutes of the 24-hour clock: 1530 h, 0200 h, etc.
- The 24-hour clock is reset at midnight (2400 h) to 0000 h.
- The AM hours begin at 0001 h (1 minute after midnight) and end at 1159 h (11:59 AM).
- The PM hours begin at 1200 h and end at 2359 h (11:59 PM).
- When saying 24-hour time, say "twelve hundred (hours)" for 1200 h. Do not say "one thousand, two hundred."

Focus on the PM hours to distinguish the major differences between the two clocks (Figure 3.9).

AM HOURS		PM HOURS	
12-hour clock AM hours	24-hour clock AM hours	12-hour clock PM hours	24-hour clock PM hours
12 AM 12 Midnight	2400 hours Midnight Reset to 0000 hours*	12 PM Noon	1200 hours Noon
1 AM	0100	1 PM	1300 hours
2 AM	0200	2 PM	1400
3 AM	0300	3 PM	1500
4 AM	0400	4 PM	1600
5 AM	0500	5 PM	1700
6 AM	0600	6 PM	1800
7 AM	0700	7 PM	1900
8 AM	0800	8 PM	2000
9 AM	0900	9 PM	2100
10 AM	1000	10 PM	2200
11 AM	1100	11 PM	2300
11:59 AM	1159h	11:59 PM	2359h

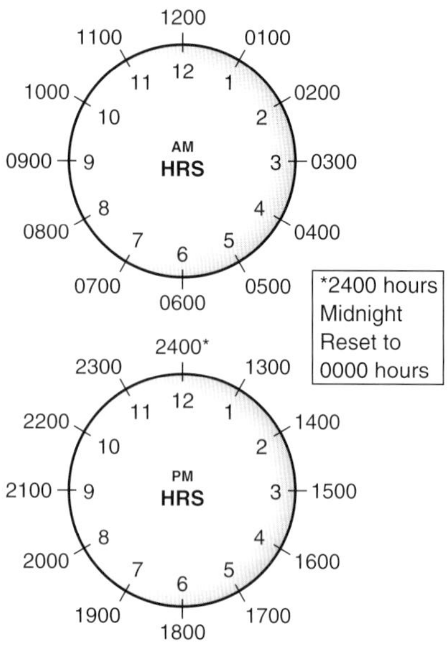

AM HRS: 12 – 1200; 1 – 0100; 2 – 0200; 3 – 0300; 4 – 0400; 5 – 0500; 6 – 0600; 7 – 0700; 8 – 0800; 9 – 0900; 10 – 1000; 11 – 1100

PM HRS: 12 – 2400*; 1 – 1300; 2 – 1400; 3 – 1500; 4 – 1600; 5 – 1700; 6 – 1800; 7 – 1900; 8 – 2000; 9 – 2100; 10 – 2200; 11 – 2300

*2400 hours Midnight Reset to 0000 hours

FIGURE 3.9 Comparison of 12- and 24-hour clock.

For faster learning, memorize these 24-hour clock times: noon (1200 h), midnight (2400 h reset to 0000 h), 1 minute after midnight (0001 h) and 1 PM (1300 h).

Examples 1159 = 1 minute before noon 2359 = 1 minute before midnight
1201 = 1 minute after noon 0001 = 1 minute after midnight

It is very helpful to study some key times in your daily schedule. Fill in the space provided in 24-hour clock time.

Your usual breakfast hour: ____________

The time your shift begins: ____________

The time your shift ends: ____________

Your usual dinner hour: ____________

Your usual bedtime hour: ____________

Noon (12 PM) ____________

Midnight (12 AM) ____________

Answers on page 97

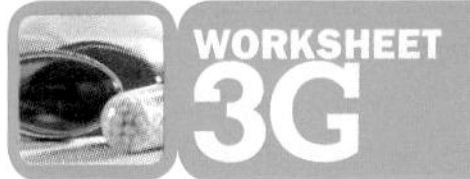

WORKSHEET 3G Converting AM/PM and 24-Hour Clock Time

Fill in the requested time in the space provided.

AM/PM Clock	24-Hour Clock (h)	24-Hour Clock (h)	AM/PM Clock
10:30 AM		1200 h	
10:30 PM		2400 h	
1:15 AM		1145 h	
1:15 PM		2345 h	
12:05 AM		0630 h	
12:05 PM		1830 h	
4:20 AM		0006 h	
7:55 AM		0910 h	
1:20 PM		0325 h	
8:40 PM		1905 h	

Understanding Medication Administration Records (MARs)

Every nursing institution has its own MAR or electronic (EMAR) forms. Similar in content but different in style, all contain the date, patient name, sex, date of birth, admission date, ID number, room number, allergies, and the name and/or signature of the primary physician. The nurse needs to be oriented to the forms of each clinical agency (Figures 3.10 and 3.11).

All MAR headings include the time span the page covers, such as one shift, three shifts, and/or 1 week or month for long-term facilities. The orders include the date of each order, dosage, route, frequency, time for administration, and the prescriber's name. MARs have codes for data entry. The nurse's entry includes the date and time each medication was administered, in addition to the accompanying code or full signature of the nurse administering the medication.

EMARs provide some additional instructions from the order or from the pharmacy, such as "Hold and report if pulse under 50," "Do not give with grapefruit juice," or "Give with at least 120 mL of water."

During orientation, a nurse who is a new employee must identify hospital policies that are not stated on the form. These policies include, for example, how to record withholding of a medication, how to handle a medication error, and how to correct an incorrect entry.

Problems noted and medication-related assessments need to be recorded on the patient record.

CLINICAL RELEVANCE

Medications are to be recorded as soon as possible after administration to avoid the event of another nurse also giving the medication.

CLINICAL ALERT!

The MAR is a confidential, legal document. It is illegal to erase, backdate, obscure, or make false entries in an MAR, or to photocopy any medical record without authorization.

Brown, John	ALLERGIES: DRUGS: *IV iodine, Aspirin*
ID# 45764304	FOODS: Denies
DOB: 01-10-50 Sex: M Rm: 406A	
Dr. Marin, Cruz	RN Verification: *Florence Dane, RN*

MAR Date: 05-07-18 0700 - 05-08-18 0659

MEDICATION: Dose Route Freq — Time of Administration, Site, and Initials

	START	STOP	0700 TO 1459	1500 TO 2259	2300 TO 0659
SCH	05-05-18 Digoxin 0.125 mg po Q AM	05-12-18	(0900) *JM* R		
SCH	05-05-18 Tylenol (acetaminophen) 500 mg po BID	05-12-18	0800 *JM*	2000	
SCH	05-05-18 Clotrimazole 1% CR TOP bid to affected area	05-12-18	0900 *JM* L	2100	

This is a pharmacy-generated MAR for a 24-hr period stated in 24-hour time beginning with the day shift, 5-7-18. The RN who signs the verification is verifying that the medication orders accurately match the provider orders and that the allergies have been noted. SCH means a regularly scheduled medication versus a PRN order. You must use the agency *code* for administration sites. A circled time denotes med NOT given. Additional documentation may need to be added elsewhere in the nurse's record. PRN meds and one-time-only meds have *separate* placeholders. You may add new orders by writing them in (refer to promethazine). This pharmacy prints instructions for diluting intravenous medications. The narcotic (morphine sulfate) has an automatic 48-hr limit and then must have a written renewal order. This hospital policy calls for a yellow highlight to denote discontinued/expired orders. All discontinued orders, automatic or other, must be renewed if it is necessary to continue them. On the SITE CODES, note that if a medication is withheld other than for NPO or surgery, the reason must be documented on the patient record, e.g.: "Alert and oriented; refused acetominophen and states it 'doesn't do anything for him.' Dr. Marin notified."

ONE TIME ONLY AND PRN MEDS

Start	Stop	Time	Initials	Full Name/Title
05-07-18 Morphine sulfate PRN 25 mg IV q6h PRN Dilute in 5 mL NS and give over 5 min	05-09-18 0700	*2300* C	*FD*	*Florence Dane, RN*
05-07-18 promethazine 25 mg IM STAT	*5/7/18*	*1900 J*	*TR*	*Tom Robbins, RN*

Sign: *Joe Mack* Initials: *JM* Sign: *Tom Robbins* Initials: *TR* Sign: *Florence Dane* Initials: *FD*

SITE CODES — **GENERAL HOSPITAL**

A	Abdomen (L)	J	Gluteus (LUQ)
B	Abdomen (R)	K	Gluteus (RUQ)
C	Arm (L)	L	Thigh (L)
D	Arm (R)	M	Thigh (R)
E	Eyes (both)	N	Ventrogluteal (L)
F	Eyes (left)	O	Ventrogluteal (R)
G	Eyes (right)	P	NPO: Lab
H	Deltoid (mid L)	Q	NPO: Surgery
I	Deltoid (mid R)	R	Withheld/See nurse's notes

FIGURE 3.10 Sample medication administration record.

CLINICAL ALERT!

Verify pharmacy data on this sheet, including dilution instructions. Remember this form is not a *copy* of the original orders. These data have been recopied into the computer.

Acct:		MR#:		M A R	MEDICATION AMINISTRATION RECORD
Admitted:	10/05/18 1630	DOB:	05-10-60 Sex: F		
Att Phys:		HT:	5'7.0" / 170.2 cm		
Diagnosis:	Gastric ulcer	WT:	224 lbs / 101.606 kg		
Allergies:	Morphine/Beta-Adrenergic blocking agts				

Start Date/Time	Stop Date/Time	RN/ LPN	Medication	0731-1530	1531-2330	2331-0730
			** ****************** PRN ****************** **			
10/05/18 2143	10/12/18 2142		Promethazine HCL (Phenergan Equiv) 25 mg = 0.5 mL IV #020 Q6H PRN PRN N/V			
			When administering IV: Must be diluted to a final concentration of 25 mg per mL. IV administration to be at a rate not to exceed 25 mg per minute.			
10/05/18 2100	10/08/18 2059		Zolpidem Tartrate (Ambien) 10 mg = 2 tablet Oral #016 At bedtime PRN for sleep **Narcotic sign-out**			Discontinue
10/05/18 2200	10/11/18 2159		Alum-Mag Hydroxide-Simethicone (Maalox Plus/Mylanta Equiv) 30 mL = 30 mL Oral #022 Q4H PRN nausea, flatulence, upset stomach Stagger one hr from other meds			

This is an example of a computer-generated MAR (cMAR) for PRN orders only. There are many similarities to the MAR in Figure 3.6 and also some differences noted: this MAR states the medication unit dose supplied; the medication nurse must enter the exact time the medication was given. In addition to dilution instructions, scheduling instructions are given with the last medication. The site code is different and the dose omission code is amplified. Even if no medication is given to a patient, the MAR must be signed by the nurse responsible for the patient each shift. Medications which are refused, withheld, or mischarted must be timed and initialed—a standard procedure that may require additional entries on the patient record if the code is not self-explanatory.

Order Date	RN INIT.	Date/Time To Be Given	One Time Orders and Pre-Operatives Medication-Dose-Route	Actual Time Given

Site Codes		
Arm	LA	RA
Deltoid	LD	RD
Ventrogluteal	LVG	RVG
Gluteal	LG	RG
Abdomen	LUQ	RUQ
Abdomen	LLQ	RLQ

Dose Omission Code
A = pt absent
H = hold
M = med absent
N = NPO
O = other
R = refused
U = unable to tolerate

INIT	Signature	INIT	Signature

60321 (8/98)A CHART

FIGURE 3.11 **A,** Example of electronic (EMAR) for PRN orders only. **B,** cMAR. (B, From Kee JL, Marshall SM: *Clinical calculations: with applications to general and specialty areas,* ed 8, St Louis, 2017, Saunders.) *N/V = Nausea/ Vomiting.

FRIDAY 10/12/18 - 0700 thru SATURDAY 10/13/18 - 0659		ST ANNE HOSPITAL MEDICATION ADMINISTRATION RECORD
Meyer, Lois M. WESOF W303-2 Age: 72 Sex: F Primary Dx: CP	Unit#: Admitted: 10/12/18 Ht: 152.40 cm Wt: kg	Acct#: Page: 1 Attending Dr: Thomas Smith, MD Run Date/Time: 10/12/18 - 2237 DOB: 06/23/1944

ALLERGIES:
Drug: PCN. ERYTHROMYCIN. IV DYE
Other: NO ALLERGIES RECORDED
Pharmacy: IODINE (INCLUDES RADIOPAQUE AGENTS W/IODINE). MACROLIDE ANTIBIOTICS, PENICILLINS

Init	IV Flushes: Routine	0700-1459	1500-2259	2300-0659
	Sodium Chloride 0.9% **IV** Flush peripheral IV lines with 5 mls 0.9 NS q 8 hours and central lines per protocol.	Time ______ Init ______ # Flushed______	Time ______ Init ______ # Flushed______	Time ______ Init ______ # Flushed______

Init	SCHED MEDS	DOSE		0700-1459	1500-2259	2300-0659
	DOCUSATE SODIUM (DOCUSATE SODIUM) START: 10/12 D/C: 11/11/18 AT 2244	**100 MG**	PO Q12 RX 002306792			
	PRAVACHOL (PRAVASTATIN SODIUM) Give at: BEDTIME START: 10/12 D/C: 11/11/18 AT 2244	**80 MG**	PO RX 002306793			
	METOPROLOL TARTRATE (METOPROLOL TARTRATE) HOLD FOR SBP<110 OR HR<55 Check apical rate and BP before drug admin. START: 10/12 D/C: 11/11/18 AT 2244	**50 MG**	PO Q12 RX 002306794			
	ACCUPRIL (QUINAPRIL HCL) HOLD FOR SBP<120 START: 10/12 D/C: 11/11/18 AT 2244	**40 MG**	PO Q12 RX 002306795			
	NITROGLYCERIN 2% (NITROGLYCERIN 2%) HOLD FOR SBP<100 START: 10/12 D/C: 11/11/18 AT 2244	**1 INCH**	TP Q6 RX 002306796			0000 0600
	ALPRAZOLAM (ALPRAZOLAM) START: 10/12 D/C: 10/14/18 AT 1601	**0.25 MG**	PO Q8 RX 002306791			0000

Init	PRN MEDS	DOSE		0700-1459	1500-2259	2300-0659
	NITROSTAT 25 TABS/BOTTLE (NITROGLYCERIN) Chest discomfort. May repeat q 5 min x 3. If no relief after 3 doses. Stat ECG & call Physician. START: 10/12 D/C: 11/11/18 at 1833	**0.4 MG**	SL STAT RX 002306718 PRN			

FIGURE 3.11, cont'd **B,** cMAR. (B, From Kee JL, Marshall SM: *Clinical calculations: with applications to general and specialty areas,* ed 8, St Louis, 2017, Saunders.) *N/V = Nausea/Vomiting.

Answers on page 97

WORKSHEET 3H Interpreting the MAR

Using the MAR in Figure 3.10, briefly answer the following questions.

1. Does the patient have a commonly seen surname? If so, why should the medication nurse take special note of this? ____________

2. Does the patient have any medication allergies? If so, which? ____________

3. This MAR indicates how many days of medication administration? ____________

4. Which drug ordered was withheld or not given as scheduled? ____________

5. By what route is Clotrimazole 1% to be administered? ____________

6. Which order has expired? ____________

7. Which drug was given at 11 PM and in which location? ____________

8. At what date and time must the morphine order be discontinued or reordered to continue administration? ____________

9. When is the next time Tylenol may be given according to the 24-hour clock? According to traditional time? ________

10. Why do you think this form requires both the initials and the full signature of the person giving the medications? ________

Medication Delivery

Hospital pharmacies stock and resupply computerized medication carts as needed. Computerized carts with bar code scanners are thought to reduce medication errors related to patient identification and wrong medication by matching the codes on the patient wristband and the medication with the electronic medical record. Provision of unit-dose (single-serving) medications reduces errors of medication selection and calculation errors. Although certain types of errors have been reduced, no system is foolproof. There are many steps in the process, starting with the medication order and ending with the administration of the medication (Figures 3.12 to 3.15).

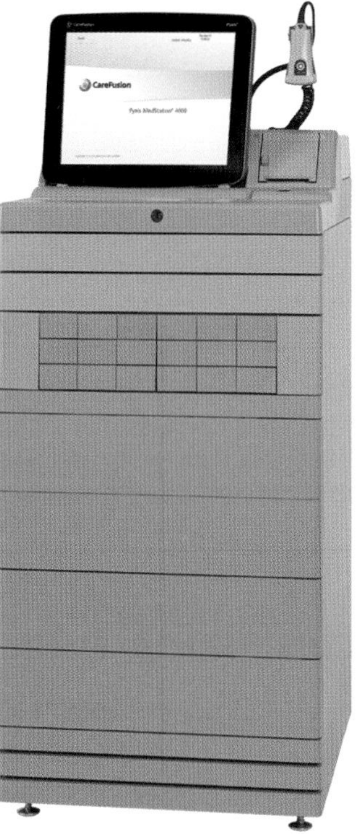

FIGURE 3.12 Computer-controlled medication ordering and dispensing system cart stocked with unit-dose (single-serving) packages supplied by the pharmacy daily, based on prescriber orders. The nurse accesses the cart using a code, a password, and/or a fingerprint, then selects the patient's name, the medication profile, and the drugs that are due to be administered. (Used with permission from Cardinal Health, San Diego, Calif.)

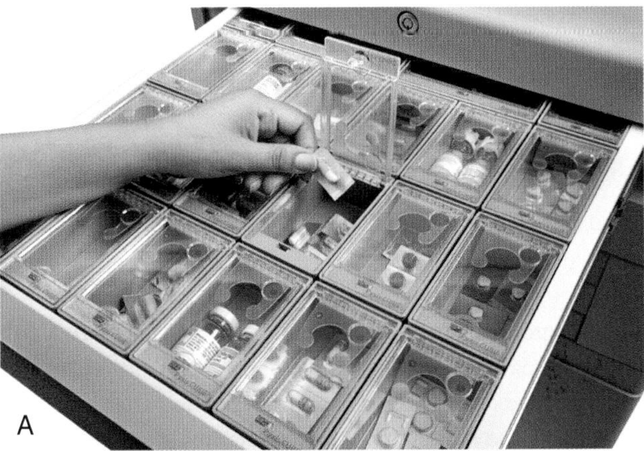

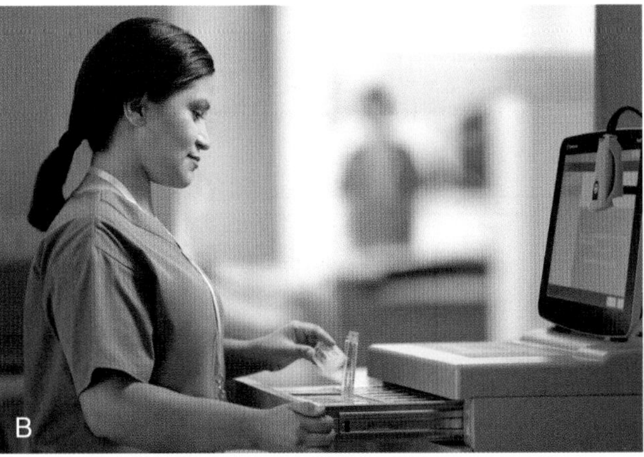

FIGURE 3.13 **A,** The nurse removes the selected medications for the specific time period. **B,** The nurse scans the bar code on each one for drug name and dose to match with the order on the computer. If there is a mismatch, the computer will issue an alert. (Used with permission from Cardinal Health, San Diego, Calif.)

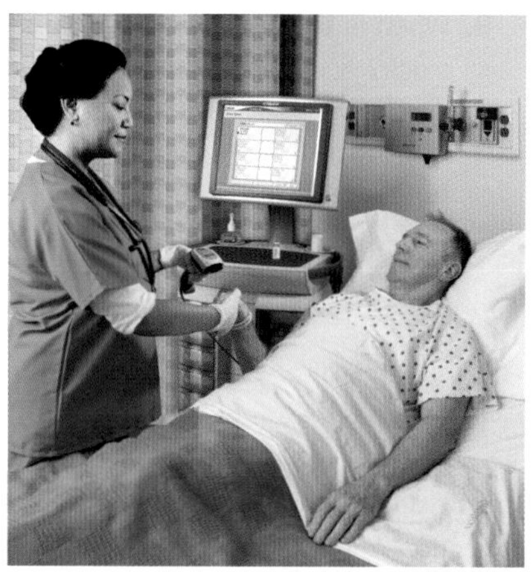

FIGURE 3.14 A nurse using the Omnicell Savvy Mobile Medication System at the patient's bedside. (From Omnicell, Inc., Mountain View, Calif.)

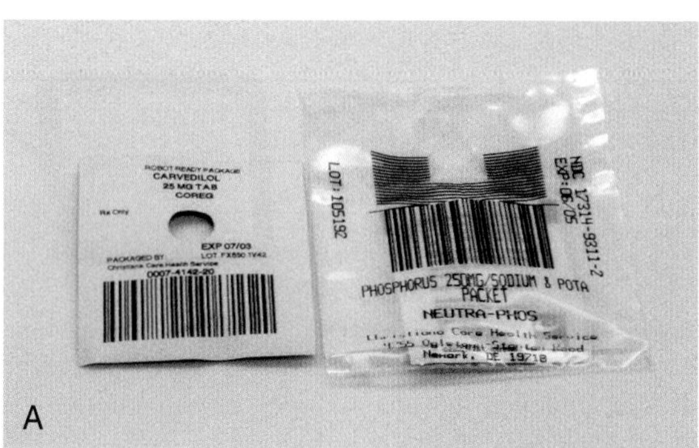

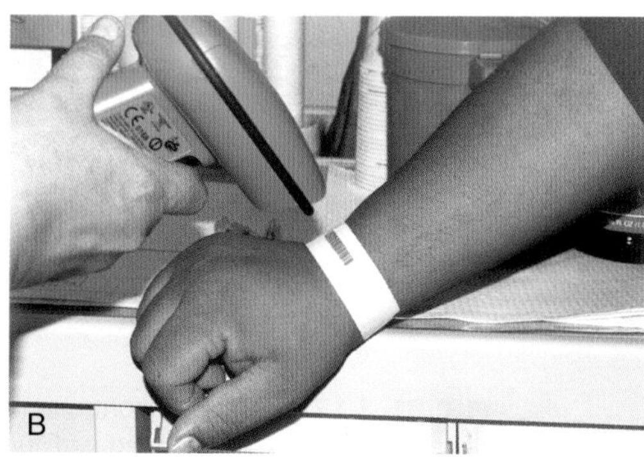

FIGURE 3.15 At the bedside, the nurse will use two permitted patient identifiers, one of which will be to scan the medication and the patient's wristband for right drug, right patient via the computer for agencies that provide this equipment. The nurse will also check the label against the complete order three times before administering the drug. (From Kee JL, Marshall SM: *Clinical calculations: With applications to general and specialty areas,* ed. 8, St. Louis, 2017, Saunders.)

Prioritizing Administration of Several Medications

Clinical experience and familiarity with guidelines are necessary when a nurse has several medications that are ordered to be given during the same time frame (e.g., pain medications, insulin, vitamins, and antibiotics). All of the drugs cannot be given at the same time to more than one patient.

Many priorities are obvious, such as medications for acute pain or medications that need to be given a certain time before or after a meal, stat medications, or preoperative medications. Others are not so obvious.

Note: It is important to take a few minutes to review the ISMP website guidelines that follow before moving on to the next chapter, and to review the guidelines periodically thereafter (http://www.ismp.org/tools/guidelines/acutecare/tasm.pdf).

CLINICAL ALERT!

Always ask for assistance if the priorities are unclear or the workload is too heavy for timely safe medication administration.

Medication incident reports are a confidential report of a medication-related incident (Figure 3.16). They are used to analyze errors, to determine error patterns and methods of error prevention, and to assess liability. They are considered to be administrative records and are not part of the patient medical record. After taking care of any immediate needs of the patient, the supervisor should be notified as well as the patient's physician. Agencies have guidelines about specific and prompt documentation for the patient medical record. Following that, the incident report is to be filled out on the same shift by the nurse *who encounters* the incident and given to the supervisor for signatures. The reports are factual

SAMPLE MEDICATION INCIDENT REPORT

Patient name: ____________________ Date of incident: __________
Time of incident: __________

Where incident occurred: Hospital: __________ Unit: __________

Admitting diagnosis: ____________________

Type of incident:

Check all that apply:

_____ Wrong drug
_____ Wrong time
_____ Wrong dose
_____ Wrong patient
_____ Wrong route
_____ Other

Medication order: ____________________

Account of incident and intervention(s) taken: ____________________

Was the physician notified? _____ Time: _____

All persons familiar with incident or involved: ____________________

Provider signature Date Supervisor signature Date

Incident reports are used to analyze errors and determine error patterns and methods of error prevention. They also assist agency insurers in assessing risk for liability for incidents. Each agency has its own forms and protocols for incidents.

FIGURE 3.16 Example of a medication incident report.

and are not supposed to be self-incriminating nor to contain causes, excuses, blame, or conjecture about prevention. *All* follow-up assessments and related actions must be recorded on the patient medication record.

CLINICAL ALERT!

During orientation to a clinical facility, be sure to check agency written policies and procedures, including what may or may not be entered into the patient medical record. Also follow the policy regarding who notifies the patient and/or the patient's family, if necessary of the error.

Medication Reconciliation (National Patient Safety Goal #3)

Measures to reduce the high rate of medication errors upon transfers, admission, and discharges are known as "Medication Reconciliation." The Joint Commission requires that all agencies that administer medications, including long-term care and home health care, provide evidence of Medication Reconciliation. The procedure includes checking allergies and all the medications the patient is taking from all providers, as well as over-the-counter (OTC) medications or herbal preparations the patient takes at home. The nurse plays a major role in this review, as do the patient, family, pharmacy, and prescribers. Check your agency's policies, forms, and computerized medical data bank, if available. Frequent updates are required if a patient leaves and returns to the unit for treatment, surgery, or other procedures.

CLINICAL ALERT!

Failure to perform Medication Reconciliation on admission, transfer, and discharge can result in serious ADE, such as double dosing and other types of wrong doses, missed drugs, incompatible medication reactions with prescription and OTC medications, as well as drugs that have been discontinued but are still being given, to name a few. Agencies have developed their own Medication Reconciliation forms and procedures to meet this challenge. Look for this procedure when you are oriented to each clinical agency. Refer to Appendix D for an example of a thorough hand-off report.

Summary of Safe Medication Practices

Interpretation

- Know the approved and prohibited abbreviations.
- Call the prescriber to clarify unclear orders. Do not guess.
- Be aware of the patient's allergies when reading medication orders.
- Phone orders are only for emergency medication orders and critical laboratory tests. Write the phone order on the record and read it back to the prescriber. Repeat numbers and doses by numeral; for example, for 30 mg say, "Three, zero, milligrams."

CLINICAL ALERT!

Beware of confusing similar-sounding drugs, such as Xanax (for anxiety) and Zantac (for gastric reflux and ulcers), Klonopin (for seizures) and Clonidine (for hypertension), and so on. There are many such examples.

Preparation

1. Clean and clear the area. Focus on the task. Avoid distractions. Do not leave a current medication preparation unfinished.
2. Recheck the patient's allergies cited on the record. Reconfirm when the medication was last given.
3. If the patient has transferred from another area or is a postoperative patient, check receiving information such as operating room, emergency department, recovery room, and nursing home transfer records to compare medication orders with those that were given, and which medications

were given and the time they were given so that the patient does not receive a double dose, skip a needed medication, or experience an interaction with new orders. (Look for a "Medication Reconciliation" form.)

4. Assess recent laboratory results for abnormal findings that may need attention.
5. Read label and package inserts, and match the label very carefully to the order. If a medication is liquid, check for dilution instructions.
6. Discard improperly labeled medication according to hospital policy.

If the dose will exceed 1 or 2 capsules or tablets, or 1 to 2 mL injectable, or more than two doses of the drug concentration supplied on the label, recheck the original order and a current pharmacology reference. Give the medication if the dose is appropriate. If there is doubt, contact your instructor, the pharmacy, or the prescriber.

Note: Oral liquid dose concentrations on the label often may exceed 1 to 2 mL, but again, the label concentration (e.g., 250 mg per 5 mL) is a guide to the "usual adult dose" ordered and is used for the calculations for "have on hand."

Check for sediment and the presence of discoloration in liquids and for intact seals on controlled substances. Discard according to agency procedures.

With single-dose medications, retain the container at least until the medication has been administered.

CLINICAL ALERT!

The drug order, dose, and label must be checked *three times* before administering the drug to the patient.

CLINICAL ALERT!

Fatal errors have occurred when a nurse miscalculated a dose and gave multiple ampules or multiple pills of a medication instead of looking up safe dose ranges (SDR) and questioning doses that exceed the single-dose amount supplied. Remember also that usual doses for adults are very different from usual doses for children, those who are very ill, or for adults who are above and below average weight.

CLINICAL ALERT!

If the clinical agency policy calls for a second independent nurse check for certain drugs, it is done *before* administering the drug to the patient. An independent check by a second nurse means "look for mistakes" (patient, drug, dose, route, time), and this is achieved by going through all the steps (except preparation) separately from the first nurse. In many cases, the preparation—for example, dilutions and mixes of high-alert drugs—may need to be observed after the order and calculations are verified.

Calculations

Learn to do your dose calculations accurately. Estimate an answer before calculating the dose; this helps to avoid major math errors. Have a reliable current pharmacology drug reference on hand to verify safe dose ranges; usual doses for the age, weight, and condition of your patients; required dilutions; recommended frequency of administration; and administration timing techniques. Call the pharmacy if there are questions.

Administration

The Joint Commission requires that two patient identifiers, such as name, hospital identification number, or birth date, always be used to check with medication records. Room or bed numbers are not valid patient identifiers. Wristbands, if used, must be on the patient, not on a table or taped to a bed. Special precautions for children, such as verification with a parent or other nurse, must be used.

CLINICAL ALERT!

Avoid asking, "Are you Mister or Ms. X?" A patient who is confused or hard of hearing or a child may mistakenly answer "Yes." Instead, ask the patient to state his or her name.

Answers on page 98

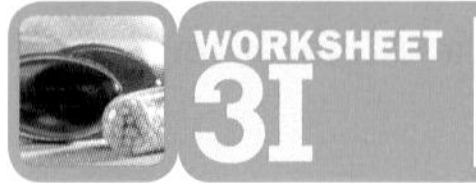

WORKSHEET 3I Multiple-Choice Practice

1. When administering a medication at the bedside, which should be the *first* priority?
   a. Make appropriate assessments.
   b. Identify the patient.
   c. Document the administration of the medication.
   d. Recheck the medication label.

2. If a medication-related problem is identified, which should be the *first* measure the nurse takes?
   a. Assess the patient for side effects.
   b. Notify the supervisor.
   c. Call the physician.
   d. Document the problem in detail on an incident report.

3. Which is the *drug concentration* for the medication shown below?
   a. 50 mg per 5 mL
   b. 1 pint
   c. 473 mL
   d. 200 mg

Vibramycin®
SYRUP Calcium
doxycycline calcium
oral suspension
50 mg / 5 ml†
1 PINT (473 ml)
†Each teaspoonful (5 ml) contains doxycycline calcium equivalent to 50 mg of doxycycline.
USUAL DOSAGE:
Adults: 200 mg on the first day (100 mg every 12 hours) followed by a maintenance dose of 100 mg a day.
Children above eight years of age: Under 100 lbs.—2 mg/lb. of body weight daily divided in two doses on the first day, followed by 1 mg/lb. of body weight on subsequent days in one or two doses. Over 100 lbs.—See adult dosage.
doxycycline U.S. Pat. No. 3,200,149
READ ACCOMPANYING PROFESSIONAL INFORMATION
RECOMMENDED STORAGE
STORE BELOW 86° F. (30° C.)
Dispense in tight, light resistant containers (USP).
CAUTION: Federal law prohibits dispensing without prescription.
Pfizer LABORATORIES DIVISION
PFIZER INC.,
NEW YORK, N.Y. 10017
MADE IN U.S.A. 2

Pfizer
NDC 0069-0971-93
6188
Vibramycin®
SYRUP Calcium
doxycycline calcium
oral suspension
50 mg/5ml†
1 PINT
(473 ml)
RASPBERRY/APPLE FLAVORED
For oral use only
SHAKE WELL BEFORE USING
IMPORTANT:
This closure is not child-resistant.

4. If a handwritten medication order is illegible or unclear, which would be the best nursing decision?
   a. Check with pharmacy.
   b. Rewrite the order to make it more legible.
   c. Give the usual unit dose and clarify.
   d. Clarify with the physician who wrote it.

5. The nurse gives a medication at 1 PM. The correct equivalent international or military time on the 24-hour clock would be:
   a. 1000
   b. 1300
   c. 1500
   d. 0100

6. Which of the following statements regarding medications is *true?*
   a. Each nurse must be able to perform accurate simple and complex medication calculations.
   b. The unit dose and the total dose in a vial are one and the same.
   c. It is wise to rely on experienced colleagues to calculate drug doses.
   d. Medication errors rarely occur in the hospital setting.

7. The Joint Commission's "Do Not Use" list (p. 61) of abbreviations specifically applies to which documents?
   a. Patient-provided history and medication records brought from home
   b. Laboratory results including x-rays and blood work
   c. All forms in a patient's record that are handwritten
   d. All orders and medication-related documentation that are handwritten or on preprinted forms or free-text computer entry

8. A tablet is ordered for a patient with a nasogastric feeding tube who is NPO. Which is the most appropriate action for the nurse to take?
   a. Crush the tablet, dilute with water, and administer via the tube.
   b. Consult with the charge nurse about the medication routine for NPO patients.
   c. Ask the patient if there have been any problems with swallowing the pill, and then give it by mouth.
   d. Clarify the route with the physician who wrote the order.

9. A physician ordered ceftazidime 1g to be given IM at 0800, 1400, and 2400 hours for a patient with an infection. The nurse administered 1 gram of cefepime IM at 0800 hours. Which patient right was violated?
   a. Right drug
   b. Right dose
   c. Right route
   d. Right time

10. An order for morphine sulfate 10 mg IM q4h prn for pain expired after 48 hours, during the previous shift. The patient continues to complain of postoperative pain and requests another pain injection. Which action is an *inappropriate* nursing action?
   a. Attempt alternative measures for pain relief such as repositioning and other comfort measures.
   b. Administer the medication because the patient has had no untoward side effects as the result of any of the prior doses.
   c. Assess the patient for unexplained sources of continued pain.
   d. Explain that the medication order has expired but that you will call for a renewed order.

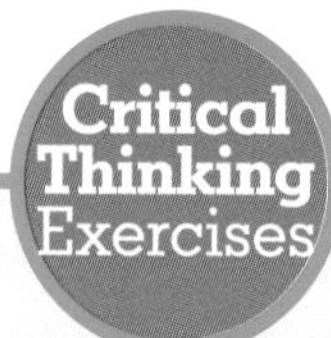

Critical Thinking Exercises provide math and medication-related patient safety issues for student discussion. Answers are not provided.

Analyze the following examples of medication errors with your peers and/or instructor and discuss the issues suggested in the left-side guidelines, using this chapter and pharmacology references. As you study the error, consider which patient rights on pages 58 to 60 have been violated. What suggestions might you have for procedural changes at the hospital to prevent this from happening again? Include those that might involve pharmacy staff, providers, nurses, and patients.

Example

1. Ordered: Tylenol #2, stat

Supplied: Tylenol in patient medication drawer and Tylenol #2 (in locked cabinet)

Given: Two Tylenol tablets

Error(s): The wrong medication was given. Two tablets of plain Tylenol were given instead of one tablet of Tylenol #2, which contains a narcotic. (If an incident report must be filed, this is the way the incident should be described in the space provided for a description of the incident.)

Potential injuries: Lack of comfort and its physiologic and emotional effects; lack of security; need for an alternative medication.

Nursing actions: Report to supervisor and provider.

Obtain orders to give additional pain medication.

Document on medical record and file incident report per hospital policy.

Assess patient periodically for side effects, and document the results.

Preventive measures: Familiarize oneself with the medications ordered and commonly used in the unit, as well as with all controlled medications supplied, including those used in emergencies.

If this common medication was known to the giver, and a lack of attention or focus was a contributing cause, techniques to avoid distractions must be addressed. If this medication was not known to the giver, a pharmacology review of commonly used medications is in order. Nurses should always look up unfamiliar medications in current pharmacology references or check with the pharmacy before administering them. Nursing students should check with an instructor or supervisor after the reference check if they are unfamiliar with a medication. It is also wise to inform the patient at the bedside exactly which medications are to be given, because the patient may question the order. An informed patient presents the last line of defense in error prevention.

2. Ordered: Aspirin 650 mg PO, two tablets at bedtime

Supplied: Aspirin 325 mg per tablet

Given: Aspirin 1300 mg by a nurse the first night; Aspirin 650 mg by another nurse the second night.

Error(s):

Potential injuries:

Nursing actions:

Preventive measures:

3. **Ordered:** Narcotic for pain q3h prn, last noted on record as given by recovery room nurse at 1445 hours

   Given: Narcotic for pain at 1545 hours by nurse who had just started evening shift and admitted patient to unit

   Error(s):

   Potential injuries:

   Nursing actions:

   Preventive measures:

4. **Ordered:** Prednisone 60 mg daily

   Given: Prednisolone 60 mg daily

   Error(s):

   Potential injuries:

   Nursing actions:

   Preventive measures:

5. **Ordered:** Percocet

   Given: 8/11 Percodan. Recorded on the medical record; patient allergic to aspirin

   Error(s):

   Potential injuries:

   Nursing actions:

   Preventive measures:

CHAPTER

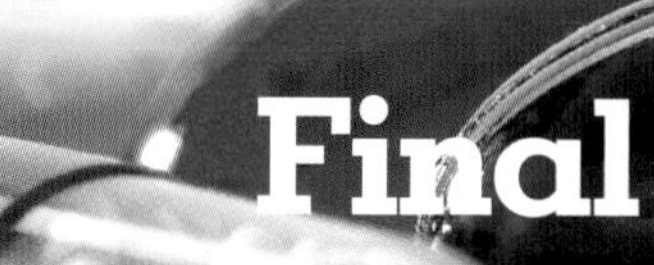

Final

1. List the patient rights stated in the text.
   a. ______
   b. ______
   c. ______
   d. ______
   e. ______
   f. ______
   g. ______
   h. ______
   i. ______
   j. ______

2. Fill in the recommended term or abbreviation in the space provided.

Term/Abbreviation	Meaning	Term/Abbreviation	Meaning
$\bar{c}$		$\bar{s}$	
po		npo	
IV		IM	
supp		bid	
tid		q6h	
prn		ad lib	
ac		pc	
subcut		ID	
SL		NG	
stat		top	

3. Write the approved abbreviation in the space provided.

Term	Abbreviation
milligram	
microgram	
gram	
kilogram	
liter	
milliliter	

4. State the comparable times in the space provided.

Traditional Time	24-Hour Clock	24-Hour Clock	Traditional Time
12 Noon (12 PM)		2100 hours	
Midnight (12 AM)		1400 hours	
1 PM		0145 hours	
9 AM		0030 hours	
5 PM		1645 hours	

5. Study the label and supply the requested information.

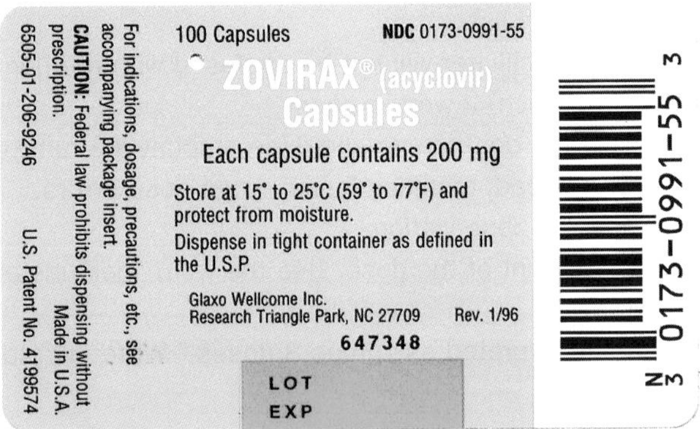

a. Generic name ______________________

b. Drug form ______________________

c. Dose per capsule ______________________

d. Single-dose or multidose container (circle one)

6. How can decimal points lead to errors in medication orders?

7. How would you write out this order: Aspirin tab 325 mg po q4h prn headache?

8. What is the purpose of The Joint Commission's "Do Not Use" list?

9. What should the nurse do if an order is unclear?

10. State nine pieces of information that the medication label may contain:

a. ______________________

b. ______________________

c. ______________________

d. ______________________

e. ______________________

f. ______________________

g. ______________________

h. ______________________

i. ______________________

Answer Key

3 Safe Medication Administration

WORKSHEET 3A (page 64)

1. Mistaken for "0," "4," or "cc"
2. Periods and O's can be mistaken for "I" (the letter I or the number 1). Do not write Q.D. or Q.I.D. Write out the abbreviations.
3. A decimal point can be missed, which may result in overdoses.
4. All medication-related documents that are handwritten, entered on a computer, and filled in on preprinted forms must abide by The Joint Commission's "Do Not Use" list.
5. The preferred abbreviation is mL. The capital L for milliliter will not be confused with the number 1 as with ml, and cc can be confused with U (units) and aa (of each) if written poorly.
6. The letter "l" can be mistaken for a number 1 if the dose name and dose amount are run together.
7. Large numbers without commas can be easily misread, resulting in very large dose errors.
8. 10 mg, with a space between the numbers and the abbreviation.
9. Slashes have been mistaken as the number 1 in front of the dose. Use the word "per" instead of the slash to avoid misinterpretation.
10. x3d meant to mean times 3 days has been misinterpreted as "times 3 doses." Write out "for 3 days."

WORKSHEET 3B (page 67)

Term	Recommended Abbreviation
capsule	cap
tablet	tab
fluid	fld, fl
solution	sol
suspension	susp
elixir	elix
teaspoon	tsp
tablespoon	tbs, Tbsp, T
liquid	liq
ounce	oz
double-strength	DS
extended release	XR
long acting	LA
sustained release	SR
controlled release	CR

WORKSHEET 3C (page 69)

Time	Abbreviation (if Applicable)	Time	Abbreviation (if Applicable)
before	a	after	p
before meals	ac	after meals	pc
daily	Write out daily	three times a day	tid
twice a day	bid	every other day	Write out every other day
every day	Write out every day	every 6 hours	q6h
every 4 hours	q4h	every 12 hours	q12h
whenever necessary	prn	as desired, freely	ad lib (fluids and activities only)
immediately, at once	stat	bedtime	Write out bedtime
with	$\bar{c}$	without	$\bar{s}$
Route	**Abbreviation (if Applicable)**	**Route**	**Abbreviation (if Applicable)**
by mouth	po	nothing by mouth	NPO
intravenous	IV	intramuscular	IM
sublingual	SL, subl	subcutaneous	subcut
intradermal	ID	suppository	supp
left eye	Write out left eye	right ear	Write out right ear
nasogastric	NG	per gastrostomy tube	GT

WORKSHEET 3D (page 70)

Metric Measurement Term	Metric Measurement Abbreviation
microgram(s)	mcg
milligram(s)	mg
gram(s)	g
kilogram(s)	kg
milliliter(s)	mL
milliequivalent(s)	mEq
unit	Write out unit
international unit	Write out international unit
liter	L
square meter	m^2
Other Measurement Term	**Abbreviation**
one half	Write out one half
teaspoon	tsp
tablespoon	tbs, Tbsp, T
pound	lb

WORKSHEET 3E (page 74)

1. **a.** NDC: 0071-0155-30
   b. Lipitor®
   c. atorvastatin calcium
   d. 10 milligrams (mg) per tablet
   e. 10 mg : 1 tablet or $\frac{10 \text{ mg}}{1 \text{ tablet}}$

2. **a.** levothyroxine sodium tablets, USP
   b. 50 mcg (0.050 mg) equivalent
   c. 50 mcg : 1 tablet or $\frac{50 \textit{ mcg}}{1 \textit{ tablet}}$

CLINICAL ALERT!

If you have a choice between an equivalent that is stated in whole numbers (e.g., 50 mcg) or one in decimals (e.g., 0.050 mg), use the whole number equivalent. It will simplify the math.

3. **a.** Liquid oral suspension
   b. 125 milligrams (mg) per 5 milliliters (mL)
   c. Usual dose: 250 mg to 500 mg every 8 hours, depending on type and severity of infection
   d. Multidose container. Contains 150 mL* in small print
   e. 150 mL is 30 times more than 5 mL
   f. 125 mg : 5 mL or $\frac{125 \text{ mg}}{5 \text{ mL}}$

4. **a.** Septra® DS
   b. Trimethoprim, 160 mg, and sulfamethoxazole, 800 mg.†
   c. Scored tablet, meaning it can be cut in half (only with a pillcutter) if half dose is ordered)
   Note: A half dose would have to be a half dose of each of the drugs in this compound.
   d. DS = "double strength"
   e. No calculation needed

5. **a.** Nitroglycerin
   b. Sublingual: administer under the tongue
   c. The nurse needs to know that the patient understands and is able to hold the tablet under the tongue until it dissolves. That enables it to be absorbed more rapidly than if it were swallowed because it bypasses the gastrointestinal tract. This medication is given promptly for chest pain to dilate coronary vessels and increase the blood flow to the heart.
   d. 0.5 mg per tablet 1/100 grain (gr) is an outdated measurement but is retained on the label to accommodate patients who have been taking this medicine for many years.

---

*Note: Check storage directions for multidose containers. Check agency policies regarding labeling before storing.
Metric measurements are not italicized. The liter abbreviation is always a capital "L." Most of the metric abbreviations are not capitalized.
†Note the prefix "sulfa" in the name denotes that drug is in the compound. It is a commonly known allergen. Check your patient for allergy to sulfa drugs before administering.

WORKSHEET 3F (page 77)

1. The route and form are not specified.

2. The dose is not specified. Aspirin is supplied in more than one dose (e.g., 325 mg per tablet, 650 mg per tablet). The number of tablets should *not* be mentioned in the order.

3. The route and form are not specified. Ampicillin can be administered by more than one route (PO, IM, IV).

4. The time or frequency is not specified—for example, stat, one time only, or more than one time.

5. The dose and form are not specified. Tylenol is supplied in tablet, liquid suspension, intravenous, and suppository forms and in a variety of doses targeted to infants, children, and adults. Teaspoons should not be mentioned in the order.

WORKSHEET 3G (page 79)

AM/PM Clock	24-Hour Clock (h)	24-Hour Clock (h)	AM/PM Clock
10:30 AM	1030h	1200 h	12 PM (Noon)
10:30 PM	2230h	2400 h	12 AM (Midnight)
1:15 AM	0115h	1145 h	11:45 AM
1:15 PM	1315h	2345 h	11:45 PM
12:05 AM	0005h	0630 h	6:30 AM
12:05 PM	1205h	1830 h	6:30 PM
4:20 AM	0420h	0006 h	12:06 AM
7:55 AM	0755h	0910 h	9:10 AM
1:20 PM	1320h	0325 h	3:25 AM
8:40 PM	2040h	1905 h	7:05 PM

CLINICAL ALERT!

"Once" means "eleven" in Spanish. The word for one is "uno" in Spanish or "una vez," one time.

WORKSHEET 3H (page 82)

1. Yes. Care must be taken in distinguishing this patient from other patients with the same or a similar name to avoid giving a medication to the wrong patient.

2. Yes. The patient is allergic to the intravenous iodine used in some contrast media tests and to products that contain aspirin. There are many.

3. One 24-hour day

4. Digoxin was withheld as denoted by a circle and the code "R."

5. Topical

6. Promethazine, a stat order

7. Morphine sulfate; left arm denoted by "C."

8. 05/09/18 at 0700

9. 05/07/18 at 2000; 8 pm

10. Having both the initials and the nurse's signature identifies the nurse who administered the medication more clearly. More than one staff member may have the same initials, or some initials may be illegible.

WORKSHEET 3I (page 88)

1. b. Correct identification of patient is always the first priority. Answers a, c, and d would all be appropriate after the patient is identified.

2. a. Answers b, c, and d would all be appropriate after the patient was assessed.

3. a. Answer b is the total amount of drug in the container. Answer c is the total volume in mL. Answer d is the usual ordered adult dosage on the first day.

4. d. Answers a, b, and c are inappropriate actions.

5. b. Refer to the international/24-hour clock on page 78.

6. a. Answers b, c, and d are false statements.

7. d. Refer to the legend below the TJC "Do Not Use" list on page 61.

8. d. The right route is usually the one that is ordered but not in this case. There is a conflict, and common sense dictates that the nurse must clarify. The patient is NPO, and there must be a written order to be able to give a medication by mouth. Some medications are totally unsuitable for nasogastric tube administration, and some just obstruct the tube. Some orders may specify to crush the tablet, dilute with water, and give via the tube.

9. a. Be very aware that there are many drugs with similar names but different uses.

10. b. Giving a medication after the expiration date, whether automatically established by the agency or written by the physician, is illegal. All other actions are appropriate.

CHAPTER 3 FINAL: SAFE MEDICATION ADMINISTRATION (page 92)

1. **a.** Right patient
   b. Right drug
   c. Right dose
   d. Right time
   e. Right route
   f. Right reason
   g. Right assessment
   h. Right documentation
   i. Right evaluation
   j. Right to refuse

2.

Term/Abbreviation	Meaning	Term/Abbreviation	Meaning
$\bar{c}$	with	$\bar{s}$	without
po, PO	by mouth	NPO	nothing by mouth
IV	intravenous	IM	intramuscular
supp	suppository	bid	twice a day
tid	three times daily	q6h	every 6 hours
prn	whenever necessary	ad lib*	freely, as desired
ac	before meals	pc	after meals
subcut	subcutaneous	ID	intradermal
SL	sublingual	NG	nasogastric
stat	immediately	top	topical

*ad lib is used for fluids and activity but not for medications.

3.

Term	Abbreviation
milligram	mg
microgram	mcg
gram	g
kilogram	kg
liter	L
milliliter	mL

4.

Traditional Time	24-Hour Clock	24-Hour Clock	Traditional Time
12 Noon (12 PM)	1200 hours	2100 hours	9 PM
Midnight (12 AM)	2400 hours	1400 hours	2 PM
1 PM	1300 hours	0145 hours	1:45 AM
9 AM	0900 hours	0030 hours	12:30 AM
5 PM	1700 hours	1645 hours	4:45 PM

5. **a.** Generic name: acyclovir
   b. Drug form: capsule
   c. Dose per capsule: 200 mg
   d. Single-dose or multidose container: multidose

6. Decimals can be missed altogether or mistaken for the number 1.

7. Aspirin tablet 325 milligrams by mouth every 4 hours as needed for headache.

8. The Joint Commission's "Do Not Use" list contains the prohibited abbreviations that have been misinterpreted and led to medication errors.

9. If an order is unclear, it should be clarified with the prescriber.

10. Generic name; proprietary, trade, or brand name; unit dose; form; total amount in container; recommended routes; preparation directions; storage directions; lot number; NDC code; and expiration date.

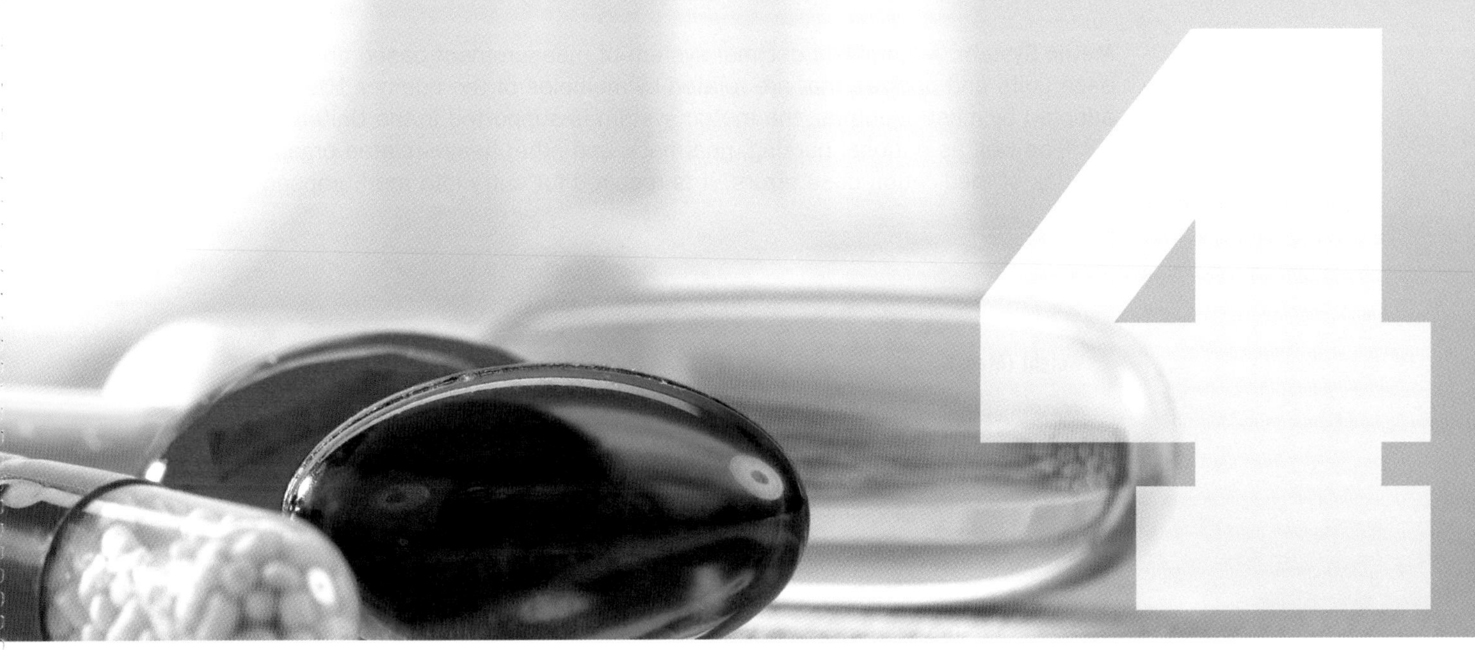

Medication Measurements and Oral Dose Calculations

Objectives

- Combine metric base units and prefixes.
- Use approved metric measurement abbreviations.
- Convert metric and household equivalents.
- Estimate and verify dose calculations.
- Solve dose calculation problems with ratio and proportion equations.
- Identify patient safety measures related to oral medication calculations and administration.
- Identify controlled (scheduled) drugs.
- Use critical thinking to analyze medication errors.

Introduction

This chapter builds on prior knowledge to solve oral medication dose calculation problems using the metric system and its equivalents. The metric system has replaced the English apothecary system and is now required for medication orders and packaging in the United States. An emphasis is placed on estimation, verification, and knowledge of the measurement-related factors needed for safe clinical practice. The focus is on understanding the calculation process and avoiding behaviors that can lead to medication errors. Mastery of this chapter will provide the reader with a thorough foundation for more complex drug dose calculations.

Vocabulary

Base Units of Metric Measurement: Three of the base units commonly used for metric measurements of medications are **gram** (g) for weight (mass), **liter** (L) for volume, and **meter** (m) for length.

Household Measurement Systems: Measuring utensils used in the home, such as teaspoons, are a safety risk for measuring medication doses because various sizes and capacities lead to inaccuracies.

Metric System: A simplified decimal system of measurement based on combinations of base units and prefixes that are related by multiples of the number 10. Modified and adopted by most countries, the metric system is supported in the United States by TJC and ISMP, as well as national nursing, pharmacy, and other health-related organizations to reduce the risk of medication dose errors. It is required for entry into the European Union.

Metric Equivalent Chart

Weight (Mass)

1000 mcg (micrograms) = 1 mg (milligram)

1000 mg = 1 g (gram)

1000 g = 1 kg (kilogram)

lb to kg conversion

2.2 lb (pound) = 1 kg

inch to cm conversion

1 inch = 2.5 cm (approximate)

Volume

1000 mL (milliliter) = 1 L (liter)

Other

1000 milliunits = 1 unit

Length

10 mm (millimeters) = 1 cm (centimeter)

100 cm = 1 m (meter)

1000 mm = 1 m (meter)

Metric Measurements: Base Units

Three base units are commonly used in the medical field. Two are used mainly for medication doses (gram and liter) and one (meter) is used occasionally for topical medications.

Memorize these three base units.

Base Units

Dimension	Metric Base Unit	Approximate English System Equivalent
Weight (or mass)	gram (g)	About 1/3 ounce dry weight
Volume	liter (L)	About 4 measuring cups, a little more than 1 quart
Length	meter (m)	About 39 inches, a little more than 1 yard

The abbreviation for the base unit liter is capitalized (L) to avoid misreading as the number 1. The base unit abbreviations for gram (g) and meter (m) are written in lowercase letters. No other abbreviations are authorized.

Metric Units Number Line

The following Metric Units Number Line illustrates the relationship of the values for selected metric prefixes.

Prefix	Abbreviation	Value
kilo-	k	1000
hecto-*	h	100
deka-*	da	10
		0 (zero)
deci-†	d	0.1
centi-	c	0.01
milli-	m	0.001
micro-	mc	0.000001

*Not seen in medication records.
†Seen in laboratory reports.

Metric Prefixes and Values

Four prefixes are commonly used for medication dose calculations:

- centi- (meaning hundredth)
- milli- (meaning thousandth)
- micro- (meaning millionth)
- kilo- (meaning a thousand times)

Table 4.1 clarifies the relationships of values among the metric measurements most frequently encountered by the nurse on medication labels and orders, laboratory test results, and medication-related literature. It is essential to understand and distinguish them from each other.

Table 4.1 Metric Measurements, Prefixes, Values, and Meanings

Prefix	Multiplier	Exponential Power of 10	Meaning	Examples	Meaning
deci- (d)	0.1	10^{-1}	tenth part of	deciliter (dL)	one tenth of a liter
centi- (c)	0.01	10^{-2}	hundredth part of	centimeter (cm)	one hundredth of a meter
milli- (m)	0.001	10^{-3}	thousandth part of	milliliter (mL)	one thousandth of a liter
				milligram (mg)	one thousandth of a gram
micro- (mc)*	0.000001	10^{-6}	millionth part of	microgram (mcg)	one millionth of a gram
kilo- (k)	1000	10^{3}	1000 times	kilogram (kg)	one thousand grams

Note: The prefix value never changes when combined with a base unit (e.g., the prefix *milli* [m] = 0.001).
1 mm = 0.001 (one thousandth of a meter).
1 mL = 0.001 (one thousandth of a liter).
1 mg = 0.001 (one thousandth of a gram).
*Note that "mc" is the only prefix abbreviation with two letters. This distinguishes it from "m" for milli.

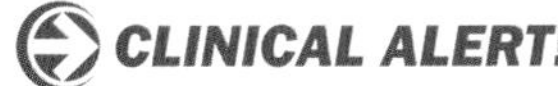

CLINICAL ALERT!

The abbreviation "mc" for the prefix "micro" is preferred over the Greek letter μ (mu). A handwritten μg can be mistaken for mg (milligrams).

Answers on page 137

WORKSHEET 4A Writing Metric Units and Abbreviations

Write the metric name and abbreviation in the space provided.

	Metric Name	Abbreviation
1. Base unit for weight/mass	______________	______________
2. Base unit for volume	______________	______________
3. Base unit for length	______________	______________
4. Prefix that means 1/1000	______________	______________
5. Prefix than means 1/100	______________	______________
6. Prefix that means 1/1,000,000	______________	______________
7. Prefix that means 1/10	______________	______________
8. Prefix that means 1000 times	______________	______________
9. Name for the base unit "m"	______________	
10. Name for the prefix "m"	______________	

Finding Equivalent Measurements Using Ratio and Proportion

There are two types of problems that are encountered in basic medication calculations. A dose can be calculated when the measurement units and values are equivalent.

1. Find an equivalent value when two measurement terms are different.
2. Calculate a dose when the terms are the same.

Metric equivalents: 1000 mcg = 1 mg **1000 mg = 1 g** **1000 g = 1 kg**

Metric Equivalent Calculation Setup

Examples **Ordered:** 1.5 g of an antibiotic. **Supplied:** 500 mg capsules. How many capsules will you give? The measurement terms are *different. They need to be the same in order to calculate the dose.*

Change the ordered 1.5 g to an equivalent amount of (unknown) (x) milligrams on hand.

Equivalent formula selected for the conversion: **1000 mg = 1 g**

Step 1: Place the known formula on the left side of the equation, and what you want to know (x mg) on the right side of the equation.

USING COLONS	**USING FRACTION CROSS PRODUCT**
KNOW WANT TO KNOW	KNOW WANT TO KNOW
1000 mg : 1 g = x mg : 1.5 g	$\frac{1000\text{ mg}}{1\text{ g}} = \frac{x\text{ mg}}{1.5\text{ g}}$

Maintain the ratio sequence: (mg : g = mg : g)

Estimate: The answer will be 1500 because the extremes (1000 × 1.5) are being multiplied by 1.

Step 2: Remove the terms, then solve for x by multiplying.

KNOW WANT TO KNOW

1000 : 1 = x : 1.5

x = 1000 × 1.5
x = 1500 mg

KNOW WANT TO KNOW

$\frac{1000}{1} \times \frac{x}{1.5}$

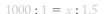

PROOF
1000 × 1.5 = 1500
1 × 1500 = 1500

Step 3: Check your estimate. Label and prove the answer.
Refer to Chapter 2, Ratio and Proportion, if review is needed.

Example 40 mg = ? g (metric equivalent problem)

KNOW WANT TO KNOW

1000 mg : 1 g = 40 mg : x g
(mg : g = mg : g)

$\frac{\cancel{1000}}{\cancel{1000}} x = \frac{4\cancel{0}}{100\cancel{0}}$

x = 0.04 g

KNOW WANT TO KNOW

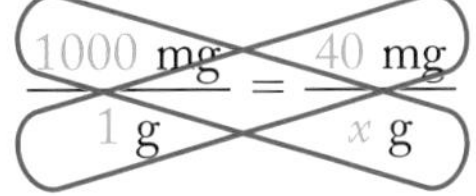

PROOF
1000 × 0.04 = 40
1 × 40 = 40

ANSWER
40 mg = 0.04 g

Answers on page 137

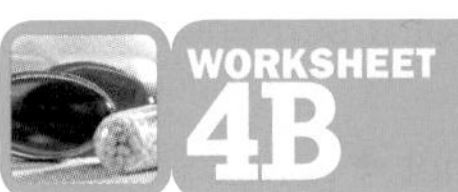

WORKSHEET 4B Metric Equivalents

Use ratio and proportion to find the following metric equivalent terms. Prove and label all answers.

remember

1000 mcg = 1 mg
1000 mg = 1 g
1000 g = 1 kg (2.2 lb)
1000 mL = 1 L (liter)

Change milligrams to grams.

1. 200 mg **2.** 250 mg **3.** 25 mg

Change grams to milligrams.

4. 2.5 g **5.** 0.5 g **6.** 0.01 g

Change micrograms to milligrams.

7. 150 mcg **8.** 500 mcg **9.** 2500 mcg

Change milligrams to micrograms.

10. 5 mg **11.** 0.1 mg **12.** 0.04 mg

Change kilograms to grams.

13. 5.5 kg **14.** 12 kg **15.** 0.5 kg

Change liters to milliliters.

16. 0.5 L **17.** 1.3 L **18.** 2.8 L

Change milliters to liters.

19. 1200 mL **20.** 800 mL

Metric Notation Review

1. Use only the approved abbreviations.*
2. Always abbreviate metric terms when they are accompanied by a number (e.g., the patient drank *2 L* of water).
3. The number comes first; the abbreviation follows.
4. Write out *metric* terms when they are *not* accompanied by a number (e.g., the patient drank a *liter* of water).
5. Leave a space between a number and metric unit (e.g., write *21 mg,* not 21mg; *21 lb,* not 21lb).
6. Capitalize *L* for liter so that it will not be misread as the numeral "1" (e.g., write *4 L,* not 4l or 4 l).
7. Metric terms are not pluralized (e.g., write *50 mL,* not 50 mLs; *5 mg,* not 5 mgs; *2 g,* not 2 gs).
8. There is no period after a metric abbreviation unless it is at the end of a sentence. Periods can be mistaken for the numeral "1."
9. Write out the word "per"; do not use a slash (e.g., write *4 g per kg,* not 4 g/kg).
10. The number 1 is implied, not written when the amount is the number 1 (e.g., write *5 mg per kg,* not *5 mg per 1 kg*).
11. Be aware that *m, u, n, v,* and *w* can look like each other, depending on how they are written.
12. The letter *c* can look like a zero or the letter *a* if the *c* is closed up (e.g., *cm* can look like *am*).

*Refer to TJC "Do-Not-Use" List and ISMP Error-Prone Abbreviations in Chapter 3.

CLINICAL ALERT!

For the sake of patient safety, the nurse must be familiar with all the metric terms, the reason for the medication order, and the safe dosage ranges for the patient's condition and the target population.

CLINICAL ALERT!

Know the 1000 times numerical difference between *mg* and g and between *mcg* and *mg.* Also, know why a patient's condition should or should not receive a smaller or larger dose.

CLINICAL RELEVANCE

Several years ago, a patient was sent for a lab test for hypothyroidism. Thyroid function is tested using a small dose (micrograms [mcg]) of radioactive iodine. Radioactive iodine is also administered in large doses milligrams (mg) to patients with overactive thyroid disease or thyroid cancer. Large doses destroy thyroid cells. The patient to be tested was given a milligram dose in error; family members at home were exposed to the radioactivity after the test, and the patient later died.

Think metric but be prepared to occasionally see unfamiliar terms. Verify questions with the pharmacist or the provider. Never guess. Document the consultation on the medical record.

Finding Metric Equivalents by Moving Decimals

The metric system is a decimal system. When the metric terms in the order and on hand are *different*, another way to verify equivalent measures for *metric* terms is to move decimals. The majority of medications are supplied in grams and milligrams; some are supplied in micrograms.

Moving Decimals for Metric Equivalents

RULE **To convert grams to milligrams, multiply by 1000.**

Examples

5 g = 5.000. mg = 5000 mg (1 g : 1000 mg = 5 g : x mg)

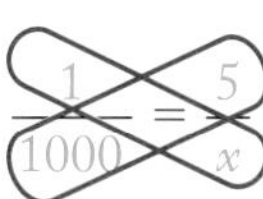

0.2 g = 0.200. mg = 200 mg

0.04 g = 0.040. mg = 40 mg

RULE **To convert milligrams to grams, divide by 1000.**

Examples

250 mg = 0.250. g = 0.25 g (1000 mg : 1 g = 250 mg : x g)

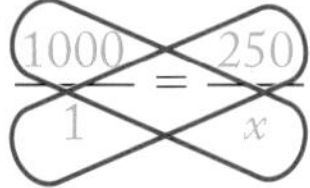

20 mg = 0.020. g = 0.02 g

5 mg = 0.005. g = 0.005 g

RULE **To convert milligrams to micrograms, multiply by 1000.**

Examples

5 mg = 5.000. mcg = 5000 mcg (1 mg : 1000 mcg = 5 mg : x mcg)

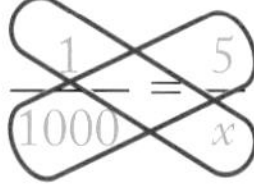

0.8 mg = 0.800. mcg = 800 mcg

0.05 mg = 0.050. mcg = 50 mcg

RULE **To convert micrograms to milligrams, divide by 1000. Figure 4.1 illustrates the decimal movement.**

Examples

2500 mcg = 2.500. mg = 2.5 mg

400 mcg = 0.400. mg = 0.4 mg

10 mcg = 0.010. mg = 0.01 mg

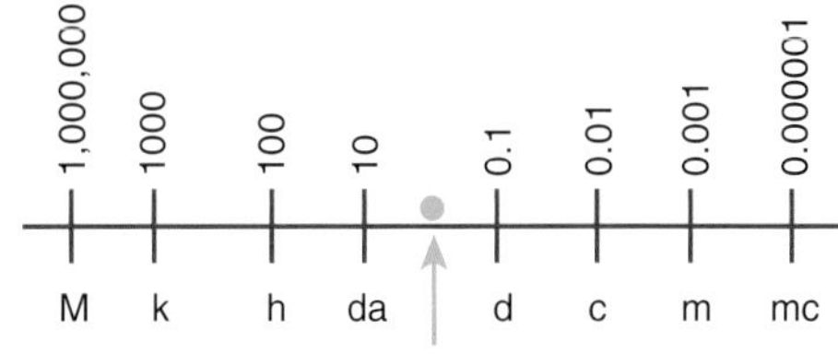

FIGURE 4.1 Metric units number line.

Answers on page 139

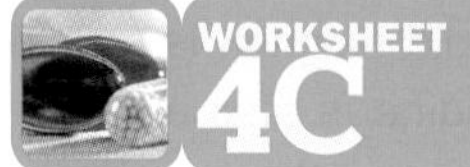

WORKSHEET 4C Metric Equivalents Practice: Micrograms, Milligrams, and Grams

Fill in the metric equivalents in the space provided.

Grams to Milligrams		Milligrams to Grams	
g	**? mg**	**mg**	**? g**
2		5000	
2.5		3500	
1.5		1200	
0.1		800	
0.5		400	
0.25		350	
0.15		200	
0.03		125	
0.015		80	
0.075		50	

Micrograms to Milligrams		Milligrams to Micrograms	
mcg	**? mg**	**mg**	**? mcg**
7500		1.5	
1200		0.8	
750		0.3	
500		0.25	
100		0.125	

- Division and multiplication by 1000 moves the decimal point three places to the left or the right.
- Always place zero in front of a decimal that is unaccompanied by a whole number.
- Do not let a decimal look like the number "1."
- Do not add "trailing" zeros to the end of decimals. They can be misread as a whole number if the decimal point is not seen. For example, 0.3 should not have a trailing zero. It could be read erroneously as 30.

Memorize

Metric Weight Equivalents	Metric-Household Weight Equivalents (Approximate)
1000 mcg = 1 mg	1 kg = 2.2 pounds (lb)
1000 mg = 1 g	
1000 g = 1 kg	

Medications in micrograms are less frequently encountered than those in milligrams and grams. That makes it all the more important to recognize and distinguish the labels for *mg* and *mcg*. There is a

1000 times difference between a microgram and a milligram. The medications ordered in such small amounts are often very powerful medications.

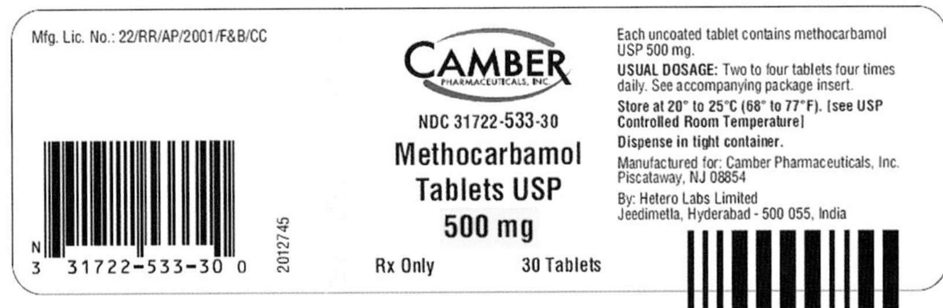

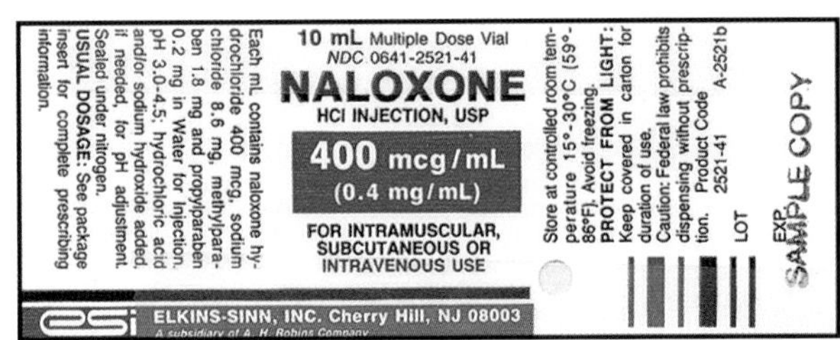

In clinical agencies, the kilogram is used for weight reporting and dose calculations. At birth, the average baby weighs 3200 g or 3.2 kg (approximately 7 lb). Low-birth-weight babies are those who weigh (less than or equal to) 2500 g (2.5 kg or 5.5 lb) at birth. Weight-based dosages for children and adults are required to be in kilograms. Oral medications contain large ranges of dosages in micrograms and millgrams, from 0.175 mg (175 mcg) to 0.5 mg, 100 mg, 250 mg, 500 mg, or 1 g or more. Calculate your own weight in pounds and kilograms.

Memorize

Metric Volume Equivalents	Metric-Household Equivalents (Approximate)
1000 mL = 1 L	5 mL = 1 teaspoon (tsp)
	15 mL = 1 tablespoon (Tbsp) or 3 teaspoons (tsp)
	30 mL = 1 ounce (oz)
	240 mL = 8 ounces (oz) = 1 cup

CLINICAL RELEVANCE

In clinical agencies, liquids are usually ordered and supplied in milliliters and liters. A calibrated metric medication teaspoon holds 5 mL of fluid. Plastic liquid medication cups are usually supplied with a capacity of 30 mL and occasionally 15 mL. Think metric: 30 mL for an ounce.

The volume of a liter is slightly greater than that of a quart (1 L = 1.06 qt; 1 qt is 0.9 L). Many intravenous solutions are delivered in one liter or half-liter containers. Examine water and beverage bottles. Drink 240 mL of water per day instead of 8 ounces or 1 "glass" or 1 "cup."

In many parts of the world, gasoline is purchased by the liter. There are approximately 4 liters to a gallon. If you normally buy 10 gallons, you would purchase about 40 liters. Although this conversion is not exact, using it when buying gasoline abroad will assist you in deciding how much to buy and give you an idea of what you will owe. Making a quick conversion is safer than saying, "Fill the tank."

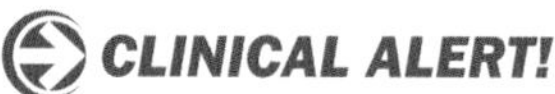

CLINICAL ALERT!

Write the abbreviation *mL* for milliliter. Do not use the abbreviation for cubic centimeter (cc), which is sometimes used to indicate milliliters. The abbreviation "cc" has been misread as two zeros (00), resulting in medication errors.

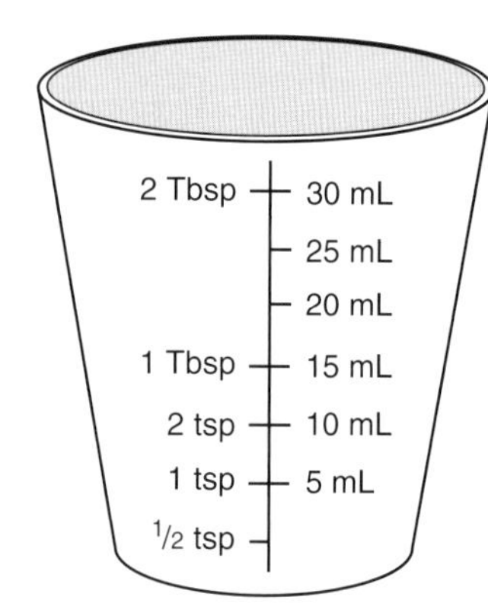

Answers on page 139

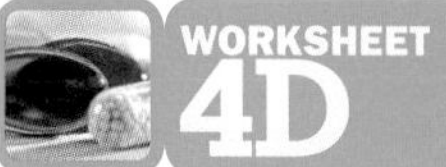

WORKSHEET 4D Equivalent Measures of Weight

1. How many micrograms are in 5 mg? ______
2. How many milligrams are in 0.5 g? ______
3. How many grams are in 5.5 kg? ______
4. How many milligrams are in 2500 mcg? ______
5. How many kilograms are in 2000 g? ______

Answers on page 140

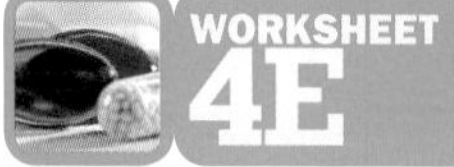

WORKSHEET 4E Equivalent Measures of Volume

1. How many mL are in one-half liter of intravenous solution? ______
2. How many mL are in 1 tablespoon (Tbsp)? ______
3. How many mL are in 8 ounces (oz)? ______
4. How many mL are in 0.25 L of an intravenous medicated solution? ______
5. It is recommended that we drink about 1.5 L of fluid per day. How many mL is the equivalent? ______

Memorize

Metric Length Equivalents (Approximate)	Metric-Household Length Equivalents
10 mm = 1 centimeter (cm)	2.5 cm = 1 inch
100 cm = 1 meter (m)	
1000 mm = 1 meter (m)	

CLINICAL RELEVANCE

In the clinical area, measurements of length are used to measure the size of wounds and sometimes to apply a specific amount of topical medication by length to wounds. Pupil size is measured for eye examinations, certain neurological examinations, and health conditions.

CLINICAL RELEVANCE

- When you are assisting with cardiopulmonary resuscitation (CPR), it is helpful to know that fully dilated pupils (10 mm, or 1 cm) can indicate that the patient has been without oxygen for more than 4 or 5 minutes. Assessment of the pupils of the eye provides a clue as to a patient's response to CPR.
- The pinpoint pupil (1 to 2 mm) may be a reaction to strong light or to certain opioids or other medications (Figure 4.2).
- Familiarity with millimeters and centimeters is also helpful when gauging the length of specified areas, such as wounds or scars, or when documenting the application of ointments in the clinical setting. Although you may be familiar with these units of measure, estimations are not precise. Always measure to ensure accuracy.

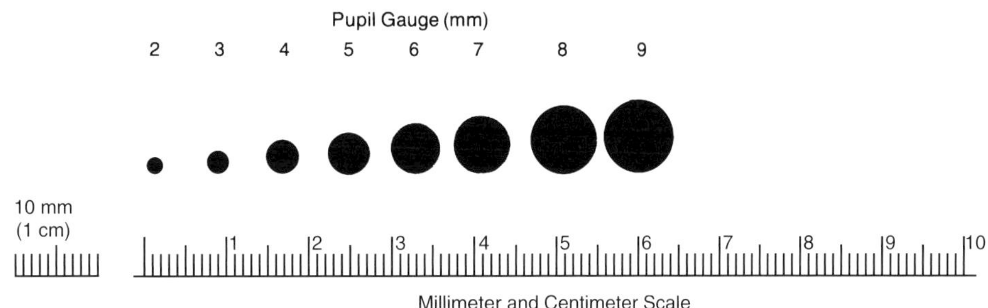

FIGURE 4.2 Pupil gauge (mm).

CLINICAL RELEVANCE

- Topical prescription ointments usually supply paper tape rulers when exact measurements are needed (Figure 4.3).
- Note that some ointments may be prescribed and measured in inches.

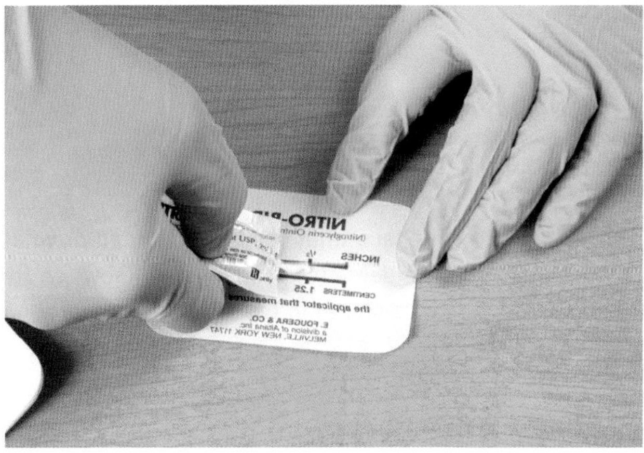

FIGURE 4.3 The nurse is wearing gloves to prevent personal absorption of the medication as well as to avoid skin contact with the patient's wound. (From Perry AG, Potter PA, Ostendort WR: *Clinical nursing skills and techniques*, ed. 9, St. Louis, 2018, Mosby.)

After you learn the major equivalent values, you can infer the equivalent values for quarters, halves, and one and a half units.

Sample Equivalent Metric Values

Row	Length	Volume	Volume	Weight	Weight	Weight	Weight	Weight	Weight
A	10 mm	500 mL	1000 mL	1000 mcg	250 mg	500 mg	1000 mg	1500 mg	1000 g
B	1 cm	0.5 L	1 L	1 mg	0.25 g	0.5 g	1 g	1.5 g	1 kg

Do not confuse micrograms with milligrams. Note the difference in value between 1 mcg and 1 mg. The metric system uses only decimals for numbers less than 1. Note the leading zeros in front of decimals and the elimination trailing zeros after numbers.

Metric Dose Calculation

When the equivalent measurement terms for the medication order and supplied medication *label* are the *same,* the dose can be calculated in one step to find the *amount* of medication to give: x tablets, x capsules, or x mL.

1. Examine the examples of the two ways to set up the ratio and proportion equation using a colon or the fraction cross-multiplication method.
2. Remove the terms and multiply. The proportion is solved in the same way as in all previous examples.

Problem Ordered: 200 mg. On hand: 100 mg per capsule.

Example

USING COLONS

HAVE ON HAND — WANT TO HAVE

100 mg : 1 capsule = 200 mg : x capsules

USING FRACTION CROSS PRODUCT

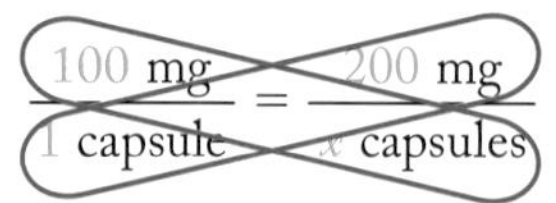

$$\frac{100 \text{ mg}}{1 \text{ capsule}} = \frac{200 \text{ mg}}{x \text{ capsules}}$$

Note: Maintain the same order in the two ratios—mg : capsule = mg : capsule

Estimate: When the terms are the same and in an equation, make a rough estimate of the answer before completing the problem. Will you give more or less than the single serving on hand? About how much more or less?

Remove the terms and multiply.

USING COLONS

100 : 1 = 200 : x

$100x = 200$

x = 2 capsules

USING FRACTION CROSS PRODUCT

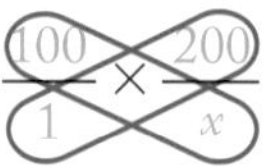

$$\frac{100}{1} \times \frac{200}{x}$$

PROOF
100 × 2 = 200
1 × 200 = 200

Example Ordered: 50 mg. Unit dose label: 25 mg per tablet.

RULE **Place what you have on hand or what you know (the label unit dose) on the left and what is ordered (want to have or know) on the right. Follow through with your math to verify your estimate as shown in the ratio and proportion examples in Chapter 2.**

KNOW — WANT TO KNOW

25 mg : 1 tablet = 50 mg : x tablets

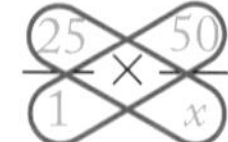

$$\frac{25}{1} \times \frac{50}{x}$$

$$\frac{25}{25} \times \frac{50}{25} = 2 \text{ or } 25x = 50$$

x = 2 tablets

PROOF
25 × 2 = 50
1 × 50 = 50

ANSWER
Give 2 tablets

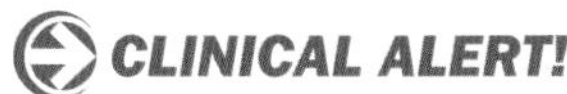

CLINICAL ALERT!

Some of these problems can be easily solved. More complex problems will be more easily solved after practice with easier problems. Always mathematically calculate a drug dosage.

Answers on page 140

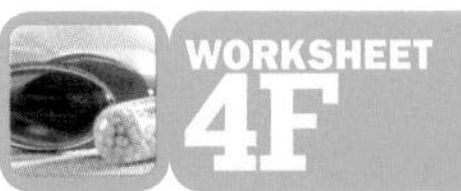

WORKSHEET 4F Oral Solid Medication Dose Practice

Estimate and calculate the dose using a ratio and proportion method.

1. Ordered: Prednisone 15 mg tablets daily po for a patient with asthma.
On hand: Prednisone 5 mg tablets.

HAVE ON HAND WANT TO HAVE

PROOF

2. Ordered: Fortovase (saquinavir) 400 mg soft gel capsule daily for a patient with an HIV infection.

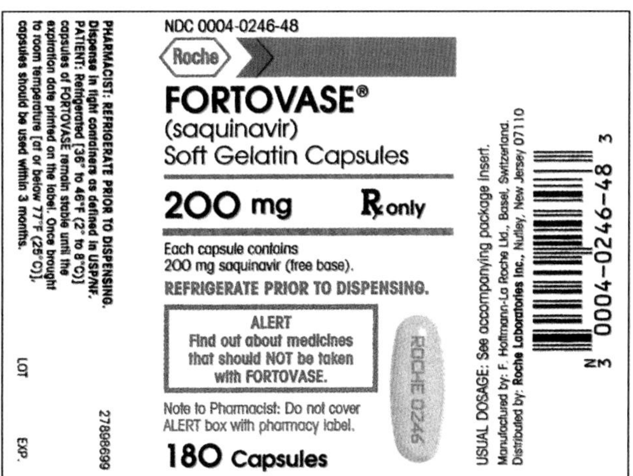

HAVE ON HAND WANT TO HAVE

PROOF

What are the refrigeration directions?

3. Ordered: Tegretol 200 mg chewable tablet po at bedtime for a patient who has seizures.

NDC 0078-0492-05 Rx only

Tegretol® 100 mg

carbamazepine USP

Chewable Tablets

100 tablets

PHARMACIST: Dispense with Medication Guide attached or provided separately.

NOVARTIS

HAVE ON HAND WANT TO HAVE

PROOF

4. Ordered: Lanoxin (digoxin) tablet 0.125 mg po daily in AM for a patient with heart failure.

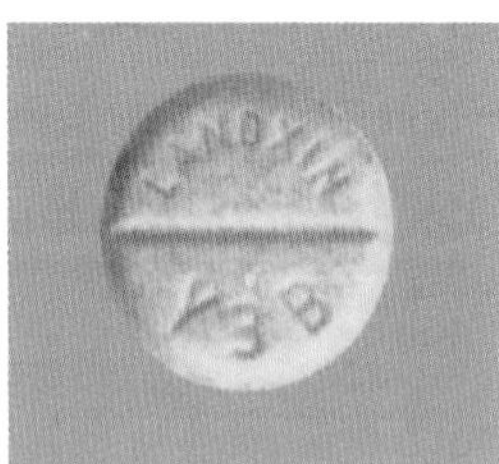

NDC 0173-0249-56

100 Tablets
(10 blisterpacks of 10 tablets each)

UNIT DOSE PACK

LANOXIN® (digoxin) Tablets

Each scored tablet contains
250 mcg (0.25 mg)

See package insert for Dosage and Administration.

Store at 25°C (77°F); excursions permitted to 15 to 30°C (59 to 86°F) [see USP Controlled Room Temperature] in a dry place.

HAVE ON HAND WANT TO HAVE

PROOF

5. Ordered: Septra DS 80 mg trimethoprim and 400 mg sulfamethoxazole tablets po daily for a patient with a urinary tract infection.

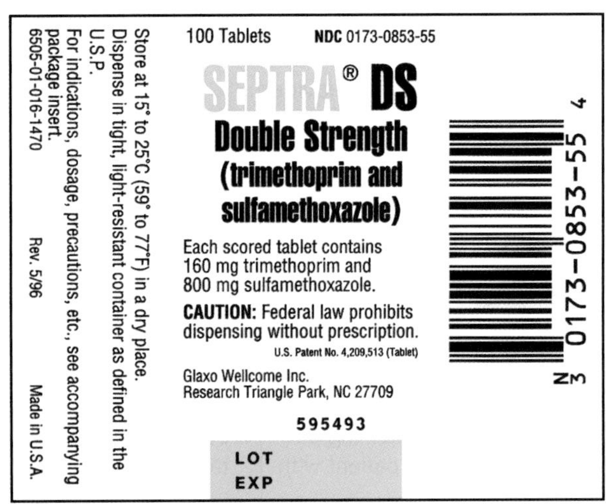

100 Tablets
NDC 0173-0853-55
SEPTRA® DS
Double Strength
(trimethoprim and sulfamethoxazole)
Each scored tablet contains 160 mg trimethoprim and 800 mg sulfamethoxazole.
CAUTION: Federal law prohibits dispensing without prescription.
U.S. Patent No. 4,209,513 (Tablet)
Glaxo Wellcome Inc.
Research Triangle Park, NC 27709
595493
LOT
EXP
Store at 15° to 25°C (59° to 77°F) in a dry place.
Dispense in tight, light-resistant container as defined in the U.S.P.
For indications, dosage, precautions, etc., see accompanying package insert.
6505-01-016-1470
Rev. 5/96
Made in U.S.A.
N 3 0173-0853-55 4

HAVE ON HAND | WANT TO HAVE

PROOF

HAVE ON HAND | WANT TO HAVE

PROOF

Note: Septra DS is a compound drug that is supplied in more than one concentration.

CLINICAL ALERT!

DS (double-strength). Do not confuse DS with extended-release or delayed-release products. Those types of products (E-R, S-R, CD, XR, XL,* etc.) are not double strength, and DS is not an abbreviation for an extended-release product.

*Refer to abbreviations on the inside front cover.

Answers on page 141

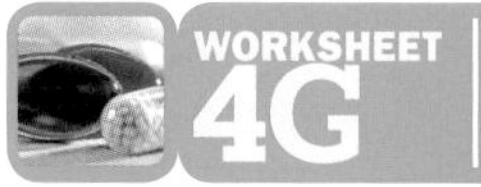

WORKSHEET 4G Oral Solid Medication Dose Practice

Compare the ordered dose with the available dose concentration supplied. Fill in the requested information in the space provided.

Ordered Type or Condition for Rx	Supplied dose	Estimate*: *More, Less, or Same as* 1 serving of the drug concentration supplied	Actual dose Solve using a ratio and proportion method
1. Rifampin (rifadin) 600 mg po daily for a patient with tuberculosis	300 mg per capsule	**a**	**b**
2. Metoprolol XL† 100 mg po at bedtime for a patient with hypertension	100 mg per XL tablet	**a**	**b**
3. Lopressor (metoprolol tartrate) 75 mg po daily at bedtime for a patient with hypertension	50 mg per scored tablet	**a**	**b**
4. Synthroid (levothyroxine) 175 mcg (0.175 mg) po daily in AM for a patient with hypothyroidism	175 mcg per tablet	**a**	**b**
5. Halcion (aprazolam) 0.125 mg po daily at bedtime for anxiety	0.25 mg tablet, unscored	**a**	**b**
Note that most of the orders for these commonly ordered drugs are between $\frac{1}{2}$ to 2 servings of the form supplied. Recheck orders that call for more than 2 servings of the supplied form.			

*An estimate can be made when the ordered dose and the dose on hand are in the same measurement terms.
†CLINICAL ALERT With XL (extra-long), E-R (extended release), SR (sustained release); the total daily dose is usually given once every 24 hours. The regular form would be given two or more times a day. Many drugs are supplied in different release forms. Be sure to double-check the form on the order and the label.

CLINICAL RELEVANCE

Examples of errors in the clinical setting include the following:*

- Giving 10 mL of a liquid drug instead of 10 mg
- Converting 1 g to 100 mg instead of 1000 mg, a tenfold error.
- Giving 20 mg instead of 200 mg for a 0.2 g order, a tenfold error
- Reading 100U as 1000 because *units* was not spelled out or a space was not left between the number and the *U*, or the *U* was closed and looked like a zero, resulting in a tenfold overdose.
- Reading 7.5 mg as 75 mg because the decimal was not seen
- Reading 100 mEq as 100 mg, two very different measurements

*For more examples of errors, refer to Appendix C.

Comparison of Metric and Approximate Household Measurements

	METRIC	HOUSEHOLD
Weight	1 kg	2.2 lb
Length	10 cm	2.5 in
	1 m	39 inches, a little more than a yard
Volume	5 mL	1 teaspoon (tsp)
	10 mL	2 teaspoons
	15 mL	1 tablespoon (T, Tbsp, TBSP, tbs) (½ oz) (3 teaspoons)
	30 mL	2 tablespoons (1 oz)
	240 mL	1 measuring cup (8 oz)
	500 mL	1 pint (16 oz) (2 cups)
	960 mL	1 quart (slightly less than 1 liter)
	4 L	1 gallon (gal) (4 quarts)

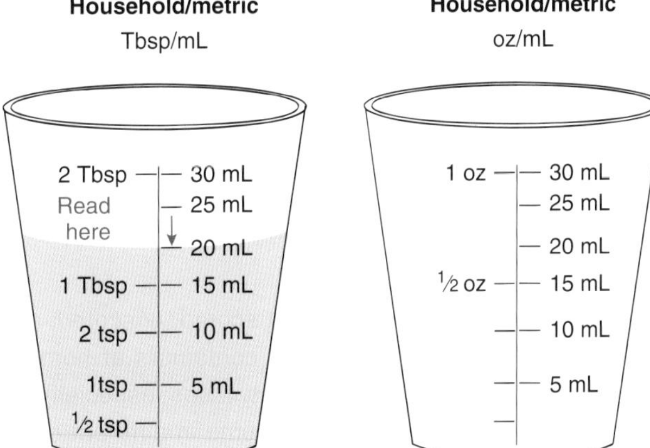

CLINICAL RELEVANCE

Always explain the importance of using the equipment that is packaged with liquid medications to the patient and/or family when you are administering medications and during discharge from the clinical facility. Many serious dose errors have been reported from use of household equipment.

Answers on page 141

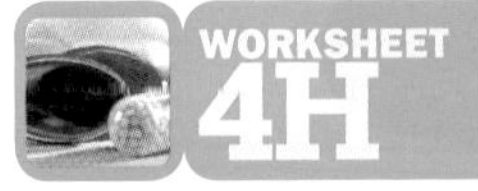

WORKSHEET 4H | Metric and Approximate Household Equivalents Review

Fill in the *approximate* equivalents for household measurements and *exact* amounts for metric equivalents in the space provided:

1. How many tsp are in a Tbsp? ______________

2. How many Tbsp are in an ounce? ______________

3. How many mL are in a metric-calibrated teaspoon? ______________

4. How many mL are in a metric-calibrated tablespoon? ______________

5. How many mL are in a metric-calibrated cup? ______________

6. How many mL are in a liter? ____________

7. How many quarts are approximately in a liter? ____________

8. How many pounds are in a kg? ____________

9. How many cm are in an inch? ____________

10. How many mm are in a cm? ____________

Rounding Oral Medication Doses

Round your answers to the nearest measurable dose based on the order and the selected equipment available.

Solids

Tablets and capsules are not rounded. Only scored tablets may be cut in half to give an ordered dose if the dose is exactly $\frac{1}{2}$ of the supplied amount. For example: Ordered—10 mg. What you have—20 mg scored tablet. Cut the 20-mg tablet in half with a pill cutter, and give the $\frac{1}{2}$ tablet (10 mg).

CLINICAL RELEVANCE

Patients who have scored-medication orders often have frequent orders for changed doses based on lab tests and response to the medication. Anticoagulant therapy is an example of various dose orders based on testing.

CLINICAL ALERT!

Remind the patient to avoid mixing scored, unscored, and half tablets in one container. They need to be kept in their original labeled containers at home and during travel to avoid errors in dose. This has become an important safety issue, especially since the patient may be switched to generics of the same brand, which may come in different colors and sizes.

Liquids

The trend is to provide oral liquids in unit-dose packaged medicine cups or prefilled oral syringes. Liquids in mL are rounded, depending on the medication order and the equipment available. Oral liquids of less than 1 or 2 mL are supplied with calibrated droppers (Figure 4.4).

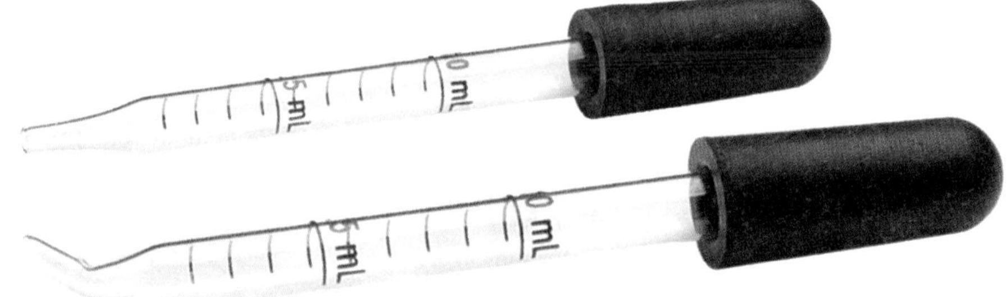

FIGURE 4.4 Calibrated droppers. (From Macklin D, Chernecky C, Infortuna H: *Math for clinical practice,* ed 2, St Louis, 2011, Mosby.)

Amounts of oral liquids less than 5 mL (1 metric teaspoon) are usually prepared in a pleasant-tasting solution to bring the total dose to 5 mL, 1 metric-calibrated teaspoon.

Oral liquids greater than 1 mL can be rounded to the nearest tenth of a milliliter.

Measuring Oral Liquid Doses

On occasion, oral liquid medications need to be prepared by the nurse from a multidose container (Figures 4.5 and 4.6).

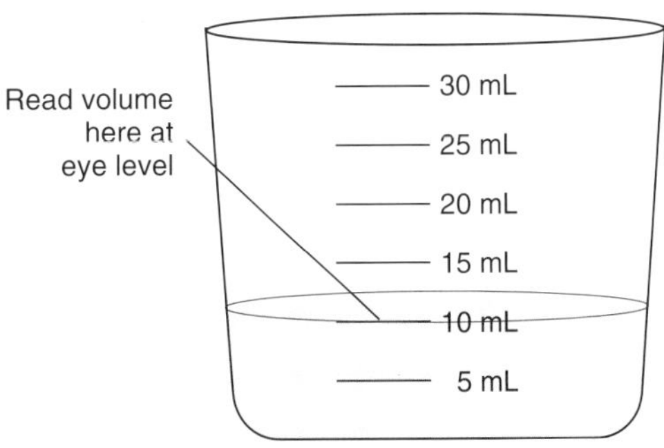

FIGURE 4.5 Pour at eye level, on a level surface, to the desired volume of liquid. Read where the meniscus is level with the line on the scale (10 mL).

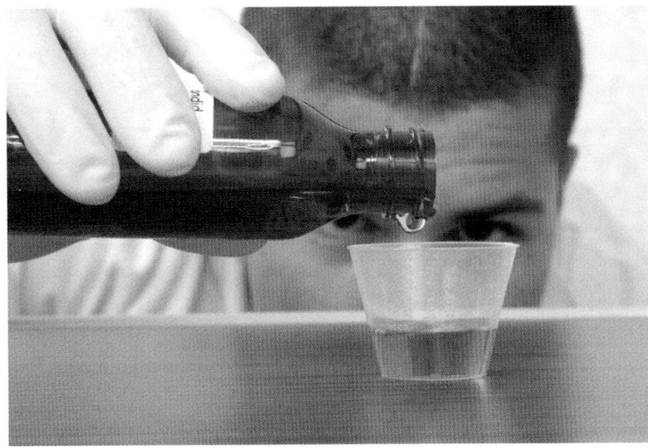

FIGURE 4.6 Measuring liquid medication on eye level on a level surface. (In Snyder JS, Collins SR, Lilley LL: *Pharmacology and nursing process,* ed. 9, St. Louis, 2020, Mosby. From Rick Brady.)

Liquids for medicine cups can be measured to the nearest tenth of a mL (Figure 4.7). This medicine cup is calibrated in multiples of 5 mL. When a liquid oral dose is not a multiple of 5 mL, fill the cup to the meniscus of the *nearest measurable* calibrated line on the cup and add the remaining precise dose with a syringe.

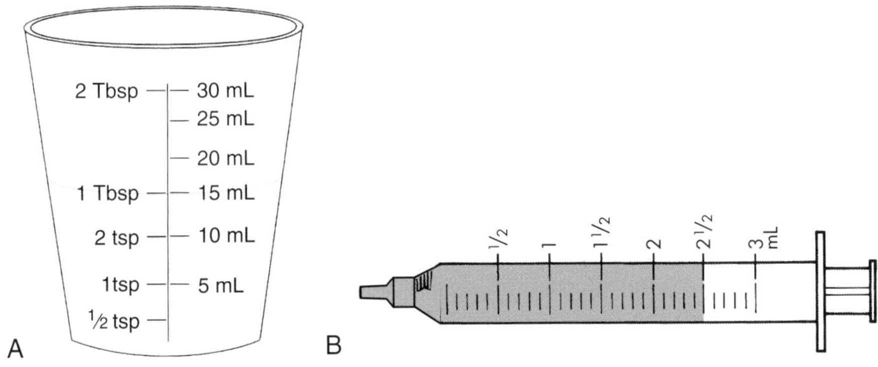

FIGURE 4.7 Total dose will be 17.5 mL. **A,** 15 mL is prepared in the medicine cup. **B,** 2.5 mL is prepared with a syringe and added to the cup.

CLINICAL ALERT!

If the oral medication is to be given with a syringe, it should be administered with an oral syringe (Figure 4.8). Chapter 5, Injectable Medication Calculations, illustrates syringe measurements.

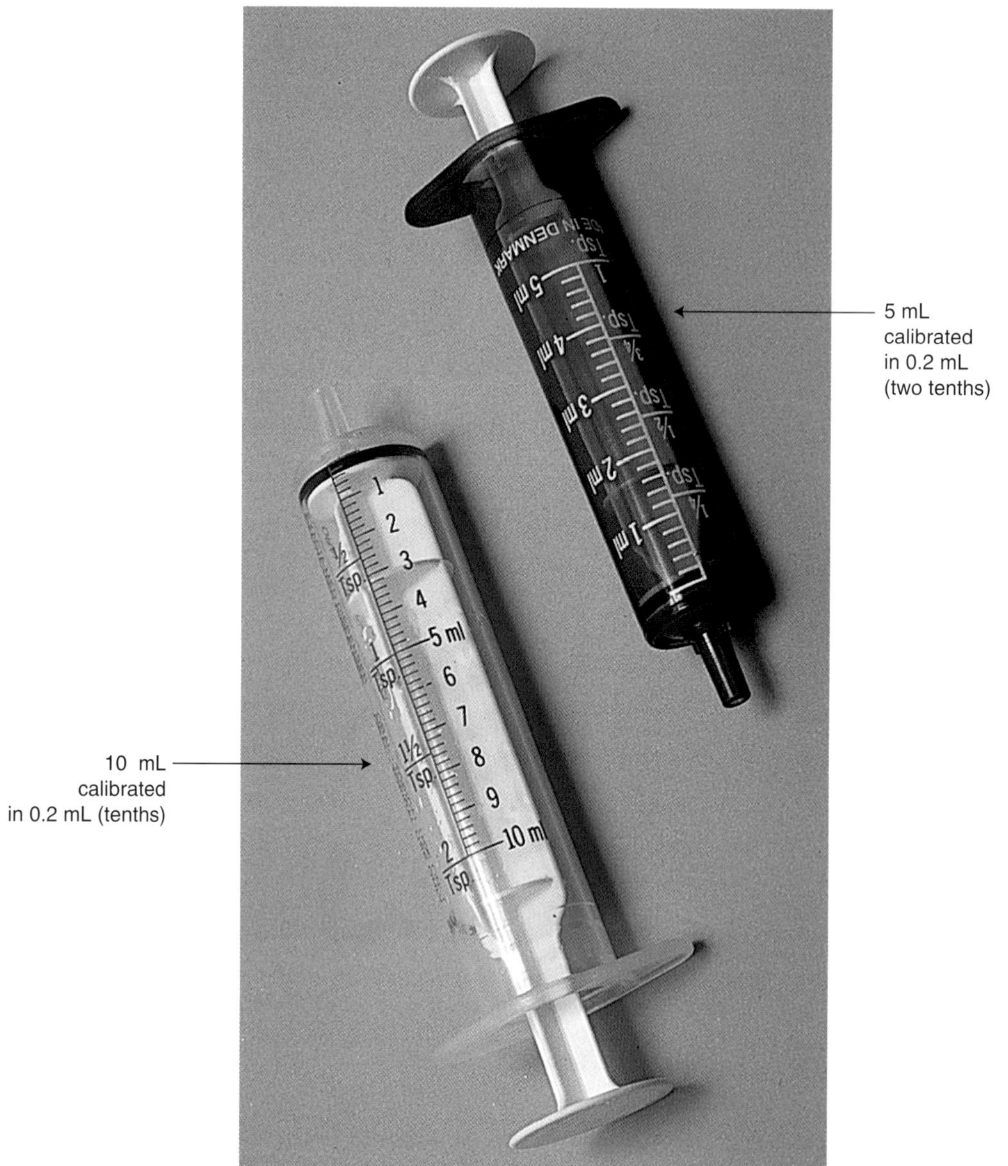

FIGURE 4.8 Oral syringes. Oral syringes are not sterile and are used only for oral medications. (From Clayton BD, Stock YN, Cooper S: *Basic pharmacology for nurses,* ed 17, St. Louis, 2017, Mosby. Courtesy of Chuck Dresner.)

CLINICAL RELEVANCE

Occasionally a small length of tubing needs to be attached to the oral syringe to deliver the medication to facilitate swallowing. Administer very slowly.

CLINICAL ALERT!

Always be aware of each patient's ability to swallow before administering oral liquids. If a question arises, check with the patient, the medical history, and the lead nurse on the unit. If no problem is known, offer a couple of sips of water first. If the patient has difficulty, hold the medication and contact the provider promptly for new orders. Document the problem and the result of the contact with the provider.

Answers on page 141

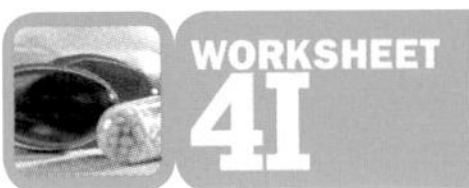

WORKSHEET 4I Liquid Oral Dose Practice

Liquid doses are calculated using the same setup as with solid medications. Estimate and solve the following liquid dose problems using ratio and proportion. Label and prove answers. Round to the nearest tenth of a mL if applicable.

1. Ordered: Morphine sulfate 5 mg oral solution po q8h for a patient with pain. How many mL will you give?

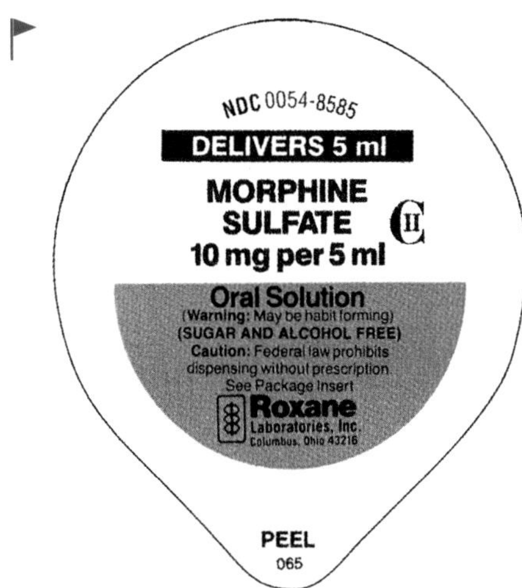

2. Ordered: Potassium chloride oral solution 10 mEq po bid for a patient with an electrolyte imbalance. How many mL will you give?

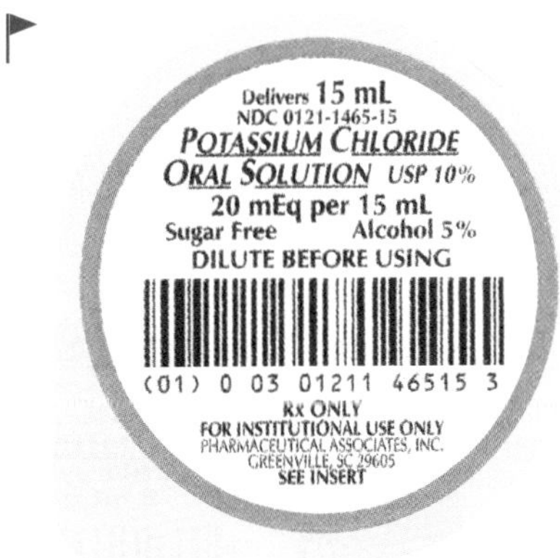

3. Ordered: Dilantin suspension 250 mg po daily in the AM for a patient with seizures. How many mL are needed?

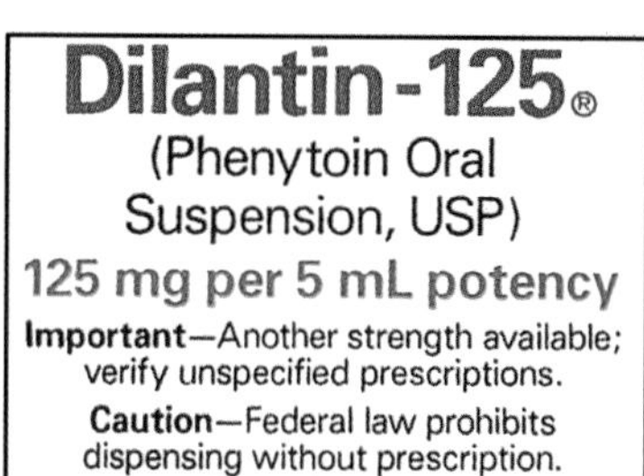

4. Ordered: Zithromax (azithromycin) syrup oral suspension 300 mg daily for a patient with an infection. How many mL should you give?

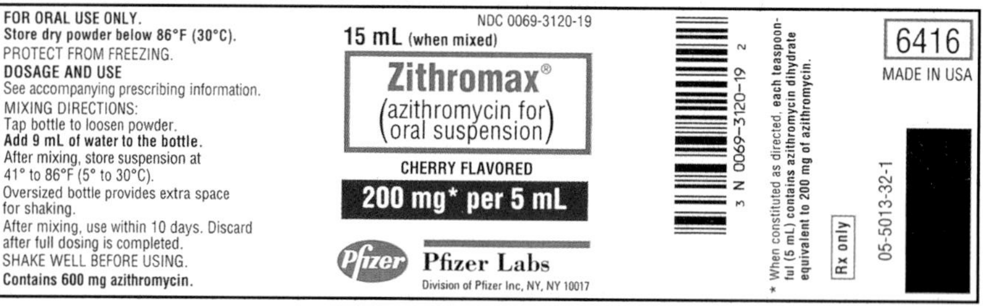

5. Ordered: Lithium citrate syrup 240 mg po bid for a patient with a bipolar disorder. How many mL will you give?

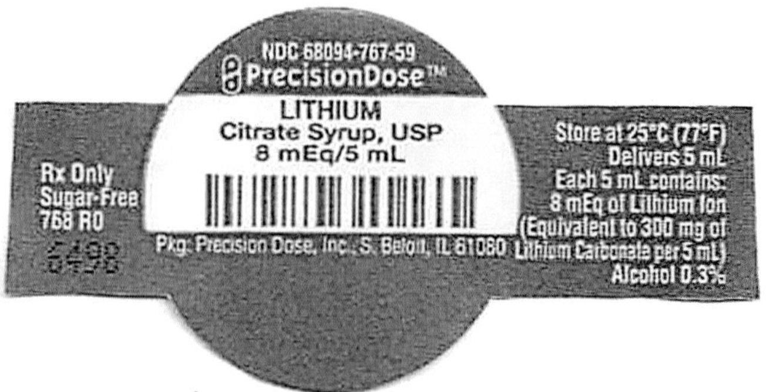

Answers on page 142

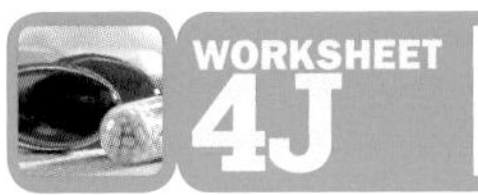

WORKSHEET 4J Liquid Oral Dose Practice

This exercise is not difficult, but it does require focus to avoid confusing the ordered dose with the dose supplied. This can happen even more easily in a busy work environment. Estimation can help prevent major math errors. Many agencies now require silence in the medication preparation area to help reduce distractions. Clinical agencies may also post signs or use identifying clothing, such as vests, to indicate that the nurse is administering medication and should not be interrupted.

Fill in the requested answers. Include an estimate of the dose to be administered.

Ordered Action or Condition for Rx	Supplied Dose	State: *More, Less, or Same amt* of mL as 1 serving of the drug concentration supplied	Actual dose in mL, calculated using ratio and proportion
1. Tylenol elixir* (acetaminophen) 200 mg q6h po prn headache	Tylenol elixir 125 mg per 5 mL		
2. Oxycodone HCl oral solution 5 mg po stat for patient with severe pain	Oxycodone oral solution 5 mg per 5 mL		
3. Zofran (ondansetron) oral sol. 8 mg po stat for a patient with nausea and vomiting (N/V) related to chemotherapy	Zofran oral sol. 4 mg per 5 mL		
4. Prozac (fluoxetine) oral sol. 30 mg po AM daily for a patient with depression	Prozac liquid 20 mg per 5 mL		
5. Milk of Magnesia 10 mg po daily bedtime prn constipation	Milk of Magnesia 30 mg per 15 mL		

*Recheck orders for elixirs if patient has known alcohol dependence. Elixirs have an alcohol base.

CLINICAL ALERT!

If there is an interruption when you are preparing medications, unless it is an emergency, complete the current preparation (and/or administration if possible) *and* the documentation of administration before attending to the interruption, such as a request for help with lifting, transport, coverage, new orders, others' conversations, etc.

Note: Do not give medications someone else has prepared.

CLINICAL ALERT!

Recheck orders and probable reason if an order is for more than one or two servings of the unit dose supplied.

Identifying Units and Milliequivalents in Medication Dosages

The following measurements in addition to micrograms, milligrams, and grams may be seen in medication orders. They may also be seen in laboratory values.

Term	Abbreviation	Meaning
unit*	write out	Is a quantity that represents a laboratory standard of measurement. It is often used as a unit of measure for products that have some or all animal or plant contents (e.g., heparin, insulin, antibiotics).
milliunit*	write out	Equals 1/1000 of a unit. Pitocin is an example of a medication ordered this way.
milliequivalent	mEq	Represents the number of grams of solute dissolved in a milliliter of solution. Electrolytes are commonly dissolved in solution and measured in milliequivalents (e.g., sodium, potassium, chlorides).
milliequivalent per liter	mEq per L	Equals one thousandth of 1 g of a specific substance dissolved in a liter of a solution. Electrolytes are frequently supplied in milliequivalents per liter for intravenous infusion (e.g., KCl 40 mEq per L).
milliequivalent per milliliter	mEq per mL	Equals one thousandth of 1 g of a specific substance dissolved in 1 mL. (The 1 is implied when a number is absent in front of mL.) 2 mEq per mL would equal two thousandths of a gram dissolved in 1 mL.

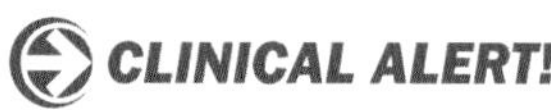

"Unit" must be written out to avoid confusion with the zero (0) or the letter "O."

Answers on page 143

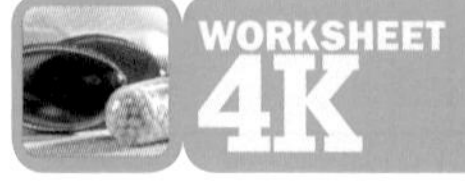

Measurements Review

1. The provider ordered 1 milligram of a medication for one patient and 1 gram for another. Which is the larger amount?

2. The provider ordered 250 milligrams of an antibiotic for one patient and 0.5 gram for another. Write the abbreviation for the larger amount. ______________

3. A patient drank 120 milliliters of juice and 2 Liters of water in 24 h. Write the abbreviation for the larger amount? ______________

4. **a.** If a patient receives 1 milligram instead of 1 microgram of a medication in an intravenous solution, is that an overdose or an underdose? ______________
   b. By how many doses is it incorrect? ______________

5. **a.** The average American consumes about 3400 mg of salt per day. How many grams is this? ______________
   b. A recommended amount of daily salt intake is less than 2300 mg per day. How many grams is this? ______________
   c. Some sources recommend limiting salt intake to 1.5 g per day. How many milligrams is this? ______________

*Refer to The Joint Commission's Do Not Use list on p. 61.

6. If a patient is supposed to have a 3-cm measured strip of an ointment applied over a wound and 3 mm were applied instead, would that be an underdose or an overdose? (circle one)

7. A popular recommendation is for an adult to drink the equivalent of about eight (8-oz) glasses of fluid per day (fluid from all sources).* One ounce is *approximately* 30 mL.
   a. How many milliliters would there be in an 8-ounce glass? ____________
   b. How many total mL would this be for a 24 hr day? ____________
   c. How many liters would this be? ____________

8. In a few words, state each of the steps in a two-step dose calculation.

   Step 1:

   Step 2:

9. An adult weighs 200 pounds. *Estimate* how many kg would be the equivalent. ____________

10. If an order was written for 15 mL of a medicine, how many metric-calibrated teaspoons would be the equivalent? ____________

*Fluid needs vary widely, depending on activity and health conditions.

Two-Step Calculation Review

Example Ordered: 100 **mg**. You have 0.05 **g** tablets on hand. How many tablets will you give?

Select the correct equivalents.
Have grams on hand. Need to change **mg** to the equivalent **g** on hand.

Equivalency tables: 1000 mcg = 1 mg
1000 mg = 1 g

Step 1 Set up a ratio and proportion problem to find the equivalent measurement.

USING COLONS

KNOW WANT TO KNOW

1000 mg : 1 g = 100 mg : x g
(mg : g = mg : g)

USING FRACTION CROSS PRODUCT

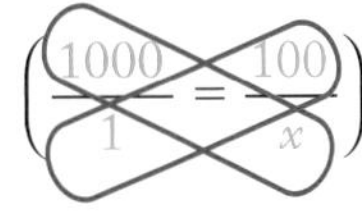

$\frac{\cancel{1000}}{\cancel{1000}} x = \frac{\cancel{100}}{\cancel{1000}} = \frac{1}{10}$ or 0.1 or $1000x = 100$
$x = 0.1$

$x = 0.1$ g My estimate is that I will give 2 tablets.

PROOF
1000 × 0.1 = 100
1 × 100 = 100

Step 2 Insert the equivalent measure from Step 1 into your ratio and proportion now that all terms of measurement are the same.

HAVE WANT TO HAVE

0.05 g : 1 tab = 0.1 g : x tab

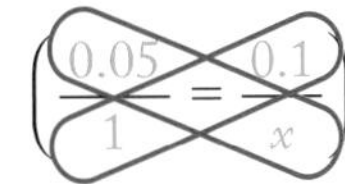

$\frac{\cancel{0.05}}{\cancel{0.05}} x = \frac{0.1}{0.05}$ or $0.05\overline{)0.1}$

$x = 2$ tabs

PROOF
0.05 × 2 = 0.1
1 × 0.1 = 0.1

Tips to Avoid Errors

1. Analyze your problem. Is it a one-step or two-step calculation? (Are the terms the same or different?)
2. Always place a zero in front of a decimal when the number is less than one. It reminds you that the next figure is a decimal, not a number 1 (0.4).
3. Eliminate trailing zeros at the end of a decimal (0.75Ø).
4. Write neatly; estimate and prove your answer. Ask yourself whether this is a reasonable amount of medication. (Close to unit dose?)
5. If you doubt your math, recalculate without looking at your original work. If still in doubt, check reliable sources.

Answers on page 143

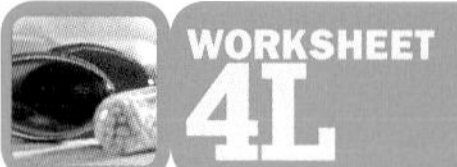

WORKSHEET 4L Additional Practice with Metric Problems

Solve the following problems using a ratio and proportion method. If the problem needs to have an equivalent equation first, fill in the measurement terms (a).

1. Ordered: Levoxyl (levothyroxine) tablets 0.35 mg po daily for a patient with hypothyroidism.

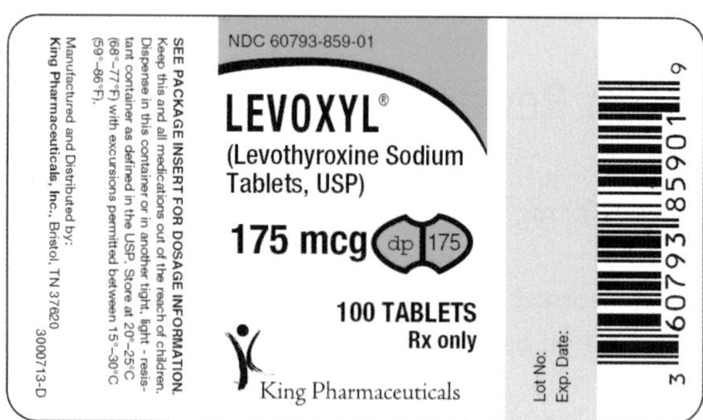

a. Equivalent: Change ________ to ________ (if needed)

b. KNOW   WANT TO KNOW

PROOF

c. HAVE   WANT TO HAVE

PROOF

2. Ordered: digoxin (Lanoxin) 250 mcg tablet po daily in the AM for a patient with heart failure.

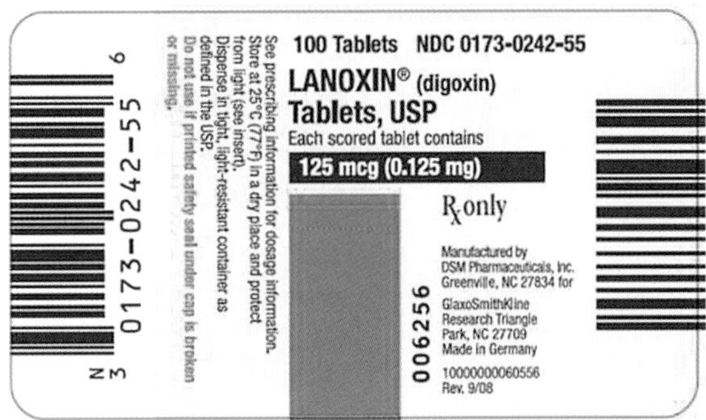

a. Equivalent: Change ________ to ________ (if needed)

b. KNOW WANT TO KNOW

PROOF

c. HAVE WANT TO HAVE

PROOF

3. Ordered: Dilantin (phenytoin) 0.2 g capsules po daily for a patient with a seizure disorder.

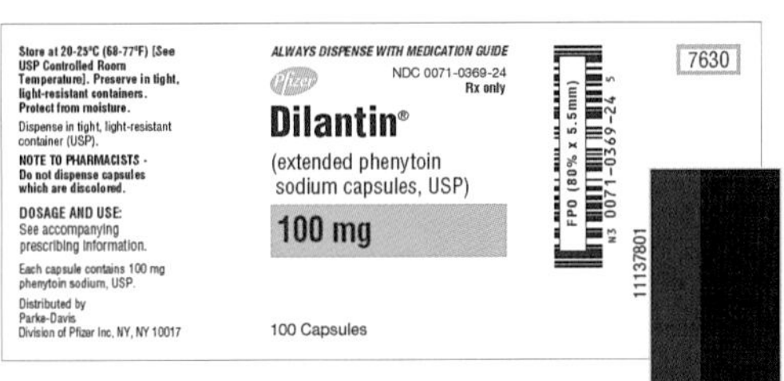

a. Equivalent: Change ________ to ________ (if needed)

b. KNOW WANT TO KNOW

PROOF

c. HAVE WANT TO HAVE

PROOF

4. Ordered: Alprazolam oral solution 750 mcg po bid for a patient with anxiety.*

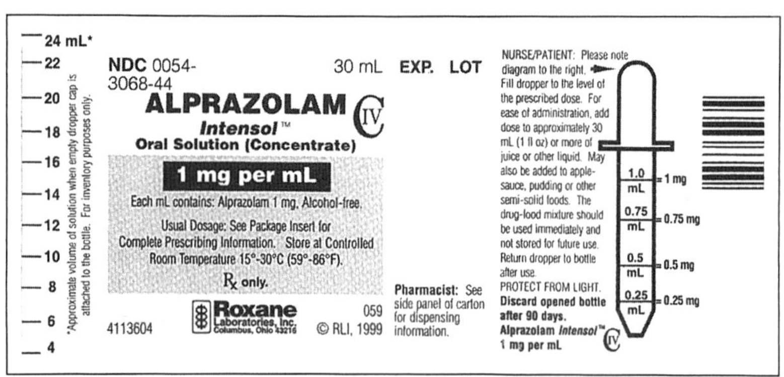

a. Equivalent: Change ________ to ________ (if needed)

b. KNOW WANT TO KNOW

PROOF

c. HAVE WANT TO HAVE

PROOF

d. mL after dilution per directions ____________________

CLINICAL RELEVANCE

Teach the patient to rinse the calibrated dropper that is packaged with the medication after using it and to continue to use the dropper with the specific medication only.

5. Ordered; Morphine Sulfate oral solution 8 mg po stat for a patient with pain.*

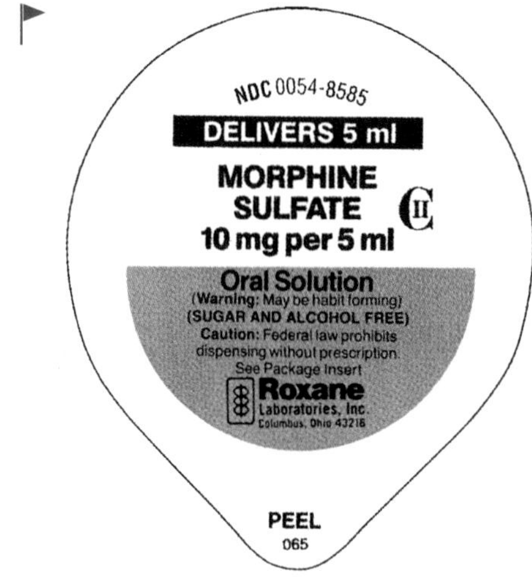

a. Equivalent: Change ________ to ________ (if needed)

b. KNOW WANT TO KNOW

PROOF

c. HAVE WANT TO HAVE

PROOF

*Note that the labels on Problems 4 and 5 each include a "C" with a Roman numeral, symbols that indicate they are controlled substances that carry potential for abuse. They are kept in a locked area separate from other medications. The schedules range from C I, indicating a high potential for abuse and dependence, to Schedule 5, drugs with a relatively lower potential for abuse and dependence.

This order will have to be measured. An oral syringe is preferred to withdraw the needed amount (Figure 4.9). The total dose may be administered with an oral syringe or a calibrated medicine cup. Refer to Figure 4.7 on page 119 for an illustration of precise measurement of oral doses for a medicine cup.

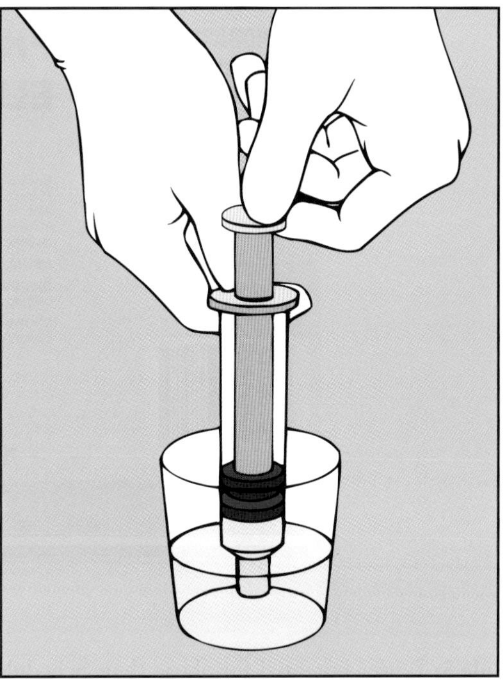

FIGURE 4.9 Transfer of liquid medications into or out of a medicine cup. (From Clayton BD, Willihnganz MJ: *Basic pharmacology for nurses,* ed. 17, St. Louis, 2017, Mosby.)

The red flag in front of the label is an icon reminder that this is an ISMP–identified high-alert drug with the potential to cause serious harm if given in error.

Controlled Drug Schedules

Alprazolam is a C IV-level and morphine is a C II-level drug. C II and C IV are the two most frequently encountered schedules in medication administration. Prescription abuse is a challenging issue for health care providers.

Schedule 1: Highest potential for abuse. These drugs (e.g., peyote and heroin) are not prescribed because they have no currently accepted medical use.

Schedule 2: High potential for abuse and do have currently accepted medical use with severe restrictions and potential for severe dependence. Examples include morphine sulfate, oxycontin, hydrocodone products, and amphetamines.

Schedule 3: Potential for abuse less than Schedule 1 and 2 and potential for moderate dependence. Examples include several codeine products and testosterone products.

Schedule 4: Lower potential for abuse than Schedules 1, 2, and 3. May lead to limited dependence relative to drugs in Schedule 3. Examples include phenobarbital, alprazolam, Halcion, Valium, and Ambien.

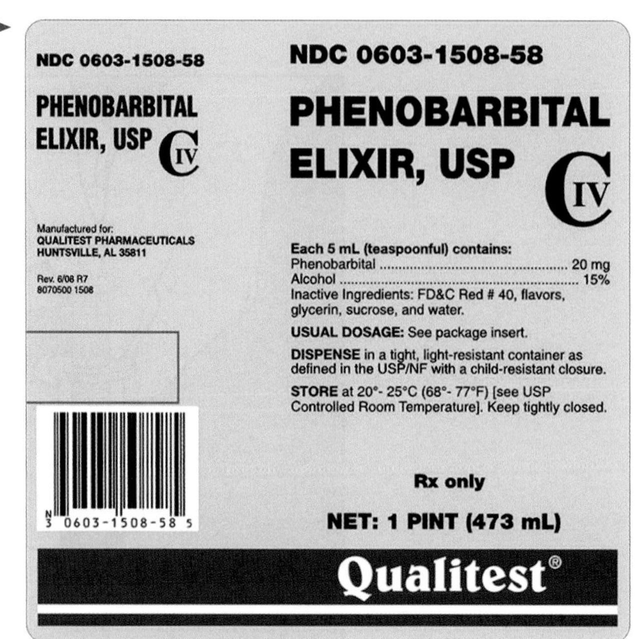

Schedule 5: Lower potential for abuse than Schedule 4. May lead to limited dependence relative to drugs in Schedule 4. This level includes cough/cold medicines with codeine.

CLINICAL ALERT!

If a portion of a controlled substance dose has to be discarded/wasted, always check and follow the clinical agency policies and procedures. Do *not* sign as a witness to any procedure unless you witnessed the *entire* medication procedure.

Answers on page 144

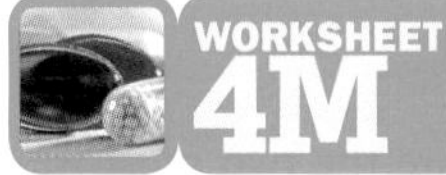

WORKSHEET 4M Multiple-Choice Practice

1. If a patient drinks 0.5 L in 4 hours, how many mL would that be? ____________
a. 25
b. 100
c. 500
d. 5000

2. The correct abbreviations for metric base units are:
a. L, m, g
b. m, c, k, mc
c. mg, mL, cc
d. mm, cm, mg, kg

3. How many mL are in 2 metric-calibrated teaspoons?
a. 2
b. 10
c. 5
d. 20

4. Select the correct equivalent in mg and mcg for 0.2 g:
a. 200 mg; 200,000 mcg
b. 2.0 mg; 2000 mcg
c. 100 mg; 2000 mcg
d. 2 mg; 200,000 mcg

5. If a current drug reference stated that an antibiotic medication of 500 mg should be given in 4 divided doses, what would you prepare?
   a. 100 mg
   b. 250 mg
   c. 125 mg
   d. 500 mg

6. Milligram to gram and microgram to milligram conversions require movement of how many decimal places:
   a. 2 decimal places to the right
   b. 3 decimal places to the right
   c. 2 decimal places to the left
   d. 3 decimal places to the left

7. Select the recommended method for preparing a liquid medication of 9 mL from a multidose bottle.
   a. Pour to 5 mL in the cup and add 4 mL with a 5 mL syringe.
   b. Pour to 10 mL in the metric measuring cup, and remove 1 mL with a sterile syringe to be returned to the bottle.
   c. Pour to approximately 9 mL between the 5-mL and 10-mL calibrations.
   d. Remove 9 mL from the bottle with a 10 mL syringe, and place in the cup.

8. A patient needs 2.5 cm of a topical medication applied to a wound. How many approximate inches would this be?
   a. 0.5
   b. 1
   c. 2
   d. 2.5

9. Which is the recommendation per TJC and ISMP to write the following medication order:
   a. Penicillin, 1,000,000 u
   b. Penicillin 1000000 units
   c. Penicillin 1,000,000 U
   d. Penicillin 1,000,000 Units

10. A patient weighs 80 pounds. Approximately how many kg would be the equivalent?
   a. 20
   b. 120
   c. 40
   d. 160

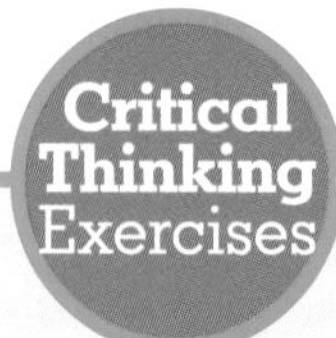

Critical Thinking Exercises provide math and medication-related patient safety issues for student discussion. Answers are not provided.

Analyze and discuss the following scenarios with a classmate.

1. Mr. R is an alert, anxious-appearing, frail gentleman, 76 years old, weighing 65 kilograms. He was admitted two days before with complaints of chest pain. His medication orders included Lanoxin 0.125 mg daily every morning. This was the only medication ordered for the morning. On hand was digoxin 0.25 mg/tablet (scored).

After you provided care for him on the evening shift, he mentioned that his doctor must have changed his orders because for 2 days he had been taking only half of a tablet in the morning; then yesterday and today, his new nurse had given him two tablets each day. His wife agreed. He wanted to know if this meant that his heart problem was getting worse.

Ordered:

Supplied:

Given:

Error(s):

Potential injuries:

Nursing actions:

Preventive measures: How could this have been avoided? If you were on a hospital committee that studies incidents, what sort of recommendations would you make for this specific incident, the nurse involved, and the pharmacy department, keeping in mind that you would not want to discourage the reporting of medication errors?

2. Mrs. D is a housewife who has been admitted to the hospital for surgery for a throat tumor. She has been taking fluoxetine (Prozac) tablets for the past year for depression. The prescriber changed her prescription to Prozac oral solution 60 mg daily because of postoperative throat discomfort. The nurse administered 60 mL (2 oz) of Prozac.

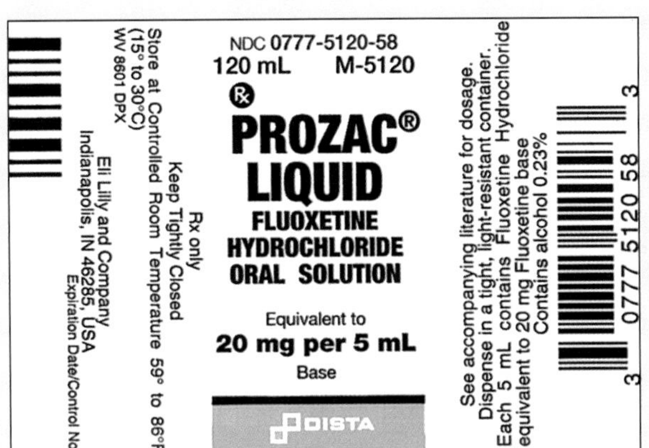

Ordered:

Supplied:

Given:

Error(s):

Potential injuries:

Nursing actions:

Preventive measures (refer to the questions in exercise No. 1):

3. Mr. Z, a 70-year-old nursing home patient who has seizures, has an order for an antiseizure drug daily. The nurse notices he complains of being very tired, sleeps most of the day, and is unwilling to walk since he has been on the new medication. The doctor reduces the order from 0.5 mg po daily at bedtime to 0.1 mg. The 0.1 mg dose has not yet been delivered. The nurse reads the new order and gives two 0.5 mg tablets to the patient. (Read the adverse effects of any antiseizure medications.)

Errors:

What is the amount of the error compared to the new order? And compared to the original order?

Potential injury to the patient:

Nursing actions:

What would you recommend to the Patient Safety Committee?

CHAPTER 4

Final

1. Write the three metric base units and their abbreviations:

   a. ______________________ __________

   b. ______________________ __________

   c. ______________________ __________

2. Write the abbreviations for the following metric terms:

   a. micrograms ______ b. milligrams ______ c. kilograms ______ d. liter ______

   e. centimeter ______ f. milli ______ g. meter ______ h. millimeter ______

3. Round the following amounts:

	Nearest tenth	Nearest hundredth
a. 4.556 mL	______________________	______________________
b. 1.928 mL	______________________	______________________
c. 0.893 mL	______________________	______________________
d. 7.467 mL	______________________	______________________
e. 0.785 mL	______________________	______________________

4. a. What kind of tablet can be cut? _______

   b. With what implement must the tablet be cut?

5. Why are increasing numbers of medications being supplied in unit-dose packaging in clinical agencies?

6. An antibiotic medication is ordered four times a day. Would you prepare a single dose or the total amount for the day?

7. Your patient has an order for 150 mL of fluid every hour for 10 hours a day. How many liters is the total amount? (Use whole numbers and decimals.) ______________________

8. Your patient has had 4 oz of juice, 8 oz of coffee, and 1 oz of liquid medication. How many mL of fluid has the patient consumed?

9. Ordered: Phenobarbital elixir 20 mg po daily in AM for seizure control. On hand is phenobarbital elixir oral liquid 16.2 mg per 5 mL. How many mL will you give?

10. Ordered: Potassium chloride sol. 25 mEq po daily. On hand is potassium chloride 40 mEq per 15 mL. How many mL will you give?

11. What is the patient-safety issue related to telling patients to use only the calibrated equipment supplied with liquid medications?

12. What is the first step that is needed for a calculation when the measurements for the ordered dose and the supplied dose are in different terms?

13. If 2.2 lb = 1 kg, how many kg does a 150-lb patient weigh to the nearest tenth of a kg?

14. Ordered: Diltiazem tablets E-R 120 mg po daily for a patient with hypertension. How many tablets will you give?

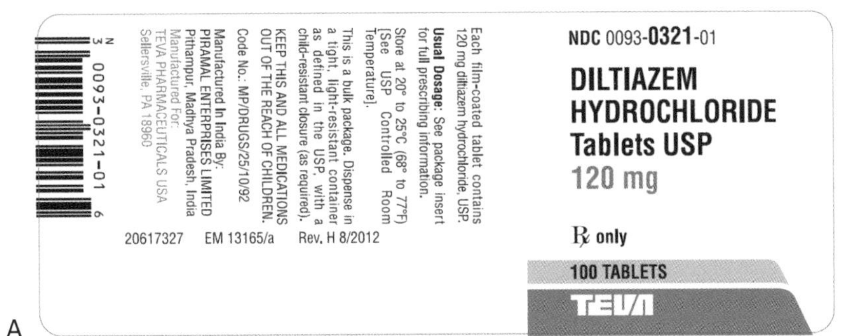

NDC 0093-0321-01
DILTIAZEM HYDROCHLORIDE Tablets USP
120 mg
℞ only
100 TABLETS
TEVA
Each film-coated tablet contains 120 mg diltiazem hydrochloride, USP.
Usual Dosage: See package insert for full prescribing information.
Store at 20° to 25°C (68° to 77°F) [See USP Controlled Room Temperature].
This is a bulk package. Dispense in a tight, light-resistant container as defined in the USP, with a child-resistant closure (as required).
KEEP THIS AND ALL MEDICATIONS OUT OF THE REACH OF CHILDREN.
Code No.: MP/DRUGS/25/10/92
Manufactured In India By: PIRAMAL ENTERPRISES LIMITED Pithampur, Madhya Pradesh, India
Manufactured For: TEVA PHARMACEUTICALS USA Sellersville, PA 18960
20617327 EM 13165/a Rev. H 8/2012
N 3 0093-0321-01 6

A

15. Ordered: Dexamethasone tablets 500 mcg po daily in AM for a patient with an inflammatory disorder. How many tablets will you give?

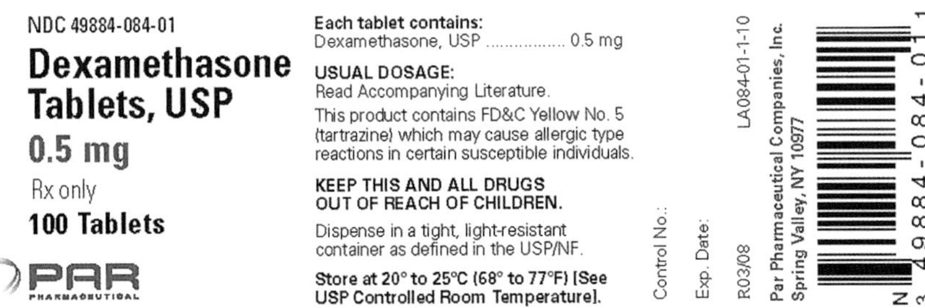

NDC 49884-084-01
Dexamethasone Tablets, USP
0.5 mg
Rx only
100 Tablets
PAR PHARMACEUTICAL
Each tablet contains:
Dexamethasone, USP .... 0.5 mg
USUAL DOSAGE:
Read Accompanying Literature.
This product contains FD&C Yellow No. 5 (tartrazine) which may cause allergic type reactions in certain susceptible individuals.
KEEP THIS AND ALL DRUGS OUT OF REACH OF CHILDREN.
Dispense in a tight, light-resistant container as defined in the USP/NF.
Store at 20° to 25°C (68° to 77°F) [See USP Controlled Room Temperature].
Control No.:
Exp. Date:
LA084-01-1-10
R.03/08
Par Pharmaceutical Companies, Inc.
Spring Valley, NY 10977
N 3 49884-084-01 1

16. Ordered: Cimetidine 0.8 g at bedtime daily for a patient with a gastric ulcer. How many tablets would you give?

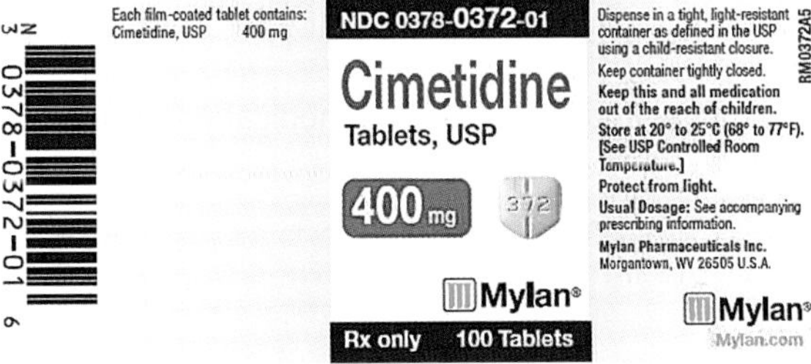

17. Ordered: Elixophylline elixir 0.04 g po for a patient with an infection. How many mL would you give?

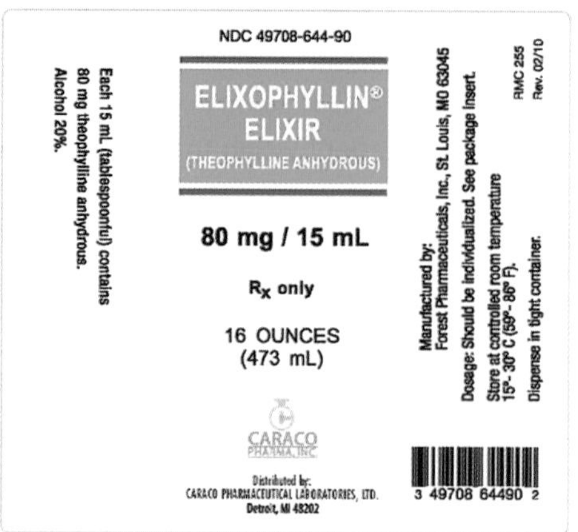

18. Ordered: Tramadol HCl 0.05 g po q12h for a patient with chronic back pain. How many tablets would you give?

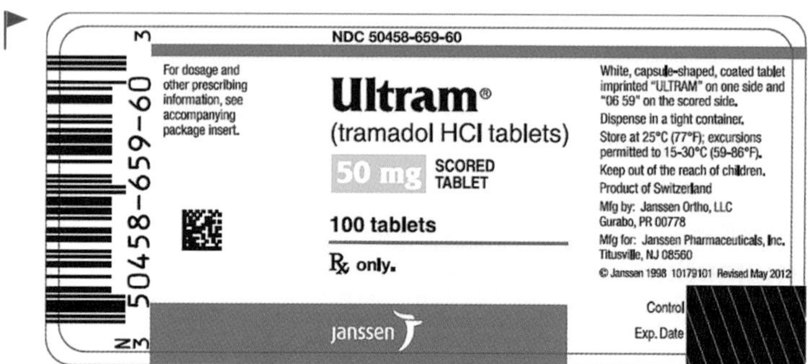

19. Name some instances in which a nurse would hold a medication and recheck the order and/or contact pharmacy or the prescriber.

a.

b.

c.

20. What actions would you take if you made or discovered a medication error?

a.

b.

c.

d.

e.

For additional practice problems, refer to the Conversions and Equivalents and Oral Dosages sections of the Elsevier's Interactive Drug Calculation Application, Version 1 on Evolve.

Answer Key

4 Medication Measurements and Oral Dose Calculations

WORKSHEET 4A (page 104)

	Metric Name	Abbreviation
1. Base unit for weight/mass	gram	g
2. Base unit for volume	liter	L
3. Base unit for length	meter	m
4. Prefix that means 1/1000	milli	m
5. Prefix than means 1/100	centi	c
6. Prefix that means 1,000,000	micro	mc
7. Prefix that means 1/10	deci	d
8. Prefix that means 1000 times	kilo	k
9. Name for the base unit "m"	meter	
10. Name for the prefix "m"	milli	

WORKSHEET 4B (page 105)

1. KNOW WANT TO KNOW

1000 mg : 1 g = 200 mg : x g

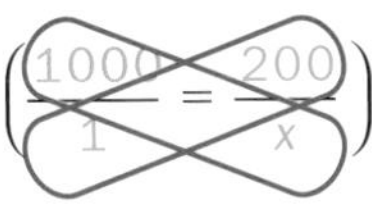

$$\frac{1000}{1000}x = \frac{200}{1000}$$

$$x = 0.2 \text{ g}$$

PROOF

$1000 \times 0.2 = 200$

$1 \times 200 = 200$

2. KNOW WANT TO KNOW

1000 mg : 1 g = 250 mg : x g

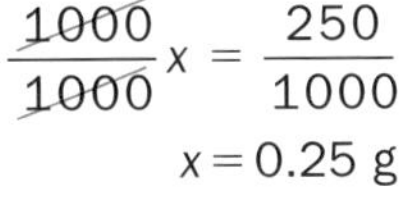

$$\frac{1000}{1000}x = \frac{250}{1000}$$

$$x = 0.25 \text{ g}$$

PROOF

$1000 \times 0.25 = 250$

$1 \times 250 = 250$

3. KNOW WANT TO KNOW

1000 mg : 1 g = 25 mg : x g

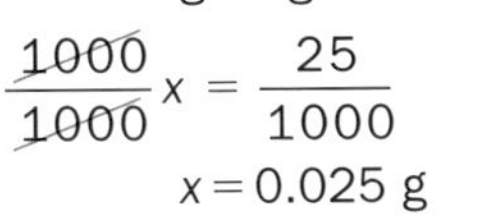

$$\frac{1000}{1000}x = \frac{25}{1000}$$

$$x = 0.025 \text{ g}$$

PROOF

$1000 \times 0.025 = 25$

$1 \times 25 = 25$

4. KNOW WANT TO KNOW

1 g : 1000 mg = 2.5 g : x mg

$x = 1000 \times 2.5$

$x = 2500$ mg

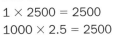

PROOF

$1 \times 2500 = 2500$

$1000 \times 2.5 = 2500$

5. KNOW WANT TO KNOW

1 g : 1000 mg = 0.5 g : *x mg*

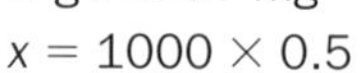

$x = 1000 \times 0.5$

$x = 500$ mg

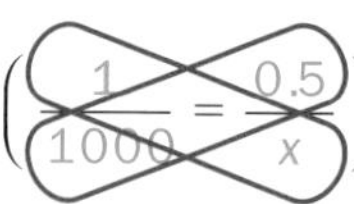

$$\frac{1}{1000} = \frac{0.5}{x}$$

PROOF

$1 \times 500 = 500$

$1000 \times 0.5 = 500$

6. KNOW WANT TO KNOW

1 g : 1000 mg = 0.01 g : *x mg*

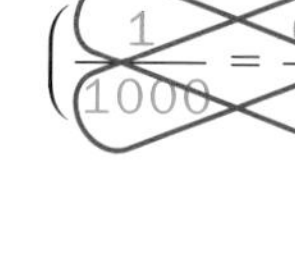

$$\frac{1}{1000} = \frac{0.01}{x}$$

$x = 1000 \times 0.01$

$x = 10$ mg

PROOF

$1 \times 10 = 10$

$1000 \times 0.01 = 10$

7. KNOW WANT TO KNOW

1000 mcg : 1 mg = 150 mcg : *x* mg

$$\frac{1000}{1000}x = \frac{150}{1000}$$

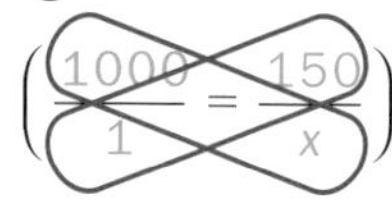

$$\frac{1000}{1} = \frac{150}{x}$$

$x = 0.15$ mg

PROOF

$1000 \times 0.15 = 150$

$1 \times 150 = 150$

8. KNOW WANT TO KNOW

1000 mcg : 1 mg = 500 mcg : *x* mg

$$\frac{1000}{1} = \frac{500}{x}$$

$$\frac{1000}{1000}x = \frac{500}{1000}$$

$x = 0.5$ mg

PROOF

1000×0.5 mg $= 500$

$1 \times 500 = 500$

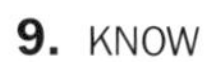

9. KNOW WANT TO KNOW

1000 mcg : 1 mg = 2500 mcg : *x mg*

$$\frac{1000}{1000}x = \frac{2500}{1000}$$

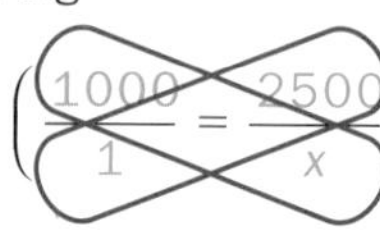

$$\frac{1000}{1} = \frac{2500}{x}$$

$x = 2.5$ mg

PROOF

$1000 \times 2.5 = 2500$

$1 \times 2500 = 2500$

10. KNOW WANT TO KNOW

1 mg : 1000 mcg = 5 mg : *x* mcg

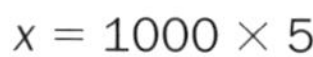

$x = 1000 \times 5$

$$\frac{1}{1000} = \frac{5}{x}$$

$x = 5000$ mcg

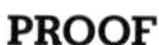

PROOF

$1 \times 5000 = 5000$

$1000 \times 5 = 5000$

11. KNOW WANT TO KNOW

1 mg : 1000 mcg = 0.1 mg : *x* mcg

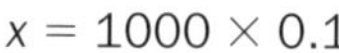

$x = 1000 \times 0.1$

$$\frac{1}{1000} = \frac{0.1}{x}$$

$x = 100$ mcg

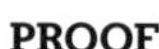

PROOF

$1 \times 100 = 100$

$1000 \times 0.1 = 100$

12. KNOW WANT TO KNOW

1 mg : 1000 mcg = 0.04 mg : *x* mcg

$x = 1000 \times 0.04$

$$\frac{1}{1000} = \frac{0.04}{x}$$

$x = 40$ mcg

PROOF

$1 \times 40 = 40$

$1000 \times 0.04 = 40$

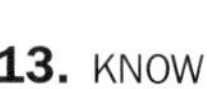

13. KNOW WANT TO KNOW

1 kg : 1000 g = 5.5 kg : *x* g

$$\frac{1}{1000} = \frac{5.5}{x}$$

$x = 1000 \times 5.5$

$x = 5500$ g

PROOF

$1 \times 5500 = 5500$

$1000 \times 5.5 = 5500$

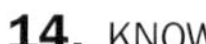

14. KNOW WANT TO KNOW

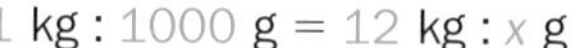

1 kg : 1000 g = 12 kg : *x* g

$$\frac{1}{1000} = \frac{12}{x}$$

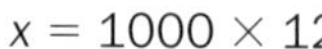

$x = 1000 \times 12$

$x = 12{,}000$ g

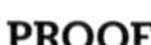

PROOF

$1 \times 12{,}000 = 12{,}000$

$1000 \times 12 = 12{,}000$

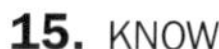

15. KNOW WANT TO KNOW

1 kg : 1000 g = 0.5 kg : *x* g

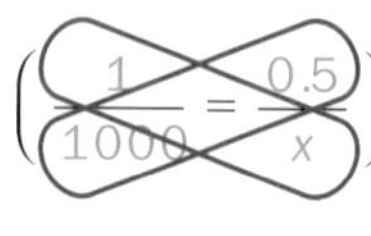

$$\frac{1}{1000} = \frac{0.5}{x}$$

$x = 1000 \times 0.5$

$x = 500$ g

PROOF

$1 \times 500 = 500$

$1000 \times 0.5 = 500$

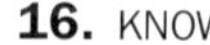

16. KNOW WANT TO KNOW

1 L : 1000 mL = 0.5 L : *x* mL

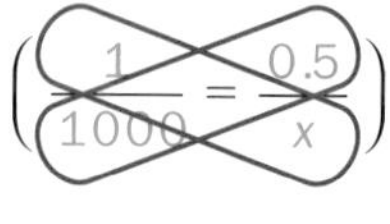

$$\frac{1}{1000} = \frac{0.5}{x}$$

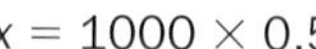

$x = 1000 \times 0.5$

$x = 500$ mL

PROOF

$1 \times 500 = 500$

$1000 \times 0.5 = 500$

17. KNOW WANT TO KNOW

1 L : 1000 mL = 1.3 L : x mL

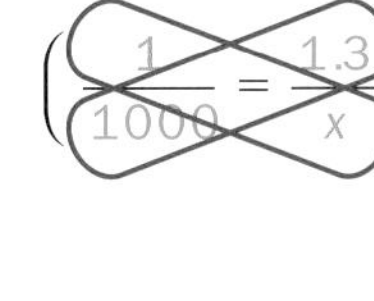

$x = 1000 \times 1.3$

$x = 1300$ mL

PROOF

$1 \times 1300 = 1300$

$1000 \times 1.3 = 1300$

18. KNOW WANT TO KNOW

1 L : 1000 mL = 2.8 L : x mL

$\frac{1}{1000} = \frac{2.8}{x}$

$x = 1000 \times 2.8$

$x = 2800$ mL

PROOF

$1 \times 2800 = 2800$

$1000 \times 2.8 = 2800$

19. KNOW WANT TO KNOW

1 L : 1000 mL = x L : 1200 mL

$\frac{1}{1000} = \frac{x}{1200}$

$\frac{1000}{1000}x = \frac{1200}{1000}$

$x = 1.2$ L

PROOF

$1 \times 1200 = 1200$

$1000 \times 1.2 = 1200$

20. KNOW WANT TO KNOW

1 L : 1000 mL = x L : 800 mL

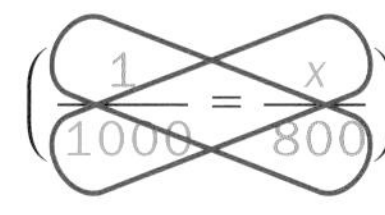

$\frac{1000}{1000}x = \frac{800}{1000}$

$x = 0.8$ L

PROOF

$1 \times 800 = 800$

$1000 \times 0.8 = 800$

WORKSHEET **4C** (page 108)

Grams to Milligrams		Milligrams to Grams	
g	**? mg**	**mg**	**? g**
2 g	2000	5000 mg	5
2.5 g	2500	3500 mg	3.5
1.5 g	1500	1200 mg	1.2
0.1 g	100	800 mg	0.8
0.5 g	500	400 mg	0.4
0.25 g	250	350 mg	0.35
0.15 g	150	200 mg	0.2
0.03 g	30	125 mg	0.125
0.015 g	15	80 mg	0.08
0.075 g	75	50 mg	0.05

Micrograms to Milligrams		Milligrams to Micrograms	
mcg	**? mg**	**mg**	**? mcg**
7500	7.5	1.5	1500
1200	1.2	0.8	800
750	0.75	0.3	300
500	0.5	0.25	250
100	0.1	0.125	125

WORKSHEET **4D** (page 110)

1. 5000 mcg
2. 500 mg
3. 5500 g
4. 2.5 mg
5. 2 kg

WORKSHEET **4E** (page 110)

1. 500 mL
2. 15 mL
3. 240 mL
4. 250 mL
5. 1500 mL

WORKSHEET **4F** (page 113)

1. HAVE WANT TO HAVE

5 mg : 1 tablet = 15 mg : x tablets

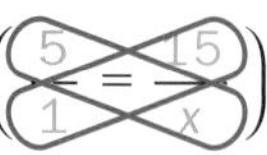

$$\frac{\not 5}{\not 5}x = \frac{15}{5}$$

x = 3 tablets

PROOF
5 × 3 = 15
1 × 15 = 15

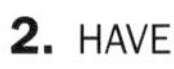

2. HAVE WANT TO HAVE

200 mg : 1 capsule = 400 mg : x capsules

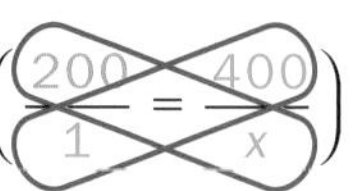

$$\frac{\not{200}}{\not{200}}x = \frac{400}{200}$$

x = 2 capsules

PROOF
200 × 2 = 400
1 × 400 = 400

Refrigeration directions: Refrigerate prior to dispensing.

3. HAVE WANT TO HAVE

100 mg : 1 tablet = 200 mg : x tablets

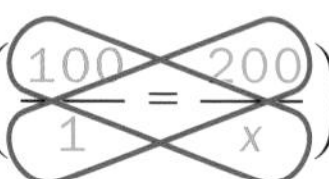

$$\frac{\not{100}}{\not{100}}x = \frac{200}{100}$$

x = 2 tablets

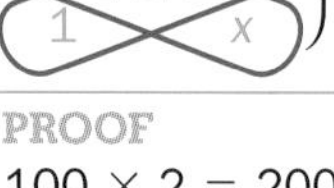

PROOF
100 × 2 = 200
1 × 200 = 200

4. HAVE WANT TO HAVE

0.25 mg : 1 tablet = 0.125 mg : x tablets

$$\left(\frac{0.25}{1} = \frac{0.125}{x}\right)$$

$$\frac{\not{0.25}}{\not{0.25}}x = \frac{0.125}{0.25}$$

$x = \frac{1}{2}$ tablet

PROOF
$0.25 \times \frac{1}{2} = 0.125$
1 × 0.125 = 0.125

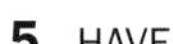

5. HAVE WANT TO HAVE

160 mg : 1 tablet = 80 mg : x tablets

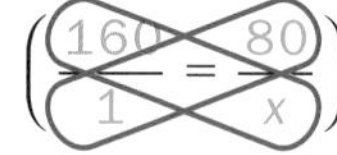

$$\frac{\not{160}}{\not{160}}x = \frac{8\not{0}}{16\not{0}}$$

x = 0.5 tablet

PROOF
1 × 80 = 80
160 × 0.5 = 80

HAVE WANT TO HAVE

800 mg : 1 tablet = 400 mg : x tablets

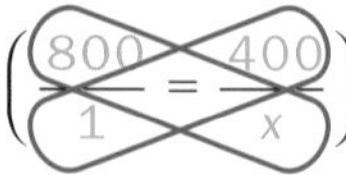

$$\frac{800}{800}x = \frac{800}{400}$$

x = 0.5 tablet

PROOF
1 × 400 = 400
800 × 0.5 = 400

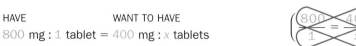

Note: ½ tablet contains the total dose for the two drugs

WORKSHEET 4G (page 116)

1. a More	**b** 2 capsules (300 : 1 = 600 : x) $\frac{300}{300}x = \frac{600}{300}$ $x = 2$	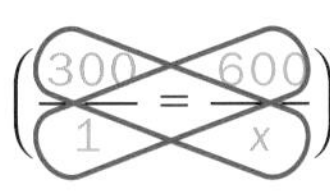
2. a Recheck tablet supplied, regular or XL; must be XL	**b** 1 XL tablet (100 : 1 = 100 : x) $\frac{100}{100}x = \frac{100}{100}$ $x = 1$	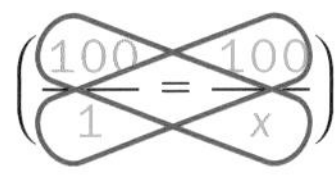
3. a More	**b** 1.5 tablets (50 : 1 = 75 : x) $\frac{50}{50}x = \frac{75}{50}$ $x = 1.5$	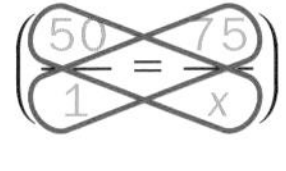
4. a Same	**b** 1 tablet (175 : 1 = 175 : x) $\frac{175}{175}x = \frac{175}{175}$ $x = 1$	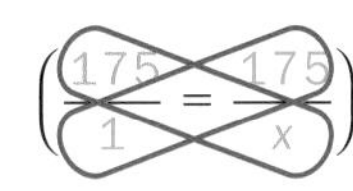
5. a Contact pharmacy.	**b** Cannot cut unscored tablets	N/A

WORKSHEET 4H (page 117)

1. 3 tsp = 1 Tbsp
2. 2 Tbsp = 1 ounce
3. 5 mL = 1 tsp
4. 15 mL = 1 Tbsp
5. 240 mL = 1 cup
6. 1000 mL = 1 L
7. 1 quart = 1 liter
8. 2.2 lb = 1 kg
9. 2.5 cm = 1 inch
10. 10 mm = 1 cm

Note: Use metric measurements for medications.

WORKSHEET 4I (page 121)

1. 2.5 mL

10 mg : 5 mL = 5 mg : x mL

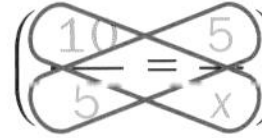

$\frac{10x}{10} = \frac{25}{10}$ $x = 2.5$ mL

PROOF 10 × 2.5 = 25
5 × 5 = 25

2. 7.5 mL

20 mEq : 15 mL = 10 mEq : x mL

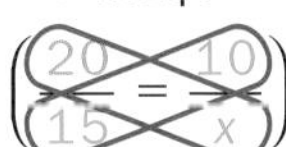

$\frac{20}{20}x = \frac{150}{20}$ $x = 7.5$ mL

PROOF 20 × 7.5 = 150
15 × 10 = 150

3. 10 mL

125 mg : 5 mL = 250 mg : x mL

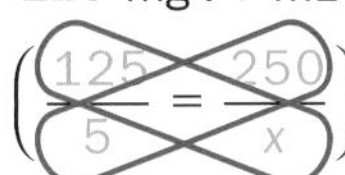

$\frac{125x}{125} = \frac{1250}{125}$ $x = 10$ mL

PROOF 125 × 10 = 1250
5 × 250 = 1250

4. 7.5 mL

200 mg : 5 mL = 300 mg : x mL

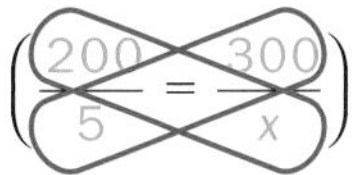

$\frac{200}{200}x = \frac{1500}{200}$ $x = 7.5$ mL

PROOF 200 × 7.5 = 1500
5 × 300 = 1500

5. 4 mL

300 mg : 5 mL = 240 mg : x mL

$$\left(\frac{300}{5} = \frac{240}{x}\right)$$

$$\frac{300x}{300} = \frac{1200}{300} \qquad x = 4 \text{ mL}$$

PROOF $300 \times 4 = 1200$
$5 \times 240 = 1200$

WORKSHEET 4J (page 123)

1. a More	**b** 8 mL (125 mg : 5 mL = 200 mg : x mL) $\left(\frac{125}{5} = \frac{200}{x}\right)$ $\frac{125}{125}x = \frac{1000}{125} \qquad x = 8 \text{ mL}$ **PROOF** $125 \times 8 = 1000$ $5 \times 200 = 1000$
2. a Same	**b** 5 mL 5 mg : 5 mL = 5 mg : x (1 mg : 1 mL = 5 mg : x mL) $\left(\frac{1}{1} = \frac{5}{x}\right) \qquad x = 5 \text{ mL}$ **PROOF** $5 \times 5 = 25$ $(1 \times 5 = 5)$ $5 \times 5 = 25$ $(1 \times 5 = 5)$
3. a More	**b** 10 mL (4 mg : 5 mL = 8 mg : x mL) $\left(\frac{4}{5} = \frac{8}{x}\right)$ $\frac{4}{4}x = \frac{40}{4} \qquad x = 10 \text{ mL}$ **PROOF** $4 \times 10 = 40$ $5 \times 8 = 40$
4. a More	**b** 7.5 mL (20 mg : 5 mL = 30 mg : x mL) $\left(\frac{20}{5} = \frac{30}{x}\right)$ $\frac{20}{20}x = \frac{150}{20} \qquad x = 7.5 \text{ mL}$ **PROOF** $20 \times 7.5 = 150$ $5 \times 30 = 150$
5. a Less	**b** 5 mL (30 mg : 15 mL = 10 mg : x mL) $\left(\frac{30}{15} = \frac{10}{x}\right)$ $\frac{30}{30}x = \frac{150}{30} \qquad x = 5 \text{ mL}$ **PROOF** $30 \times 5 = 150$ $15 \times 10 = 150$

WORKSHEET 4K (page 124)

1. 1 g
2. g
3. L
4. a. overdose b. 1000 times overdose
5. a. 3.4 g b. 2.3 g c. 1500 mg
6. underdose
7. a. 240 mL b. 1920 mL c. 1.92 L
8. Step 1: Find equivalent terms. Step 2: Calculate the dose using the equivalent terms.
9. 100 kg (divide lb by 2)
10. 3 metric teaspoons

WORKSHEET 4L (page 126)

1. a. Change mg to mcg

   b. KNOW WANT TO KNOW

   1000 mcg : 1 mg = x mcg : 0.35 mg

   $x = 1000 \times 0.35$

   $x = 350$ mcg

   PROOF
   $1000 \times 0.35 = 350$
   $1 \times 350 = 350$

   c. HAVE WANT TO HAVE

   175 : 1 tablet = 350 : x tablets

   $$\frac{175}{175}x = \frac{350}{175}$$

   $x = 2$ tablets

   PROOF
   $2 \times 175 = 350$
   $1 \times 350 = 350$

2. a. Change mcg to mg

   b. KNOW WANT TO KNOW

   1000 mcg : 1 mg = 250 mcg : x mg

   $$\frac{1000}{1000}x = \frac{250}{1000}$$

   $x = 0.25$ mg

   PROOF
   $1000 \times 0.25 = 250$
   $1 \times 250 = 250$

   Alternate Solution:
   Since label also gives mcg

   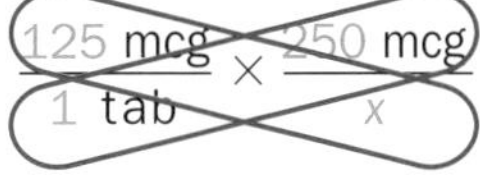

   $$\frac{125 \text{ mcg}}{1 \text{ tab}} \times \frac{250 \text{ mcg}}{x}$$

   PROOF
   $1 \times 250 = 250$
   $2 \times 125 = 250$

   $125x = 250$

   $x = 2$ tablets

   c. HAVE WANT TO HAVE

   0.125 mg : 1 scored tablet = 0.25 mg : x tablets

   $$\frac{0.125x}{0.125} = \frac{0.25}{0.125}$$

   $x = 2$ tablets

   PROOF
   $0.125 \times 2 = 0.25$
   $1 \times 0.25 = 0.25$

3. The order does not specify the extended release form.

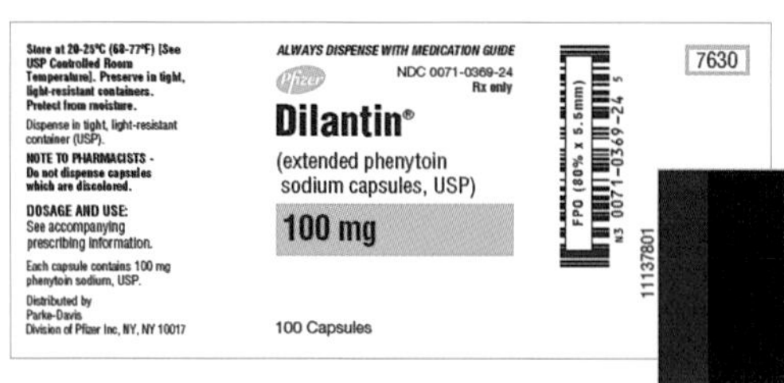

a. Not needed. The order needs to be rechecked with the record and with pharmacy.

The prescriber may need to be contacted to confirm the order.

Document the clarification.

4. a. Change mcg to mg

b. KNOW WANT TO KNOW

1000 mcg : 1 mg = 750 mcg : x mg

$$\frac{1000}{1000}x = \frac{750}{1000}$$

x = 0.75 mg

PROOF
1000 × 0.75 = 750
1 × 750 = 750

c. HAVE WANT TO HAVE

1 mg : 1 mL = 0.75 mg : x mL

x = 0.75 mL

PROOF
1 × 0.75 = 0.75
1 × 0.75 = 0.75

d. 30 mL

CLINICAL RELEVANCE

Teach the patient to rinse and reuse the equipment that is packaged with this medication.

5. a. Conversion not needed.

b. KNOW WANT TO KNOW

N/A

PROOF
N/A

c. HAVE WANT TO HAVE

10 mg : 5 mL = 8 mg : x mL

10x = 40

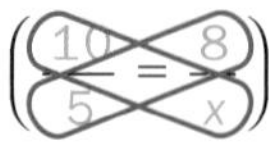

$$\frac{10}{10}x = \frac{40}{10}$$

x = 4 mL

PROOF
10 × 4 = 40
8 × 5 = 40

WORKSHEET **4M** (page 130)

1. c. 1000 mL : 1 L = x mL : 0.5 L

x = 1000 × 0.5

x = 500 mL

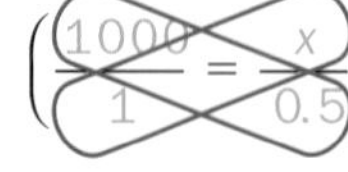

2. a. 1000 mg = 1 g

3. b. (5 mL per teaspoon)

4. a. 1000 mg = 1g 200 mg = 0.2 g 1000 mcg = 1 mg; 200,000 mcg = 200 mg
Note: it helps to write the metric base equivalents in mg and mcg

5. c. 500 mg ÷ 4 = 125 mg per dose. Only the current dose is prepared.

6. d. 3 places to the left

7. a. Excess medication needs to be discarded. The other methods risk wasting medication.

8. b. 2.5 cm = 1 inch

9. d. Units needs to be written out with a capital "U" and commas.

10. c. 2.2 lb = 1 kg. Dividing pounds by 2 gives a rough estimate of the equivalent for the kg.

CHAPTER 4 FINAL: MEDICATION MEASUREMENTS AND ORAL DOSE CALCULATIONS (page 134)

1. a. (weight/mass) gram (g) **b.** (volume) liter (L) **c.** (length) meter (m)

2. a. mc + g = mcg **b.** m + g = mg **c.** k + g = kg
d. L (capitalized) (small l's look like a number 1) **e.** c + m = cm
f. m **g.** m **h.** m + m = mm

3.	**Nearest tenth**	**Nearest hundredth**
a.	4.6	4.56
b.	1.9	1.93
c.	0.9	0.89
d.	7.5	7.47
e.	0.8	0.79

4. a. scored tablet **b.** a pill cutter

5. Unit-dose packaging reduces underdose and overdose errors and reduces waste that occurs with multidose containers.

6. You would only calculate and/or prepare a single dose, not the daily dose.

7. 1500 mL; 1.5 L

8. 120 + 240 + 30 = 390 mL have been consumed. (1 oz = 30 mL)

9. 6.17 rounded to 6.2 mL (16.2 mg : 5 mL = 20 mg : x mL) 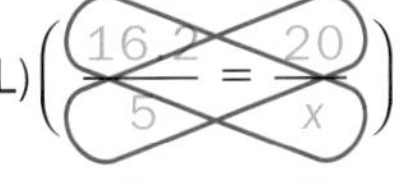

10. 9.37 rounded to 9.4 mL (40 mEq : 15 mL = 25 mEq : x mL) 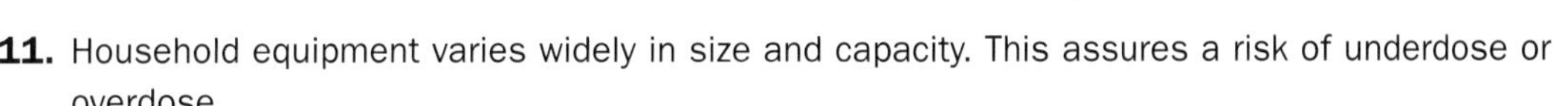

11. Household equipment varies widely in size and capacity. This assures a risk of underdose or overdose.

12. Obtain equivalent terms first. Then calculate the dose.

13. 68.18 rounded to 68.2 kg (2.2 lb : 1 kg = 150 lb : x kg) 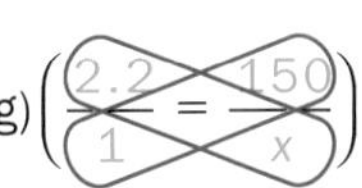

14. The label does not state extended release (E-R or S-R). Hold the medication. Recheck the order. If the patient has been taking the medication at home, get some information from the patient, if possible, about type and how many times a day the medication has been taken. Recheck the order with pharmacy and/or the prescriber. Note: Color of pills changes if manufacturer of brand or generic company is changed.

15. 1 tablet (1000 mcg : 1 mg = 500 mcg : x mg) (0.5 mg : 1 tablet = 0.5 mg : x tablets)

Note: What you have on hand is the first entry, on the left, in the dose calculation equation step.

16. 2 tablets (1000 mg : 1 g = x mg : 0.8 g) (400 mg : 1 tablet = 800 mg : x tablets)

17. 7.5 mL (1000 mg : 1 g = x mg : 0.04 g) (80 mg : 15 mL = 40 mg : x mL)

18. 1 tablet (1000 mg : 1 g = x mg : 0.05 g) (50 mg : 1 tablet = 50 mg : 1 tablet)

19. **a.** order or label unclear

b. patient states allergic to the medication or similar medications

c. patient states medication looks different from what was being taken

d. patient is complaining of new issue (rash, diarrhea, nausea, etc.), which could be result of a side effect of this particular medication

e. patient refuses the medication

20. **a.** Assess patient and attend to immediate needs with help if necessary to take corrective action

b. Notify supervisor promptly and prescriber (many agency policies have the supervisor notify the prescriber if it is necessary).

c. Follow agency policy about what is to be recorded on the patient MAR.

d. Document frequent follow-up assessments on the MAR in a timely manner.

e. Fill out an incident report according to agency policy the same day, and give it to the supervisor or appropriate department.

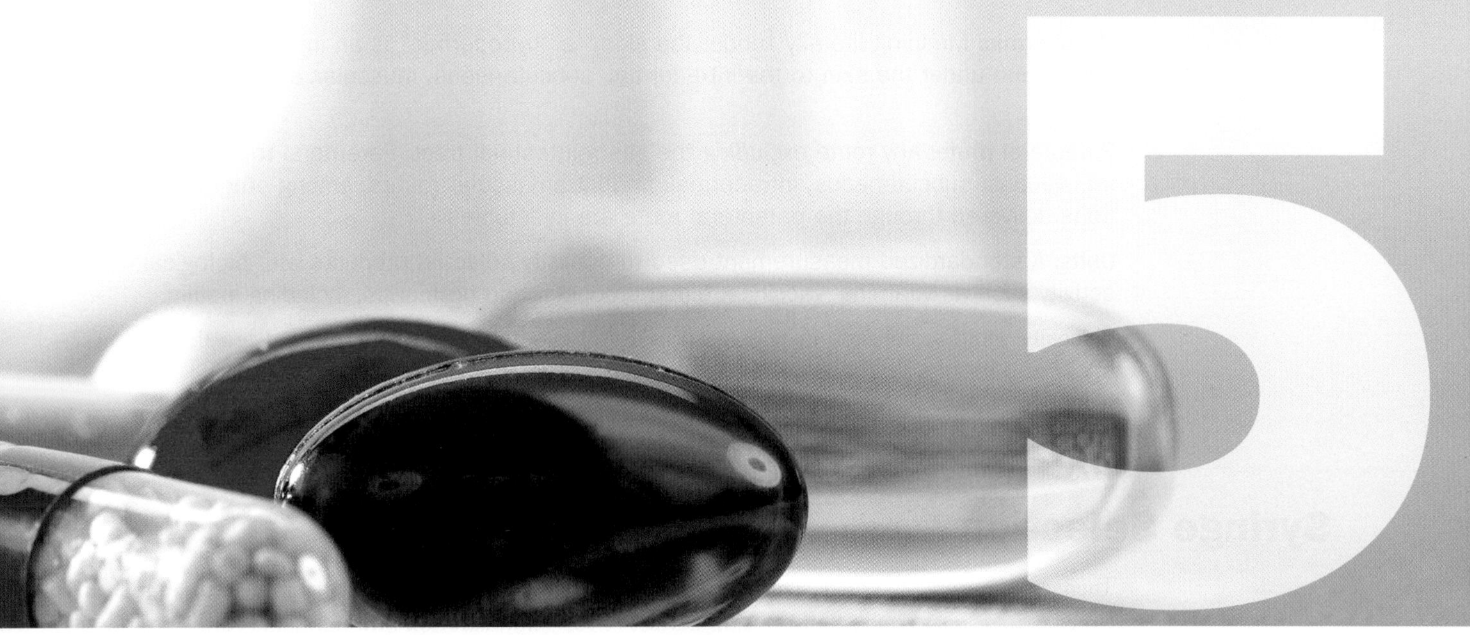

Injectable Medication Calculations

Objectives

- Read and measure syringe capacities and volumes.
- Identify the lowest measurable dose on various syringes.
- Identify critical information on injectable labels.
- Calculate injectable doses.
- Differentiate tuberculin and insulin syringes.
- State three criteria for needle selection.
- State safety measures to protect the patient from injectable medication errors.
- State safety measures to protect the nurse from needlestick injuries.

Introduction

The trend for pharmacies to supply unit-dose injectable medications reduces contamination, dose errors, and waste. This chapter focuses on intradermal, subcutaneous, and intramuscular routes.* The medications that may be encountered for these routes include vaccines, antidiabetic agents, insulin products, anticoagulants, pain medications, and emergency drugs, as well as a variety of medications that are to be given relatively infrequently or for a short period. Injectable medications that have to be given frequently are often given by the intravenous route to avoid the emotional and/or physical trauma of multiple needlesticks.

Dose calculations for injectable medications are the same as for oral liquid medications.

Vocabulary

Calibration: A set of gradations on a scale to indicate values, such as seen on a ruler or a syringe.

cc: An abbreviation for cubic centimeter (ccm) occasionally used interchangeably with milliliter. May be seen on some syringes. *Write mL.* Do not write cc.† It has been misinterpreted as aa or two zeros, 00, when not written carefully.

---

*Intravenous medications are covered in later chapters.
†See ISMP Error-Prone Abbreviations in Appendix B.

Hypodermic: Meaning literally "under the skin," a "hypodermic" is an injection that delivers medication under the skin to the intradermal, subcutaneous, muscular, and intravenous layers.

Parenteral route: Any route excluding the gastrointestinal tract. Parenteral routes include intravenous, subcutaneous, intradermal, and intramuscular routes, among others. Medications delivered through the parenteral route are injectables.

Units: A standardized measurement used to quantify selected products with biological activity such as vitamins, vaccines, blood products, and hormones, including insulin.

Viscosity: Fluid resistance to flow seen in some injectable medications that are thick or sticky and require larger-diameter needles.

Syringe Selection

There are a variety of syringe sizes available—from 1 mL, 3 mL, 5 mL, and 10 mL up to 60 mL. The larger syringes may be used for infusion devices or for administration into the spinal cord (intrathecal) and other special procedures. The nurse most frequently uses the 1-, 3-, 5-, and 10-mL syringe sizes (Figure 5.1).

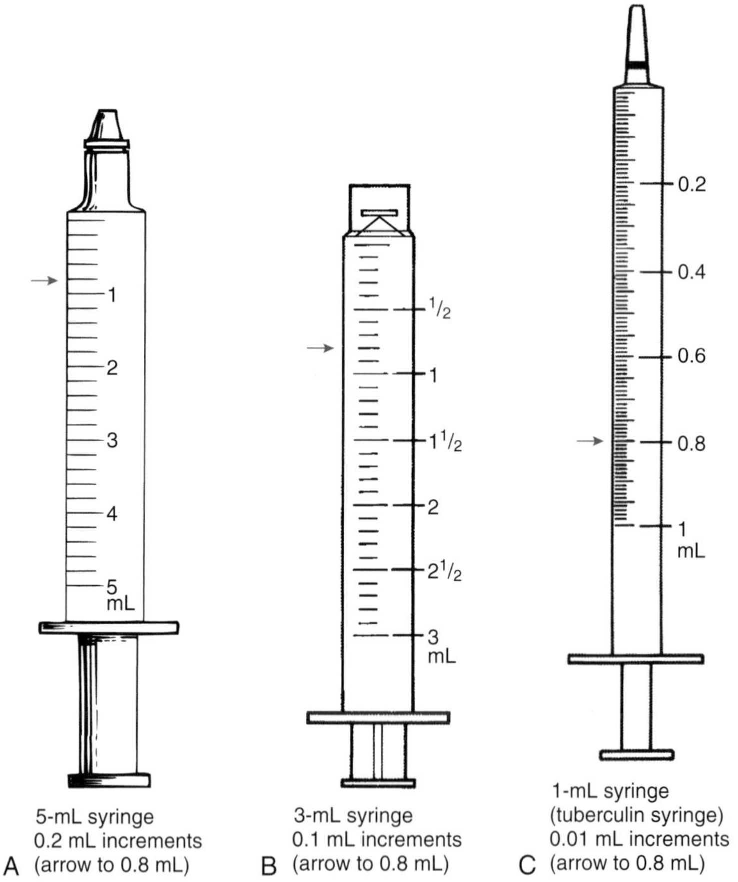

FIGURE 5.1 Comparison of syringe sizes and calibrations. Note the red arrows are where the 0.8-mL dose is measured. **A,** 5-mL syringe. **B,** 3-mL syringe. **C,** 1-mL tuberculin syringe.

A 5-mL syringe 0.2 mL increments (arrow to 0.8 mL)

B 3-mL syringe 0.1 mL increments (arrow to 0.8 mL)

C 1-mL syringe (tuberculin syringe) 0.01 mL increments (arrow to 0.8 mL)

The selection of a syringe depends on several practical factors:

- The *volume* of the medication to be administered and the capacity of the syringe so that the nearest measurable dose ordered can be given. For a medication dose of 3 mL, you would not select three (1-mL) syringes or a 10-mL syringe.

CLINICAL ALERT!

If the syringe is at full capacity, be aware there is risk of disconnection of the plunger from the syringe. Figure 5.2 illustrates a syringe with the plunger in partial extensions.

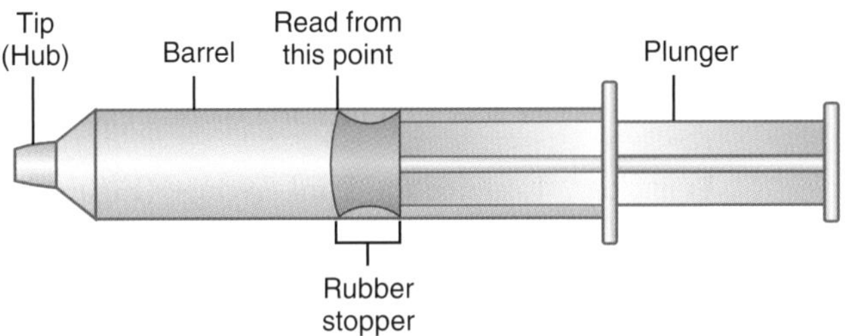

FIGURE 5.2 Parts of a syringe. (From Kee JL, Marshall SM: Clinical calculations: with applications to general and specialty areas, ed 8, St Louis, 2017, Saunders.)

CLINICAL RELEVANCE

Check agency policies regarding slight, gentle withdrawal of the plunger after the needle is inserted to check for blood return. Blood return may indicate that the needle is in a blood vessel. The procedure is standard for administration of intravenous injections, but the benefits are controversial for subcutaneous and intramuscular injections.

- The *calibrations* on the syringe. If you need to give 2.7 mL, the syringe size has to have 0.1 increments to measure the portion of the dose.
- The *route* to be administered. Larger-barrel syringes deliver with lower pressure than narrow barrels. This is important when delivering viscous medications or delivering directly into veins or narrow tubing.
- The *viscosity* of the medication ordered. Very thick medications need to be administered in a syringe that is large enough to accommodate more pressure without the needle detaching from the syringe. Syringes are usually chosen on the basis of the volume of the medication and the syringe capacity in order to give the nearest measurable dose of the medication for intradermal, intramuscular, and subcutaneous routes. Some syringes are selected based on the route.

  To measure doses and read syringe volumes, examine the illustrated syringes in this *suggested order:*

Steps for Reading and Measuring Amounts in a Syringe

1. **Identify the *total liquid capacity* of the syringe and the capacity between two adjacent bold calibrations.** The major calibrations are bolder with longer lines. Different-sized syringes will have different capacities between the calibrations.
2. **Divide the measured capacity by the number of spaces within two adjacent bold lines.** This gives you the **capacity *per calibration*—the lowest measurable dose, which will be in increments of 0.01 mL, 0.1 mL, 0.2 mL, 1 mL, or larger.**
3. **Identify the minimum and maximum range** of doses that may be given with the syringe.

Note the 3-mL syringe illustration (Figure 5.3). The 3-mL syringe is frequently used for subcutaneous and intramuscular injections, depending upon the size of the patient.

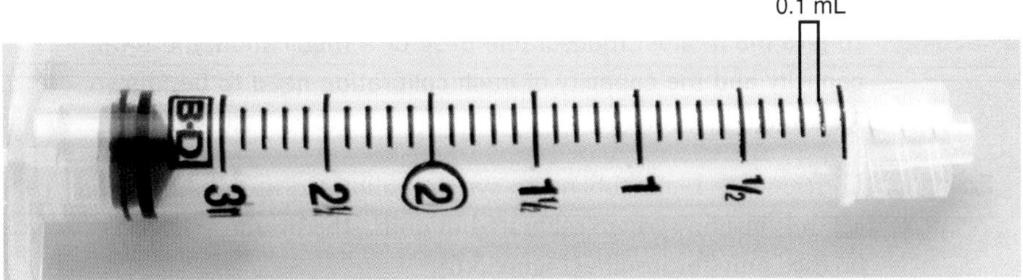

FIGURE 5.3 3-mL syringe calibrated in 0.1-mL increments.

Total Capacity:	3 mL
Capacity between 2 adjacent bold calibrations:	0.5 mL
Lowest measurable dose (capacity each calibration):	0.1 mL (1 mL ÷ 10 spaces)
Minimum/maximum dose range:	0.1 mL to 3 mL in increments of tenths of a mL

Doses in tenths of a milliliter, such as 1.4 mL or 2.8 mL up to 3 mL, may be given. Doses of *less than 0.1 mL* or more than 3 mL *cannot* be measured on this syringe. Doses of hundredths of a milliliter, such as 1.04 mL or 2.07 mL, cannot be measured.

Examples Examine the 5-mL syringe (Figure 5.4). This syringe is used for intramuscular injections.

Total Capacity:	5 mL
Capacity between 2 adjacent bold calibrations:	1 mL
Lowest measurable dose (capacity each calibration):	0.2 mL (1 mL ÷ 5 spaces)
Minimum/maximum dose range:	0.2 mL to 5 mL in 0.2-mL increments

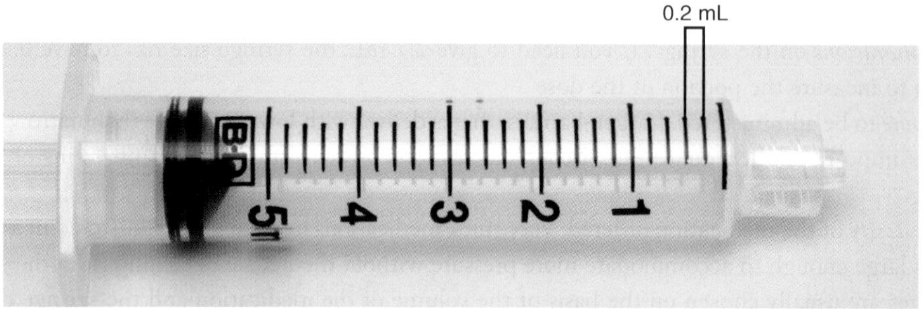

FIGURE 5.4 5-mL syringe calibrated in 0.2-mL increments.

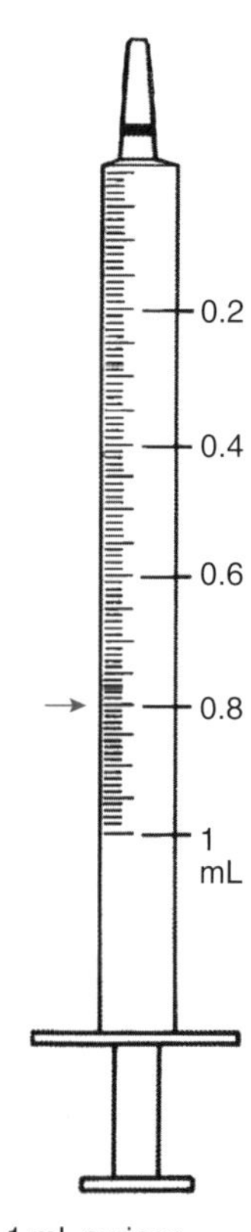

1 mL syringe (tuberculin syringe) 0.01 mL increments (arrow to 0.8 mL)

FIGURE 5.5 1-mL syringe.

Doses that end with an even number, such as 1.2 mL or 3.6 mL, can be measured. Odd-numbered doses cannot be measured.

The 1 mL tuberculin syringe is used for skin tests and injectable volumes of 1 mL or less.

Total Capacity:	1-mL tuberculin syringe
Capacity between 2 adjacent bold calibrations:	0.2 mL
Lowest measurable dose (capacity each calibration):	0.01 mL (0.2 mL ÷ 20 spaces)
Minimum/maximum dose range:	0.01 mL to 1 mL in increments of 0.01 mL

Doses of less than and up to 1 mL can be given in hundredths and tenths of a milliliter. For example, doses such as 0.05 mL, 0.36 mL, 0.8 mL, and 0.91 mL can be given. Doses that exceed 1 mL cannot be given.

remember **To give the nearest measurable dose of a medication, the total capacity and the capacity of each calibration need to be known for syringe selection.**

Example Differentiate 1-mL tuberculin syringe calibrated in milliliters from a 1-mL insulin syringe calibrated in units. The insulin syringe is to be used only for insulin (Figure 5.6).

Prefilled syringes are thought to reduce medication dose errors by simplifying home use, delivering precise doses, and minimizing medication waste. Some need to be attached to compatible equipment as shown in Figure 5.7, *A* to *D*. Others are provided as a syringe and may have a needle attached (Figure 5.7, *E* and *F*).

Prefilled Auto-injector syringes contain a hidden fine needle that is released immediately when the barrel contacts the skin. Figure 5.7, *F* is an example of a single-use autoinjector pen.

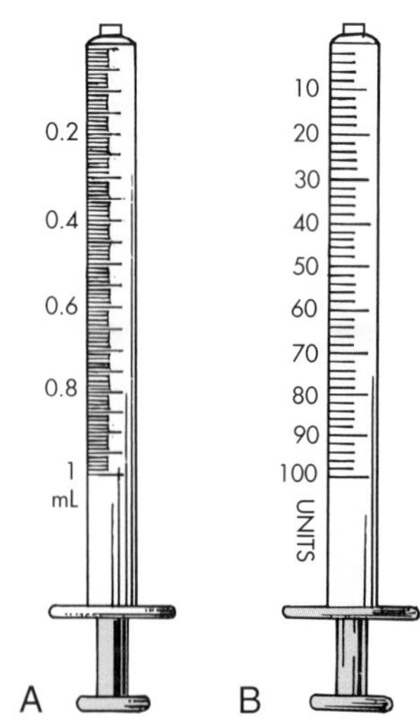

FIGURE 5.6 **A,** 1-mL tuberculin syringe. **B,** 100-unit 1-mL insulin syringe. (From Perry AG, Potter PA, Ostendorf WR: *Clinical nursing skills and techniques,* ed 9, St Louis, 2018, Mosby.)

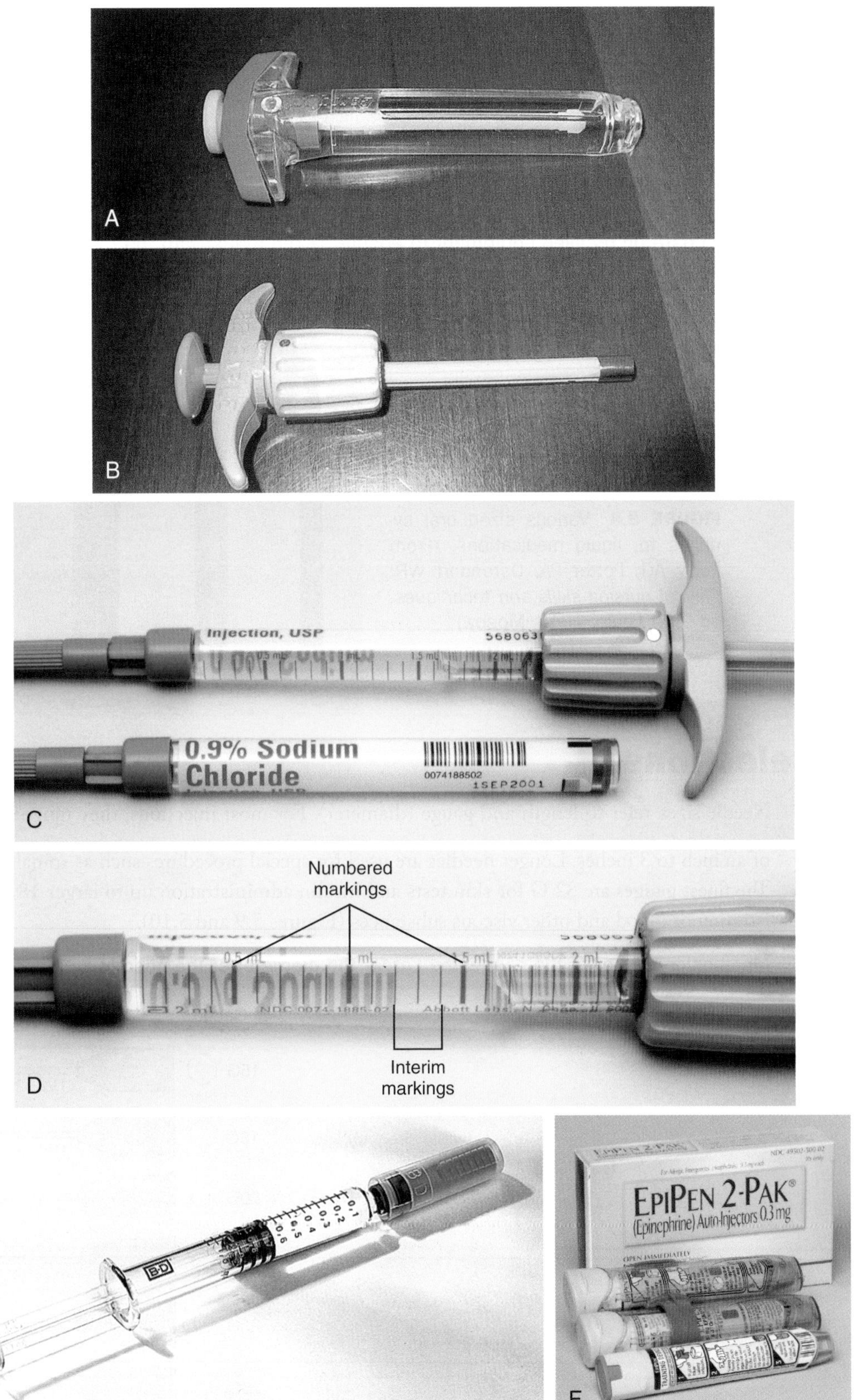

FIGURE 5.7 **A,** Carpuject syringe holder. **B,** Tubex syringe holder. **C,** Tubex prefilled cartridge syringe in holder. **D,** Tubex prefilled cartridge syringe with calibrations (enlarged). **E,** B-D Hypak prefilled syringe. **F,** Epipen—a prefilled autoinjector containing epinephrine (Adrenalin) for treatment of extreme emergency allergic reactions (anaphylactic shock). (**A** and **B** From McCuistion LE, DiMaggio K, Winton MB, Yeager JJ: *harmacology: A patient-centered nursing process approach*, ed 9, St Louis, 2018, Saunders. **C** and **D** From Macklin D, Chernecky C, Infortuna MH: *Math for clinical practice*, ed. 2, St Louis, 2011, Elsevier/Mosby. **E** From Becton, Dickinson and Company, Franklin Lakes, New Jersey. **F** From Mylan Specialty, I.P., Basking Ridge, New Jersey.)

CLINICAL RELEVANCE

The trend is to supply more prefilled autoinjector medications. There is no plunger on an autoinjector. This design permits faster administration and is simpler for use by a caretaker or for self-administration than a standard syringe with a plunger. There are also autoinjector insulin syringe pens that have been designed for multiple use for patients with diabetes.

CLINICAL ALERT!

As with all medication, the nurse needs to carefully examine the label, calibrations, dose, and expiration date on prefilled equipment to ensure a safe match with the medication order.

CLINICAL ALERT!

Distinguish injectable from oral syringes. Oral syringes are not to be connected to injectable equipment (Figure 5.8).

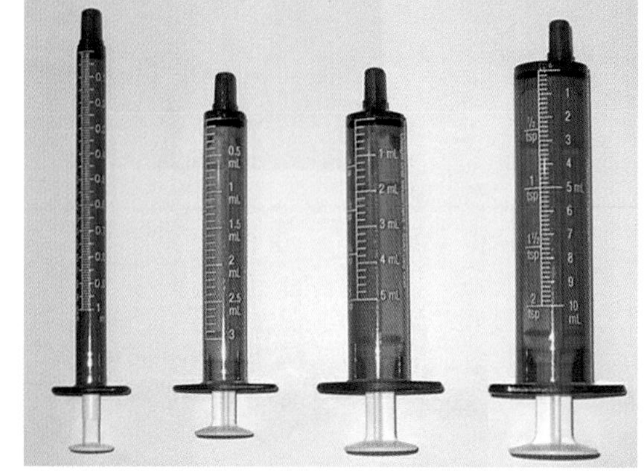

FIGURE 5.8 Various sized oral syringes for liquid medications. (From Perry AG, Potter PA, Ostendorf WR: *Clinical nursing skills and techniques*, ed 9, St Louis, 2018, Mosby.)

Needle Selections

Needle sizes refer to length and gauge (diameter). For most injections, they range in length from $\frac{3}{8}$ of an inch to 3 inches. Longer needles are used for special procedures such as spinal taps and biopsies. The finest gauges are 32 G for skin tests and insulin administration up to larger 18 G for the administration of blood and other viscous substances (Figures 5.9 and 5.10).

remember **Mnemonic: The Lower the gauge, the Larger the diameter of the needle.**

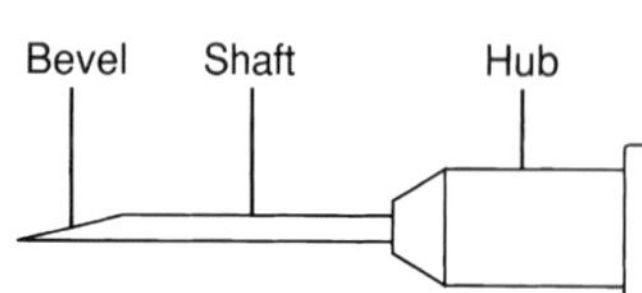

FIGURE 5.9 Parts of a needle. (From McCuistion LE, DiMaggio K, Winton MB, Yeager JJ: *Pharmacology: A patient-centered nursing process approach*, ed 9, St Louis, 2018, Saunders.)

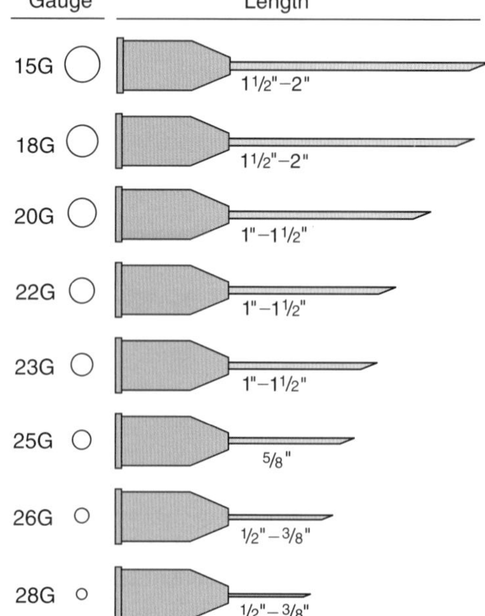

FIGURE 5.10 Needle length and gauge. (From Clayton BD, Willihnganz M: *Basic pharmacology for nurses*, ed 17, St Louis, 2017, Mosby.)

Selection of needles varies widely and depends upon the following criteria:

- Patient size
- Location to be administered
- Condition of skin
- Development of muscle
- Type and viscosity of medication
- Equipment available
- Route by which to administer the injection: intramuscular, subcutaneous, or intradermal

Intramuscular injections may consist of larger volumes than injections to the subcutaneous or intradermal layers of the skin. Older children and adults can tolerate larger amounts of medication in one site than babies or frail, underweight, malnourished people.

The following chart shows examples of syringe and needle sizes and syringe medication volumes.*

	Intradermal	Subcutaneous	Intramuscular
Length	3/8″ to 1/2″	1/2″ to 5/8″	1″ to 2″
Gauge	25 to 27	26 to 32	20 to 23
Usual syringe size	1 mL	3 mL	3 mL
Volume	0.01 to 1 mL	0.5–1 to 2 mL	0.5 to 3 mL

Comfort during an injection depends on prior experiences, feelings about injections, length and gauge of the needle, sharp polishing (finishing) of the needle, and skill of the nurse who administers the injection.

CLINICAL ALERT!

Fear of injections is not uncommon. Try to obtain a history of previous injection experiences. Patients sometimes faint from injections. Give injections with the patient lying down or seated to avoid injury.

CLINICAL RELEVANCE

Injections are emotionally and/or physically traumatic for many patients, young and old. Do not give false reassurance, such as "You won't feel a thing." Prepare the patient for a little discomfort. It is better to prepare the patient seconds before administration to avoid having the patient suddenly move. Do the preparation of the injection out of sight of the patient. Good technique takes supervised practice. Provide some distraction if needed and an empathetic physical or verbal pat on the shoulder before leaving to document the medication.

*Lengths, sizes, best location, and angles of injection are highly indivualized.

CLINICAL ALERT!

Avoid needlestick injuries and contact with blood. Keep the syringe pointed down, away from you, visitors, and bedside curtains. Dispose of the syringe and needle immediately in the nearest sharps container (Figures 5.11 and 5.12).

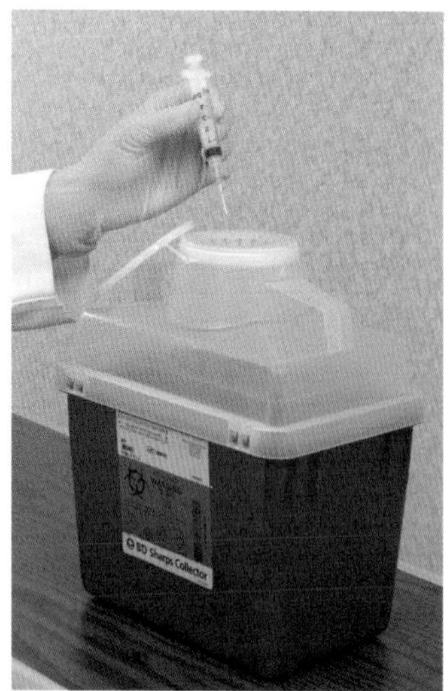

FIGURE 5.11 Sharps container. (From Snyder JS, Collins SR, Lilley LL: *Pharmacology and nursing process,* ed 9, St Louis, 2020, Mosby.)

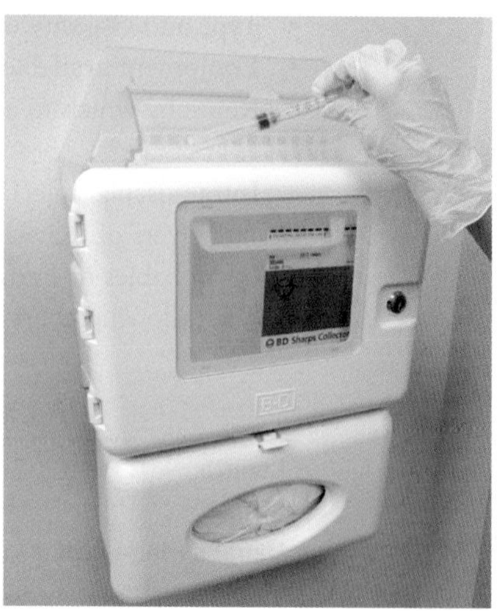

FIGURE 5.12 Sharps disposal using only one hand. (From Perry AG, Potter PA, Stockert, PA, Hall, AM: *Fundamentals of nursing*, ed 9, St Louis, 2017, Elsevier.)

CLINICAL ALERT!

The major cause of needlestick injuries is the recapping of needles. Figure 5.13 illustrates a needless vial access adapter.

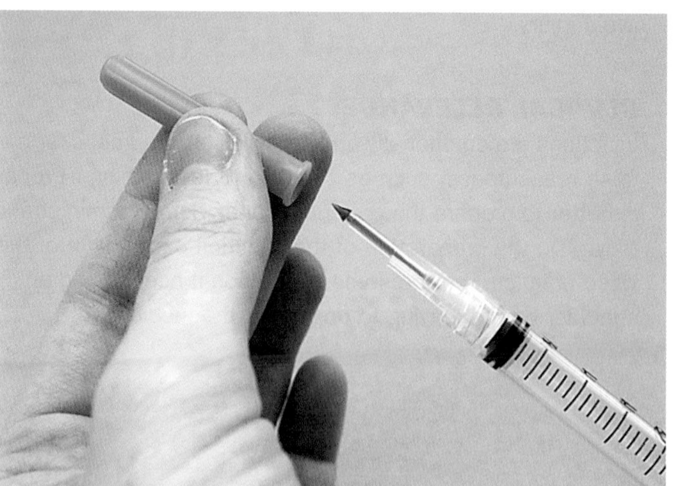

FIGURE 5.13 Syringe with a needless vial access adapter. (From Potter PA, Perry AG, Stockert P, Hall A: *Fundamentals of nursing*, ed. 9, St. Louis, 2017, Mosby.)

CLINICAL ALERT!

Needlestick injuries and the handling of blood-contaminated syringes or sponges can result in the transmission of blood-borne illnesses such as hepatitis B and C and HIV (human immunodeficiency virus). Do not add or force syringes or needles into a sharps container that is almost full. Do not *reuse* needles. It dulls the point and can cause injuries and breakage.

CLINICAL ALERT!

Be very careful when clearing an area where a procedure using needles, such as a spinal tap, has been carried out. Needlestick injuries have occurred from unseen needles under linens.

The incidence and dangers of needlestick injuries have resulted in production of an increasing variety of safety syringes. The trend to create and provide needleless equipment is growing. There are syringes manufactured with various types of covers that reduce the chance of needlesticks (Figure 5.14).

The Luer-Lok syringe tip locks the needle in the syringe (Figure 5.14, *E*).

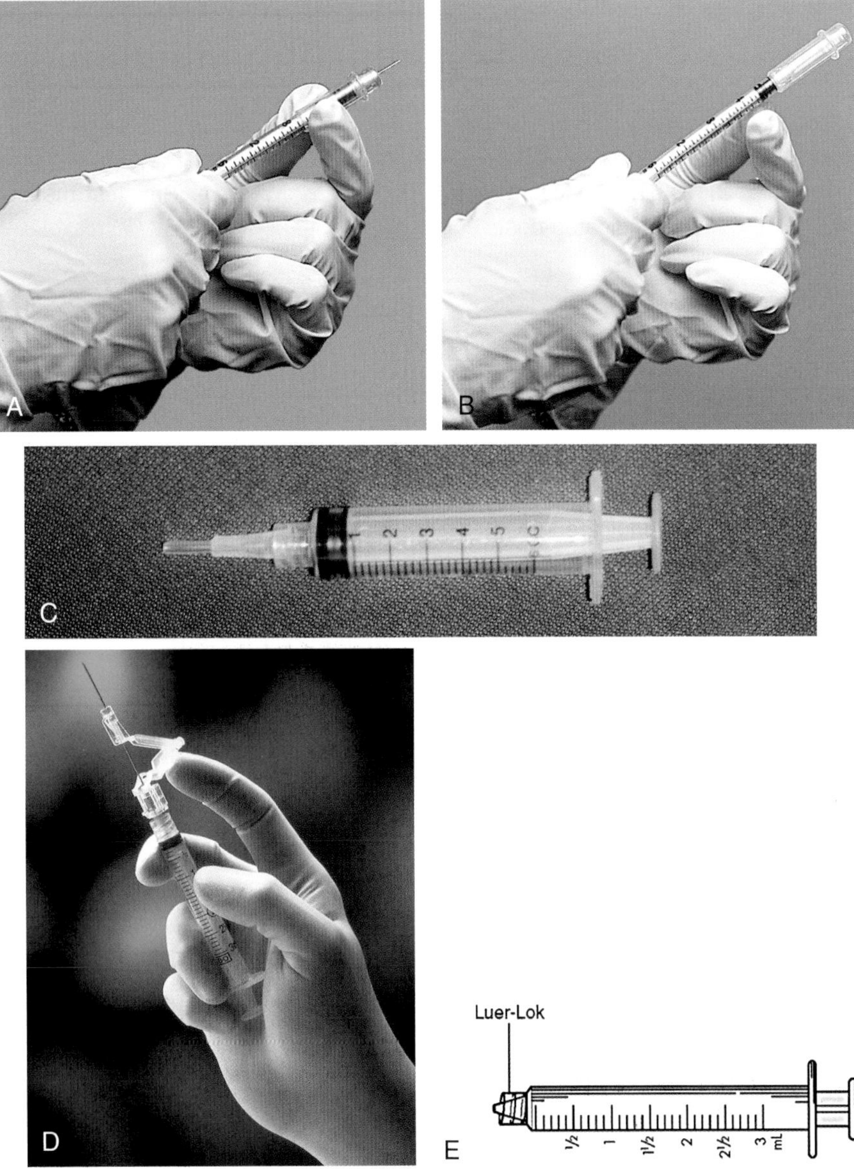

FIGURE 5.14 Safety syringes. **A** and **B,** Safety guard before and after. **C,** Needle-less 5-mL syringe. **D,** Safety glide. **E,** 3-mL Luer-Lok syringe. (**A** and **B** From Perry AG, Potter PA, Stockert, PA, Hall, AM: *Fundamentals of nursing*, ed 9, St Louis, 2017, Elsevier. **C** From McCuistion L, DiMaggio K, Winton MB, Yeager JJ: *Pharmacology: A patient-centered nursing process approach, ed 9, St Louis, 2018, Saunders.* **D** From Becton Dickinson and Company, Franklin Lakes, New Jersey. **E** From Potter PA, Perry AG, Stockert P, Hall A: *Fundamentals of nursing,* ed. 9, St. Louis, 2017, Mosby.)

Answers on page 173

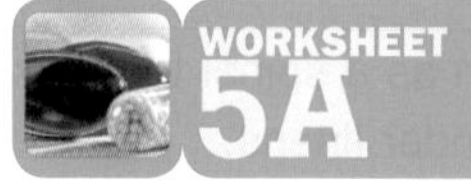

WORKSHEET 5A Reading Syringe Measurements

Examine the following syringes. Note the total capacity and the 1 mL markings. Indicate the filled-in dose measurements in the space provided.

1. **a.** Total capacity: _________ mL **b.** Smallest measurable dose:_________ mL
c. Indicated dose: _________

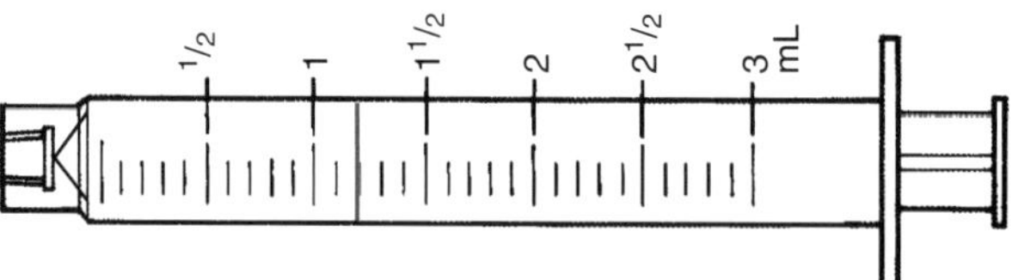

2. **a.** Total capacity: _________ mL **b.** Smallest measurable dose:_________ mL
c. Indicated dose: _________

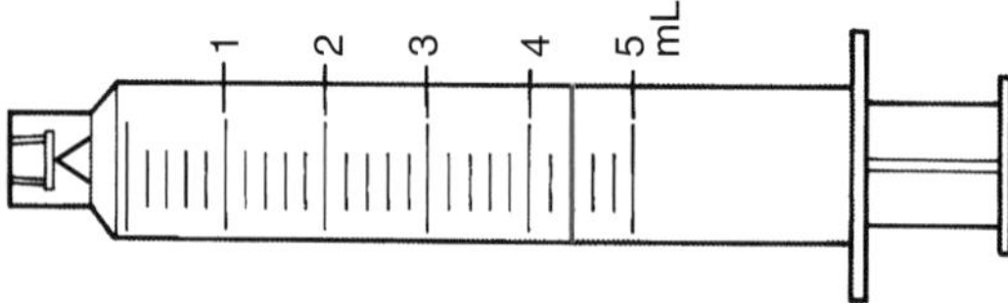

3. **a.** Total capacity: _________ mL **b.** Smallest measurable dose:_________ mL
c. Indicated dose: _________

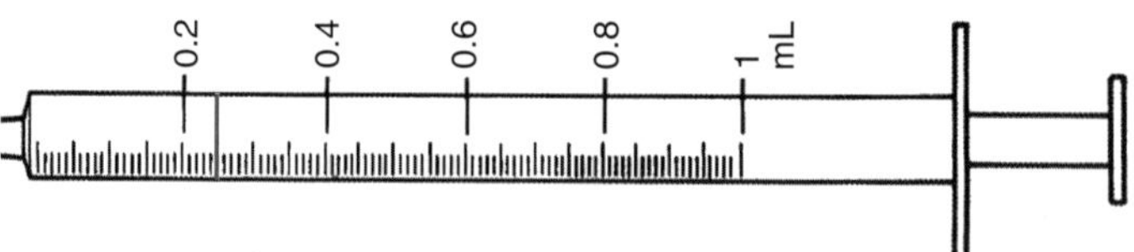

4. **a.** Total capacity: _________ mL **b.** Smallest measurable dose:_________ mL
c. Indicated dose: _________

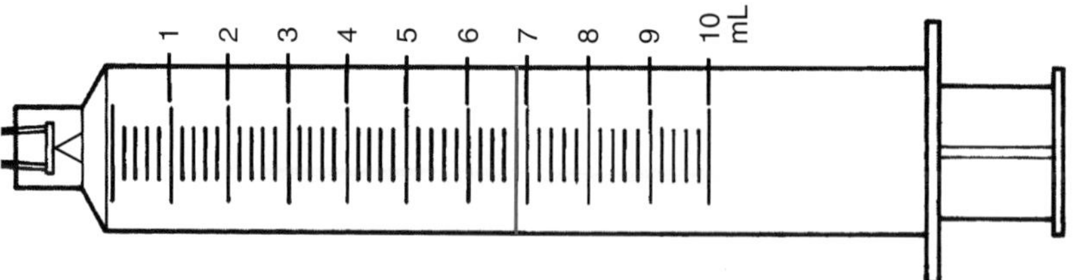

5. **a.** Total capacity: _________ mL **b.** Smallest measurable dose:_________ mL
c. Indicated dose: _________

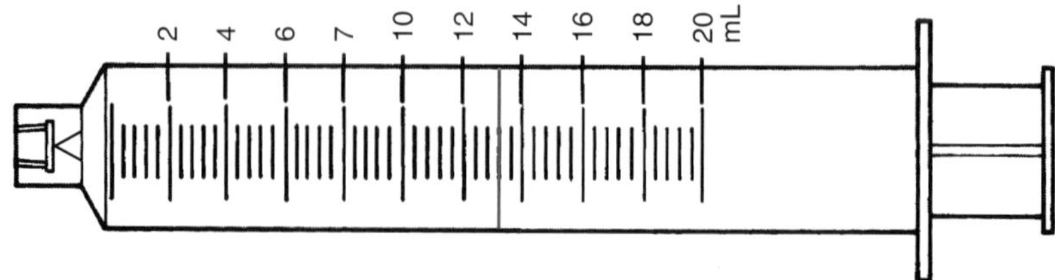

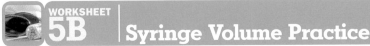

Answers on page 174

WORKSHEET 5B

Syringe Volume Practice

Examine the following syringes. Note the total capacity and the 1 mL and 0.5 mL markings. Fill in the blanks and the dose on the syringe. If possible, practice with real syringes.

1. Total capacity: _________ mL. Calibrated in 0.1, 0.2, or 0.01 of a milliliter? (Circle one)
Indicated dose _________

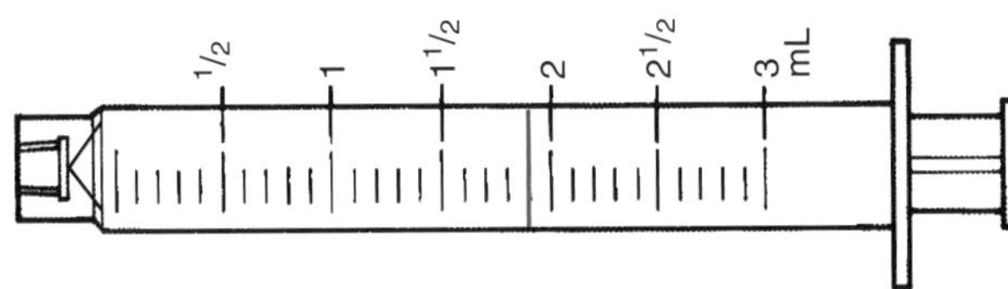

2. Total capacity: _________ mL. Calibrated in 0.1, 0.2, or 0.01 mL increments? (Circle one)
Indicated dose _________

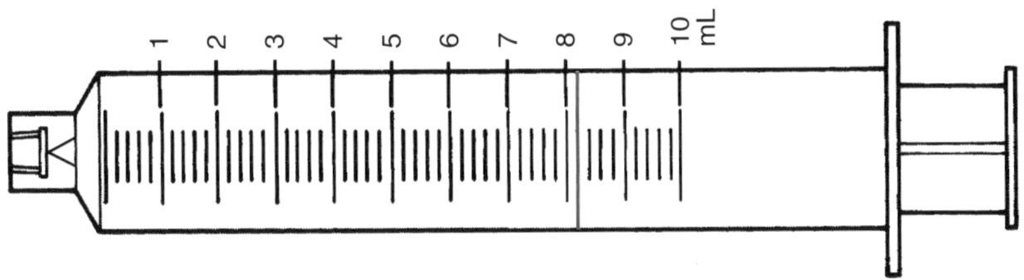

3. Total capacity: _________ mL. Calibrated in 0.1, 0.2, or 0.01 mL increments? (Circle one)
Indicated dose _________

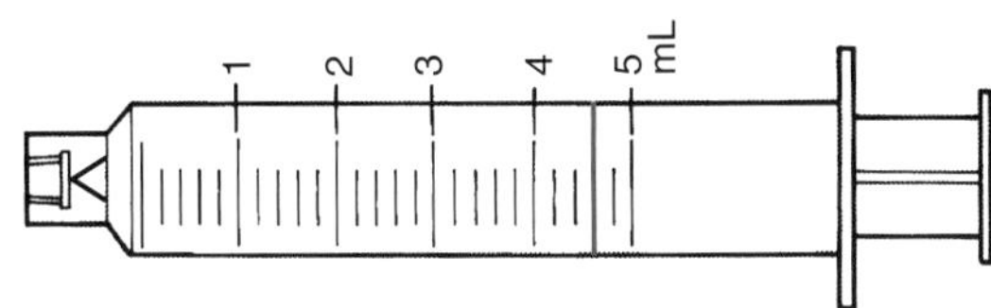

4. Total capacity: _________ mL. Calibrated in 0.1, 0.2, or 0.01 mL increments? (Circle one)
Indicated dose _________

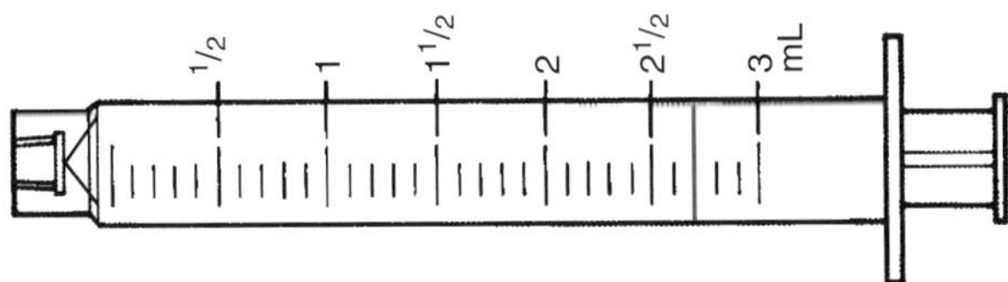

5. Total capacity: _________ mL. Calibrated in 0.1, 0.2, or 0.01 mL increments? (Circle one)
Indicated dose _________

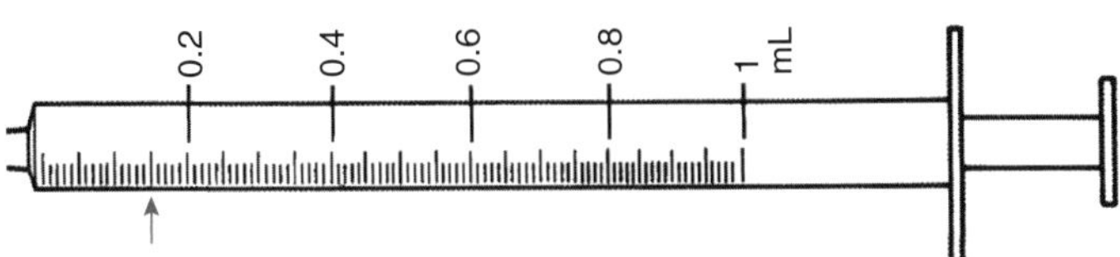

Answers on page 174

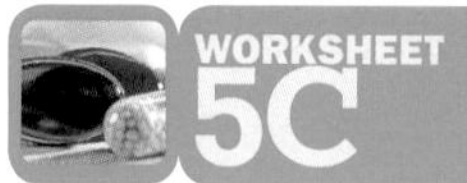

WORKSHEET 5C Additional Syringe Volume Practice

Examine the following syringes. Note the total capacity and the 1 mL and 0.5 mL markings. Fill in the blanks and shade the syringe to the volume requested. If possible, practice with real syringes.

1. Total capacity: _________ mL. Calibrated in tenths or hundredths of a milliliter? (Circle one)
Indicate 1.6 mL.

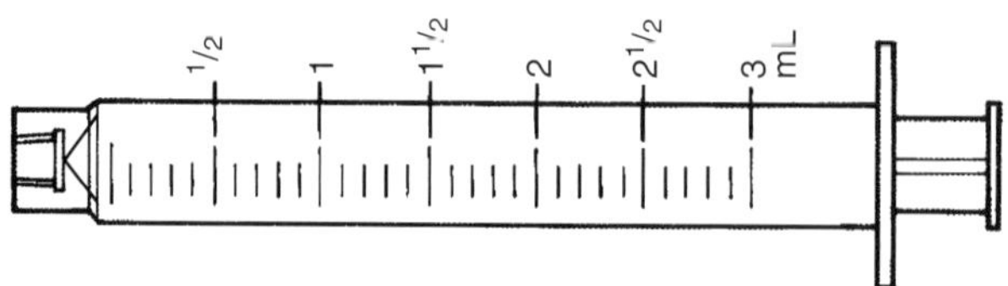

2. Total capacity: _________ mL. Calibrated in 0.1, 0.2, or 0.1 mL increments? (Circle one)
Indicate 4.6 mL.

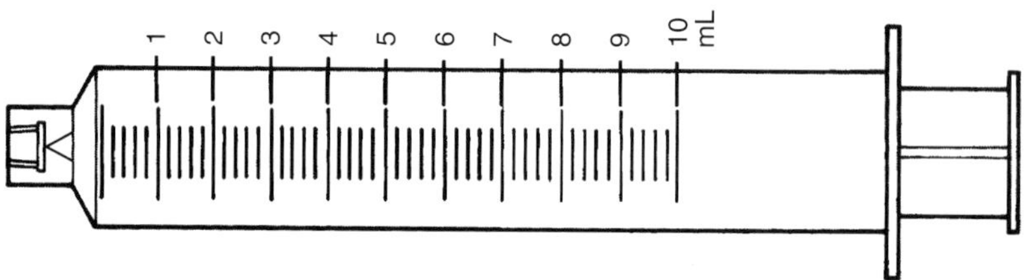

3. Total capacity: _________ mL. Calibrated in 0.1, 0.2, or 0.1 mL increments? (Circle one)
Indicate 3.4 mL.

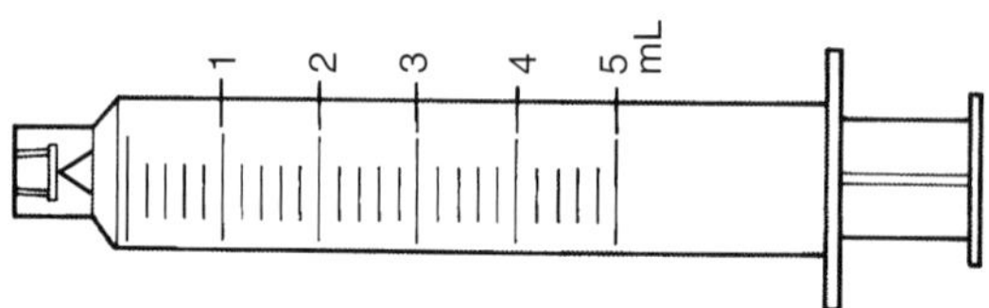

4. Total capacity: _________ mL. Calibrated in tenths or hundredths of a milliliter? (Circle one)
Indicate 2.5 mL.

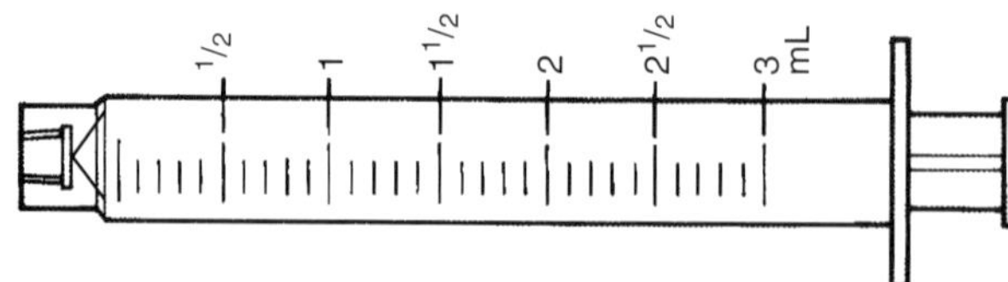

5. Total capacity: _________ mL. Calibrated in tenths or hundredths of a milliliter? (Circle one)
Indicate 0.75 mL.

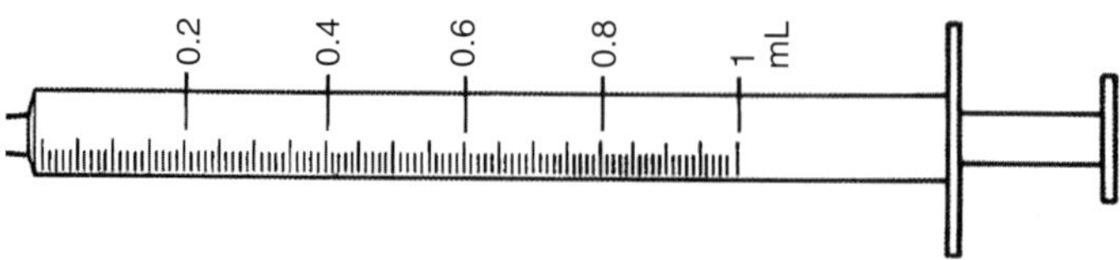

Ampules are containers made of glass with narrow necks and require special care. The tops are snapped off to access the medication. Amber-colored containers, such as the ampule shown in Figure 5.15, *A*, are used for medications that are unstable in light. Vials are rubber-topped containers with a metal or plastic cover. They may hold liquid or dry medication and can be single- or multiple-dose containers.

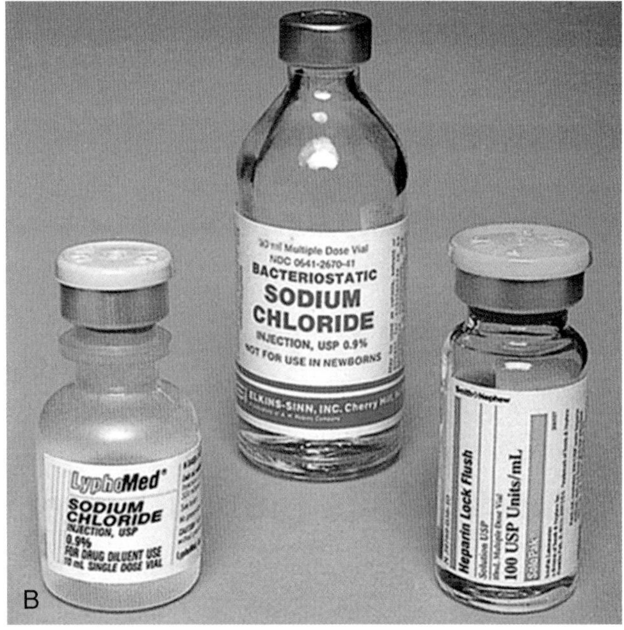

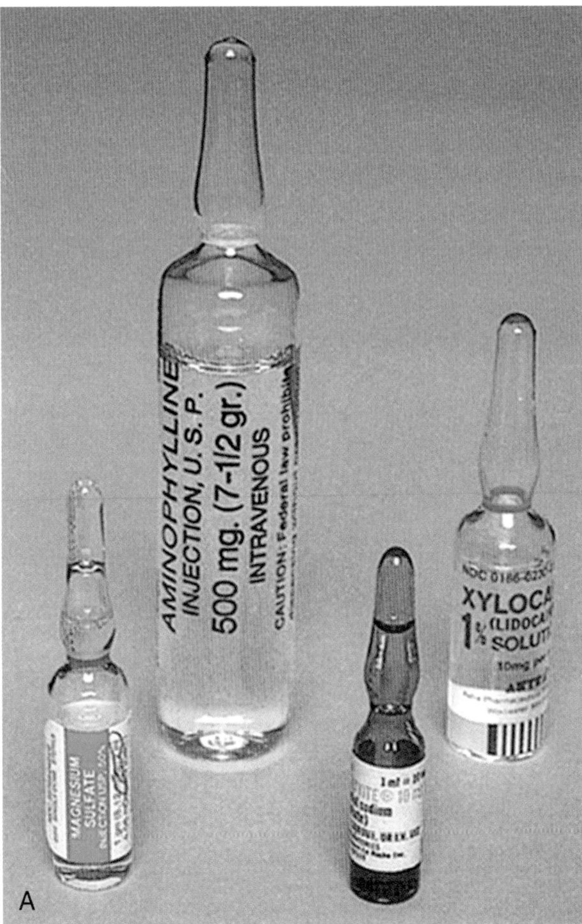

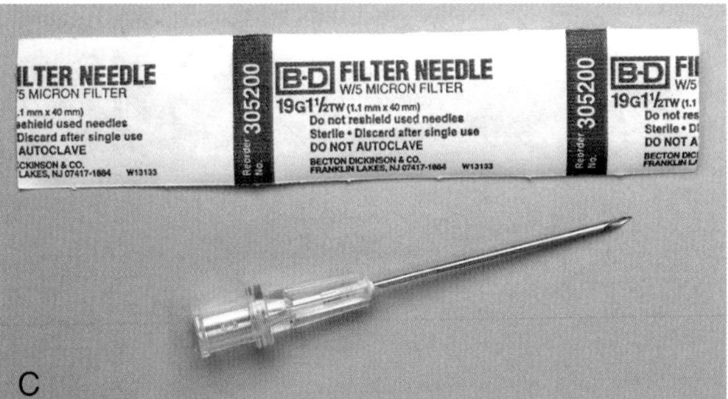

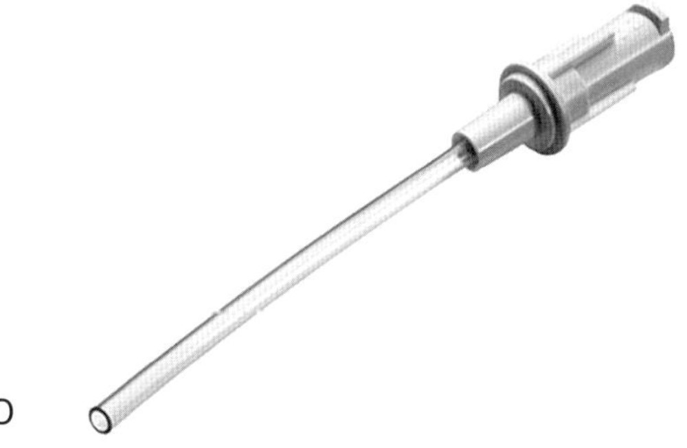

FIGURE 5.15 **A,** Injectable liquid supplied in ampules. **B,** Injectable liquid supplied in vials. **C,** Filter needle. **D,** Filter straw. (**A & B** From Potter PA, Perry AG, Stockert P, Hall A: *Fundamentals of nursing*, ed. 9, St. Louis, 2017, Mosby. **C** From Becton, Dickinson and Company, Franklin Lakes, NJ.)

Filter needles (Figure 5.15, *C*) and are used to withdraw medications from glass ampules and multidose vials. They filter out particles of glass and rubber that might be withdrawn into the syringe. Filter straws (Figure 5.15, *D*) are also used to withdraw medication from ampules.

CLINICAL ALERT!

Vials with rubber latex stoppers may also contain latex in the medication if it has been in contact with the stopper. Allergic reactions to even very small amounts of an allergen can be very serious.

Manufacturers are being asked to include latex on the vial label when it is present. Be sure to check the patient for latex allergy and document it on the chart. Latex allergy may be overlooked because it is not a medicine.

CLINICAL ALERT!

The filter needles *must be removed* and *replaced* with a traditional needle *before* administering the medication. Otherwise, the filtered glass or particles would be injected into the patient.

Parenteral Routes

Injectable medication routes known as parenteral (outside the gastrointestinal [GI] tract) include the routes mentioned below as well as the intravenous route, which is covered in a later chapter.

Many injectables are provided in ampules and vials and prefilled syringes.

Intradermal (ID) Injections

These are small-volume injections usually administered as skin tests. The usual dose for a skin test administered with a 1-mL syringe and a 25- to 30-gauge needle is 0.1 mL (Figure 5.16).

Subcutaneous (subcut) Injections

Nonirritating substances up to 1 mL may be injected into subcutaneous fatty tissue sites usually with a 25- to 30-gauge needle. Insulin and anticoagulants are examples of medications that may be delivered by this route. The most common sites for subcutaneous injections are noted in Figure 5.17.

A 2-inch zone around the umbilicus (illustrated in white in Figure 5.17) is to be avoided when giving abdominal subcutaneous injections.

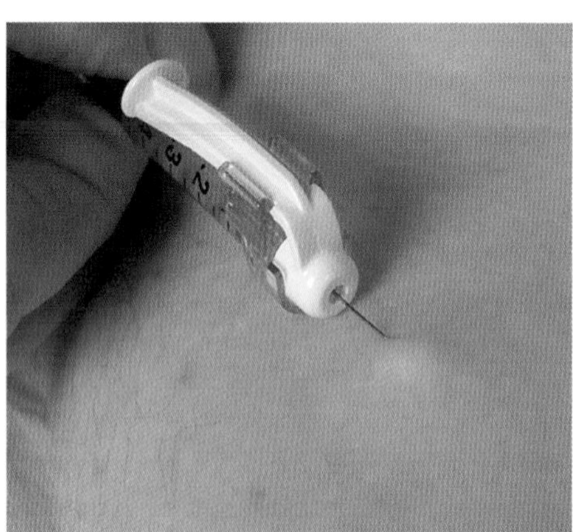

FIGURE 5.16 During intradermal injection, note formation of small bleb (blister-like raised area) on the skin's surface. (From Potter PA, Perry AG, Stockert P, Hall A: *Fundamentals of nursing*, ed. 9, St. Louis, 2017, Mosby.)

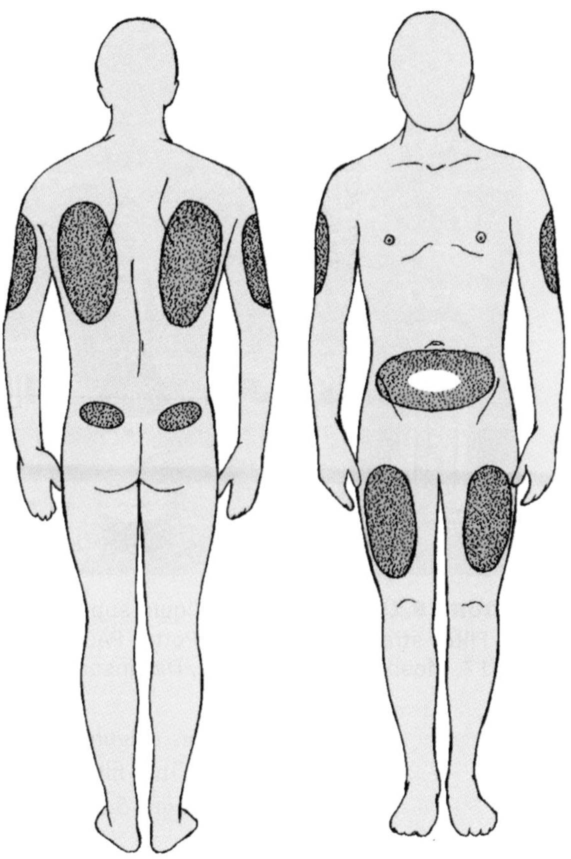

FIGURE 5.17 Sites recommended for subcutaneous injections. (From Potter PA, Perry AG, Stockert P, Hall A: *Fundamentals of nursing*, ed. 9, St. Louis, 2017, Mosby.)

Intramuscular (IM) Injections

Intramuscular (IM) injections are selected to deliver medications for faster absorption. They tolerate more concentrated substances than subcutaneous sites. Doses up to 3 mL may be injected into a single site, depending on the patient's skin integrity and muscle size. The most common sites are noted in Figure 5.18. The angle of injection is shown in Figure 5.19.

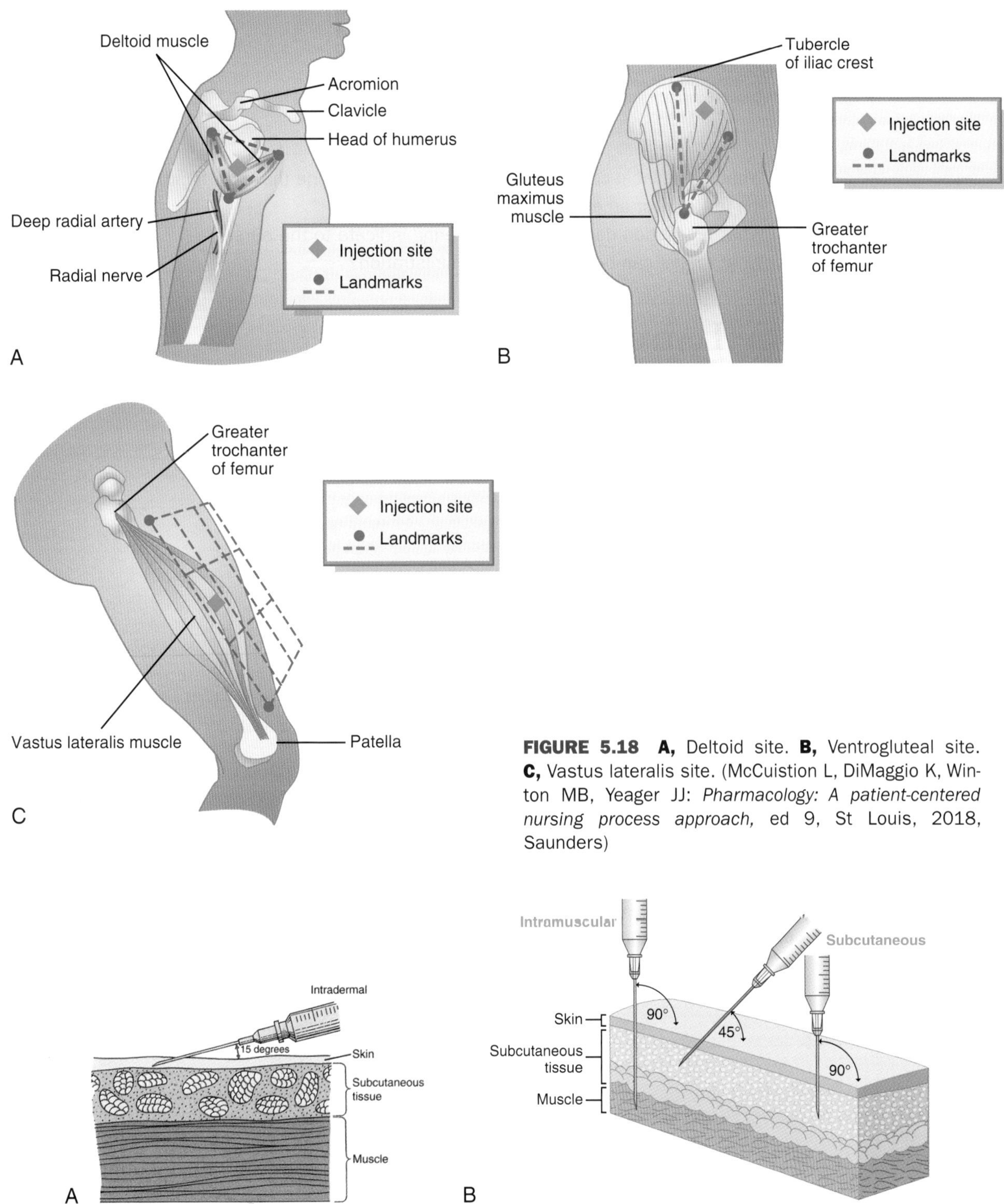

FIGURE 5.18 **A,** Deltoid site. **B,** Ventrogluteal site. **C,** Vastus lateralis site. (McCuistion L, DiMaggio K, Winton MB, Yeager JJ: *Pharmacology: A patient-centered nursing process approach,* ed 9, St Louis, 2018, Saunders)

FIGURE 5.19 Angles of injection. **A** From Potter PA, Perry AG, Stockert P, Hall A: *Fundamentals of nursing*, ed. 9, St. Louis, 2017, Mosby. **B** From Kee JL, Marshall SM: *Clinical calculations,* ed. 7, St. Louis, 2013, Saunders.)

Answers on page 175

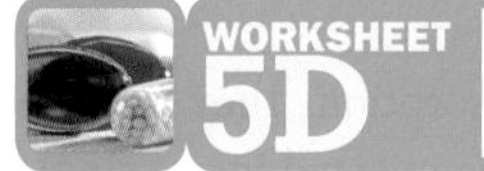

WORKSHEET 5D Injectable Label Interpretation

1.

MethylPREDNISolone Sodium Succinate for Injection, USP
FOR IM OR IV USE
40 mg*
Rx ONLY
Recommended Diluent Contains Benzyl Alcohol as a Preservative.

NDC 55390-209-10 Single Dose Vial
Reconstitute with 1.2 mL of Bacteriostatic Water for Injection with benzyl alcohol.
*Each 1 mL (when mixed) contains: Methylprednisolone sodium succinate equiv. to 40 mg methylprednisolone.
Lyophilized in container.
Protect from light.
Manufactured for: Bedford Laboratories™ Bedford, OH 44146 **MPNL-V01**

a. What is the label concentration of this male hormone (have on hand), to be entered on the left side of an equation for this product?
b. What precaution does the label lettering indicate to the nurse?
c. What routes can be ordered for administration?

2.

LOT **506572A** EXP
LOVENOX®
(enoxaparin sodium) Injection
40 mg/0.4 mL
Syringe
RHÔNE-POULENC RORER PHARMACEUTICALS INC. COLLEGEVILLE, PA 19426
Made in France L-5560A

a. What is the label concentration of this anticoagulant?
b. How is the medication "packaged"?

3.

BICILLIN® C-R 900/300
(900,000 units penicillin G benzathine and 300,000 units penicillin G procaine injectable suspension)
1,200,000 UNITS per 2 mL
Not for the Treatment of Syphilis
FOR DEEP **IM** INJECTION **ONLY**
WARNING: NOT FOR INTRAVENOUS USE
Mfg. by: King Pharmaceuticals, Inc., Bristol, TN
3000970 (01)00360793602028
Lot: Exp:

a. What is the label concentration of this antibiotic?
b. What does the unit of measurement mean: "units"?
c. What are the three warnings for this product?
d. What does C-R mean?

4. 

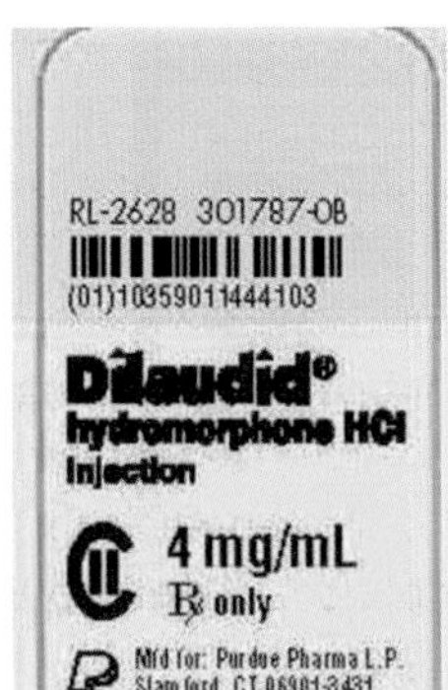

a. What is the drug concentration?*
b. What does *C II* mean?
c. How many mcg are equal to the mg per mL concentration?
d. Will this product be in a regular medicine drawer or a locked drawer?
e. State briefly what the meaning of an ISMP-identified high-alert drug is.

5.

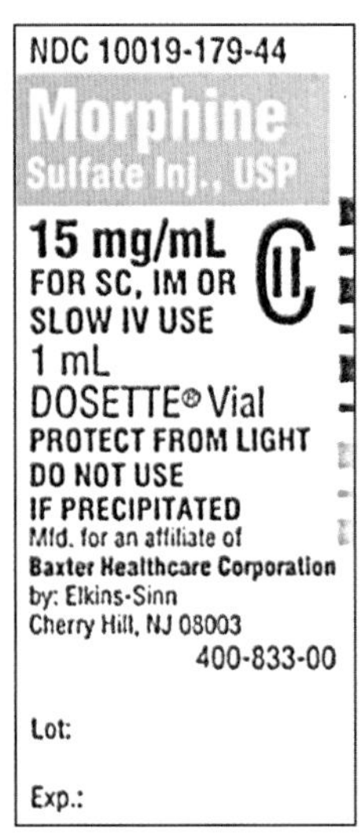

a. What is the drug concentration?†
b. How is this narcotic packaged?

6.

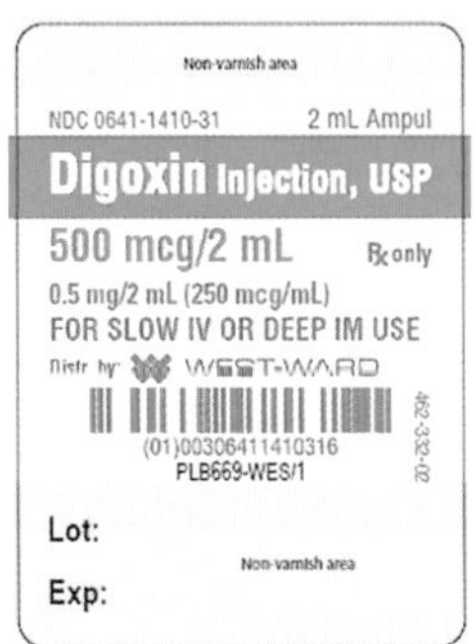

a. What is the drug concentration in mcg?
b. What is the drug concentration in mg?
c. What are the warnings on the label?

*Note: The estimated potency of Dilaudid to morphine is a ratio of 7.5 to 1.
†Note: Concentrations are not comparable among products of same or different types. For example, 4 mg of morphine per mL is not equal to 4 mg of Dilaudid.

7. 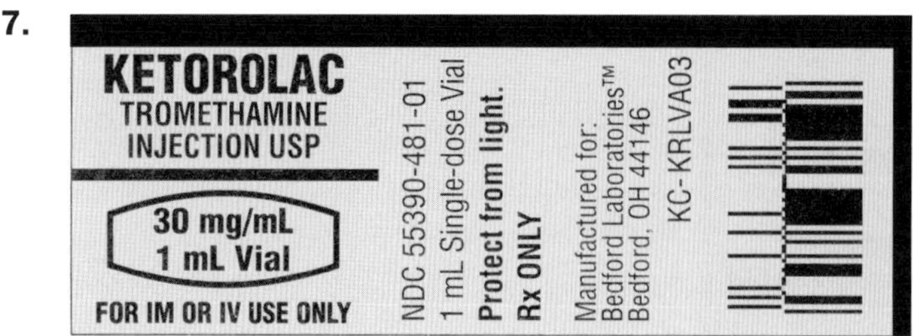

a. What is the concentration of this nonsteroidal antiinflammatory drug?
b. Which routes are specified for this medication?
c. What is the warning on the label?

8. 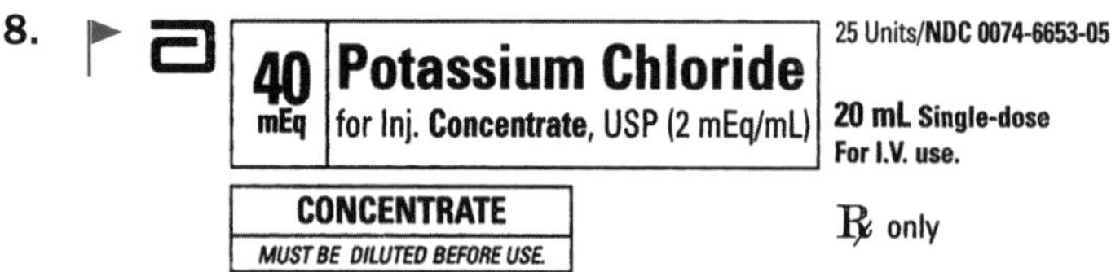

a. What is the concentration of this high-alert electrolyte medication?
b. What does the word *concentrate* convey to the nurse?
c. What route is specified for this medication?
d. Is this a reusable container?

9. 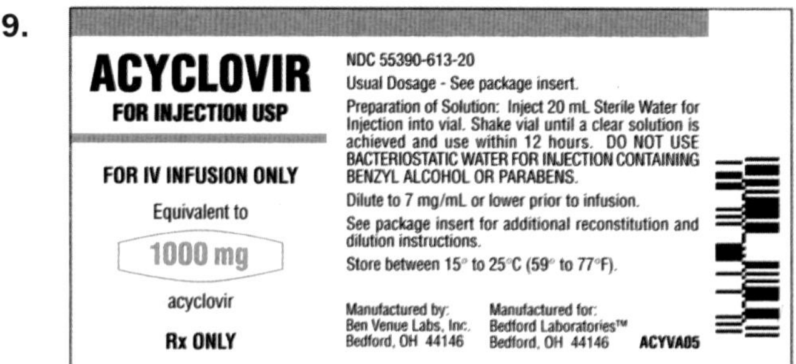

Method of Preparation: Each 10 mL vial contains acyclovir sodium equivalent to 500 mg of acyclovir. Each 20 mL vial contains acyclovir sodium equivalent to 1000 mg of acyclovir. The contents of the vial should be dissolved in Sterile Water for Injection as follows:

Contents of Vial	Amount of Diluent
500 mg	10 mL
1000 mg	20 mL

The resulting solution in each case contains 50 mg acyclovir per mL (pH approximately 11). Shake the vial well to assure complete dissolution before measuring and transferring each individual dose. DO NOT USE BACTERIOSTATIC WATER FOR INJECTION CONTAINING BENZYL ALCOHOL OR PARABENS.

a. What is the concentration in mg per mL after dilution?
b. What is the specified route?
c. What is the warning on the label?

10. 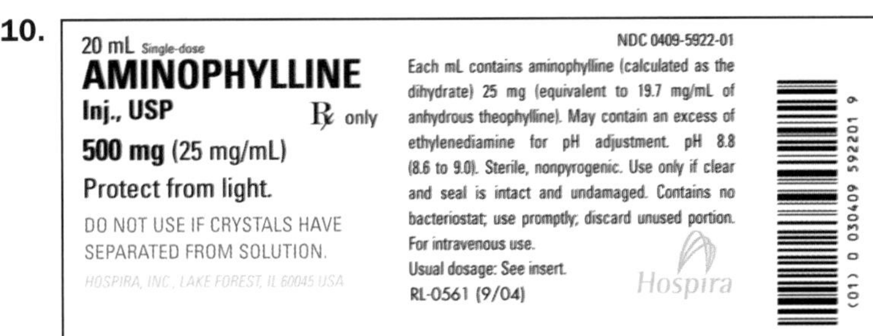

a. What is the concentration of mg per mL?
b. What are the two warnings on the label?

Answers on page 176

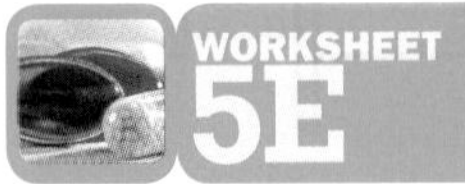

WORKSHEET 5E Injectable Dose Calculation

Estimate an answer. Use a ratio and proportion method to calculate the dose. Label and prove the answer. Indicate the dose on the syringe.

1. Ordered: Diazepam 7.5 mg IM stat for a patient with agitation. How many mL will you administer?

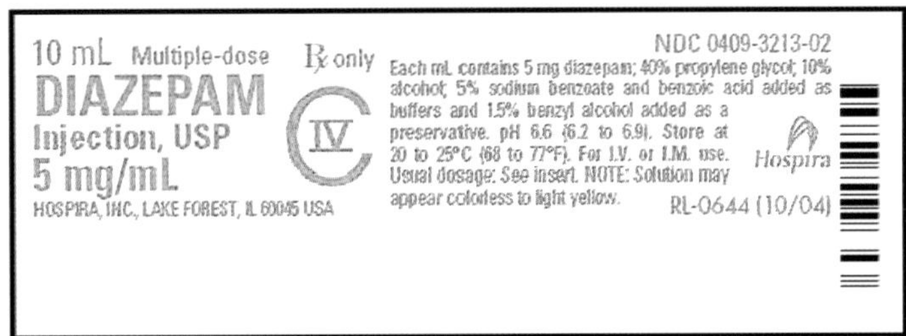

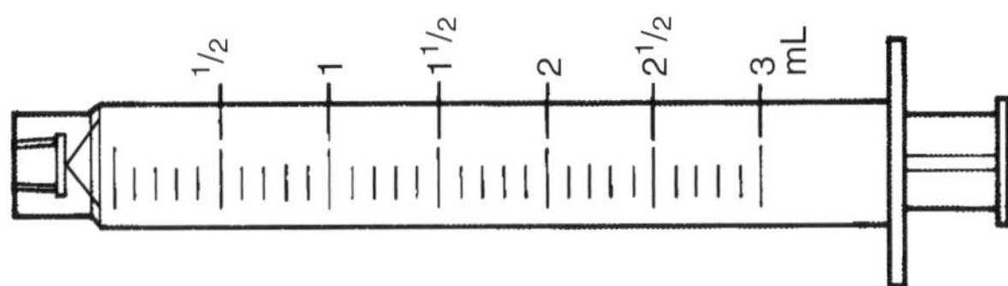

2. Ordered: Solu-Cortef (hydrocortisone sodium succinate) 0.2 g IM for a patient with a severe allergic reaction. How many mL will you administer?

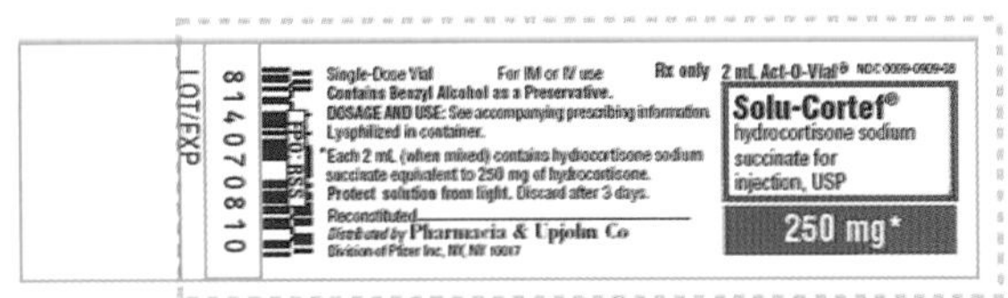

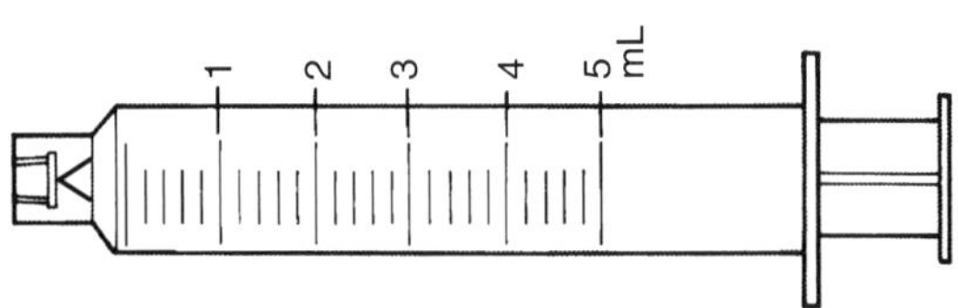

3. Ordered: Diphenhydramine HCl Injection 0.1 g IM for a patient with nausea.* How many mL will you administer?

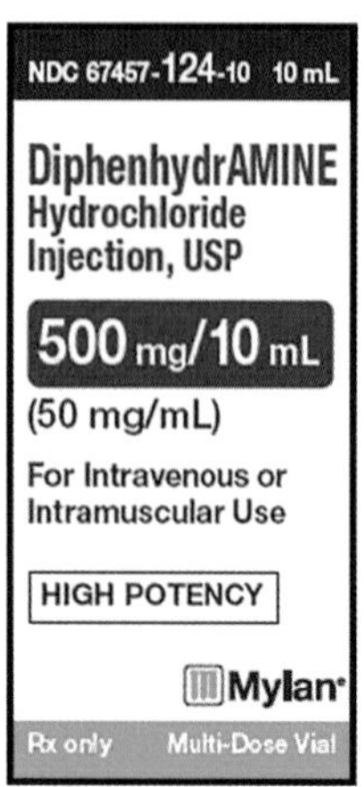

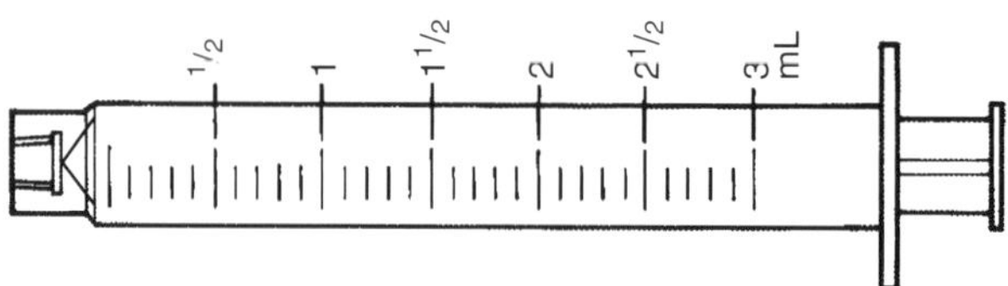

4. Ordered: Naloxone 1 mg IM stat for an adult with a heroin overdose. How many mL will you administer?†

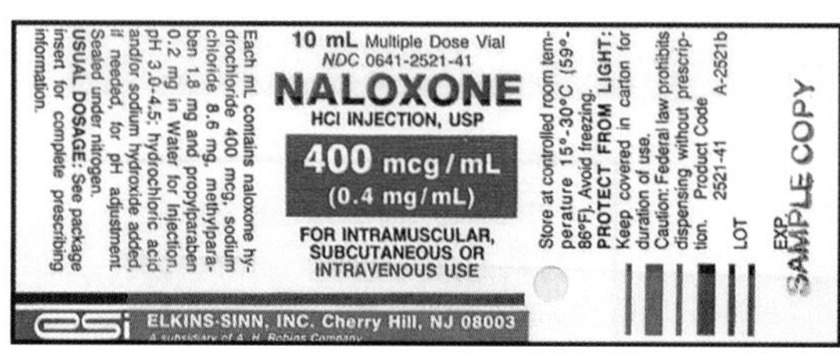

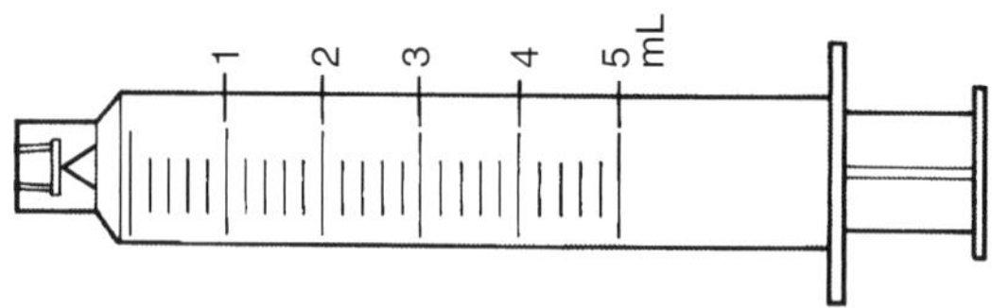

5. Ordered: Aranesp (darbepoetin alfa) 0.45 mcg per kg subcut for a patient with anemia related to chemotherapy. Pt wt is 80 kg.

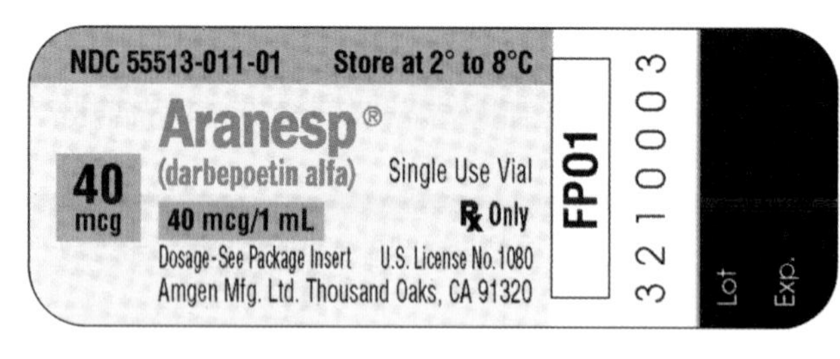

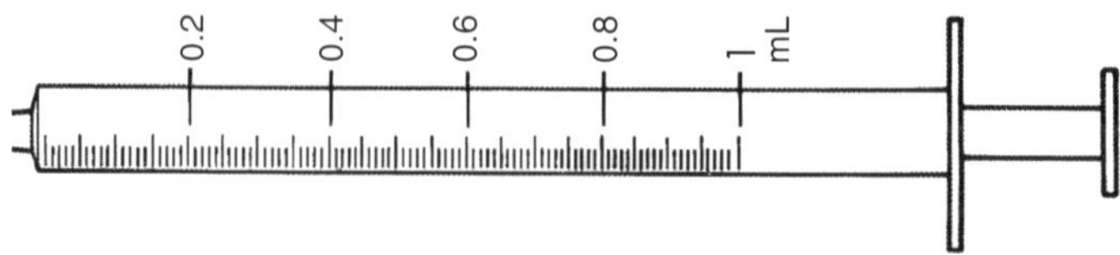

*Note the Tall Man letters on this label. The tall letters help differentiate the product from a look-alike, sound-alike drug—dimenhyDRINATE—to reduce the chance of medication error.

†A multidose vial is supplied because more than one dose may have to be given every few minutes up to a maximum of 10 mg to reverse the overdose.

Answers on page 178

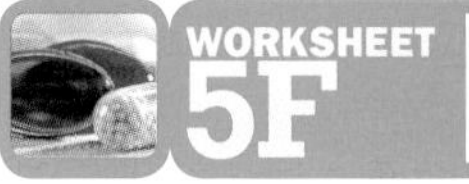

WORKSHEET 5F

Multiple-Choice Practice

1. What are the increments of the calibrations on a 1-mL syringe?

a. 1
b. 0.1
c. 0.01
d. 0.001

2. Which of the following statements about needle gauge is true?

a. The lowest-gauge needles have the largest diameters.
b. An 18-gauge needle would be used for intradermal skin tests.
c. The needles for intramuscular injections have the smallest diameters.
d. The gauge of the needle selected is determined by the length of the needle to be used.

3. Which site is to be avoided for intramuscular injections, particularly for infants and toddlers, because of potential injury to the sciatic nerve and blood vessels in the area?

a. deltoid
b. dorsogluteal
c. vastus lateralis
d. ventrogluteal

4. Which size syringe would you select for an intramuscular injection of 3.1 mL?

a. A 3-mL syringe with 0.1 mL calibrations
b. A 5-mL syringe with 0.1 mL calibrations
c. A 5-mL syringe with 0.2 mL calibrations
d. A 10-mL syringe with 0.2 mL calibrations

5. Which is a major cause of needlestick injuries and serious blood-borne diseases?

a. Recapping the needle
b. Failure to wear gloves
c. Lack of cooperation of the patient
d. Poor injection technique

6. Which of the following situations would necessitate a lower-gauge syringe?

a. Viscous medications
b. Large-size patients
c. Undeveloped muscle
d. Intradermal medication

7. Which is the first important nursing responsibility before preparing an injection mix of more than one medication?

a. Check the dilution instructions.
b. Inspect the patient's previous injection sites.
c. Clear and clean the area of preparation.
d. Check the medications' compatibility.

8. If a patient states that there has been some kind of previous problem with a medication the nurse plans to administer, what action should the nurse take next?

a. Give the medication and monitor the patient for side effects.
b. Give half the dose and monitor the patient for side effects.
c. Hold the medication and call the provider for another order.
d. Hold the medication and find out what kind of problem occurred.

9. Which of the following reactions to a new or recently changed medication indicates a possible allergic reaction and reason to hold the medication?
   a. Skin color changes, swollen joints, and/or chest pain
   b. Blurred vision, ringing in the ears (tinnitus), white patches on the tongue
   c. Rash, respiratory difficulty, diarrhea
   d. Brittle nails, hair loss, flaking skin

10. Which of the following statements is *true* about the use of filter needles?
   a. They should be used with the preparation of all injectable medications.
   b. They need to be placed on the syringe before injecting the medication in the patient.
   c. Filter needles are to be used to withdraw medication from glass ampules and multidose vials with rubber stoppers.
   d. The filter needle can be reused because it doesn't come in contact with the patient.

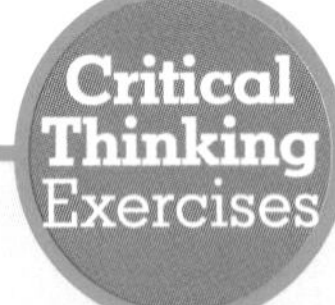

Critical Thinking Exercises provide math and medication-related patient safety issues for student discussion. Answers are not provided.

1. Ordered: Phenergan 50 mg IM stat for a patient who has nausea.

On hand:

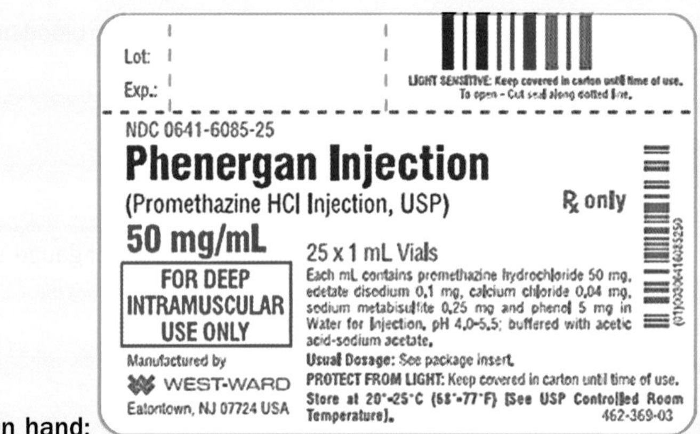

Lot:
Exp.:
LIGHT SENSITIVE: Keep covered in carton until time of use.
To open - Cut seal along dotted line.
NDC 0641-6085-25
Phenergan Injection
(Promethazine HCl Injection, USP)
℞ only
50 mg/mL
25 x 1 mL Vials
FOR DEEP INTRAMUSCULAR USE ONLY
Each mL contains promethazine hydrochloride 50 mg, edetate disodium 0.1 mg, calcium chloride 0.04 mg, sodium metabisulfite 0.25 mg and phenol 5 mg in Water for Injection, pH 4.0-5.5; buffered with acetic acid-sodium acetate.
Usual Dosage: See package insert.
PROTECT FROM LIGHT: Keep covered in carton until time of use.
Store at 20°-25°C (68°-77°F) [See USP Controlled Room Temperature].
Manufactured by
WEST-WARD
Eatontown, NJ 07724 USA
462-369-03

Given: Phenergan 50 mg IM using a 1-inch needle in a patient weighing 109.1 kg (240 lb).

Error:

Potential problem for patient:

Recommendations for the Patient Safety Committee for this nurse:

2. Ordered: Glycopyrrolate 0.2 mg IM stat preop for an operative patient to reduce secretions during surgery.

On Hand:

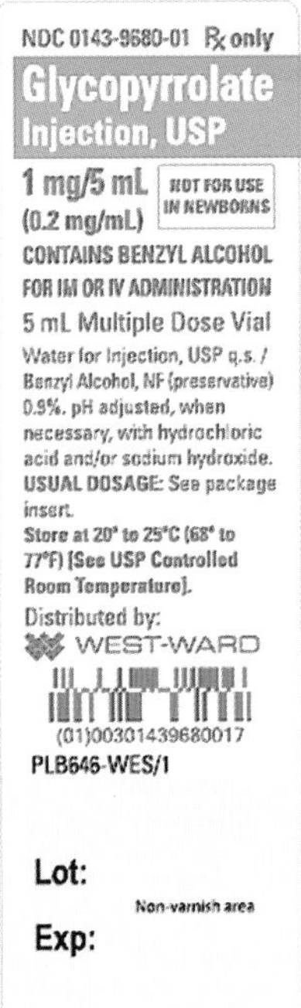

Given: Glycopyrrolate 2 mL

Error:

Potential injury to patient:

Recommendations for the Patient Safety Committee for this nurse:

3. Ordered: Cyanocobalamin 0.5 mg IM for a frail patient with vitamin B-12 deficiency. Patient weight 40 kg. The patient developed a sciatic nerve injury.

On Hand:

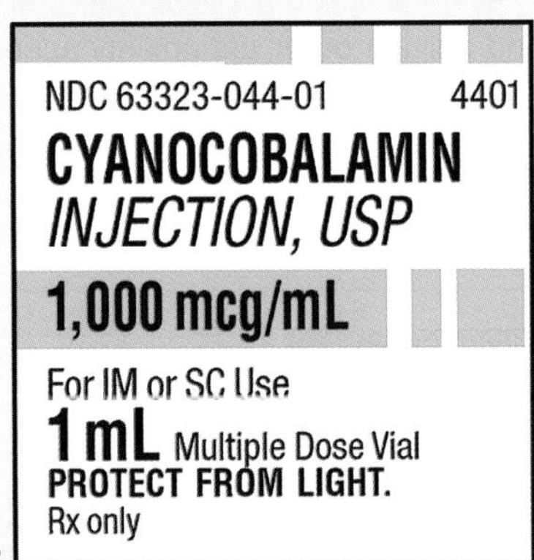

Given: 0.5 mg IM in the dorsogluteal muscle.

Error:

Recommendations for the Patient Safety Committee for this nurse:

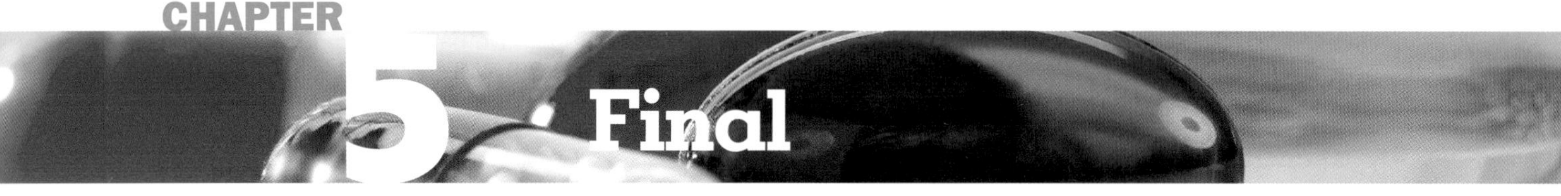

CHAPTER 5 Final

Directions: Solve the problems using a ratio and proportion method. Estimate, label, and prove your answer. Indicate the dose on the syringe.

1. Ordered: Lorazepam 2 mg deep IM stat, a sedative and antianxiety agent, for an agitated patient. Note: Ativan is a very irritating substance and should be given undiluted deep IM.

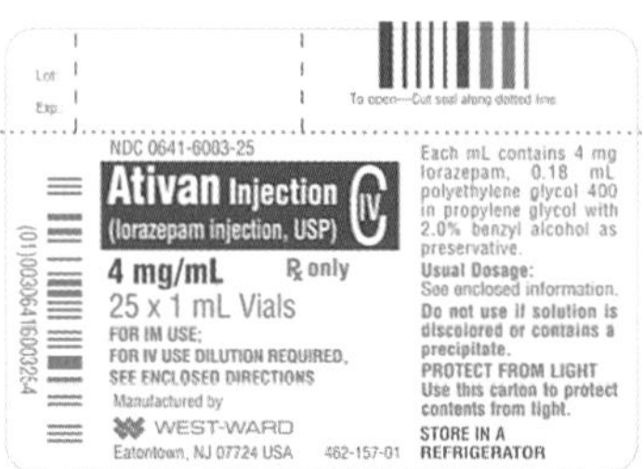

a. Drug concentration ________

b. Route ________

c. How many mL will you prepare? ________

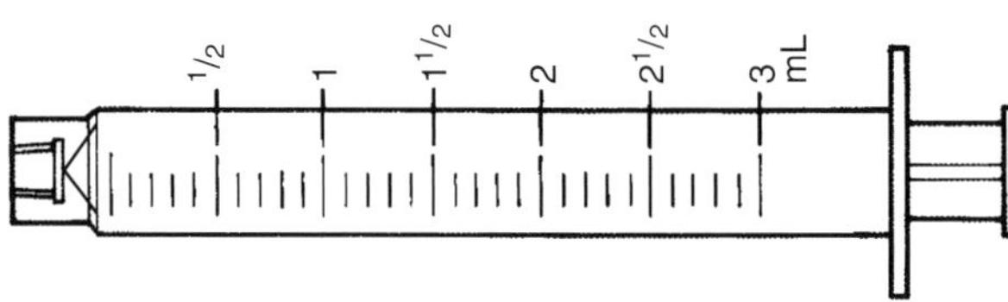

Note that Ativan (lorazepam) is labeled C IV (controlled substance Schedule IV). Drugs in this category have less potential for abuse or addiction than Schedule I, II, or III drugs. Schedule IV drugs include phenobarbital and certain other antianxiety agents.

2. Ordered: Atropine 0.1 mg subcut on call to OR. How many mL will you prepare? Indicate the dose on the syringe.

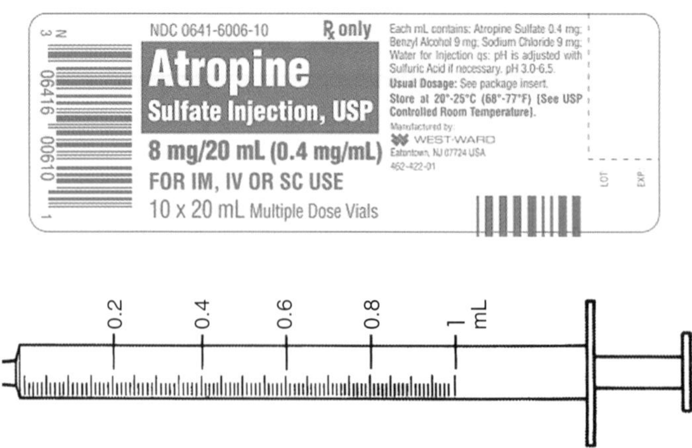

3. Ordered: Lanoxin (digoxin), a cardiotonic, 0.25 mg deep IM daily for three days for a patient with heart failure.

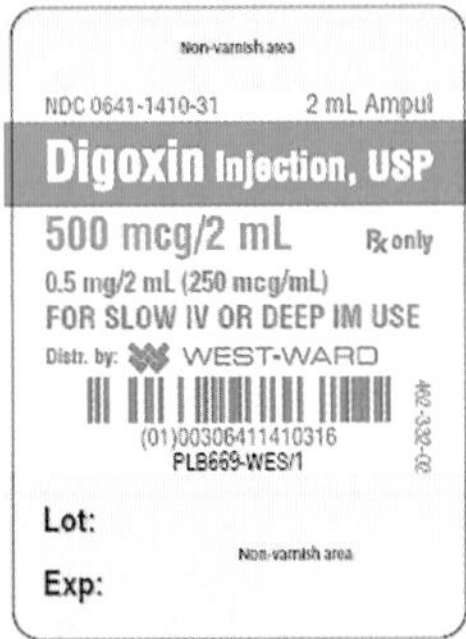

How many mL will you prepare? _________

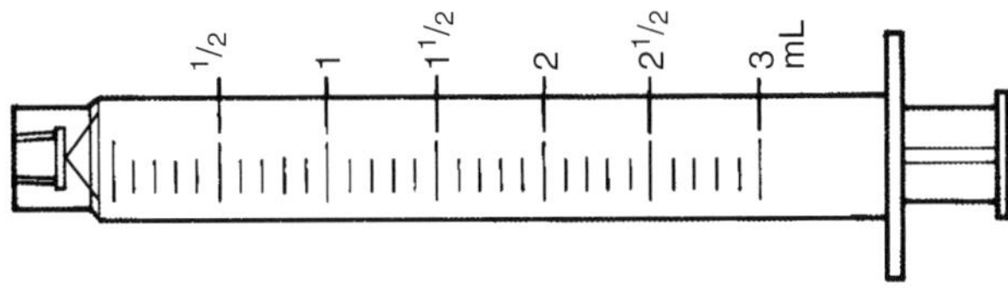

4. Ordered: Meperidine HCL 50 mg IM stat for a patient allergic to other analgesics. hydroxyzine 30 mg

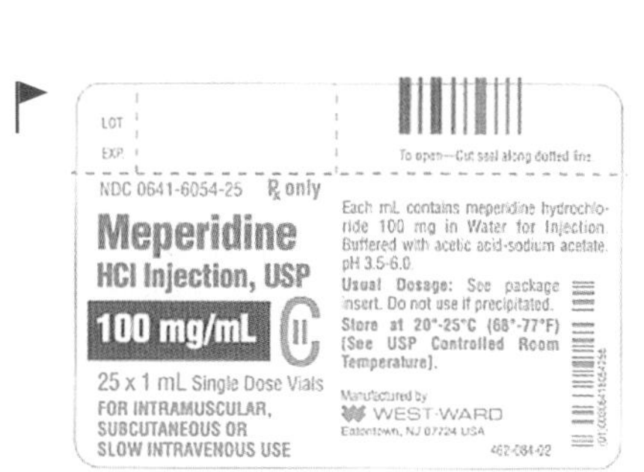

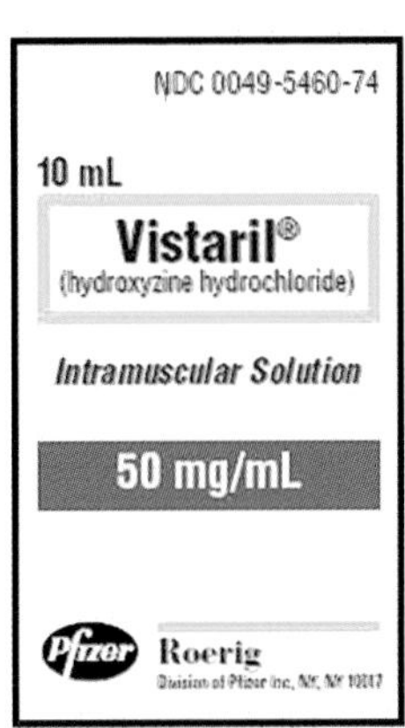

a. How many mL of meperidine will you prepare? _________

b. How many mL of hydroxyzine will you prepare? _________

Indicate the combined dose on the syringe.

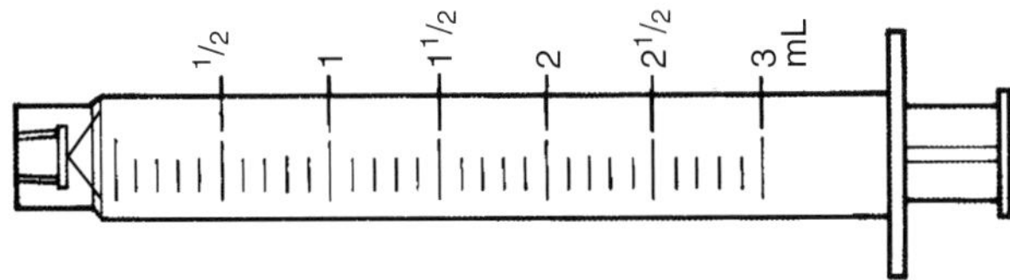

Note: Combined injectables are seldom ordered. If they are, it's best to prepare each dose in a separate syringe and then add them together in one of the two syringes.

CLINICAL ALERT!

Always check a current reliable reference for incompatibility when a mixture of solutions is to be administered. If a question arises, check with pharmacy.

5. Ordered: Furosemide 34 mg IM stat for a patient with heart failure and edema. Draw an arrow pointing to the nearest measurable dose on the syringe provided.

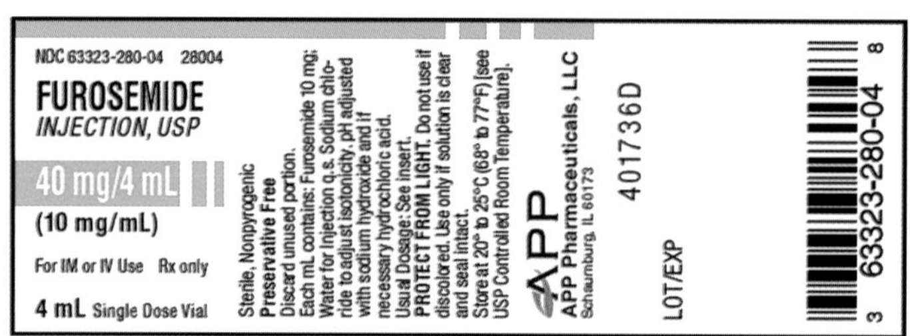

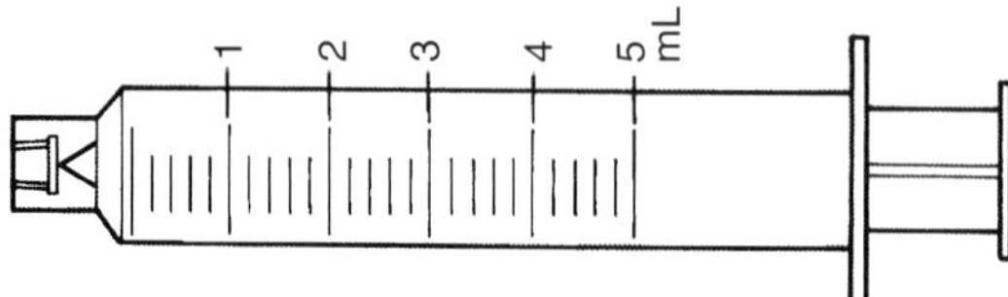

6. Ordered: Tuberculin skin test ID for an adult patient. The volume for this test is 0.1 mL. Draw an arrow pointing to the nearest measurable dose on the syringe provided.

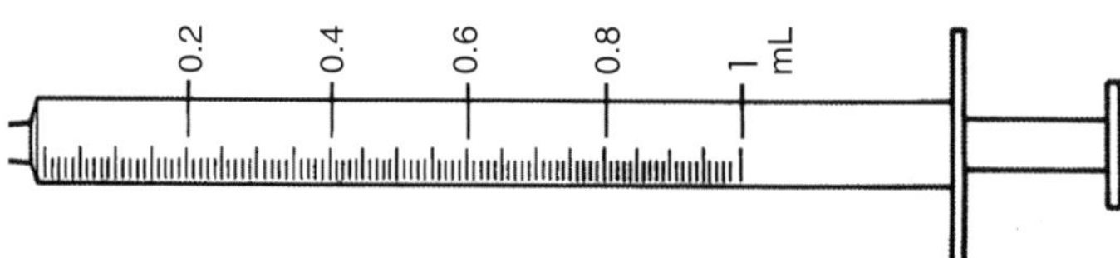

7. Ordered: Imitrex (sumaTRIPtan) 10 mg subcut bid prn for a patient with acute migraine headaches. Available: Imitrex vial 12 mg per mL.

a. How many mL will you prepare for the nearest measurable dose?

b. Indicate the dose with an arrow on the syringe provided.

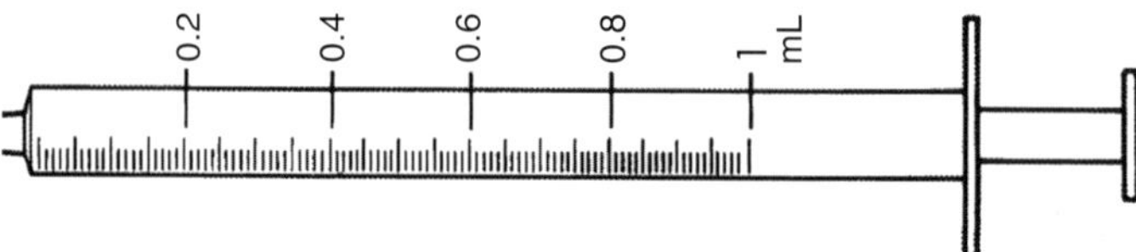

8. Indicate 4.7 mL on the syringe.

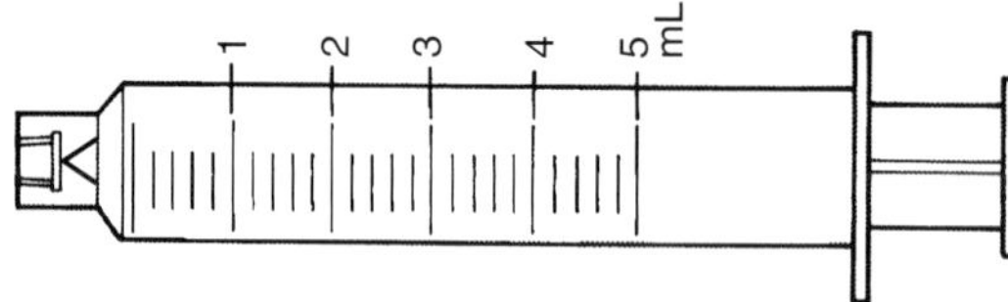

9. State the volume prepared in the syringe.

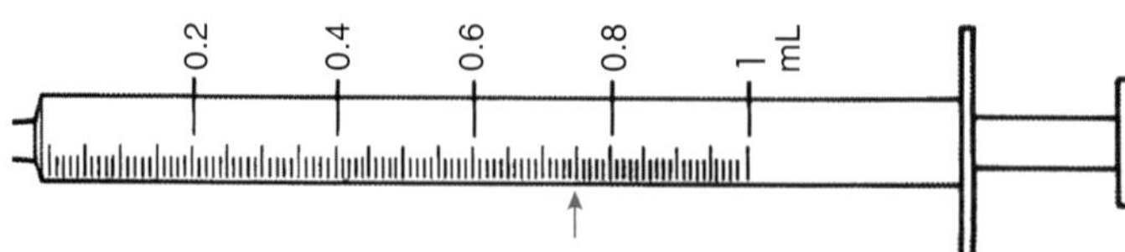

10. State three practices that can protect the nurse from needlestick injuries.

For additional practice problems, refer to the Parenteral Dosages section of the Elsevier's Interactive Drug Calculation Application, Version 1 on Evolve.

Answer Key

5 Injectable Medication Calculations

WORKSHEET **5A** (page 156)

1. **a.** 3 mL
   b. 0.1 mL
   c. 1.2 mL

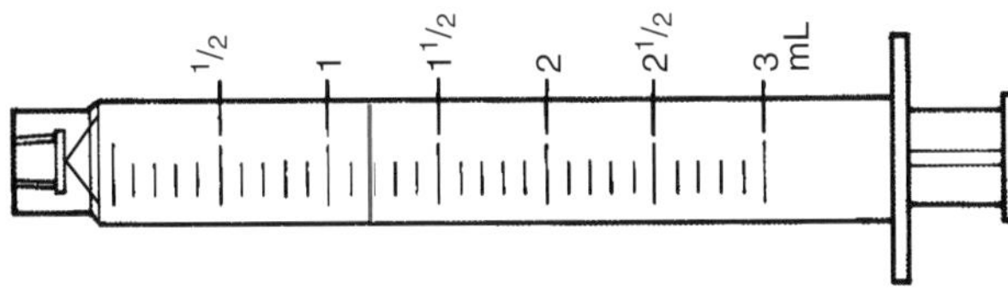

2. **a.** 5 mL
   b. 0.2 mL
   c. 4.4 mL

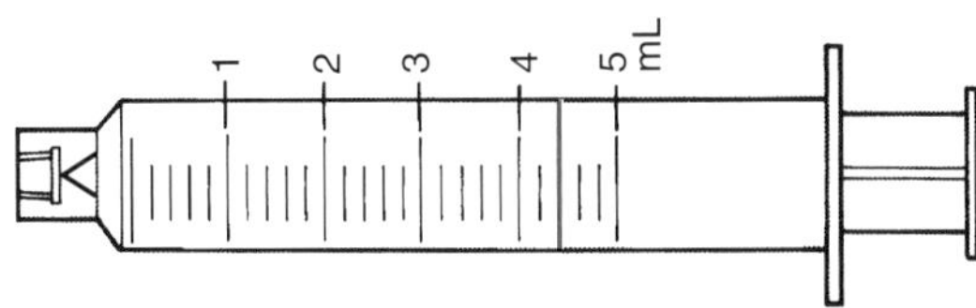

3. **a.** 1 mL
   b. 0.01 mL
   c. 0.25 mL

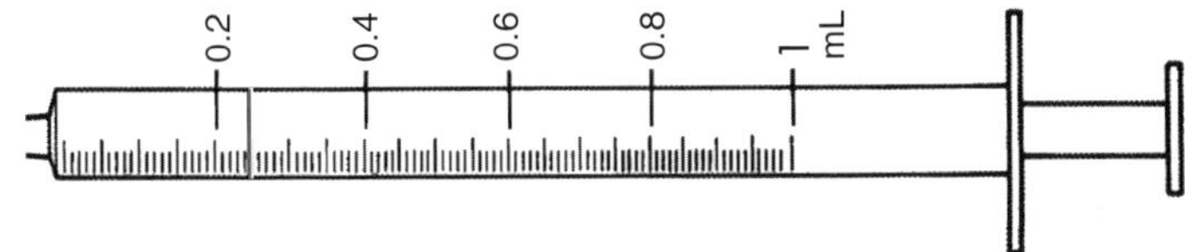

4. **a.** 10 mL
   b. 0.2 mL
   c. 6.8 mL

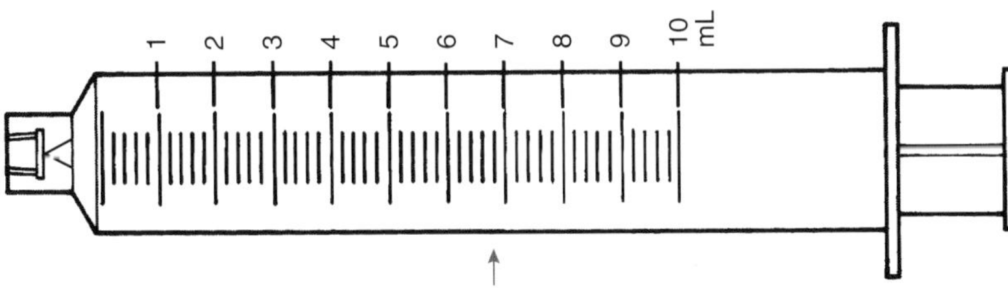

5. **a.** 20 mL
   b. 0.4 mL
   c. 13.2 mL

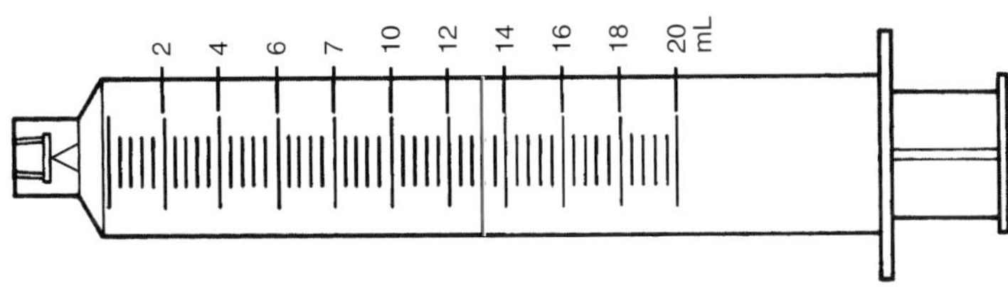

WORKSHEET 5B (page 157)

1. 3 mL, 0. 1, 1.9 mL
2. 10 mL, 0.2, 8.2 mL
3. 5 mL, 0.2, 4.6 mL
4. 3 mL, 0.1, 2.7 mL
5. 1 mL, 0.01, 0.15 mL

WORKSHEET 5C (page 158)

1. **a.** 3 mL
   b. tenths

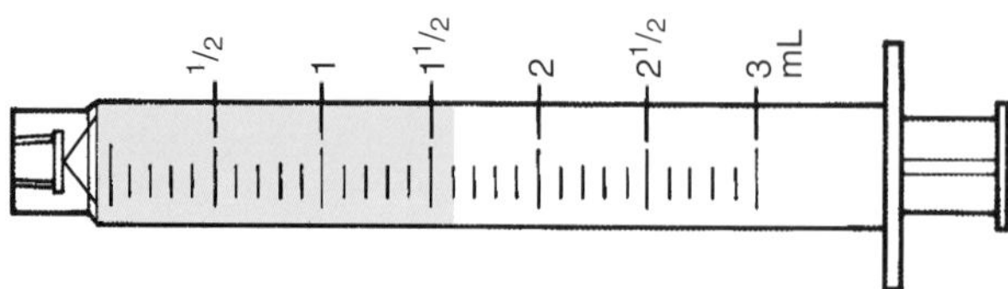

2. **a.** 10 mL
   b. 0.2

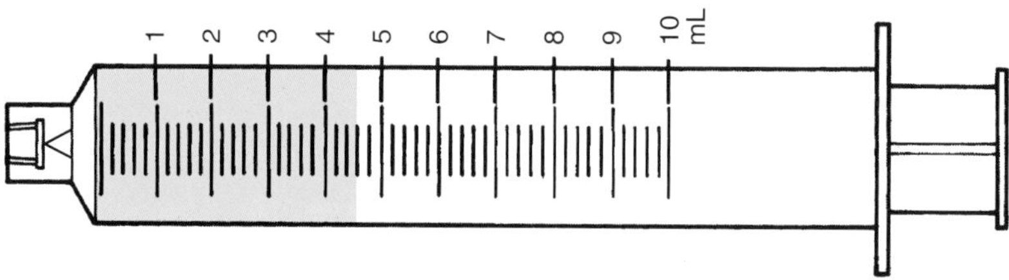

3. **a.** 5 mL
   b. 0.2

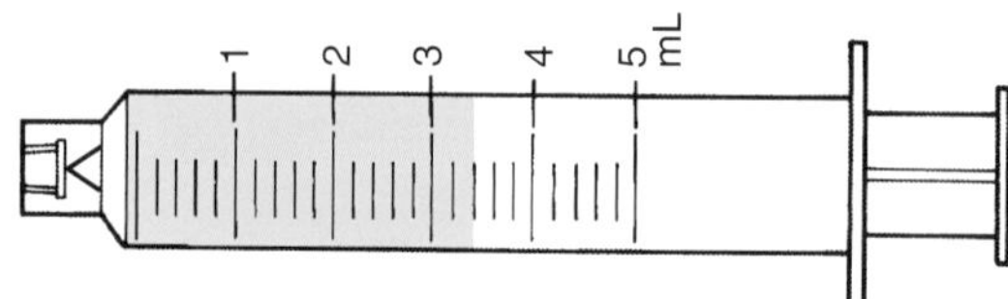

4. **a.** 3 mL
   b. tenths

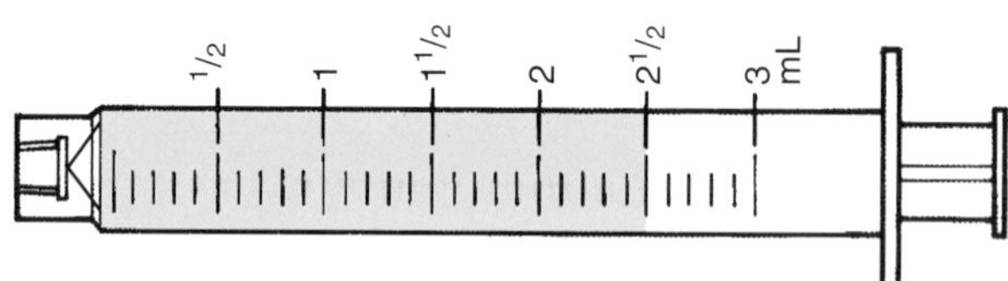

5. **a.** 1 mL
   b. hundredths

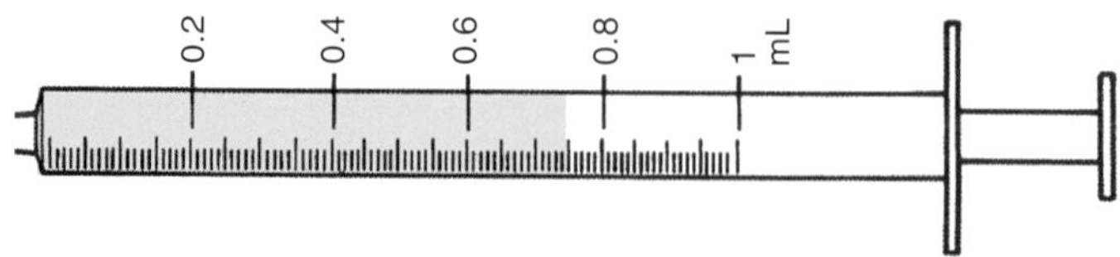

WORKSHEET **5D** (page 162)

Reading labels carefully is a critical patient-safety responsibility, in addition to knowing why the medication was ordered for the patient. The nurse who administers the medication provides the last protection from a medication error for the patient.

1. a. 40 mg per mL

b. There are other medications with similar names that may be confused with this name, so special care must be taken when identifying the order, including matching the patient condition with the drug activity and reason for the order.

c. IM or IV

2. a. 40 mg per 0.4 mL

b. In a syringe

3. a. 1,200,000 Units per 2 mL

b. Units are standardized measure used to quantify the biological activity of selected products, including vitamins, hormones, vaccines, and blood products (see Vocabulary section).

c. Not for treatment of syphilis; for deep IM injection only; not for intravenous use

d. Controlled-release product (see Abbreviations on inside front cover)

4. a. 4 mg per mL of this high-alert narcotic

b. A federally controlled substance. Schedule II drugs have a high potential for abuse and physical and/or psychological dependence.

c. 4000 mcg per mL

d. Locked drawer

e. High-alert drugs have the potential to cause serious harm if given in error.

5. a. 15 mg per mL of this high-alert narcotic

b. 1 mL Dosette vial

6. a. 500 mcg per 2 mL

b. 0.5 mg per 2 mL

c. For *slow* IV or *deep* IM route

7. a. 30 mg per mL

b. For IM or IV use

c. Protect from light. Product is unstable when exposed to light.

8. a. 2 mEq per mL

b. *Concentrate* alerts the nurse to be sure to look for dilution instructions on the label or in the accompanying literature or in a current drug reference if the label does not specify dilution.

c. For IV route

d. No single dose

9. a. 50 mg per mL

b. IV route

c. WARNING re: dilution with Sterile Saline or Sterile Water for Injection. It is very important to note that Sterile Saline and Sterile Water for injection are NOT interchangeable. Sterile Saline and Sterile Water for injection containing *preservatives* are also NOT interchangeable with the non-preservative equivalents. A label with preservatives will usually say BACTERIOSTATIC. It may contain phenol and/or other products.

ALWAYS check dilution solution labels and literature for preservatives. The label with preservatives will usually say *bacteriostatic*. Injectables with preservatives *cannot* be administered via the intravenous or spinal, epidural, or any central nervous system route. The preservatives are usually harmless via the subcutaneous and intramuscular route. Sterile saline for injection is most commonly used for injection dilutions because it is an isotonic solution. Sterile water for injection is used *only* for specific purposes because it is hypotonic. Recheck with Pharmacy if there are any questions.

10. a. 25 mg per mL

b. Protect from light. Do not use if crystals have separated from solution.*

WORKSHEET **5E** (page 165)

1. 1.5 mL

HAVE WANT TO HAVE

5 mg : 1 mL = 7.5 mg : x mL

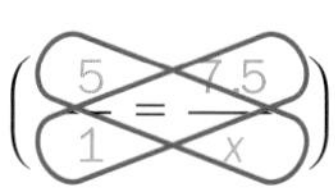

Estimate: Will give more than the unit dose on hand

$$\frac{\not{5}}{\not{5}}x = \frac{7.5}{5}$$

x = 1.5 mL

Answer supports the estimate.

PROOF
5 × 1.5 = 7.5
1 × 7.5 = 7.5

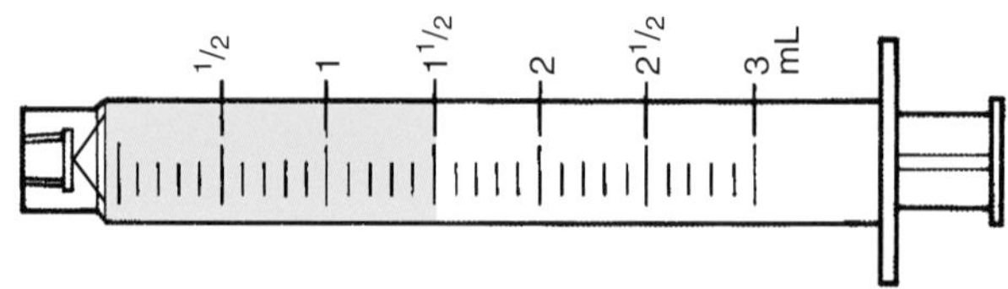

*Always check fluids for discoloration and crystals and foreign bodies. Hold them up to a good light. If problems are noted, return fluids to pharmacy and obtain a replacement.

2. 1.6 mL

KNOW WANT TO KNOW

1000 mg : 1 g = x mg : 0.2 g

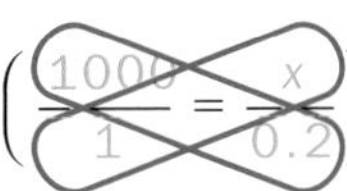

x = 200 mg

HAVE WANT TO HAVE

250 mg : 2 mL = 200 mg : x mL

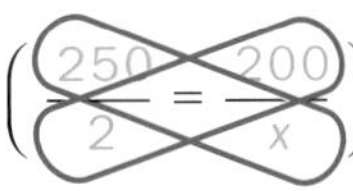

Estimate: Will give less than the unit dose 2 mL on hand.*

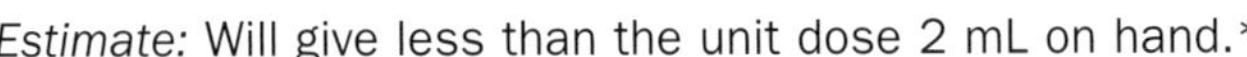

$$\frac{250}{250}x = \frac{400}{250}$$

x = 1.6 mL

Answer supports the estimate.

PROOF
255 × 1.6 = 400
2 × 200 = 400

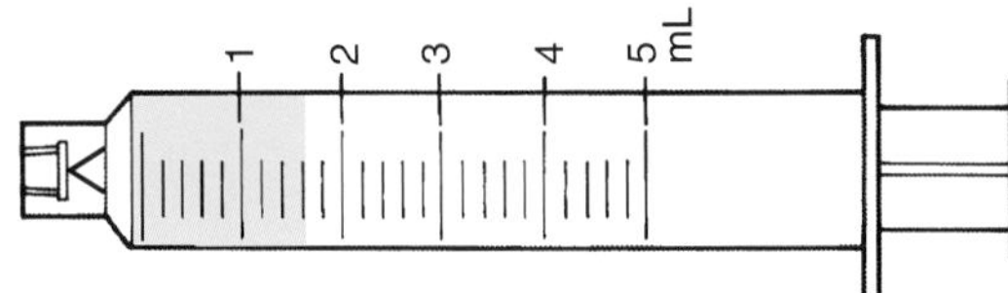

3. 2 mL

KNOW WANT TO KNOW

1000 mg : 1 g = x mg : 0.1 g

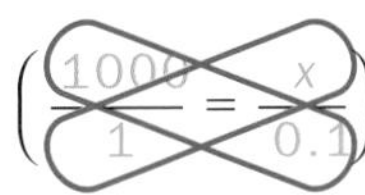

x = 100 mg

Estimate: Will give 2 times the unit dose on hand.

HAVE WANT TO HAVE

50 mg : 1 mL = 100 mg : x mL

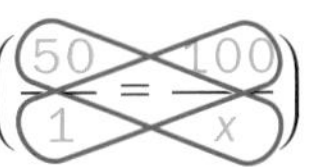

$$\frac{50}{50}x = \frac{100}{50}$$

x = 2 mL

Answer supports the estimate.

PROOF
50 × 2 = 100
1 × 100 = 1

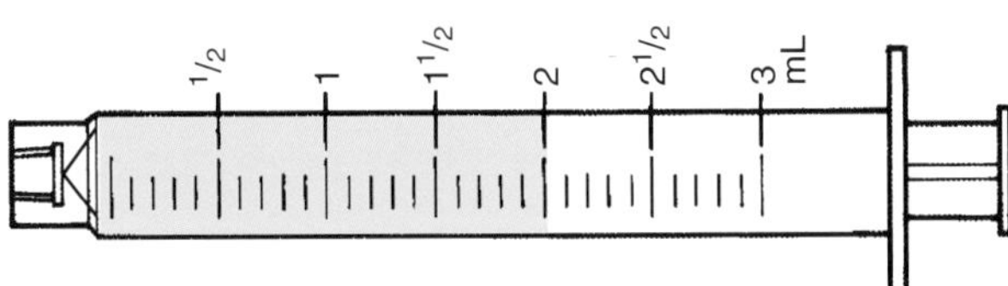

---

*Make your estimate when the terms are equal.

4. KNOW WANT TO KNOW

1000 mcg = 1 mg = x mcg : 1 mg

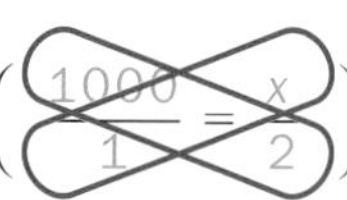

x = 1000 mcg

HAVE WANT TO HAVE

400 mcg : 1 mL = 1000 mcg : x mL

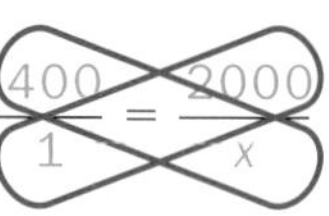

Estimate: Will give about $2\frac{1}{2}$ times more than 1 mL.

400 x = 2000

x = 2.5 mL

Answer supports the estimate.

PROOF
400 × 2.5 = 1000
1 × 1000 = 1000

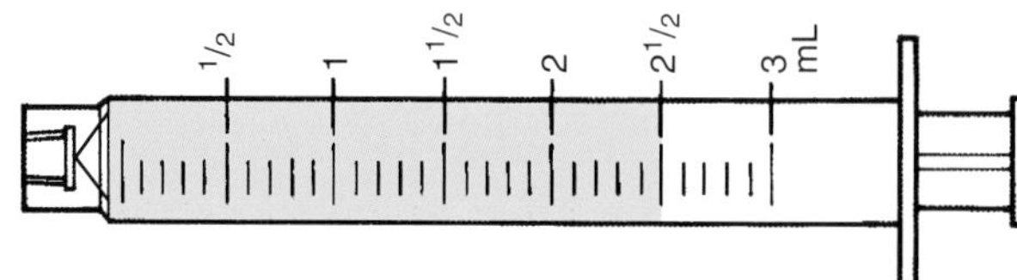

5. 0.9 mL

KNOW WANT TO KNOW

0.45 mcg : 1 kg = x mcg : 80 kg

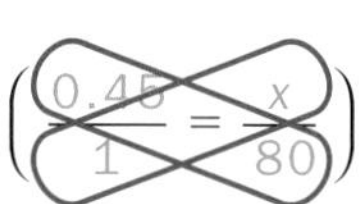

x = 36 mcg

HAVE WANT TO HAVE

40 mcg : 1 mL = 36 mcg : x mL

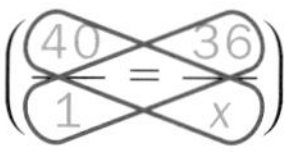

Estimate: Will give slightly less than 1 mL.

$$\frac{\cancel{40}}{\cancel{40}} x = \frac{36}{40}$$

x = 0.9 mL

Answer supports the estimate.

PROOF
40 × 0.9 = 36
1 × 36 = 36

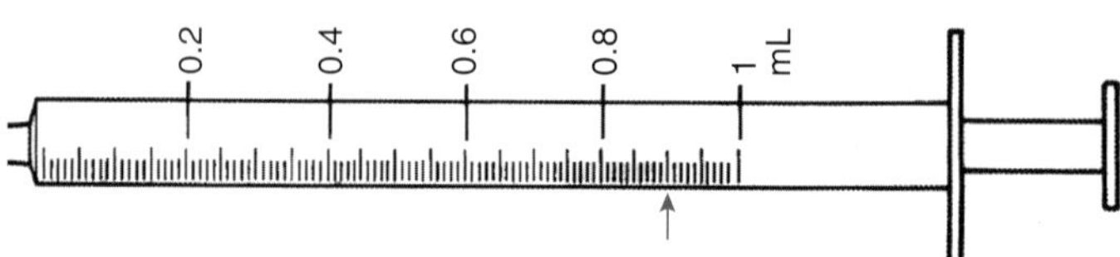

WORKSHEET **5F** (page 167)

1. c
2. a
3. b
4. b
5. a
6. a
7. d
8. d
9. c*
10. c

*All of the choices present a reason to hold the medication and contact the prescriber.

CHAPTER 5 FINAL (page 170)

1. **a.** 4 mg per mL
   b. Deep IM
   c. 0.5 mL

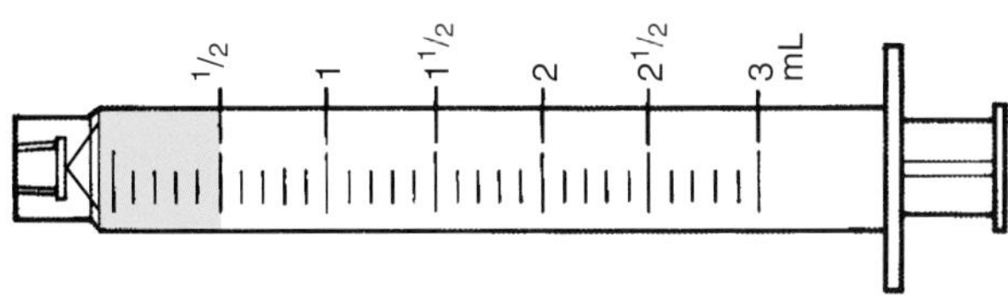

2. **a.** 0.25 mL

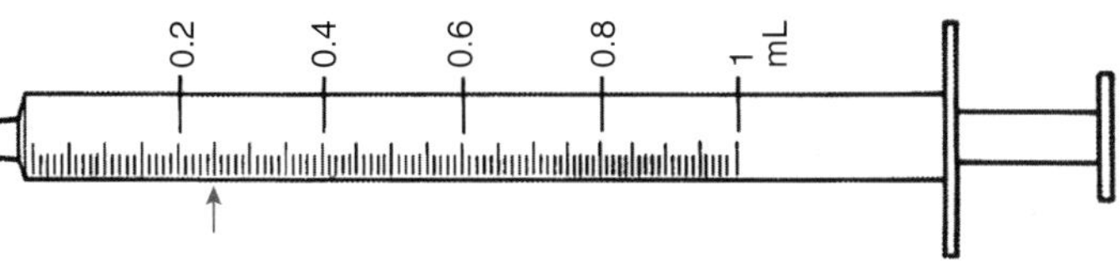

3. **a.** 1 mL

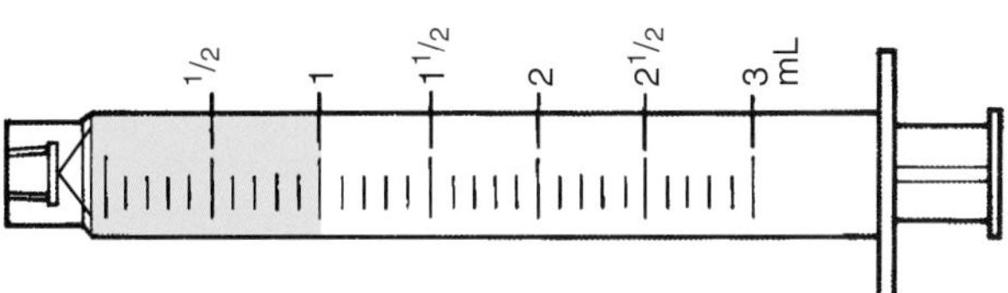

4. **a.** 0.5 mL meperidine
   b. 0.6 mL Vistaril

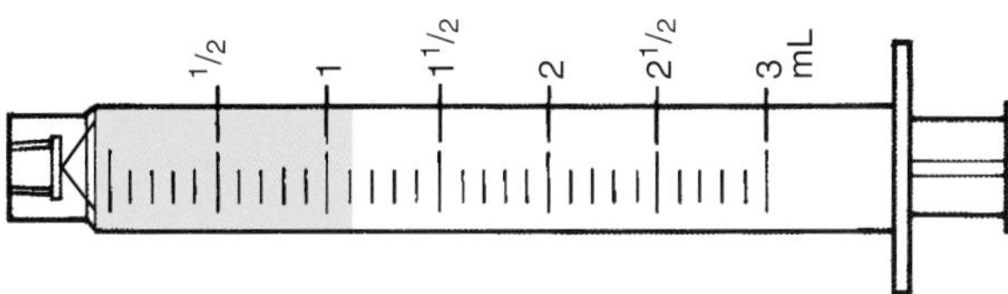

5. 3.4 mL

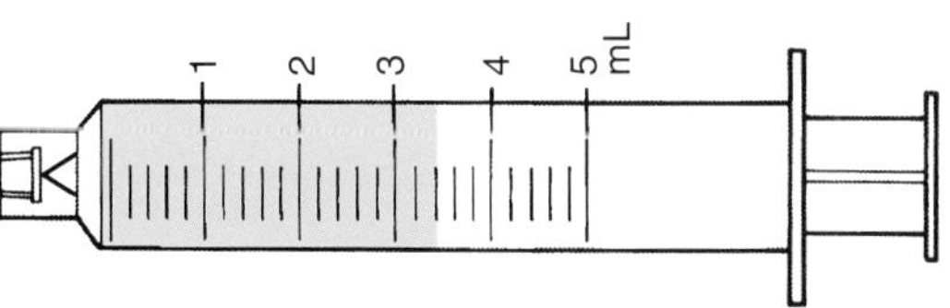

6.

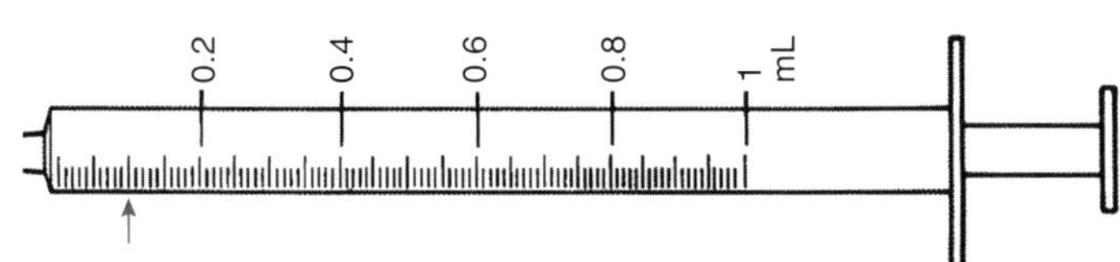

7. 0.83 mL

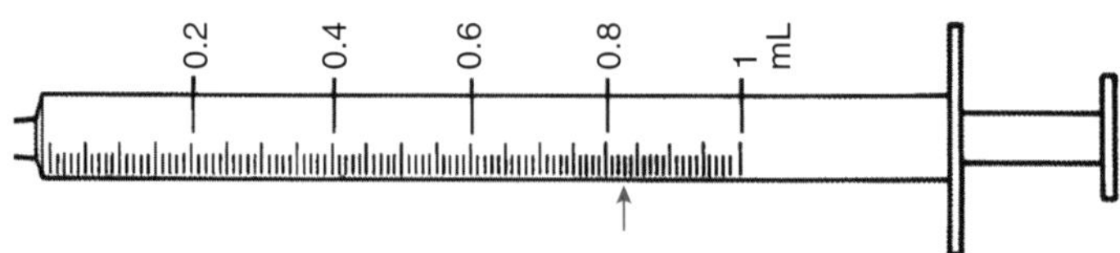

8.

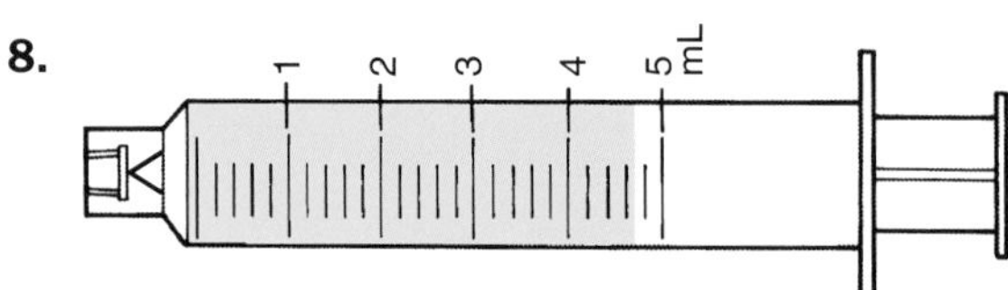

9. 0.75 mL

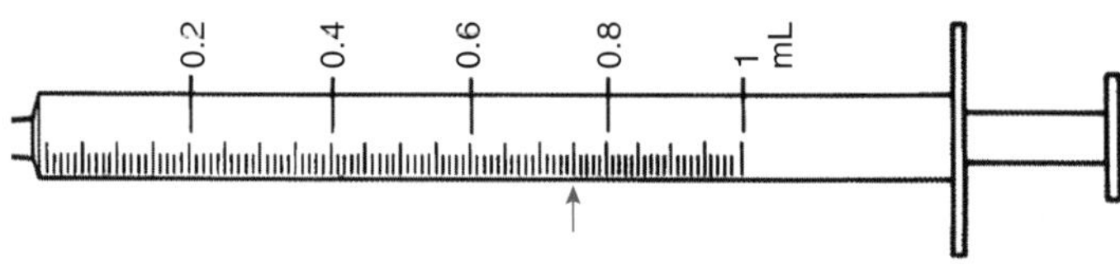

10. **a.** Dispose of used needles and syringes immediately in the nearest hazardous waste container.

b. Use safety syringes and needles if available.

c. Take care in handling the linens and equipment of bedside procedures that involve injections.

d. Wear gloves with any procedure involving injections and/or potential contact with blood.

Note: Report any incident of potential contamination immediately according to agency procedure. Do not wait to see if a problem arises.

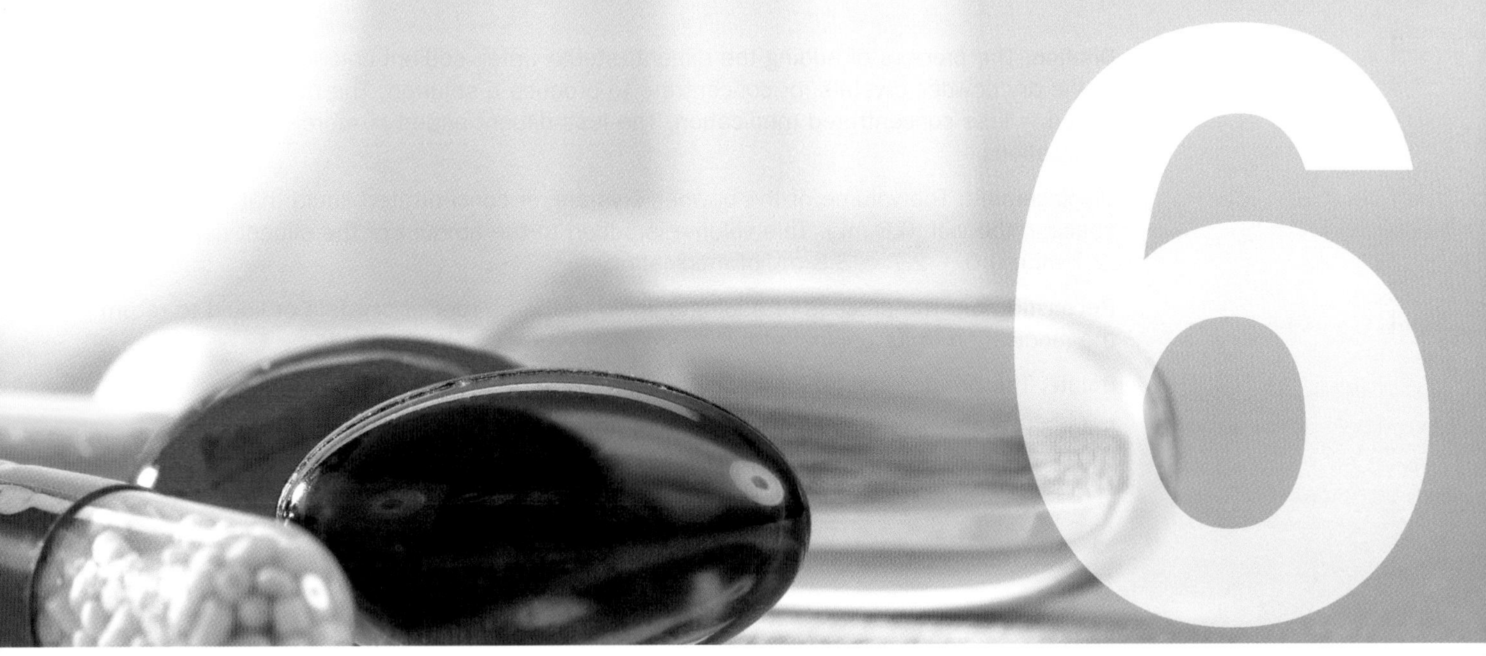

Reconstitution of Medications From Powders and Crystals: Oral and Intramuscular

Objectives

- Accurately determine the specific diluents, diluent amounts, specific doses, conditions for storage, and expiration dates as identified on labels of medications that require reconstitution.
- Reconstitute oral and injectable medications from powders and crystals.
- State the importance of writing the date and time of reconstitution on the medication vial or bottle on multidose medications and initialing.
- Reconstitute and measure liquid medications using a medicine cup and oral syringe.
- Determine the best dilution strength to use for multiple-dosage-strength vials.
- Calculate doses in milligrams, grams, and milliliters for oral and parenteral routes.

Introduction

Preparation of reconstituted medications, often antibiotics, from powders and crystals is usually the nurse's responsibility. The medications are reconstituted by adding a diluent (liquid) recommended by the manufacturer as the vehicle for administration. The shelf life of reconstituted medications is usually short; therefore careful consideration must be given as to how they are stored, the date and time of reconstitution (initialed by the nurse), the expiration date, and the route of administration. This chapter covers the steps for safely and accurately preparing medications from powders and crystals for administration. The dosage used in the problem setups would be first confirmed in the provider's orders.

Vocabulary

Diluent (Solvent): The liquid that is added to the powder or liquid concentrate. The type and amount of diluent (solvent) used is indicated by the manufacturer and found on the medication label. If this information is not printed on the label or accompanying literature, consult the pharmacist, the Physicians' Desk Reference (PDR), the hospital formulary, or the manufacturer's website.

Dilution: The process of adding the diluent (sterile water, sodium chloride, or other liquid) to the dry powder, crystals, or concentrate to produce a solution. The more diluent added = less concentrated medication. The less diluent added = more concentrated medication.

Displacement: The volume of the powder, crystals, or concentrated liquid that occupies space in the vial (0.6 mL). This volume is added to the amount of the diluent used (2.7 mL). 0.6 + 2.7 = 3.3 mL of medication.

Reconstitution: The process of adding a liquid to the powder or crystals or liquid to return the medication to its original state.

Solute: The powder, crystal, or liquid concentrate to be diluted or dissolved.

Solution: The liquid medication that results after the diluent has been added.

Reconstitution

Reconstitution is necessary for medications that are in powdered or crystal form. These medications must be diluted with a liquid (diluent) before they can be administered. Most medications should be reconstituted just before administration. Medications that require reconstitution are stable for only a short time after a diluent is added. In their powdered or crystal form, medications are stable, but when a diluent is added, such as sterile water, normal saline, or an accompanying diluent provided by the manufacturer, the medication begins its "shelf life." That is the time the medication will be stable and able to be used. Labels will indicate whether the reconstituted medication needs to be refrigerated or can be stored at room temperature. The label will also state the number of days the medication will be stable, or able to be used. If multiple doses are prepared, the label must be clearly marked with the diluent used, the strength prepared, the date and time of reconstitution, the preparer's initials, and the date the medication must be discarded to avoid giving an ineffective medication.

CLINICAL RELEVANCE

Reconstituted medications are expensive, as most have a short shelf life. Therefore it is important for the nurse to check that the medication order is current and has not been discontinued before reconstituting. Reconstituted medications are cost effective if all doses are used.

Parenteral reconstituted medication labels will state for intravenous (IV), intramuscular (IM), or subcutaneous (subq) use. Oral medications will be reconstituted with tap water or sterile water. If the directions for reconstitution are unclear, consult the pharmacist, the hospital drug formulary, the Physicians' Desk Reference (PDR), or the manufacturer's website.

Reconstitution: Medication Labels

Labels for medications that require reconstitution contain information about the amount of diluent to use and the resulting concentration. The important information is as follows:

- Strength-reconstitution directions
- Usual dose
- Route
- Name—generic and proprietary
- Expiration date
- Storage conditions/shelf life

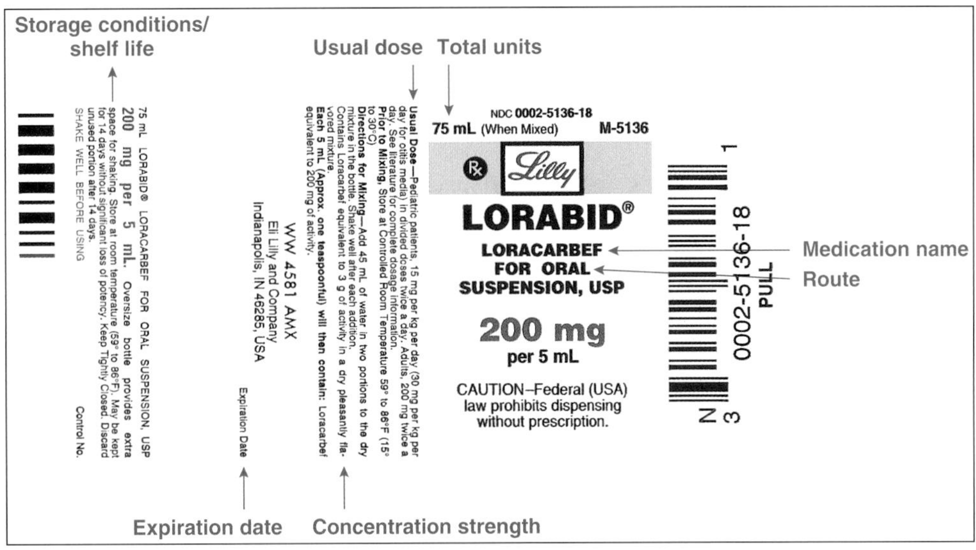

Storage conditions/ shelf life
Usual dose
Total units
NDC 0002-5136-18
75 mL (When Mixed)
M-5136
Lilly
LORABID®
LORACARBEF
FOR ORAL
SUSPENSION, USP
200 mg
per 5 mL
CAUTION–Federal (USA) law prohibits dispensing without prescription.
Medication name
Route
0002-5136-18
PULL
Expiration date
Concentration strength

CLINICAL ALERT!

If the vial is a multiple-dose vial, the nurse must note on the label the date, time, amount of diluent used, and his or her initials.

Many solutions are unstable after being reconstituted. Read labels carefully for directions on storing the solution in the refrigerator or in a dark place. There is usually a time limit or expiration date on the vial. It is important to date, label, and initial all reconstituted medications.

Measuring Liquid Medications

When measuring a liquid medication, put the transparent measuring device on a flat surface, then measure at eye level. The curved surface of the liquid is called *the meniscus* (Figure 6.1). The meniscus is caused by the surface tension of the medication against the side of the medication cup. All liquid medication is measured at the meniscus level.

Medications can be measured in a medicine cup and transferred to an oral syringe for ease in administration and accuracy (Figure 6.2).

However, liquid medications can be measured more accurately in a syringe than in a medicine cup (Figure 6.3).

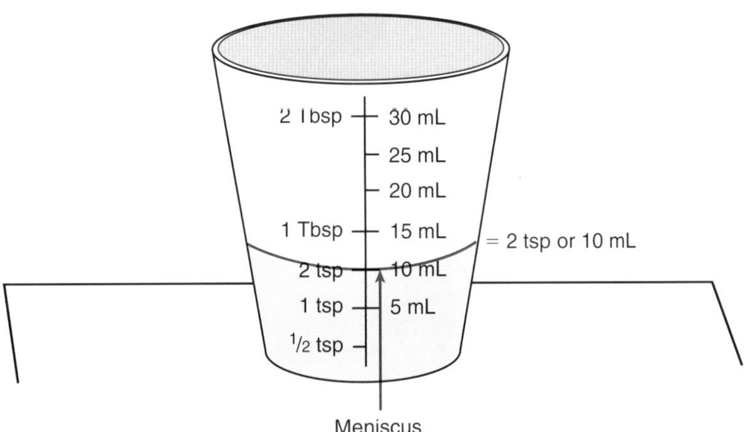

FIGURE 6.1 Measuring cup showing meniscus. Meniscus is the lowest level. Always measure the meniscus on a flat surface.

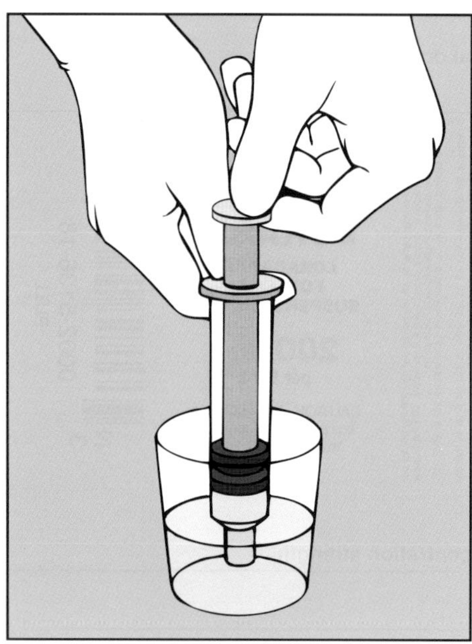

FIGURE 6.2 Filling a syringe directly from medicine cup. (From Clayton BD, Willihnganz M: *Basic pharmacology for nurses*, ed 17, St Louis, 2017, Mosby.)

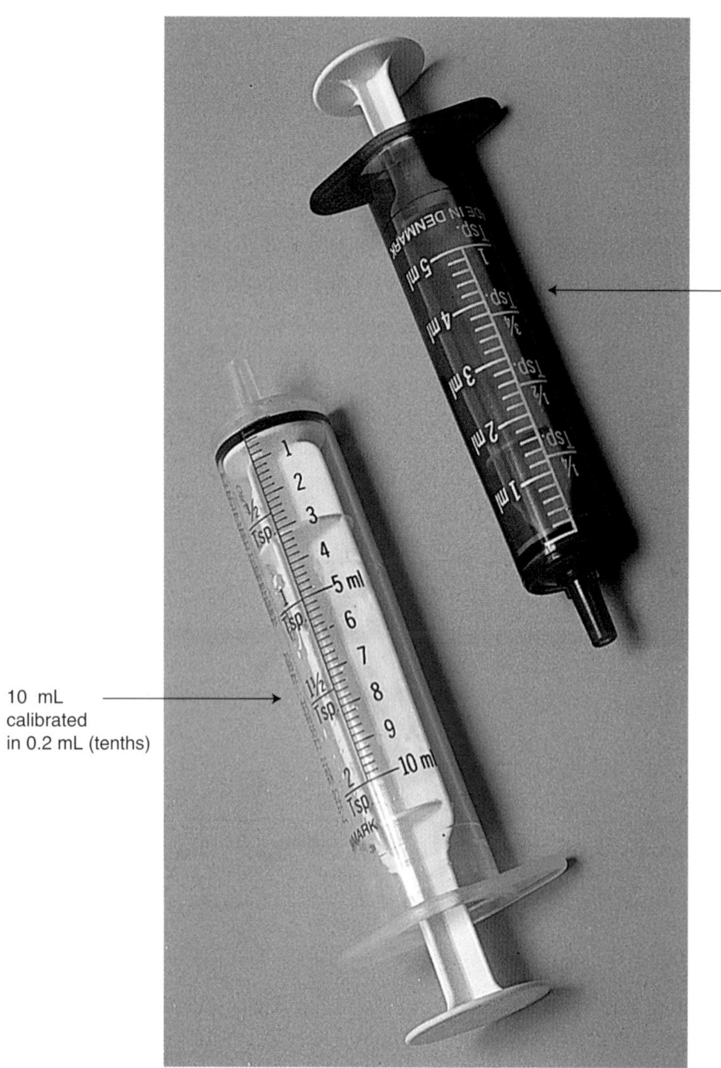

FIGURE 6.3 Oral syringes. Oral syringes are not sterile and are used only for oral medications. (From Clayton BD, Willihnganz M: *Basic pharmacology for nurses*, ed 17, St Louis, 2017, Mosby.)

Answers on page 215

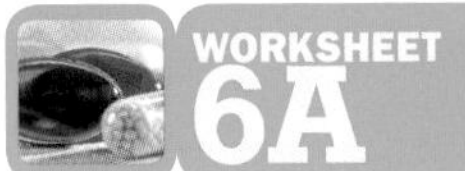

WORKSHEET 6A Practice in Reconstituting and Measuring Liquid Medications for Administration

Show your calculations and proofs in the following problems. Shade in the correct dose on the medicine cup. Draw a line on the syringe showing the correct dose. Which should be used to administer the medication and why?

1. Ordered: Biaxin 300 mg po bid for lung infection.
Follow mixing directions on the label.

a. How many total milliliters of water are needed?

b. How many total milligrams of Biaxin are in the bottle?

c. How many milliliters will provide 300 mg of Biaxin? Draw the amount you will give on the medicine cup and the syringe.

d. How many doses are in the bottle?

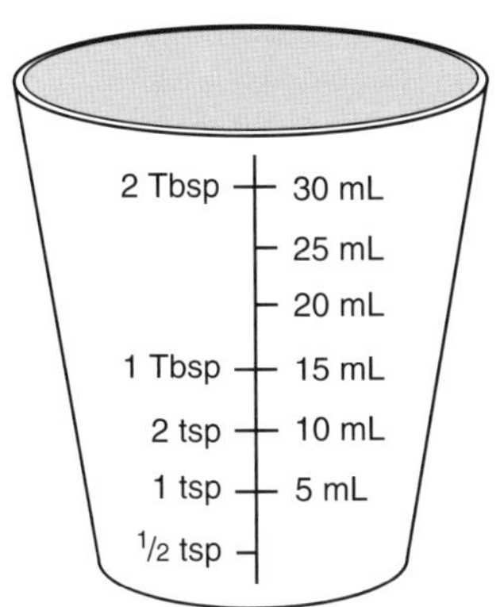

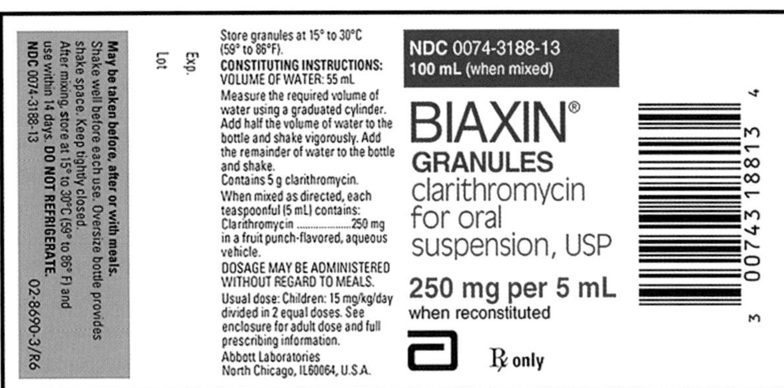

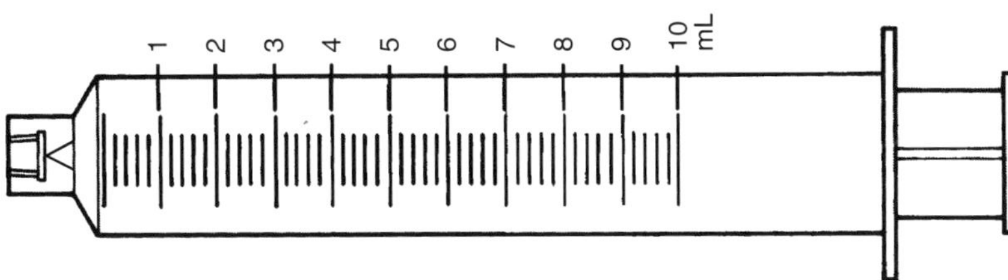

2. Ordered: Cefprozil 300 mg po stat, then 125 mg every 6 hours for a urinary tract infection.
   a. How many milliliters of water will you add?
   b. How many milliliters will you administer for the stat dose?
   c. How many doses are remaining after administering the stat dose?

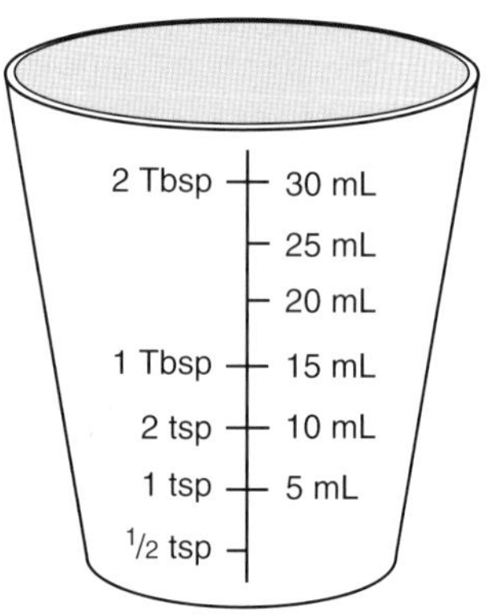

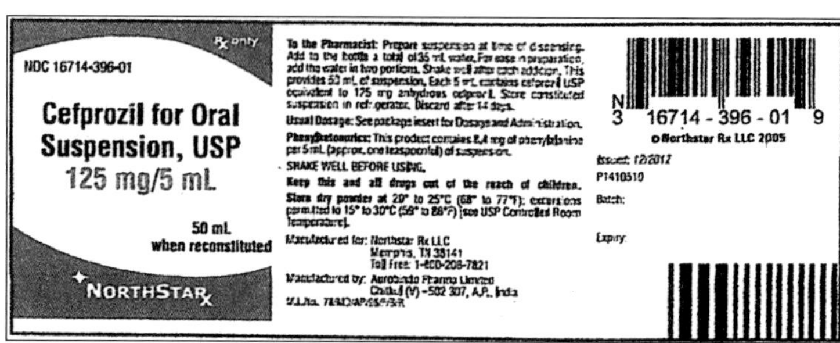

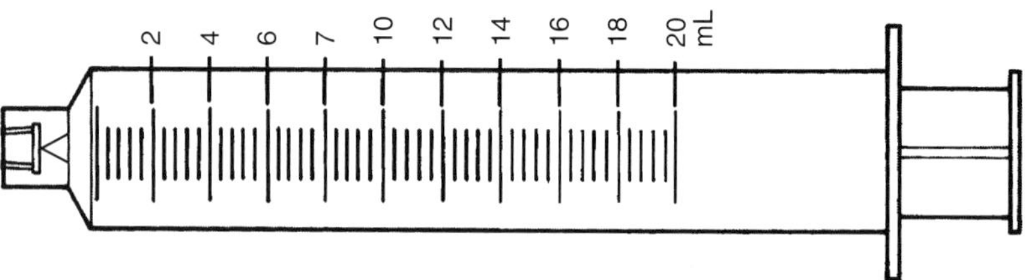

3. Ordered: 350 mg of clarithromycin suspension bid po for mastoiditis.
   a. How many milligrams are in the bottle?
   b. How many milliliters will you administer? Draw the amount you will give on the medicine cup and syringe.

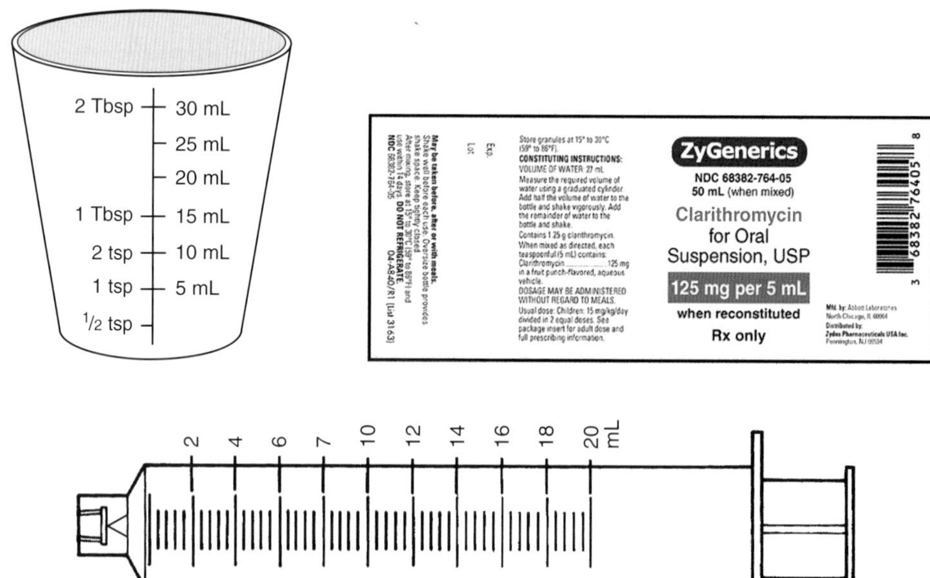

4. Ordered: cefadroxil suspension 200 mg po q8h for acute sinusitis.
   a. How many milliliters of water will you add?
   b. How many total milliliters are in the bottle?
   c. How many milliliters of cefadroxil will you administer? Draw the amount you will give on the medicine cup and syringe.

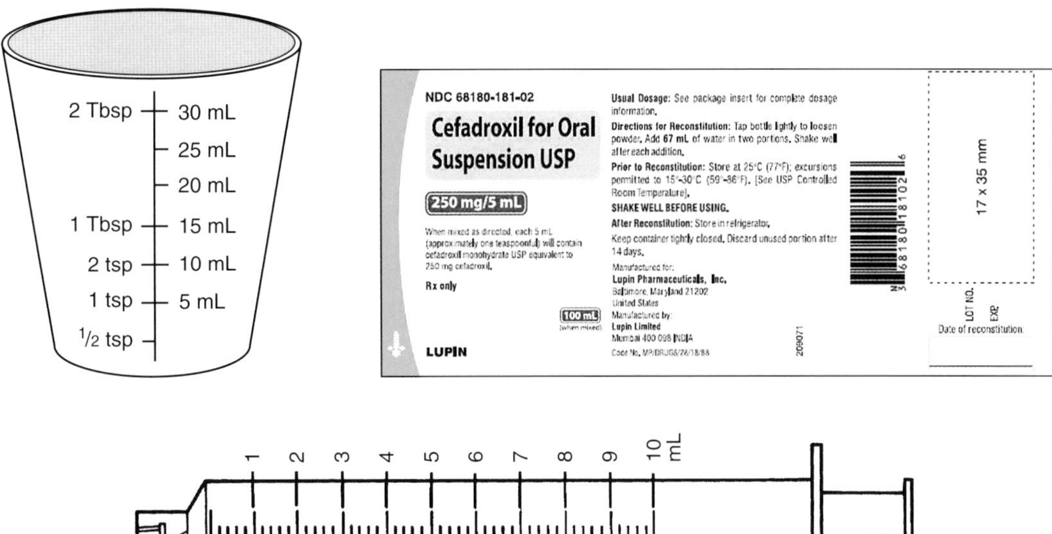

5. Ordered: Lorabid 400 mg po q12h times 14 days 1 hour ac for pneumonia. Follow mixing directions on the label.
   a. How many total milliliters of water are needed?
   b. How many total milligrams of Lorabid are in the bottle?
   c. How many milliliters will provide 400 mg? Draw the amount you will give on the medicine cup.
   d. How many doses are in the bottle?

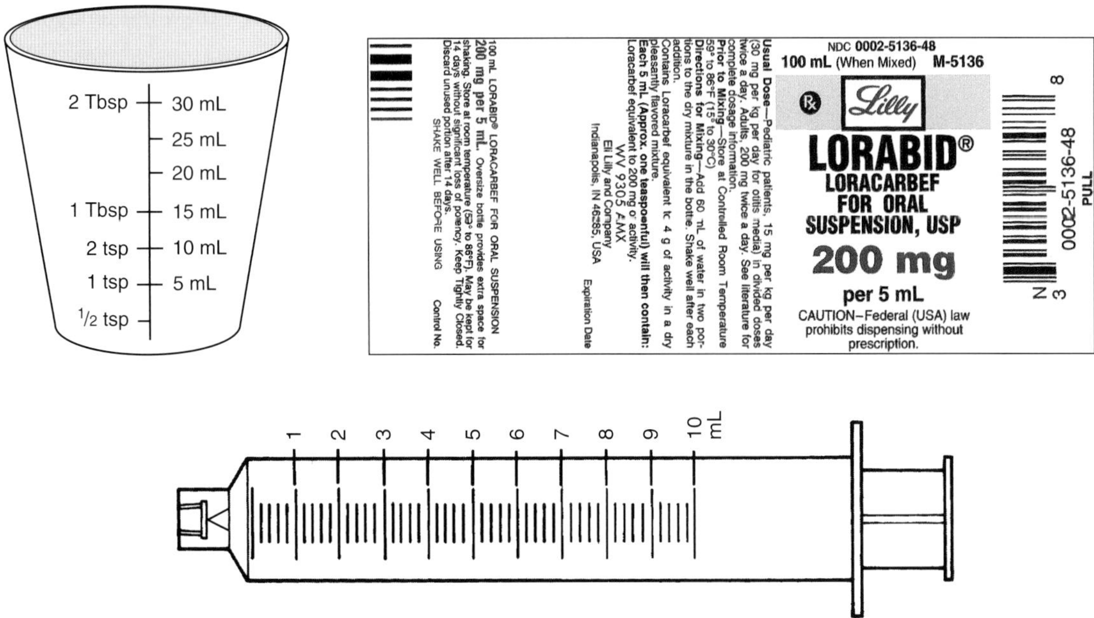

6. Ordered: 40 mg Pepcid po four times a day for a duodenal ulcer.
   a. How many milliliters of diluent will you add?
   b. How many total milliliters of Pepcid are in the bottle?
   c. How many milliliters will you administer?
   d. How many doses are in the bottle?

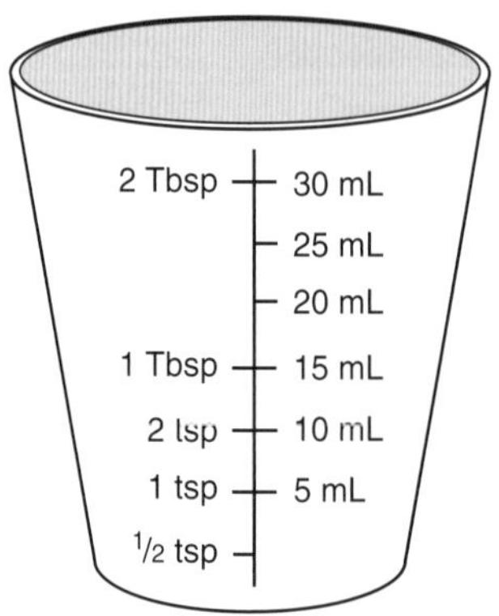

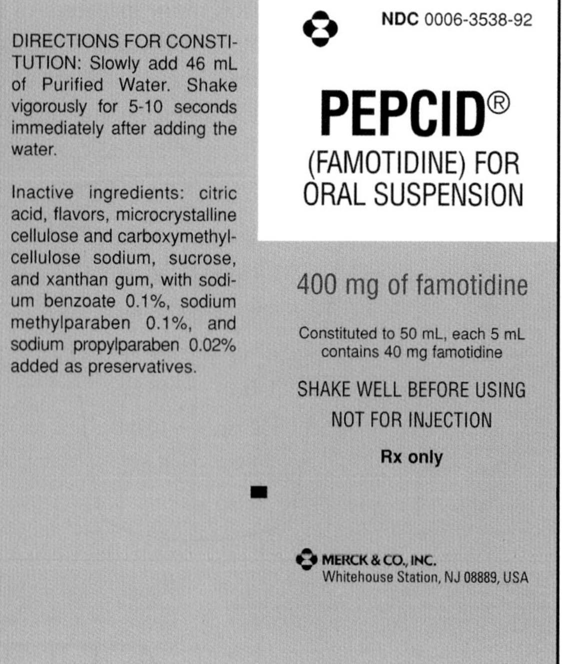

DIRECTIONS FOR CONSTITUTION: Slowly add 46 mL of Purified Water. Shake vigorously for 5-10 seconds immediately after adding the water.
Inactive ingredients: citric acid, flavors, microcrystalline cellulose and carboxymethylcellulose sodium, sucrose, and xanthan gum, with sodium benzoate 0.1%, sodium methylparaben 0.1%, and sodium propylparaben 0.02% added as preservatives.
NDC 0006-3538-92
PEPCID®
(FAMOTIDINE) FOR ORAL SUSPENSION
400 mg of famotidine
Constituted to 50 mL, each 5 mL contains 40 mg famotidine
SHAKE WELL BEFORE USING
NOT FOR INJECTION
Rx only
MERCK & CO., INC.
Whitehouse Station, NJ 08889, USA

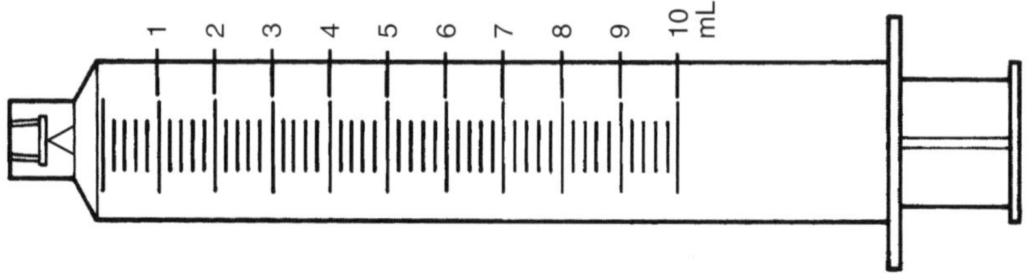

7. Ordered: cefaclor 350 mg po every 8 hours for otitis media. Follow mixing directions on the label.
   a. How many milliliters of water are needed?
   b. How many total milligrams of cefaclor are in the bottle?
   c. How many doses are in the bottle?
   d. How many milliliters of cefaclor will provide 350 mg? Draw the amount you will give on the medicine cup and syringe.

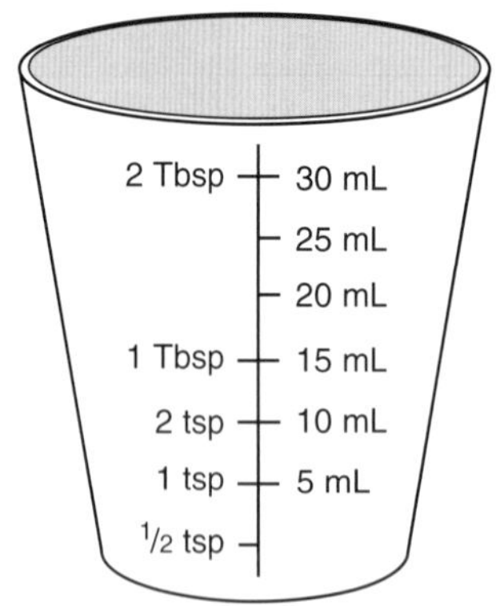

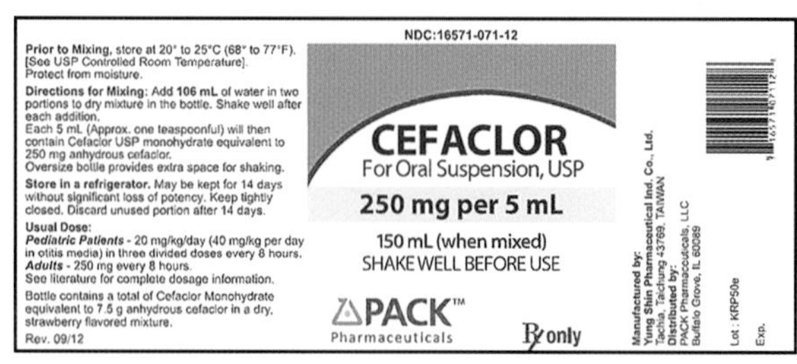

Prior to Mixing, store at 20° to 25°C (68° to 77°F). [See USP Controlled Room Temperature]. Protect from moisture.
Directions for Mixing: Add 106 mL of water in two portions to dry mixture in the bottle. Shake well after each addition.
Each 5 mL (Approx. one teaspoonful) will then contain Cefaclor USP monohydrate equivalent to 250 mg anhydrous cefaclor.
Oversize bottle provides extra space for shaking.
Store in a refrigerator. May be kept for 14 days without significant loss of potency. Keep tightly closed. Discard unused portion after 14 days.
Usual Dose:
Pediatric Patients - 20 mg/kg/day (40 mg/kg per day in otitis media) in three divided doses every 8 hours.
Adults - 250 mg every 8 hours.
See literature for complete dosage information.
Bottle contains a total of Cefaclor Monohydrate equivalent to 7.5 g anhydrous cefaclor in a dry, strawberry flavored mixture.
Rev. 09/12
NDC:16571-071-12
CEFACLOR
For Oral Suspension, USP
250 mg per 5 mL
150 mL (when mixed)
SHAKE WELL BEFORE USE
PACK™
Pharmaceuticals
℞ only
Manufactured by:
Yung Shin Pharmaceutical Ind. Co., Ltd.
Tachia, Taichung 43769, TAIWAN
Distributed by:
PACK Pharmaceuticals, LLC
Buffalo Grove, IL 60089
Lot : KRP50e
Exp.

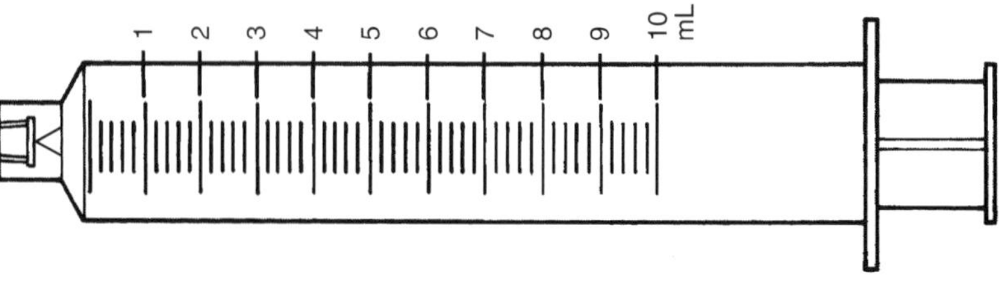

8. Ordered: Augmentin 450 mg po every 8 hours for 24 hours then 250 mg twice a day for 4 days for endocarditis prophylaxis.
   a. How many milliliters of diluent will you add?
   b. How many milliliters will you administer per dose for 24 hours? Draw the amount you will give on the medicine cup and syringe.
   c. How many milliliters are left after the 24 hr doses?
   d. Will you have enough medication for the next 4 days?

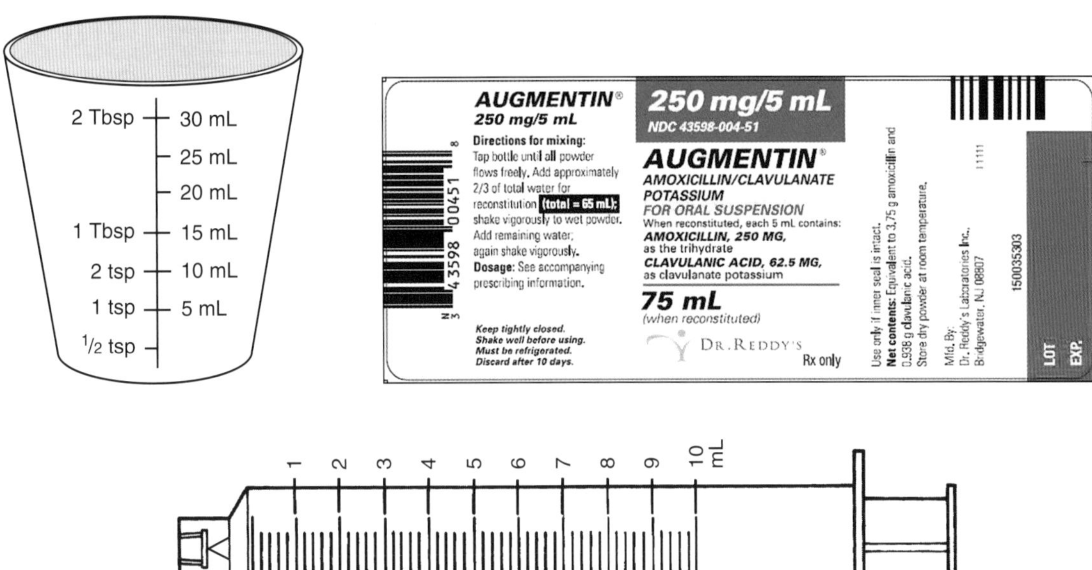

CLINICAL ALERT!

For accuracy, read the medication's level at the meniscus.

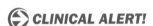

9. Ordered: Fluconazole 50 mg po twice a day as a prophylaxis of candidiasis.
   a. How many mL of distilled water will be added to the powder?
   b. How many mL will you administer?
   c. How many 50-mg doses are in the bottle?

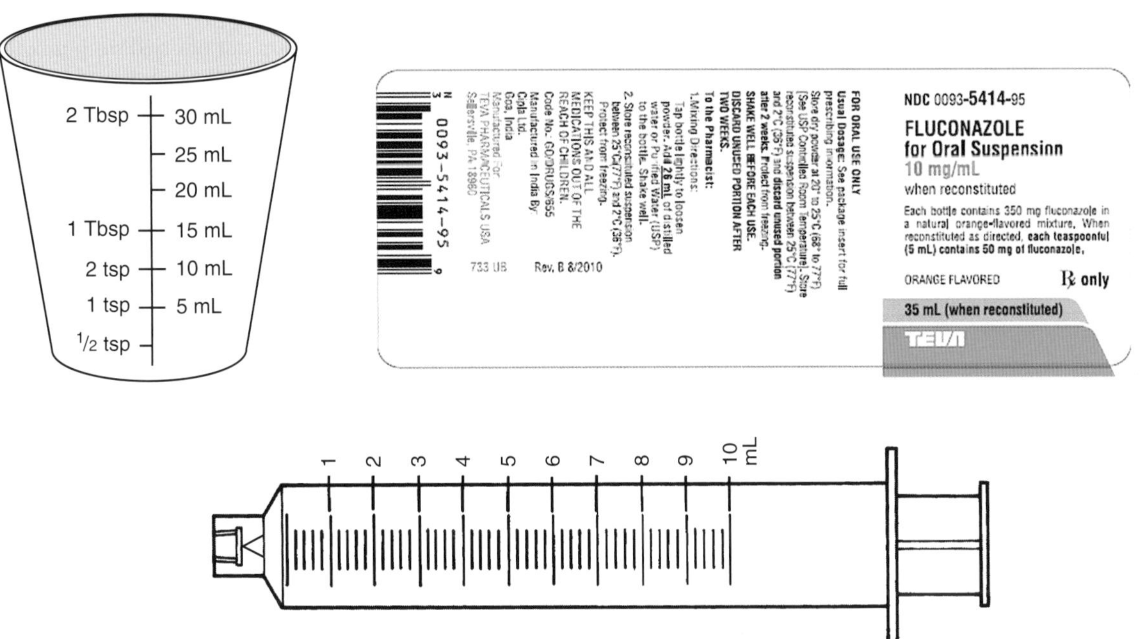

10. Ordered: 200 mg of Biaxin po two times a day for laryngitis.
    a. How many mL of water should be added?
    b. How many mL will you administer?
    c. How many doses are in the bottle?

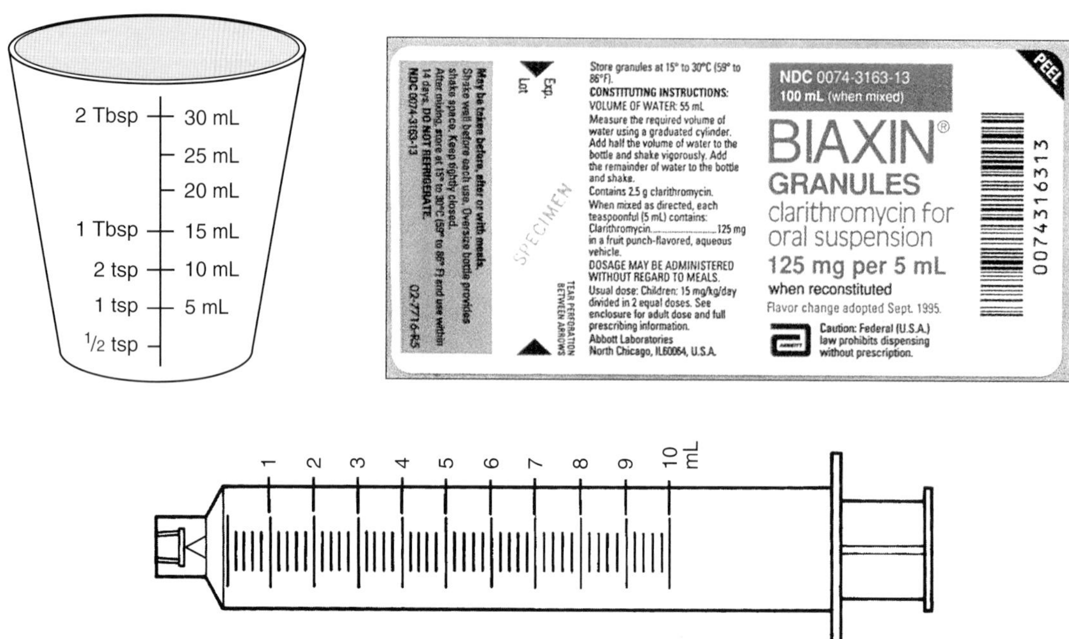

Reconstituting Medications for Parenteral Use: Multiple Strength Decisions

For some medications requiring reconstitution, various amounts of diluent or liquid can be added to produce various strengths of the medication. Medications labels provide directions as to the amount of diluent to be added to produce a specific strength of the medication. As the amount of diluent added changes the strength, the nurse determines the closest strength to the provider's order and adds that amount of diluent. Once the medication is reconstituted, the medication label will provide how many units, grams, milligrams, or micrograms are in each milliliter of the reconstituted drug. The nurse then calculates the correct dosage and prepares the medication for administration.

To understand this concept, consider preparing a cup of soup out of dried soup mix from a package. When more liquid, or diluent, is used, the soup becomes weaker. The less liquid or diluent used, the stronger the soup. The main point is that the amount of dried soup remains constant; only the amount of liquid (diluent) changes to make a stronger or weaker dilution. Reconstituting medications works in the same manner.* There is always a certain amount of powder or crystals in the container before the diluent is added. The drug manufacturer tells you what the displacement factor is. This amount is added to the amount of diluent to give the total number of milliliters (volume). The label on the medication vial states the strength (amount) of medication in the vial. That amount never changes. The only thing that can change is the amount of diluent (liquid) that is added.

*Directions for dissolving medications in vials can be found in the accompanying literature. What will be given is the volume of the powder after it is dissolved in the specified diluent. For instance, the directions may read: *Add 1.4 mL NS to make 2 mL of reconstituted solution.* These directions tell the user that the powder takes up 0.6 mL of space. The displacement factor is 0.6 mL.

1.4 mL + 0.6 mL = 2 mL of medication

Types of Diluents

It is important to use the type of diluent described in the directions for reconstitution. The diluents used to reconstitute powders vary based on the chemical properties of the powder. For example, erythromycin must be reconstituted with sterile water. If normal saline (NS) is used, the powder clumps and will not go into solution. The bacteriostatic agent used in bacteriostatic water is benzyl alcohol. If sterile water is used instead of bacteriostatic water, it may cause some products to clump instead of going into solution. The choice of diluent is based on the pH and the physical properties of the product (medication).

Dibasic sodium is added to some powders to correct the final pH of the product.

Lidocaine is added to ease pain during IM administration. The amount of lidocaine added to the medication would not affect vasoconstriction.

CLINICAL ALERT!

Always use the diluent recommended for reconstitution.

Two-Vial Reconstitution Method

When parenteral drugs are supplied with two vials, one vial will have the diluent and the other the powdered medication. Both vials are cleaned with alcohol swabs. The amount of diluent needed is stated on the medication label. The required amount of the diluent is withdrawn from its vial (Figure 6.4) and injected into the powdered-drug vial. The mixture is then rotated until it is thoroughly mixed.

Example Read the medication label to find out how many units, grams, milligrams, or micrograms are in each milliliter of the reconstituted drug.

Begin by adding 2.7 mL of air to the sterile water for injection (diluent) vial, and then invert the vial to withdraw the 2.7 mL of diluent. Add the 2.7 mL of diluent to the oxacillin sodium vial to make 500 mg of medication in 3 mL.

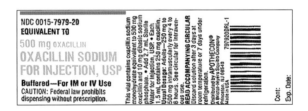

Ordered: 250 mg oxacillin sodium IM q6h.

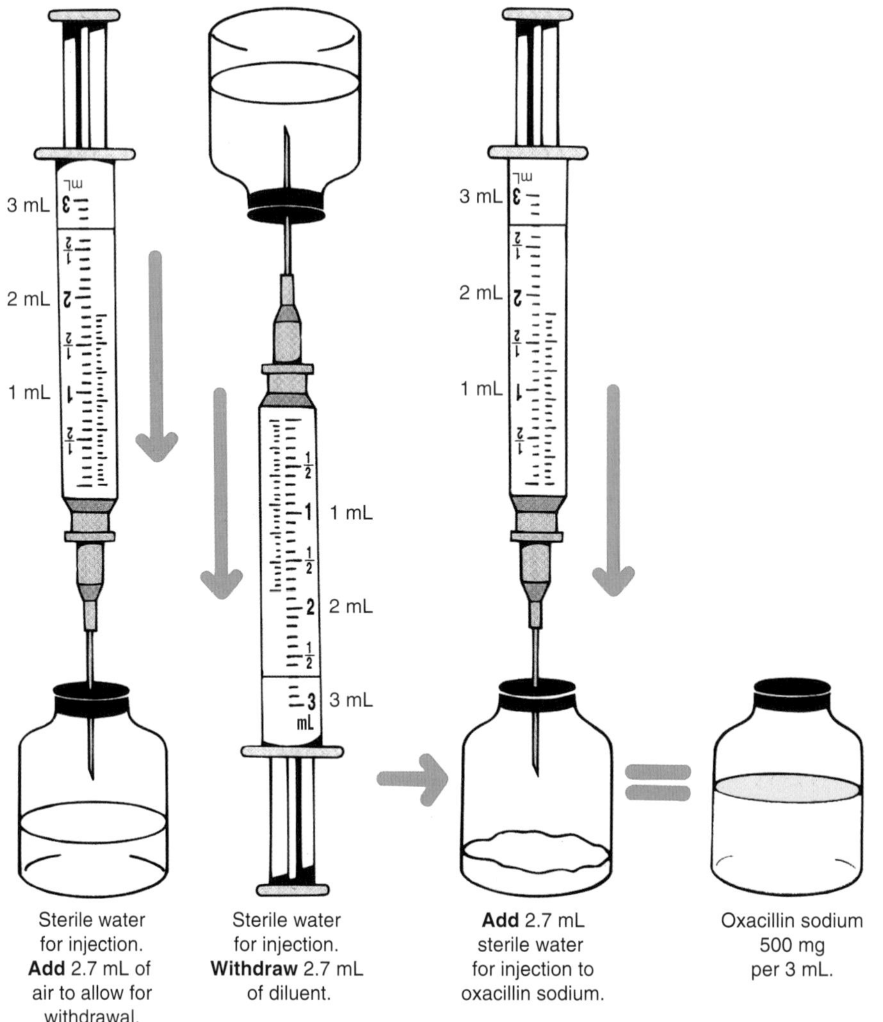
3 mL
2 mL
1 mL
1 mL
2 mL
3 mL
3 mL
2 mL
1 mL
Sterile water for injection. Add 2.7 mL of air to allow for withdrawal.
Sterile water for injection. Withdraw 2.7 mL of diluent.
Add 2.7 mL sterile water for injection to oxacillin sodium.
Oxacillin sodium 500 mg per 3 mL.

FIGURE 6.4 Diluting oxacillin sodium in sterile water for injection.

Use either ratio and proportion or fraction cross product.

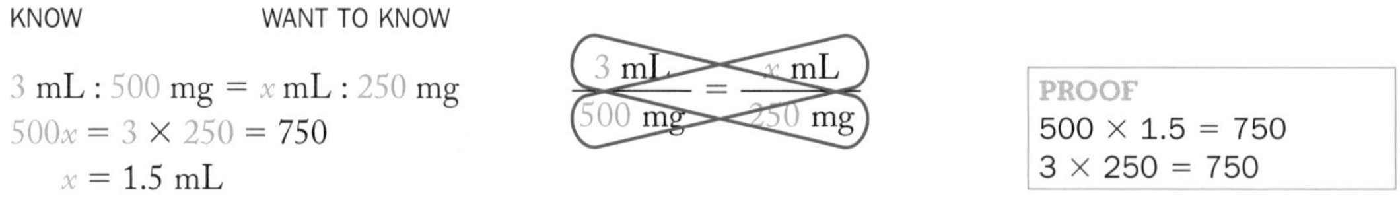

KNOW WANT TO KNOW

3 mL : 500 mg = x mL : 250 mg

$500x = 3 \times 250 = 750$

$x = 1.5$ mL

$$\frac{3 \text{ mL}}{500 \text{ mg}} = \frac{x \text{ mL}}{250 \text{ mg}}$$

PROOF
500 × 1.5 = 750
3 × 250 = 750

Give 1.5 mL of reconstituted solution for each 250 mg.

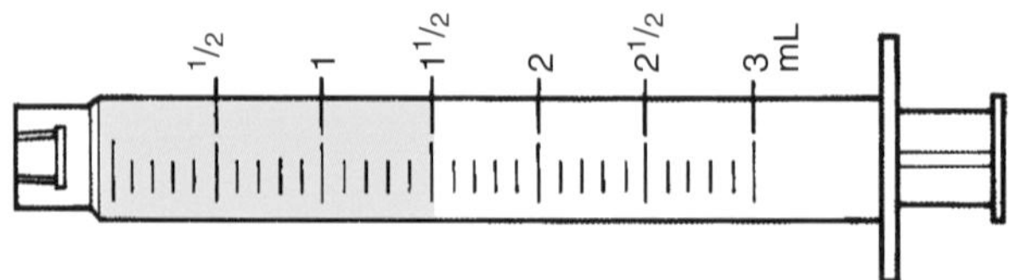
1/2
1
1 1/2
2
2 1/2
3
mL

CLINICAL ALERT!

When giving intramuscular injections, current evidence supports not aspirating prior to administering IM injections. However, there are other studies that support aspirating depending on the physical condition of the patient. Therefore the nurse must always assess the patient and aspirate prior to injecting the medication if there is a possibility the medication may enter a blood vessel. If blood is returned, discard the dose.

Prefilled Vials and Syringes

When medications to be reconstituted are packaged with the diluent attached, the sterility and accuracy of the reconstituted powder are ensured (Figure 6.5). Some medications are reconstituted by the manufacturer and are delivered in prefilled cartridges or syringes. With this technique there is less chance for contamination.

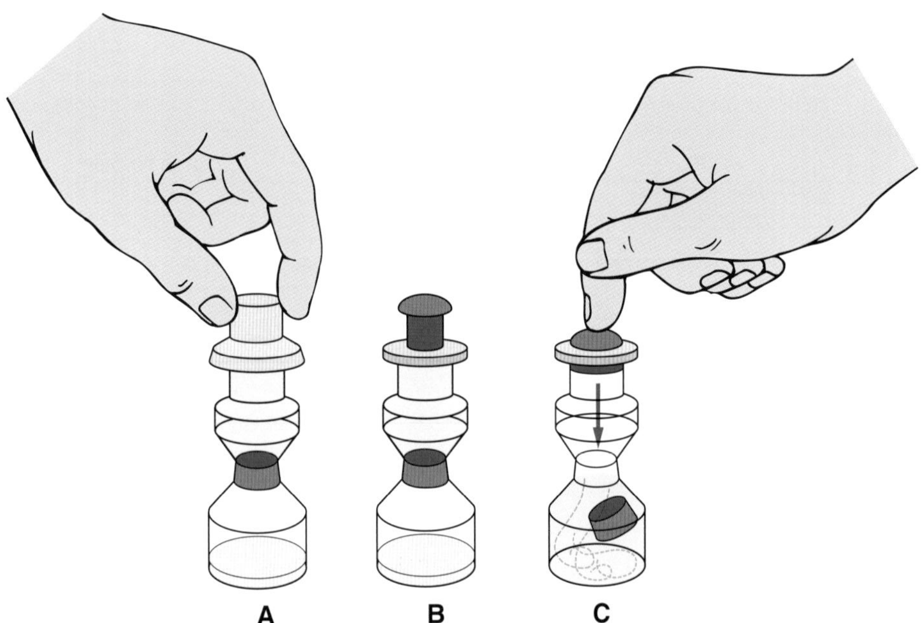

FIGURE 6.5 Mix-o-vial directions. **A,** Remove lid protector. **B,** Powdered medication is in lower half; diluent is in upper half. **C,** Push firmly on the diaphragm-plunger. Downward pressure dislodges the divider between the two chambers. (From Clayton BD, & Willihnganz *Basic pharmacology for nurses,* ed 17, St Louis, 2017, Mosby. Courtesy of Chuck Dresner.)

Most reconstituted medications are antibiotics and have similar-sounding generic and trade names. The following chart is an example of some common sound-alike and look-alike drugs.

Generic Name	Trade Name
Cefaclor	Ceclor
Cefprozil	Cefzil
Cefuroxime	Ceftin
Cephalexin	Keflex
Cephazolin	Kefzol
Ciprofloxacin	Cipro
Gatifloxacin	Tequin
Gemifloxacin	Factive

Figure 6.6 is a pharmacy-generated MAR for 24 hours stated in military time for 8-hour shifts beginning at 0700. At the top, the orders must be signed by an RN indicating that the original order has been verified and is correct and allergies have been noted. SCH is a regularly scheduled medication. The start and stop dates are printed. PRN orders and One Time Only Meds are written in a separate space. Narcotic orders must be rewritten q48h. Discontinued orders are highlighted according to hospital policy and must be renewed if it is necessary to continue them. Site codes are in alpha order. Withheld meds use the code R circled with a nurse's note on the chart. The nurses giving the meds must initial each dose and sign the bottom of the MAR to identify their initials.

Doe, John
ID# 45764304
Age: 50 Sex: M Rm: 406A
Dr. Marin, Cruz

ALLERGIES: DRUGS: Codeine
FOODS: none

RN Verification: *Mary Smith*

Date: *11-09-18* **(Beg)**
11-13-18 **(End)**

MEDICATION: Dose Route Freq

Time of Administration, Site, and Initials

	START	STOP	0700 TO 1459	1500 TO 2259	2300 TO 0659
SCH	*11-09-18 Kefzol* *300 mg IM q8h*	*11-13-18*	*0700* *N MS*	*1500* *O IB*	*2300* *N JB*

Each health care agency will have a protocol for charting injection sites. This is one example

ONE TIME ONLY AND PRN MEDS

Start	Stop	Time	Initials	Full name/title
Lasix 11-16-18 *40 mg IV STAT*		*2000*	*IB*	*Irene Butler, RN*

Sign: *Mary Smith* Initials: *MS* Sign: *Irene Butler* Initials: *IB* Sign: *Jill Beck* Initials: *JB*

SITE CODES

GENERAL HOSPITAL

A	Abdomen (L)	J	Gluteus (LUQ)
B	Abdomen (R)	K	Gluteus (RUQ)
C	Arm (L)	L	Thigh (L)
D	Arm (R)	M	Thigh (R)
E	Eyes (both)	N	Ventrogluteal (L)
F	Eyes (left)	O	Ventrogluteal (R)
G	Eyes (right)	P	NPO: Lab
H	Deltoid (mid L)	Q	NPO: Surgery
I	Deltoid (mid R)	R	Withheld/see nurse's notes

FIGURE 6.6 Medication administration record (MAR).

CLINICAL RELEVANCE

Ask patients who are receiving antibiotics if they have ever had an allergic reaction to antibiotics. If the answer is yes, ask which medication and what type of reaction they had. Report any previous reactions to the physician before administering the medication.

CLINICAL RELEVANCE

When all of the medication in a prefilled syringe is not used, the unused portion must be discarded, and this action must be witnessed by another health professional. The syringe is intended only for a one-time injection.

Answers on page 220

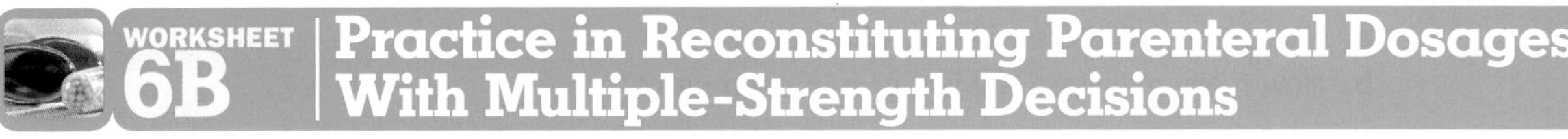

WORKSHEET 6B Practice in Reconstituting Parenteral Dosages With Multiple-Strength Decisions

Show your calculations and proofs in the following problems. Shade in the correct doses on the syringes.

1. Ordered: Pfizerpen (penicillin G potassium) 300,000 units IM bid to prevent bacterial endocarditis. Available: 1 million units.
   Calculate the strength closest to the ordered amount.
   a. How many milliliters of diluent will you add?
   b. How many milliliters will you administer?
   c. How many doses are in the multidose vial?

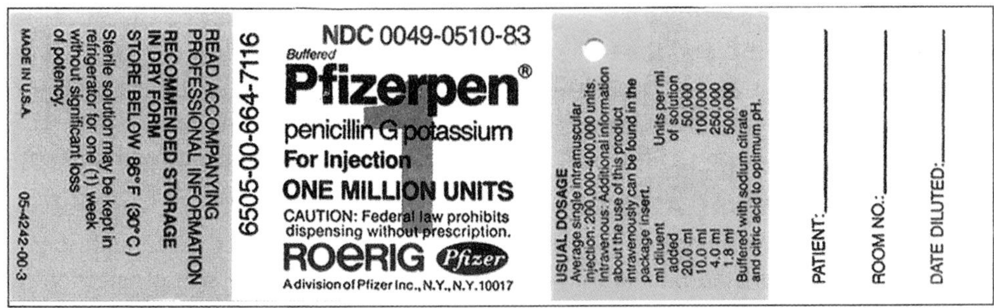

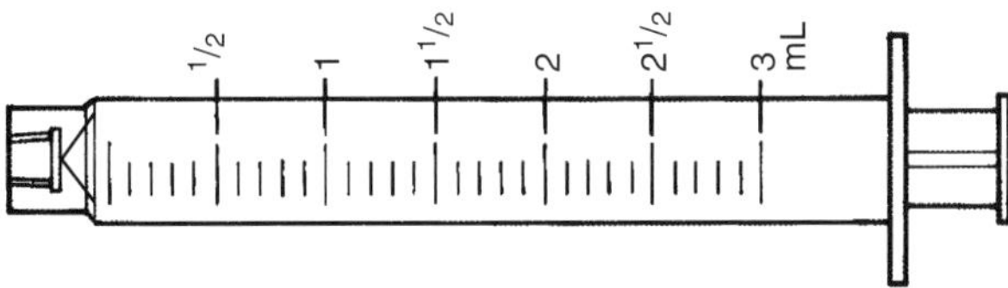

2. Ordered: Ceftriaxone 0.5 g IM q4h for gonorrhea.
   a. How many milliliters of diluent will you add?
   b. How many milligrams per milliliter will this make?
   c. How many milliliters will you administer?
   d. How many 350 mg doses are in the vial?

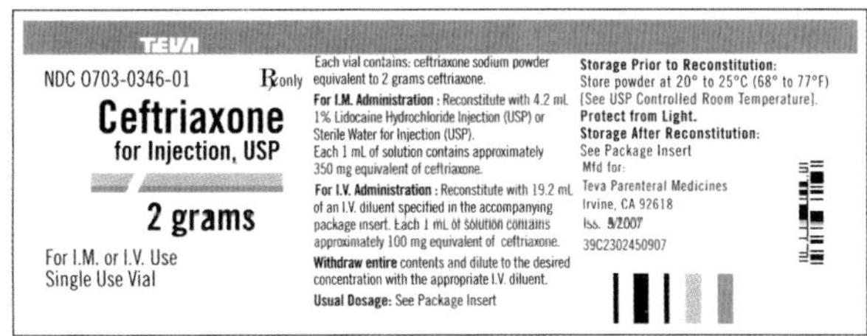

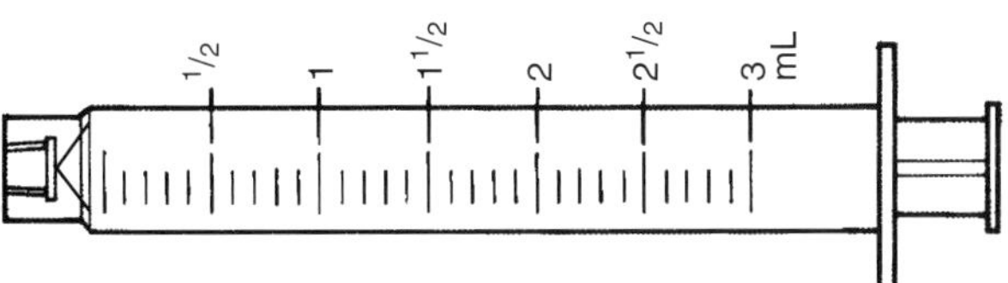

3. Ordered: Ampicillin 1000 mg q6h IM for tonsillitis. Available: Ampicillin 1 g.

a. How many milliliters will you administer?

b. How many milliliters will you give in each site?

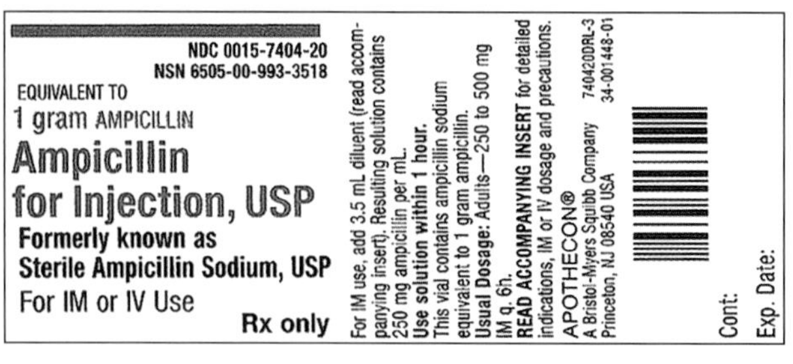

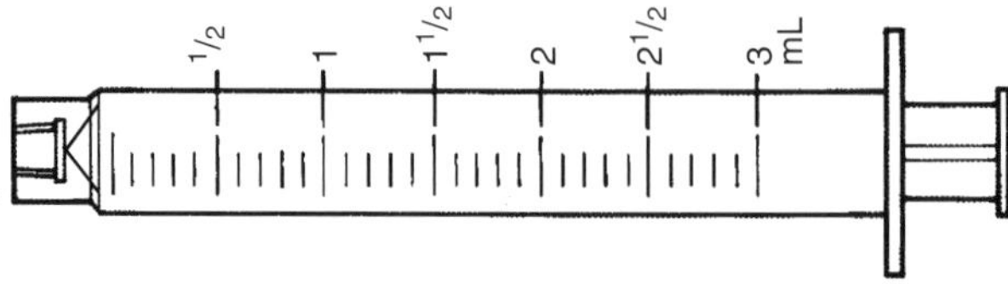

CLINICAL ALERT!

The maximum single injection for adults is 3 mL. Not all patients can tolerate a 3-mL injection. Assess the patient for adequate muscle mass at the site of injection to determine the ability for absorption, which aids in patient comfort as well as therapeutic value.

4. Ordered: Oxacillin sodium 500 mg IM for a leg infection. Available: A multidose vial.

a. How many mL of diluent will you add?

b. How many mL of oxacillin will you administer?

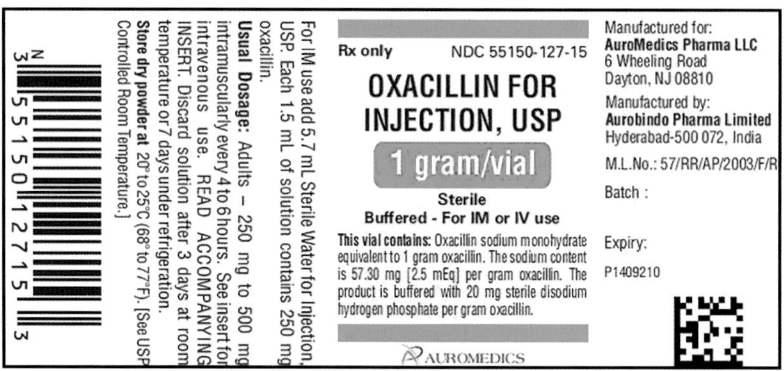

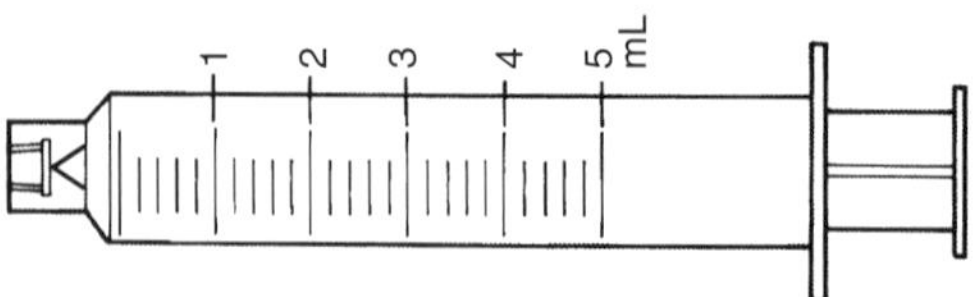

5. Ordered: Cefobid 1000 mg IM q12h for pelvic inflammatory disease. Available: Cefobid 1 g. Reconstitute IM doses with 2.2 mL of bacteriostatic water for injection (taken from insert). The powder displaces 0.4 mL. How many milliliters will be administered?

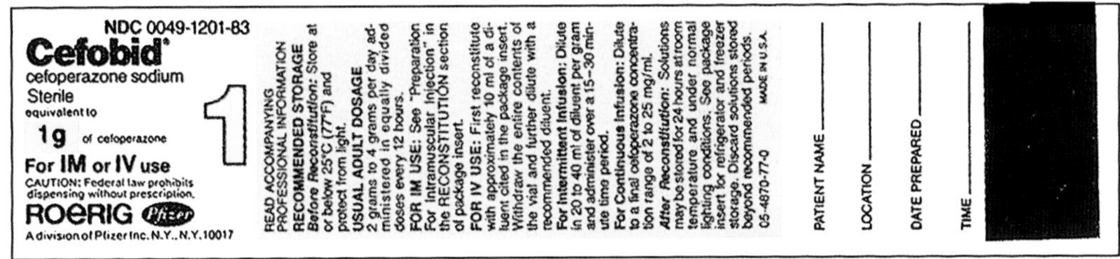
NDC 0049-1201-83
Cefobid®
cefoperazone sodium
Sterile
equivalent to
1 g of cefoperazone
1
For IM or IV use
CAUTION: Federal law prohibits dispensing without prescription.
ROERIG Pfizer
A division of Pfizer Inc. N.Y., N.Y. 10017
READ ACCOMPANYING PROFESSIONAL INFORMATION
RECOMMENDED STORAGE
Before Reconstitution: Store at or below 25°C (77°F) and protect from light.
USUAL ADULT DOSAGE
2 grams to 4 grams per day administered in equally divided doses every 12 hours.
FOR IM USE: See "Preparation For Intramuscular Injection" in the RECONSTITUTION section of package insert.
FOR IV USE: First reconstitute with approximately 10 ml of a diluent cited in the package insert. Withdraw the entire contents of the vial and further dilute with a recommended diluent.
For Intermittent Infusion: Dilute in 20 to 40 ml of diluent per gram and administer over a 15–30 minute time period.
For Continuous Infusion: Dilute to a final cefoperazone concentration range of 2 to 25 mg/ml.
After Reconstitution: Solutions may be stored for 24 hours at room temperature and under normal lighting conditions. See package insert for refrigerator and freezer storage. Discard solutions stored beyond recommended periods.
05-4870-77-0
MADE IN U.S.A.
PATIENT NAME
LOCATION
DATE PREPARED
TIME

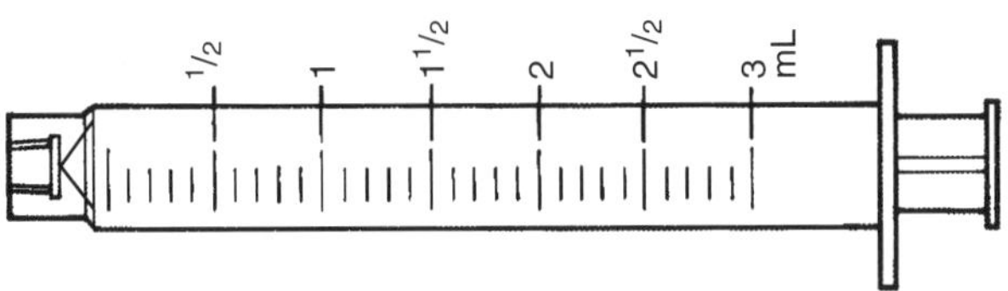

6. Ordered: Ceftriaxone 450 mg IM twice a day times 3 days for meningitis. Available: A vial containing 500 mg.

a. How many mL of 1% Lidocaine will you add?

b. What amount will you administer?

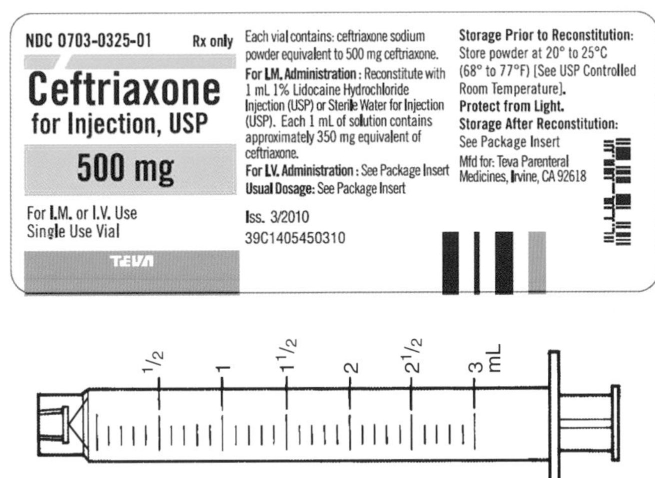

7. Ordered: Tazicef 250 mg IM q8h for otitis media.
Available: Tazicef 1 g for IM or IV use.
Follow insert directions for reconstitution directions.
   a. How many mL of diluent will be added to the powder?
   b. How many mg/mL will this make?
   c. How many mL will you administer IM?

RECONSTITUTION

Single Dose Vials:
For I.M. injection, I.V. direct (bolus) injection, or I.V. infusion, reconstitute with Sterile Water for injection according to the following table. The vacuum may assist entry of the diluent. SHAKE WELL.

Table 5

Vial Size	Diluent to Be Added	Approx. Avail. Volume	Approx. Avg. Concentration
Intramuscular or Intravenous Direct (bolus) Injection			
1 gram	3.0 ml.	3.6 ml.	280 mg./ml.
Intravenous Infusion			
1 gram	10 ml.	10.6 ml.	95 mg./ml.
2 gram	10 ml.	11.2 ml.	180 mg./ml.

Withdraw the total volume of solution into the syringe (the pressure in the vial may aid withdrawal). The withdrawn solution may contain some bubbles of carbon dioxide.

NOTE: **As with the administration of all parenteral products, accumulated gases should be expressed from the syringe immediately before injection of 'Tazicef'.**

These solutions of 'Tazicef' are stable for 18 hours at room temperature or seven days if refrigerated (5C.). Slight yellowing does not affect potency.

For I.V. infusion, dilute reconstituted solution in 50 to 100 ml. of one of the parenteral fluids listed under COMPATIBILITY AND STABILITY.

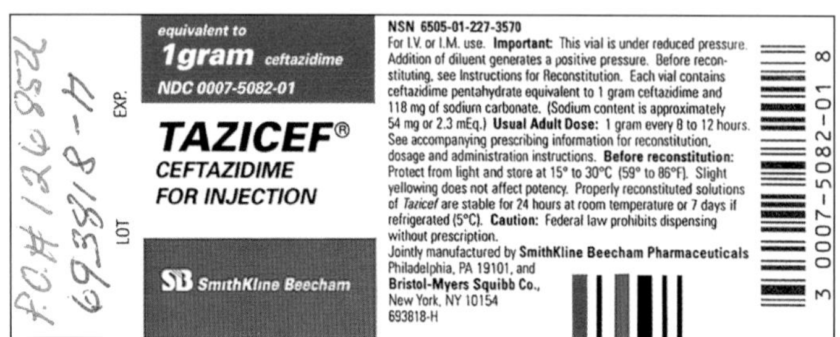

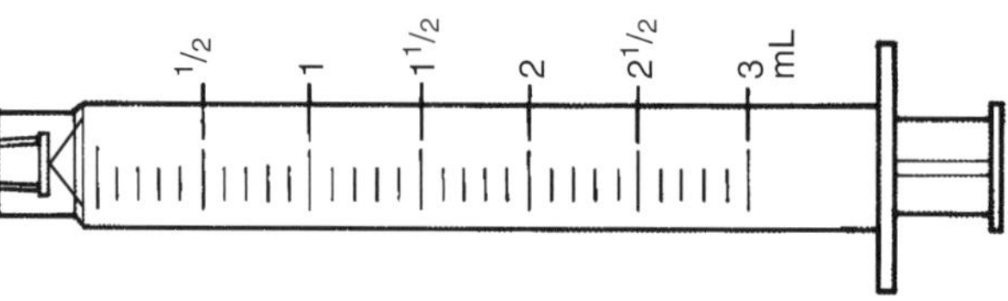

8. Ordered: 100 mg ampicillin IM q12h to treat a skin ulcer.
   a. How many milliliters of diluent will be added?
   b. What is the shelf life after reconstitution?
   c. What is the total amount of medication in the vial?
   d. How many milliliters of ampicillin will you administer?

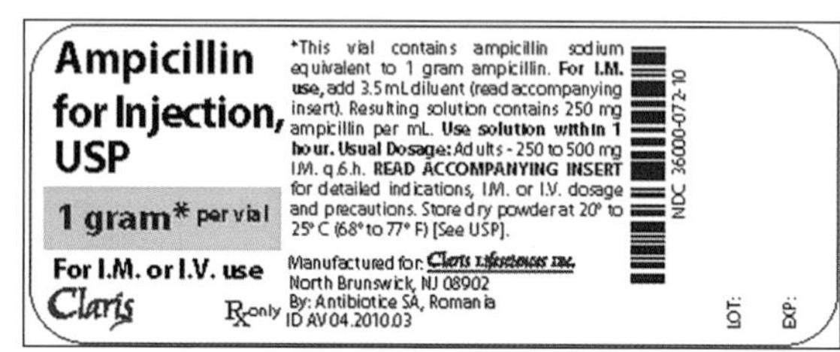
Ampicillin for Injection, USP
1 gram* per vial
For I.M. or I.V. use
Claris
Rx only
*This vial contains ampicillin sodium equivalent to 1 gram ampicillin. For I.M. use, add 3.5 mL diluent (read accompanying insert). Resulting solution contains 250 mg ampicillin per mL. Use solution within 1 hour. Usual Dosage: Adults - 250 to 500 mg I.M. q.6.h. READ ACCOMPANYING INSERT for detailed indications, I.M. or I.V. dosage and precautions. Store dry powder at 20° to 25° C (68° to 77° F) [See USP].
Manufactured for:
North Brunswick, NJ 08902
By: Antibiotice SA, Romania
ID AV04.2010.03
NDC 36000-072-10
LOT:
EXP:

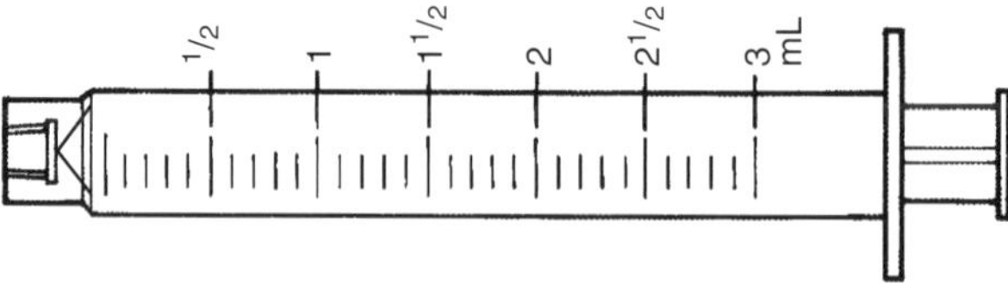

9. Ordered: Cefadyl 700 mg IM q6h for bronchitis. Available: Cefadyl 1 g. Follow directions on label.

a. How many milliliters will you administer per injection?

b. How many milligrams will the patient receive in 24 hours?

c. How many vials will you need for a 24-hour period?

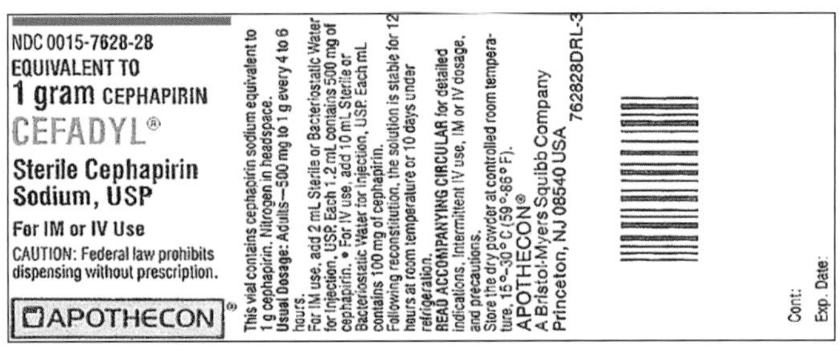

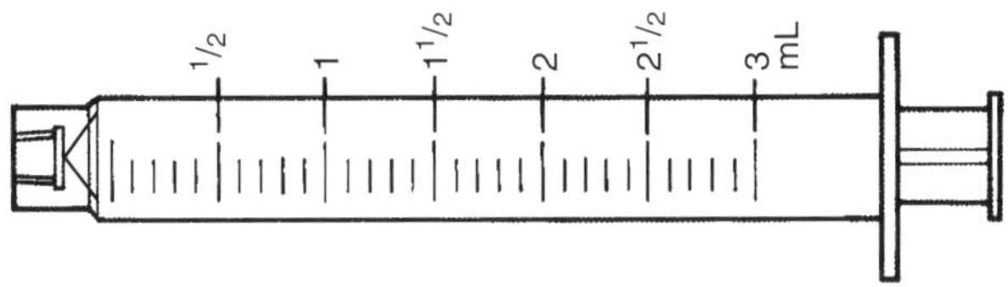

CLINICAL ALERT!

Do not confuse units of medication with milligrams.

10. Ordered: Cefobid 2 g IM q12h for a respiratory tract infection. Available: Cefobid 2 g vial. Reconstitution for IM use is found on the package insert. Directions read: Add 3.4 mL of sterile water for injection. The Cefobid powder displaces 0.6 mL. Administer the entire dose.

a. How many milliliters will you give for the first dose?

b. How many injections will you administer?

c. What sites will you select?

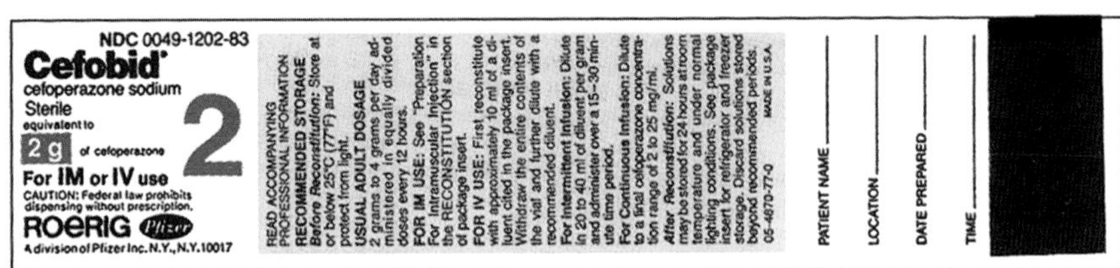

Answers on page 223

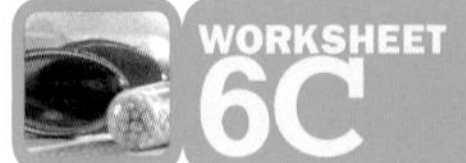

WORKSHEET 6C Additional Practice in Reconstituting Parenteral Dosages With Multiple-Strength Decisions

Answer the questions in the following problems. Show your calculations and proofs; then shade in the correct dose on the syringes.

1. Ordered: Streptomycin 0.5 g IM q12h for a patient with *Klebsiella* pneumonia.

a. If you add 1.8 mL of diluent, what mg per mL concentration will you have?

b. How many mL will you give?

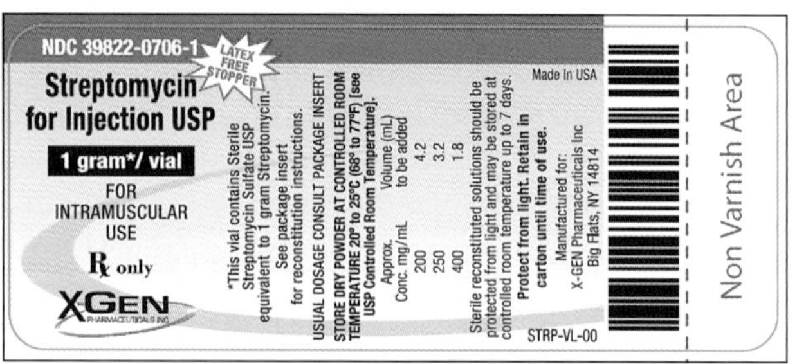
NDC 39822-0706-1
LATEX FREE STOPPER
Streptomycin for Injection USP
1 gram*/ vial
FOR INTRAMUSCULAR USE
℞ only
XGEN PHARMACEUTICALS INC
*This vial contains Sterile Streptomycin Sulfate USP equivalent to 1 gram Streptomycin.
See package insert for reconstitution instructions.
USUAL DOSAGE CONSULT PACKAGE INSERT
STORE DRY POWDER AT CONTROLLED ROOM TEMPERATURE 20° to 25°C (68° to 77°F) [see USP Controlled Room Temperature].
Approx. Conc. mg/mL | Volume (mL) to be added
200 | 4.2
250 | 3.2
400 | 1.8
Sterile reconstituted solutions should be protected from light and may be stored at controlled room temperature up to 7 days.
Protect from light. Retain in carton until time of use.
Manufactured for: X-GEN Pharmaceuticals Inc Big Flats, NY 14814
Made In USA
STRP-VL-00
Non Varnish Area

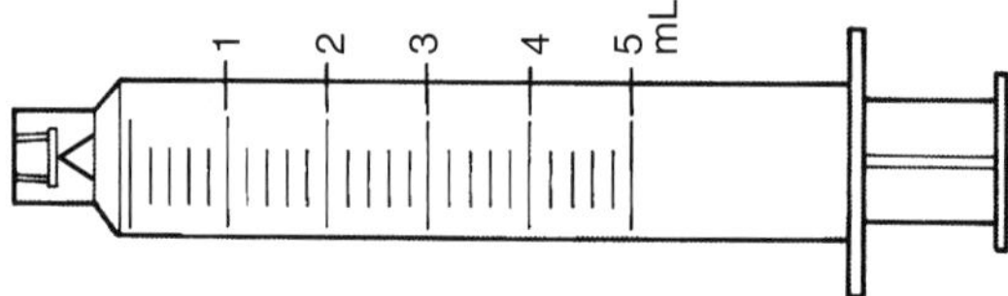

2. Ordered: Cefadyl (cephapirin) 500 mg IM q6h for infected bone (leg).

a. How many milliliters of sterile water will you add?

b. How many mg/per 1.2 mL will you have?

c. How many milliliters will you administer?

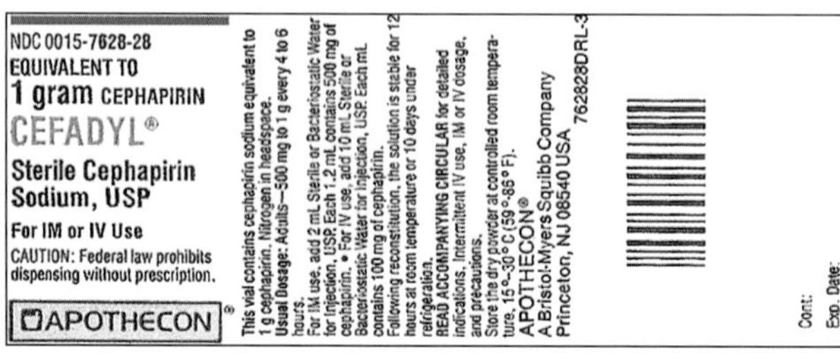
NDC 0015-7628-28
EQUIVALENT TO
1 gram CEPHAPIRIN
CEFADYL®
Sterile Cephapirin Sodium, USP
For IM or IV Use
CAUTION: Federal law prohibits dispensing without prescription.
APOTHECON®
This vial contains cephapirin sodium equivalent to 1 g cephapirin. Nitrogen in headspace.
Usual Dosage: Adults—500 mg to 1 g every 4 to 6 hours.
For IM use, add 2 mL Sterile or Bacteriostatic Water for Injection, USP. Each 1.2 mL contains 500 mg of cephapirin. • For IV use, add 10 mL Sterile or Bacteriostatic Water for Injection, USP. Each mL contains 100 mg of cephapirin.
Following reconstitution, the solution is stable for 12 hours at room temperature or 10 days under refrigeration.
READ ACCOMPANYING CIRCULAR for detailed indications, Intermittent IV use, IM or IV dosage, and precautions.
Store the dry powder at controlled room temperature, 15°–30° C (59°–86° F).
APOTHECON®
A Bristol-Myers Squibb Company
Princeton, NJ 08540 USA
762828DRL-3
Cont:
Exp. Date:

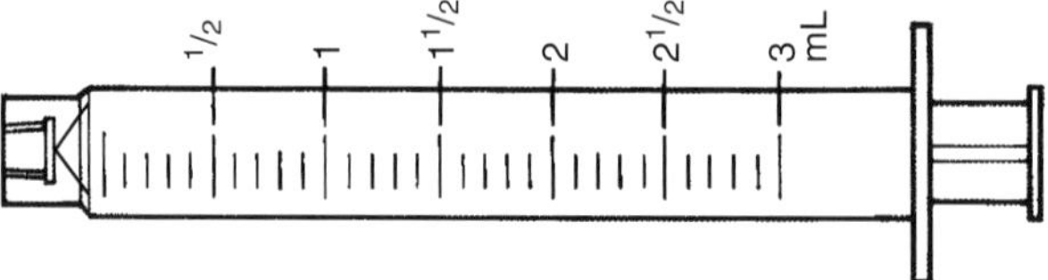

3. Ordered: Ceftriaxone 500 mg IM bid for a urinary tract infection.
Directions: For IM use, add sterile water for injection according to directions. Withdraw entire contents to yield 500 mg. Give deep in a large muscle. Aspirate before giving. Calculate both dosages to determine which amount is appropriate for your patient.

Vial Dose Size	Amount of Diluent to Be Added
	1.8 mL ——— 250 mg/mL
500 mg	1 mL ——— 350 mg/mL

Which concentration did you choose? Measure it on the syringe.

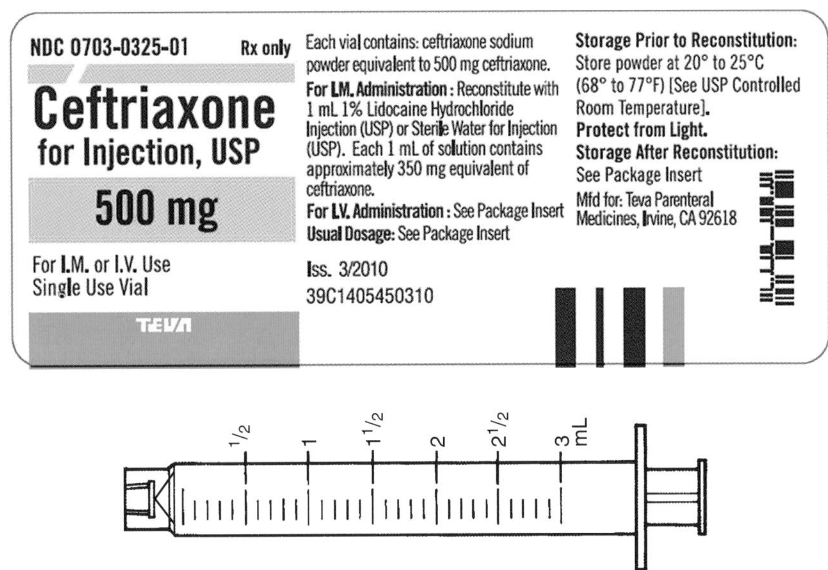

CLINICAL ALERT!

Check patient's medication history of drug sensitivity before administration of antiinfectives. Keep epinephrine, an antihistamine, and resuscitation equipment nearby in the event of an anaphylactic shock reaction.

4. Ordered: 400,000 units Pfizerpen IM q6h for pneumococcal pneumonia.
Available: Pfizerpen 1 million units with mixing options.
Choose between adding 4 mL and adding 1.8 mL of diluent.
   a. How many units/mL will you administer if you use 4 mL of diluent? Mark the syringe.
   b. How many units/mL will you administer if you use 1.8 mL of diluent? Mark the syringe.

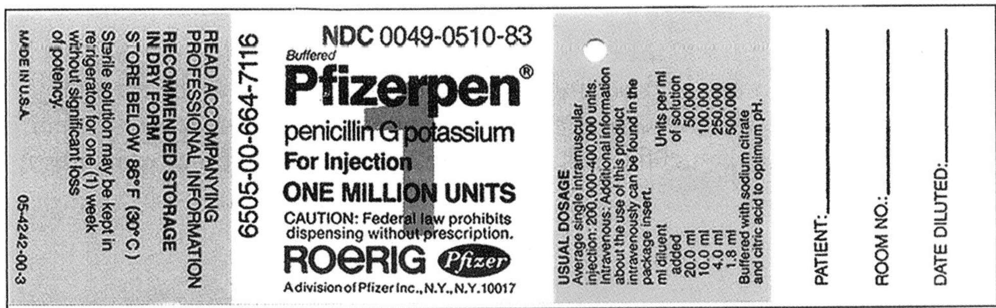

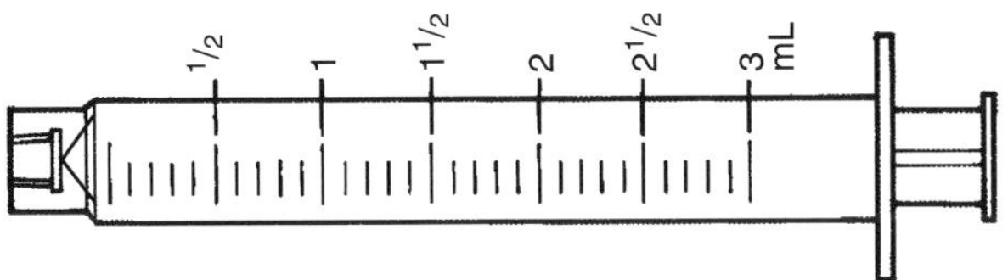

5. Ordered: Methylprednisolone 125 mg IM q6h for ulcerative colitis.
   a. How many milliliters of diluent will you add?
   b. How many milligrams per milliliters will this make?
   c. How many milliliters will you give?
   d. How many doses are in the vial?
   e. The medication has to be used within how many hours after reconstituting?
   f. Will all of the doses for this order be given within the recommended time frame?

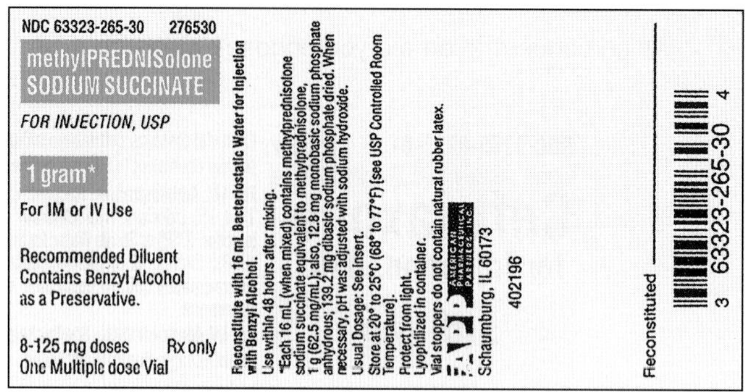
NDC 63323-265-30 276530
methylPREDNISolone
SODIUM SUCCINATE
FOR INJECTION, USP
1 gram*
For IM or IV Use
Recommended Diluent
Contains Benzyl Alcohol
as a Preservative.
8-125 mg doses Rx only
One Multiple dose Vial
Reconstitute with 16 mL Bacteriostatic Water for Injection with Benzyl Alcohol.
Use within 48 hours after mixing.
Schaumburg, IL 60173
402196
Reconstituted
3 63323-265-30 4

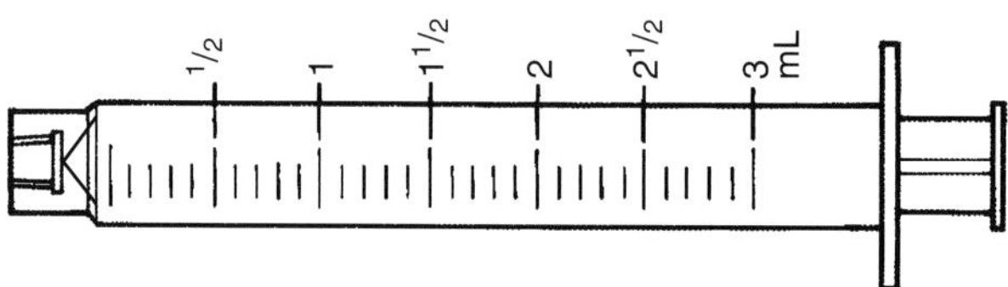

6. Ordered: Pfizerpen 400,000 units IM every 12 hours for a patient with a streptococcal infection.
   a. Which strength will you prepare for your patient. Show the different calculations.
   b. How many mL's will you give? How will you determine which strength to give?

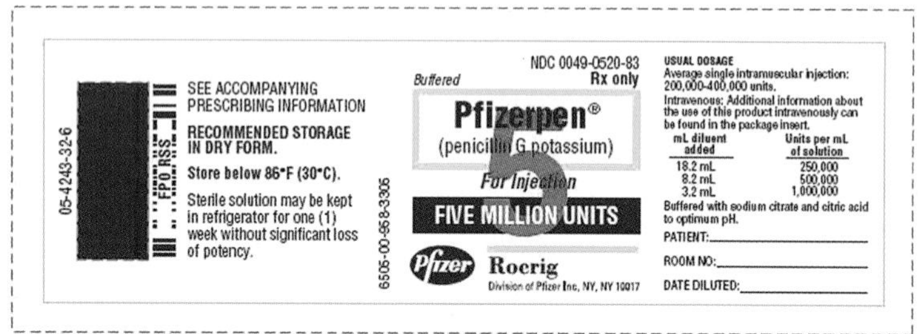
SEE ACCOMPANYING
PRESCRIBING INFORMATION
RECOMMENDED STORAGE
IN DRY FORM.
Store below 86°F (30°C).
Sterile solution may be kept in refrigerator for one (1) week without significant loss of potency.
NDC 0049-0520-83
Buffered
Rx only
Pfizerpen®
(penicillin G potassium)
For Injection
FIVE MILLION UNITS
Pfizer
Roerig
USUAL DOSAGE
mL diluent added
Units per mL of solution
18.2 mL 250,000
8.2 mL 500,000
3.2 mL 1,000,000
PATIENT:
ROOM NO:
DATE DILUTED:

3 Strengths to Determine Dosage
18.2 mL = 250,000 units/mL
8.2 mL = 500,000 units/mL
3.2 mL = 1,000,000 units/mL

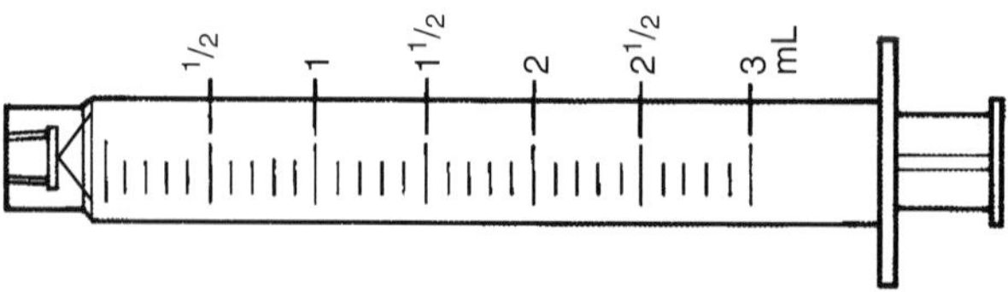

7. Ordered: Ticar 750 mg IM q8h for peritonitis.

a. How many milliliters of diluent will be added?

b. 2.6 mL of Ticar contains how many grams?

c. What is the shelf life of the medication?

d. What is the total amount of medication in the vial?

e. How many milliliters will you administer?

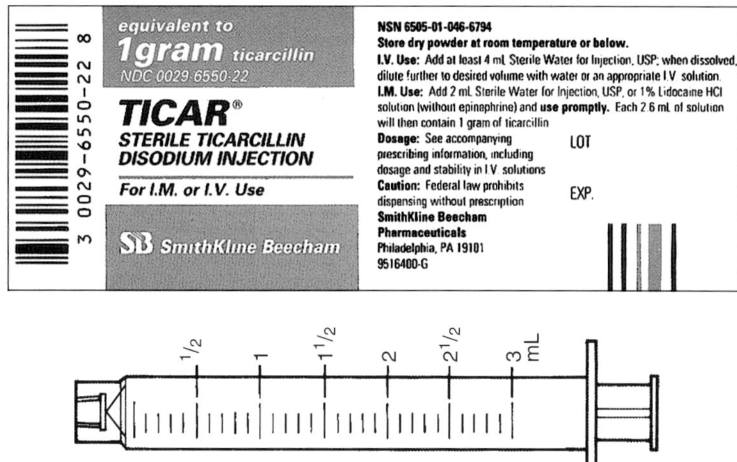

8. Ordered: ampicillin 0.5 g IM q6h for a patient with an URI (upper respiratory infection).

a. How many milliliters of diluent will you add?

b. What is the resulting concentration?

c. How many milliliters of medication will you administer?

d. What is the shelf life?

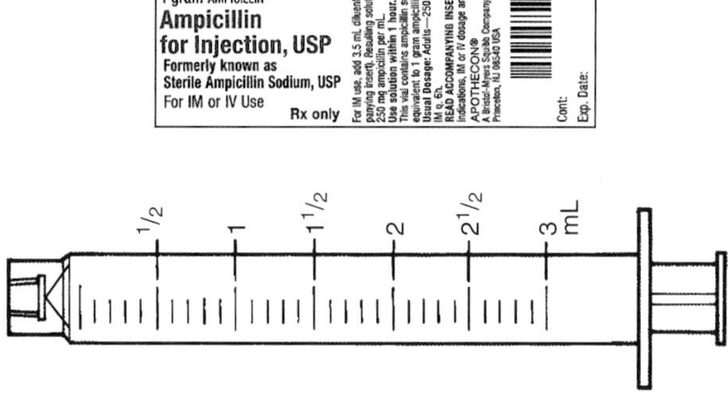

9. Ordered: Ampicillin 500 mg IM q6h times 3 days for a streptococcal throat infection.

a. How many milliliters of diluent are needed to reconstitute the medication?

b. How many mg/mL will it make?

c. What is the shelf life of the medication?

d. How many milliliters will you administer?

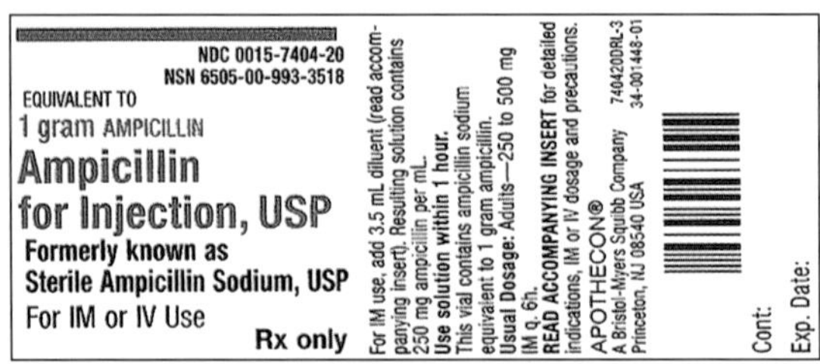

NDC 0015-7404-20
NSN 6505-00-993-3518
EQUIVALENT TO
1 gram AMPICILLIN
Ampicillin
for Injection, USP
Formerly known as
Sterile Ampicillin Sodium, USP
For IM or IV Use
Rx only
For IM use, add 3.5 mL diluent (read accompanying insert). Resulting solution contains 250 mg ampicillin per mL.
Use solution within 1 hour.
This vial contains ampicillin sodium equivalent to 1 gram ampicillin.
Usual Dosage: Adults—250 to 500 mg IM q. 6h.
READ ACCOMPANYING INSERT for detailed indications, IM or IV dosage and precautions.
APOTHECON®
A Bristol-Myers Squibb Company
Princeton, NJ 08540 USA
7404200RL-3
34-001448-01
Cont:
Exp. Date:

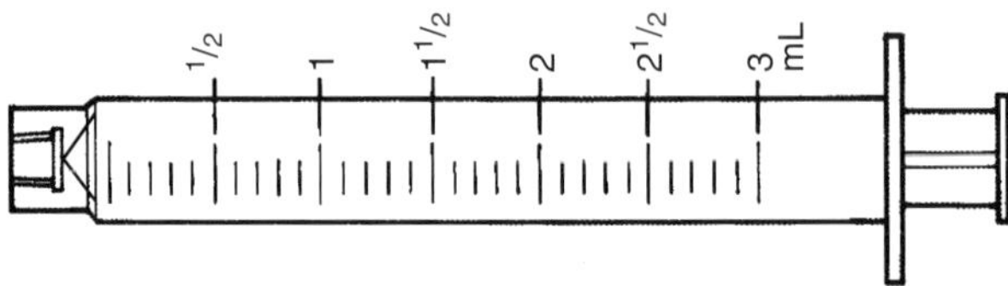

10. Ordered: Oxacillin sodium 450 mg IM q6h for actinomycosis.

a. How many milliliters of sterile water will be used for reconstitution?

b. How many mg/mL will it make?

c. What is the shelf life of the medication after reconstitution?

d. What is the total amount of medication in the vial?

e. How many milliliters will you administer?

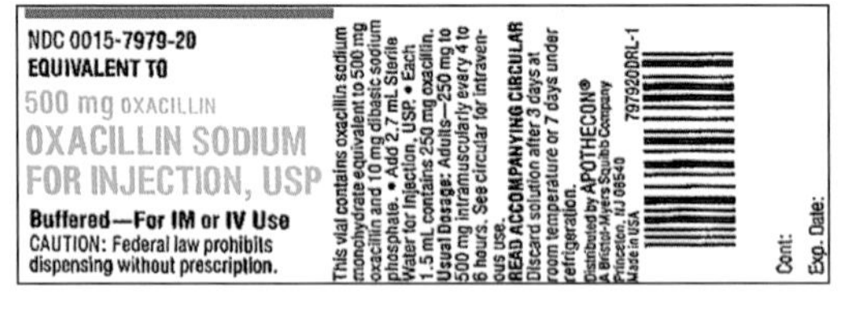

NDC 0015-7979-20
EQUIVALENT TO
500 mg OXACILLIN
OXACILLIN SODIUM
FOR INJECTION, USP
Buffered—For IM or IV Use
CAUTION: Federal law prohibits dispensing without prescription.
This vial contains oxacillin sodium monohydrate equivalent to 500 mg oxacillin and 10 mg dibasic sodium phosphate. • Add 2.7 mL Sterile Water for Injection, USP. • Each 1.5 mL contains 250 mg oxacillin.
Usual Dosage: Adults—250 mg to 500 mg intramuscularly every 4 to 6 hours. See circular for intravenous use.
READ ACCOMPANYING CIRCULAR
Discard solution after 3 days at room temperature or 7 days under refrigeration.
Distributed by APOTHECON®
A Bristol-Myers Squibb Company
Princeton, NJ 08540
Made in USA
7979200RL-1
Cont:
Exp. Date:

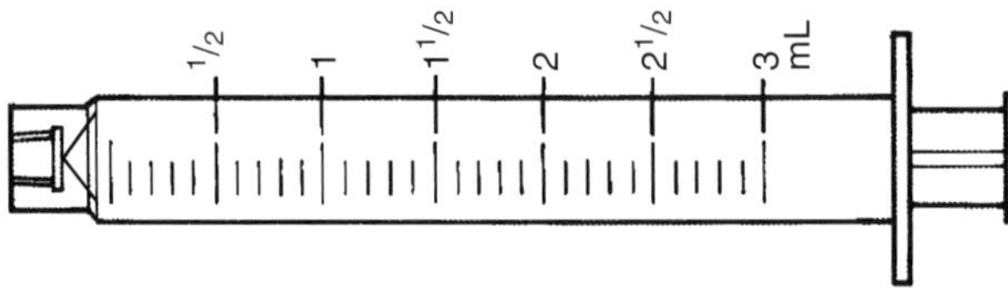

CLINICAL ALERT!

Always make sure that the patient's body mass is adequate for the amount of medication that will be given intramuscularly.

Answers on page 227

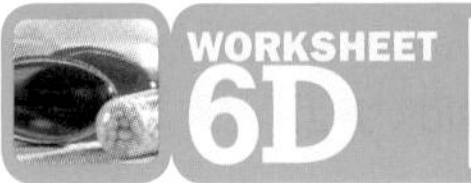

WORKSHEET 6D Multiple-Choice Practice

1. Ordered: Levothyroxine 60 mcg IM for a thyroid condition.
How many milliliters will you administer?

a. 2 mL **b.** 1.5 mL **c.** 2.2 mL **d.** 2.5 mL

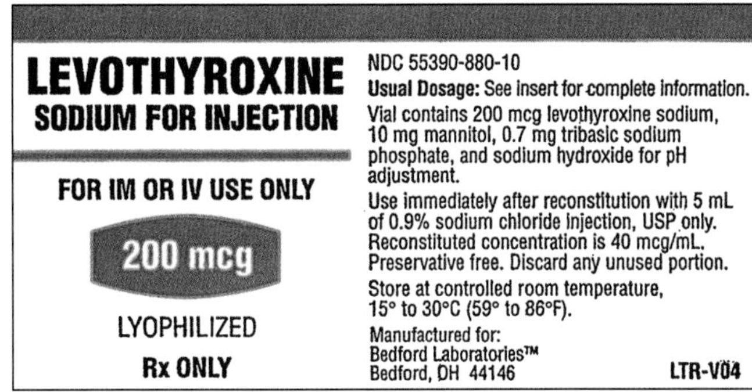

2. Ordered: Ampicillin 250 mg IM q12h to treat an infected surgical site.
Available: Ampicillin 125 mg.
How many milliliters of diluent will you add?

a. 2 mL **b.** 1.2 mL **c.** 3 mL **d.** 1.5 mL

How many vials will you need in 24 hours?

a. 1 vial **b.** 2 vials **c.** 3 vials **d.** 4 vials

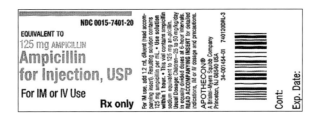

3. Ordered: Methylprednisolone 35 mg IM every day times 3 days for arthritis.
Available: Methylprednisolone 40 mg/mL.
How many milliliters of bacteriostatic water will you add?

a. 2.1 mL **b.** 12 mL **c.** 3.1 mL **d.** 1.2 mL

How many milliliters will you administer?

a. 1.5 mL **b.** 1 mL **c.** 0.8 mL **d.** 0.9 mL

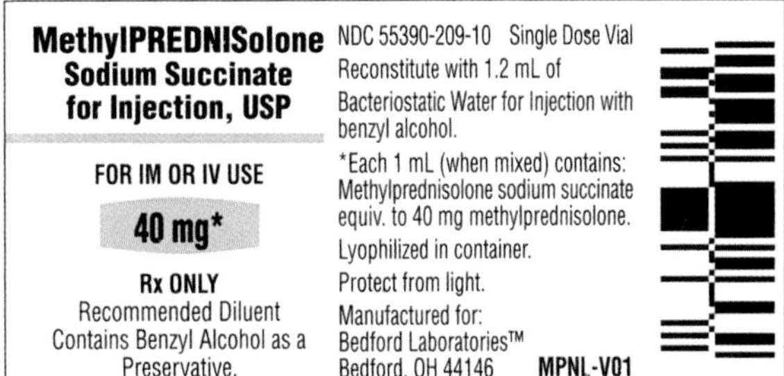

4. Ordered: Cefobid 1.5 g IM q12h for bacterial endocarditis.
Available: Cefobid 1 g vial.
Directions read: Add 1.4 mL of sterile water for injection. Each 2 mL yields 1 g.
How many milliliters will you administer?

a. 2.5 mL b. 3 mL c. 2 mL d. 1.5 mL

How many vials will you need for 24 hours?

a. 2 vials b. 2.5 vials c. 3.5 vials d. 3 vials

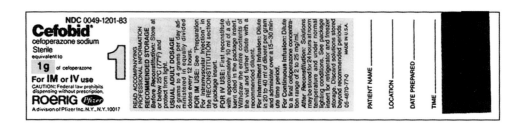

5. Ordered: Cefobid 1g IM q12h for a respiratory tract infection.
Available: Cefobid 2 g vial.
Directions for IM use read: Add 3.4 mL of sterile water for injection. Each 4 mL yields 2 g.
How many milliliters will you administer?

a. 3.5 mL b. 4 mL c. 2 mL d. 2.5 mL

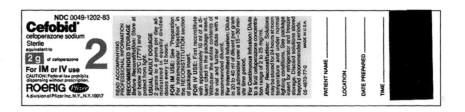

6. Ordered: Ticar 500 mg IM tid for a pseudomonas infection.
Available: Ticar 1 g.
Directions read: Add 2 mL of sterile water for injection.
How many milliliters will you administer?

a. 2.6 mL b. 2 mL c. 1.3 mL d. 3 mL

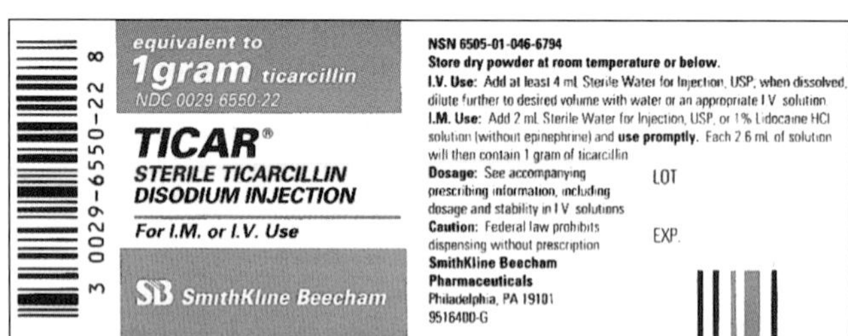

7. Refer to question 6.
How many vials of Ticar will be needed in 24 hours?

a. 3 vials b. 4 vials c. 2 vials d. 5 vials

8. Ordered: Pfizerpen 400,000 units IM bid to treat diphtheria.
Available: Pfizerpen (penicillin G potassium) 1 million units.
How many milliliters of diluent will you add?

a. 5 mL **b.** 10 mL **c.** 1.8 mL **d.** 20 mL

How many milliliters will you administer?

a. 2 mL **b.** 2.5 mL **c.** 1.6 mL **d.** 0.8 mL

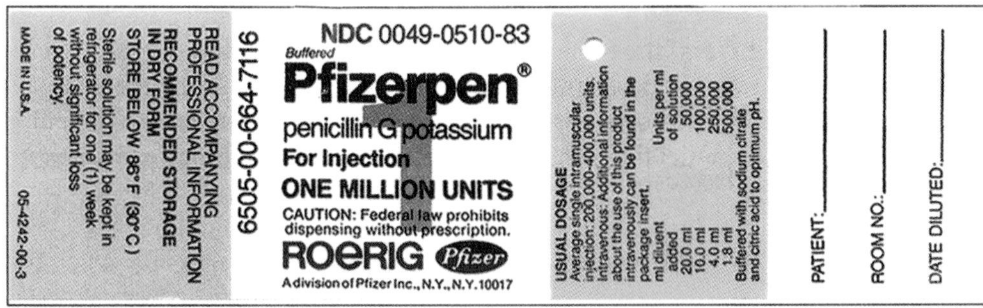

9. Ordered: Streptomycin 500 mg IM bid for meningitis.
Available: Streptomycin sulfate 5 g.
What is the concentration after dilution?

a. 500 mg/mL **b.** 1 g/mL **c.** 400 mg/mL **d.** 0.5 g/mL

How many milliliters will you administer?

a. 1.3 mL **b.** 1 mL **c.** 2.2 mL **d.** 1.8 mL

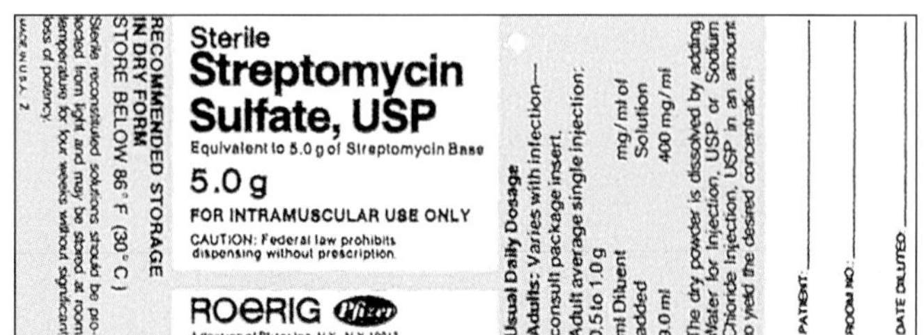

10. Ordered: Ancef 250 mg IM q6h for a urinary tract infection.
Available: Ancef 1 gram for reconstitution.
How many mL will you administer?

a. 2 mL **b.** 0.5 mL **c.** 0.8 mL **d.** 4.5 mL

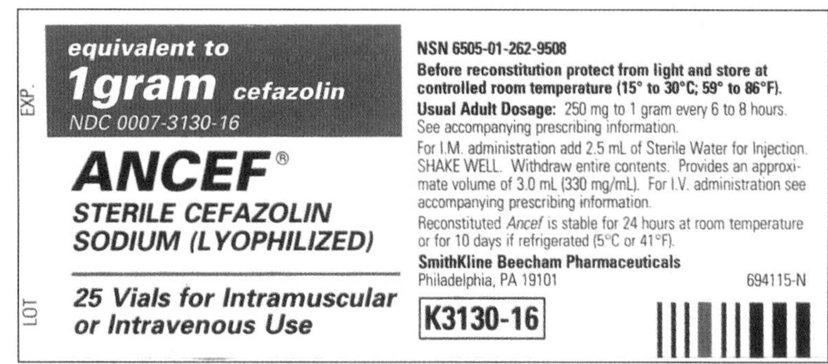

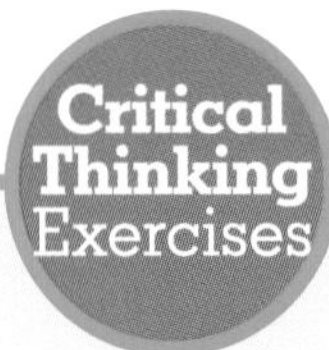

Critical Thinking Exercises provide math and medication-related patient safety issues for student discussion. Answers are not provided.

Analyze the following scenarios.

1. A 1-million-unit multiple-dose vial of penicillin G potassium has these directions for reconstitution:

Add Diluent	**Concentration of Solution**
9.6 mL	100,000 units/mL
4.6 mL	200,000 units/mL
1.6 mL	500,000 units/mL

The medication was reconstituted with 9.6 mL of diluent and 200,000 units per mL circled.

Ordered: Penicillin G potassium 200,000 units IM q6h

Given: Penicillin G potassium 1 mL IM q6h

Error(s):

Potential injuries:

Discussion

How many units of penicillin G potassium were given?

What were the potential injuries?

Which concentration would have provided the ordered amount in 1 mL?

How could this error have been prevented?

2. Ordered: Cefadyl 250 mg IM every 12 hours times 4 doses for dermatitis.

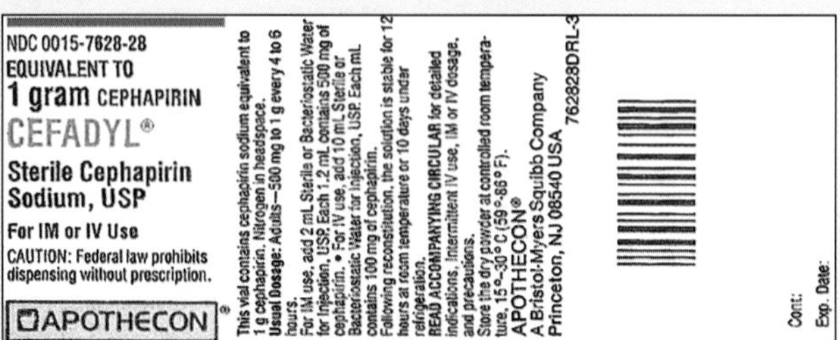

The Cefadyl (cephapirin) vial was reconstituted with 2 mL of sterile water for injection. The vial was labeled with the date, time, amount of diluent (2 mL of sterile water) circled, and the nurse's initials. The nurse gave the first injection (0.6 mL) of Cefadyl IM at 0800 hours. The next nurse gave the 250 mg dose (0.3 mL) at 2000 hours. The next dose of 250 mg (0.3 mL) was given at 0800 hours. The nurse noted that the vial was empty and discarded it.

How many doses of 250 mg were in the 1 gram vial?

How many doses were given?

What should you do if you found that a medication error had been made by another nurse?

Was the patient's safety jeopardized in any way?

How could this error have been prevented?

3. Multiple-dose vials have various reconstitution directions for both IM and IV administration along with different shelf life and storage requirements.

Discuss how each of these steps for reconstitution of drugs could cause potential harm to a patient if not followed properly.

a. Adding the wrong diluent

b. Adding the wrong amount of diluent

c. Administering the wrong amount of reconstituted medication

d. Administering via the wrong route

e. Storing the medication in the wrong place after reconstitution

f. Keeping the medication longer than the recommended shelf life

g. Not labeling the date and time and initialing the label

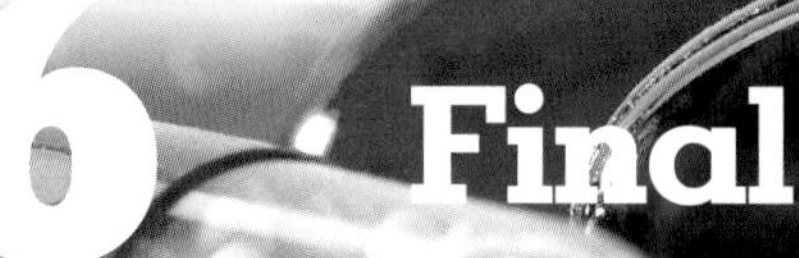

1. Ordered: Biaxin 150 mg po twice a day for helicobacter gastritis.
   Shade in medicine cup or the syringe to indicate the ordered dose for accurate measurement.
   a. How much diluent will you add?
   b. When reconstituted, how many milligrams per milliliter will be in the bottle?
   c. How many milliliters will you administer?

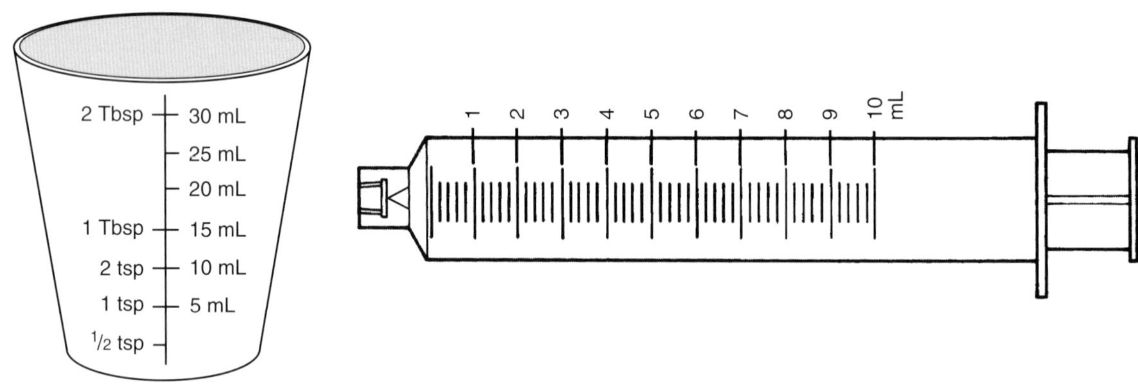

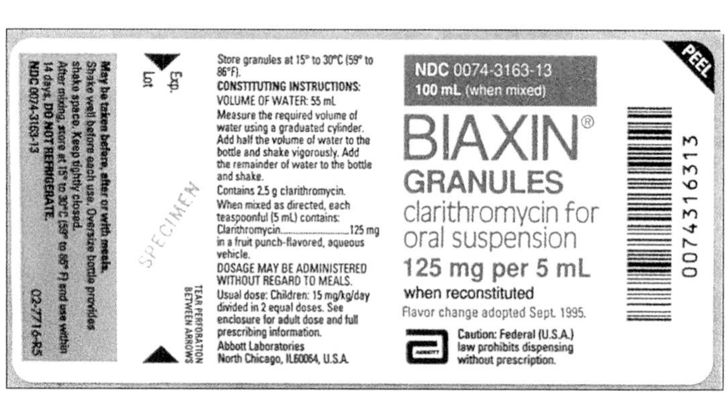

2. Ordered: Vibramycin 200 mg the first day followed by a maintenance dose of 100 mg for 5 days for a patient with an intestinal infection.

a. How many mg will the patient receive during the course of treatment?

b. What is the generic name for Vibramycin?

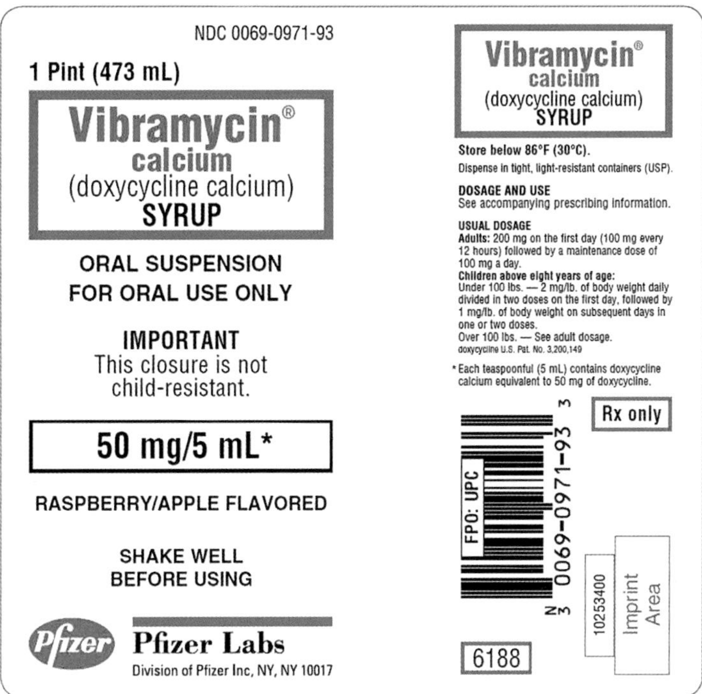

3. Ordered: Ampicillin 250 mg IM q4h for endocarditis prophylaxis.

a. How much diluent will you add?

b. How many milliliters will you administer? Shade in the amount on the syringe.

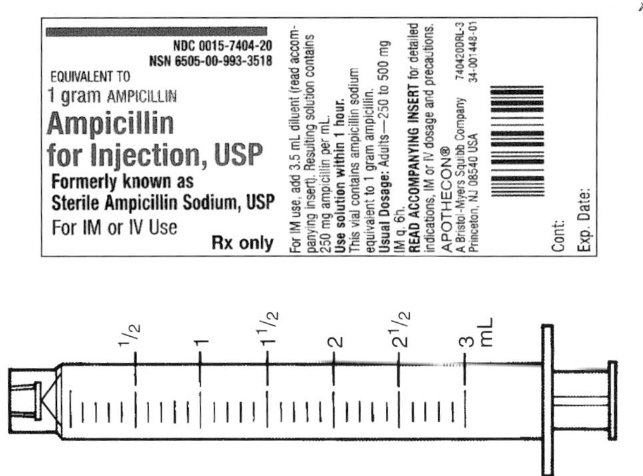

4. Ordered: Ticar 0.5 g IM q6h for salpingitis.

a. How much diluent will you add?

b. How many milliliters will you administer? Shade in the amount on the syringe.

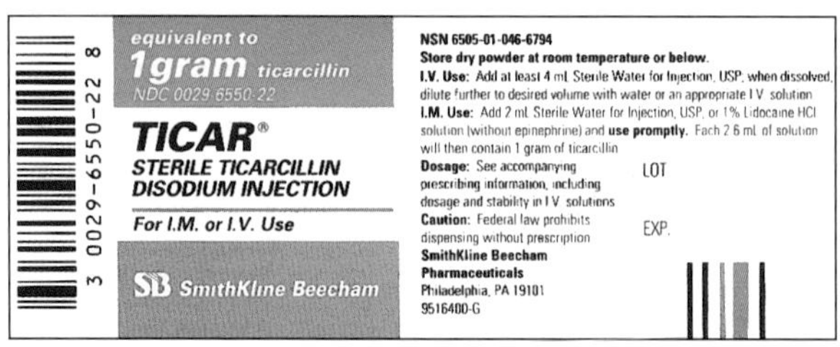

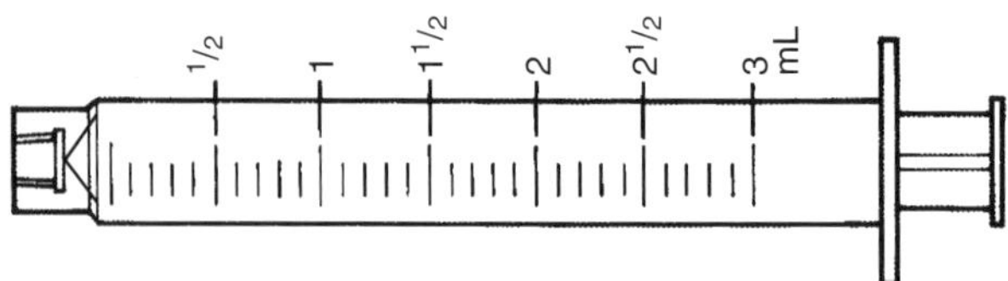

5. Ordered: Pfizerpen 300,000 units IM q12h for chronic obstructive pulmonary disease.
Available: Pfizerpen 5 million units.
If you add 18.2 mL of diluent to the Pfizerpen:

a. How many units/mL will this yield?

b. How many milliliters will you administer?

c. How many doses are in the multidose vial?

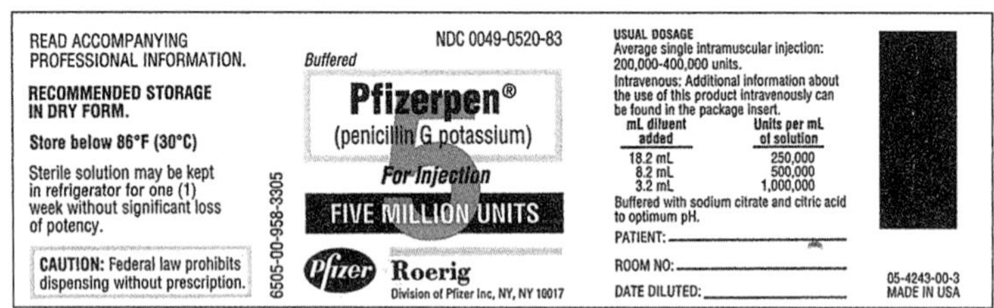

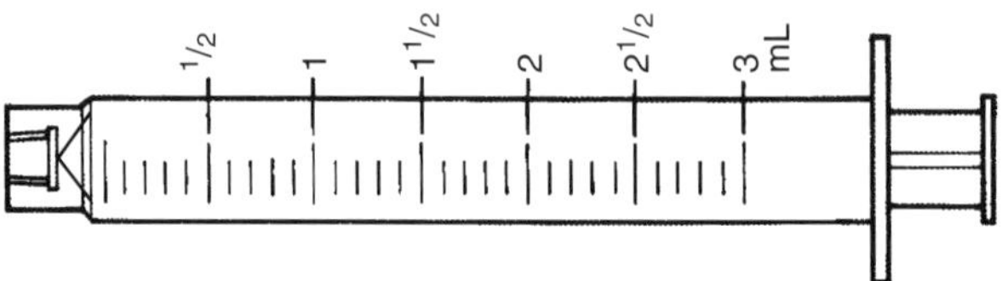

6. Ordered: Carbenicillin 750 mg IM q8h for endocarditis.
Available: Geopen (carbenicillin) 5 g for reconstitution.

a. How many mL of diluent will you add?

b. How many mL will you administer? Shade in the syringe.

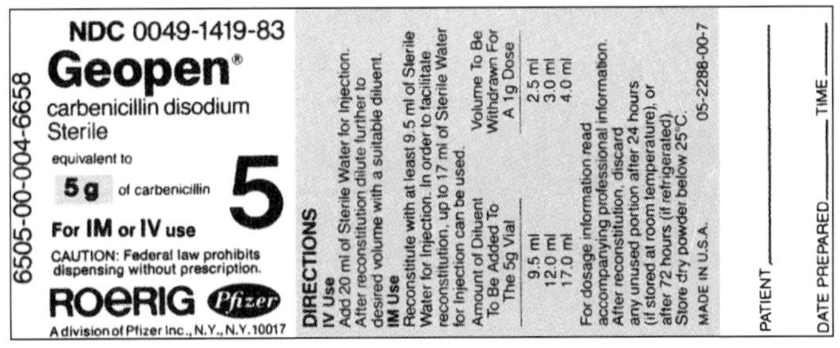

NDC 0049-1419-83
Geopen®
carbenicillin disodium
Sterile
equivalent to
5 g of carbenicillin
5
For IM or IV use
CAUTION: Federal law prohibits dispensing without prescription.
ROERIG Pfizer
A division of Pfizer Inc., N.Y., N.Y. 10017
6505-00-004-6658
DIRECTIONS
IV Use
Add 20 ml of Sterile Water for Injection. After reconstitution dilute further to desired volume with a suitable diluent.
IM Use
Reconstitute with at least 9.5 ml of Sterile Water for Injection. In order to facilitate reconstitution, up to 17 ml of Sterile Water for Injection can be used.
Amount of Diluent To Be Added To The 5g Vial
Volume To Be Withdrawn For A 1g Dose
9.5 ml 2.5 ml
12.0 ml 3.0 ml
17.0 ml 4.0 ml
For dosage information read accompanying professional information. After reconstitution, discard any unused portion after 24 hours (if stored at room temperature), or after 72 hours (if refrigerated). Store dry powder below 25°C.
MADE IN U.S.A.
05-2288-00-7
PATIENT
DATE PREPARED
TIME

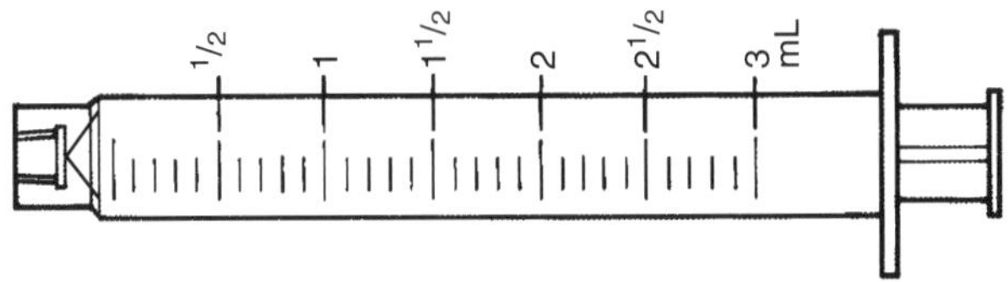

7. Ordered: Ceftazidime 0.5 g IM, an antibiotic, for a patient with *Klebsiella* pneumonia.

a. How much diluent will you add for an IM injection?

b. What is the concentration per mL after dilution.

c. How many mL will you give?

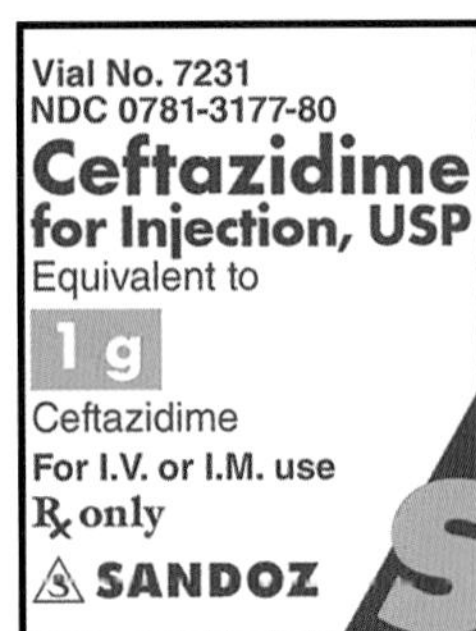

RECONSTITUTION

Single Dose Vials:
For I.M. injection, I.V. direct (bolus) injection, or I.V. infusion, reconstitute with Sterile Water for injection according to the following table. The vacuum may assist entry of the diluent. SHAKE WELL.

Table 5

Vial Size	Diluent to Be Added	Approx. Avail. Volume	Approx. Avg. Concentration
Intramuscular or Intravenous Direct (bolus) Injection			
1 gram	3.0 ml.	3.6 ml.	280 mg./ml.
Intravenous Infusion			
1 gram	10 ml.	10.6 ml.	95 mg./ml.
2 gram	10 ml.	11.2 ml.	180 mg./ml.

Withdraw the total volume of solution into the syringe (the pressure in the vial may aid withdrawal). The withdrawn solution may contain some bubbles of carbon dioxide.

NOTE: As with the administration of all parenteral products, accumulated gases should be expressed from the syringe immediately before injection of 'Tazicef'.

These solutions of 'Tazicef' are stable for 18 hours at room temperature or seven days if refrigerated (5C.). Slight yellowing does not affect potency.

For I.V. infusion, dilute reconstituted solution in 50 to 100 ml. of one of the parenteral fluids listed under COMPATIBILITY AND STABILITY.

8. Ordered: Penicillin G potassium 100,000 units IM q4h for pneumonia. The directions read: *Sterile solution may be kept in refrigerator for 7 days without significant loss of potency. Add diluent 9.6 mL for 100,000 units/mL concentration of solution; add diluent 4.6 mL for 200,000 units/mL; add diluent 1.6 mL for 500,000 units/mL.*

a. Which dilution will you use? Why?

b. How many milliliters will you administer? Shade in the amount on the syringe.

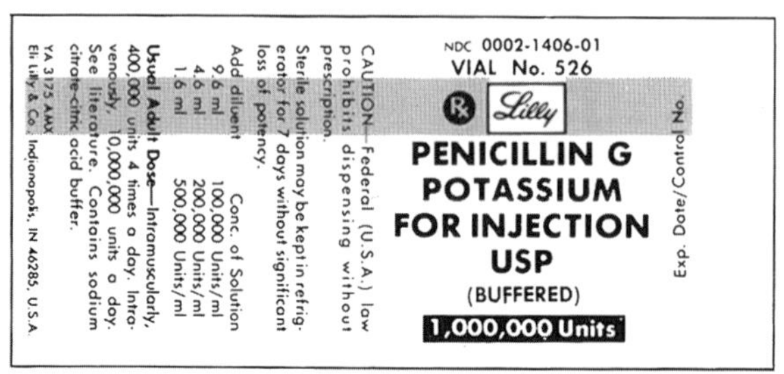

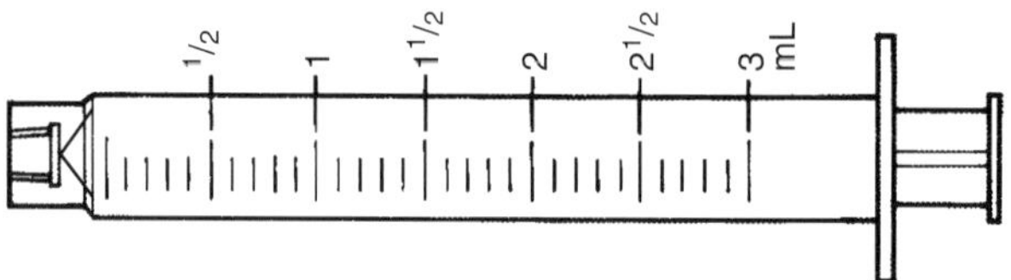

9. Ordered: Oxacillin sodium 250 mg IM q4h for a urinary tract infection (UTI).

a. How many milliliters of diluent will you add?

b. How many milliliters of oxacillin sodium will you administer? Shade in the amount on the syringe.

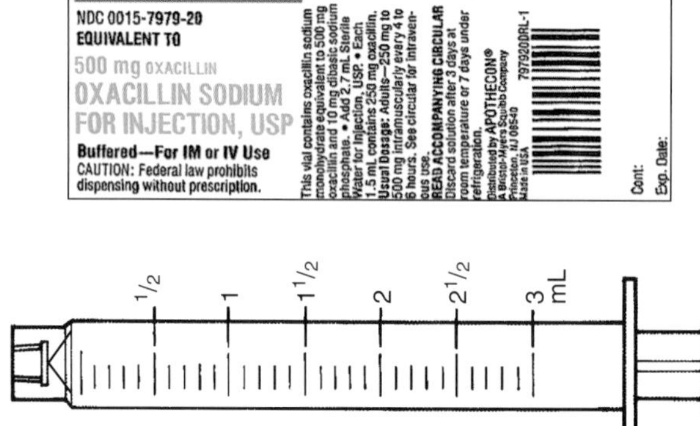

10. Ordered: Keflin 400,000 units IM q12h for a kidney infection.
Available: a vial with 600,000 units/mL. How many milliliters will you administer? Shade in the amount on the syringe.

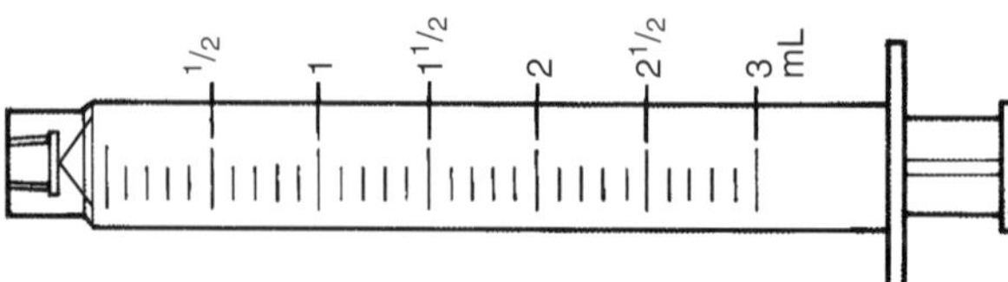

For additional practice problems, refer to the Oral Dosages and Parenteral Dosages sections of the Elsevier's Interactive Drug Calculation Application, Version 1 on Evolve.

Answer Key

6 Reconstitution of Medications From Powders and Crystals: Oral and Intramuscular

WORKSHEET **6A** (page 185)

1. a. Add 55 mL of water, half at a time.

b. 5000 mg

c. 6 mL

KNOW / WANT TO KNOW	PROOF	CROSS FRACTION
250 mg : 5 mL = 300 mg : x mL	5 × 300 = 1500	$\frac{25 \text{ mg}}{5} = \frac{30}{x \text{ mL}}$
250x = 5 × 300 = 1500 x = 6 mL	6 × 250 = 1500	25x = 5 × 30 = 150 x = 6 mL

d. 16.6 doses per bottle

KNOW / WANT TO KNOW	PROOF	CROSS FRACTION
6 mL : 1 dose = 100 mL : x dose	1 × 100 = 100	$\frac{6 \text{ ml}}{1} = \frac{100 \text{ mL}}{x}$
6x = 100 x = 16.6	16.6 × 6 = 99.6 = 100	6x = 100 x = 16.6

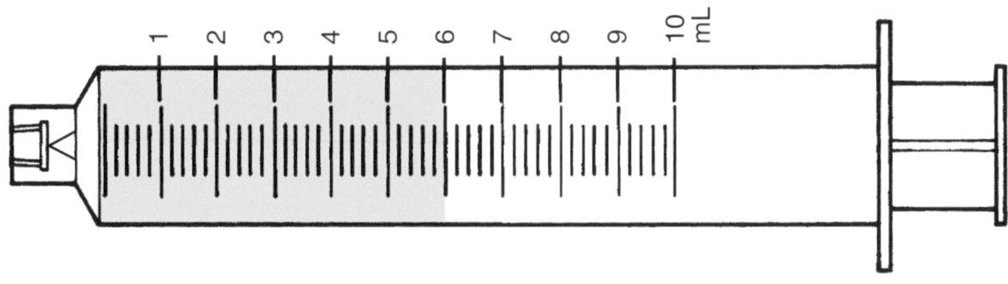

2. a. Add 35 mL of water, half at a time.

b. 12 mL stat dose

KNOW	WANT TO KNOW	PROOF	CROSS FRACTION
125 mg : 5 mL = 300 mg : x mL		$5 \times 300 = 1500$	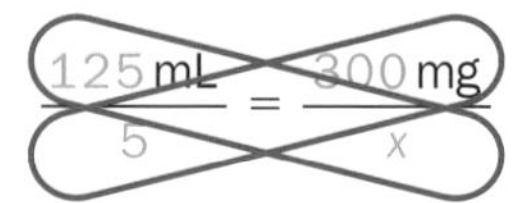
$125x = 5 \times 300 = 1500$		$12 \times 125 = 1500$	$125x = 1500$
$x = 12$ mL			$x = 12$ mL

c. 7.6

KNOW	WANT TO KNOW	PROOF	
5 mL : 1 dose = 38 mL : x doses		$1 \times 38 = 38$	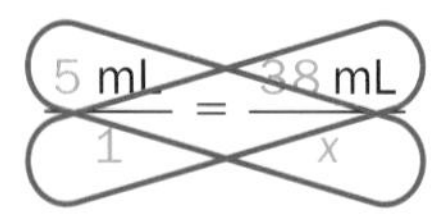
$5x = 38$		$5 \times 7.6 = 38$	$5x = 38$
$x = 7.6$ doses			$x = 7.6$ doses

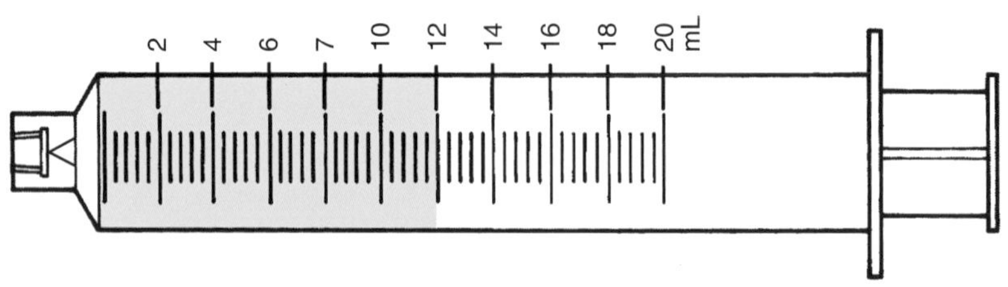

3. a. 1250 mg

KNOW	WANT TO KNOW	PROOF	CROSS FRACTION
5 mL : 125 mg = 50 mL : x mg		$1250 \times 5 = 6250$	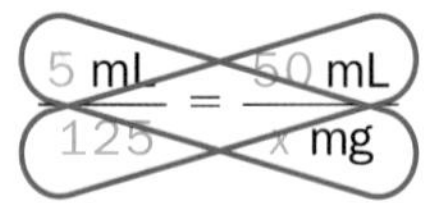
$5x = 125 \times 50 = 6250$		$125 \times 50 = 6250$	$5x = 125 \times 50 = 6250$
$x = 1250$ mg			$5x = 6250$
			$x = 1250$ mg

b. 14 mL.

KNOW	WANT TO KNOW	PROOF	
5 mL : 125 mg = x mL : 350 mg		$14 \times 125 = 1750$	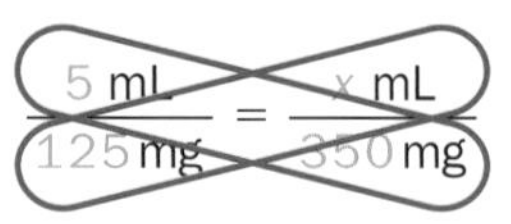
$125x = 5 \times 350 = 1750$		$5 \times 350 = 1750$	$125x = 5 \times 350 = 1750$
$x = 14$ mL			$x = 14$ mL

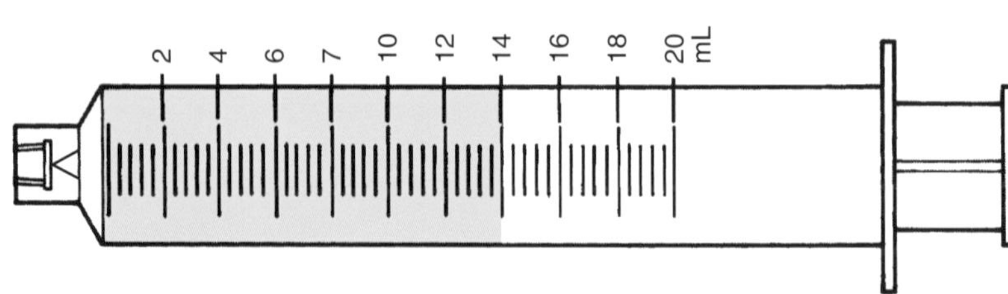

8. a. 65 mL total

b. 9 mL

KNOW	WANT TO KNOW	PROOF	CROSS FRACTION
250 mg : 5 mL = 450 mg : x mL		9 × 250 = 2250	$\frac{25}{5} = \frac{45}{x}$
$25x = 5 \times 45 = 225$		5 × 450 = 2250	$25x = 225$

$x = 9$ mL per dose times 3 doses = 27 mL per day for 24 hr — $x = 9$ mL

c.
  75 mL total in the bottle
− 27 mL initial dose for 24 hours
  48 mL left in the bottle

d. Yes

KNOW	WANT TO KNOW	PROOF
250 mg : 5 mL = 250 mg : x mL		250 × 5 = 1250
$250x = 1250$		5 × 250 = 1250

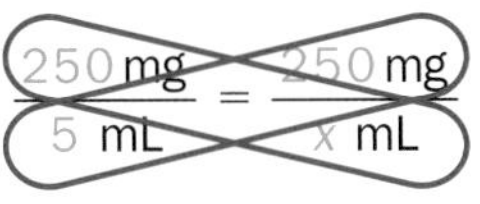

$x = 5$ mL

$x = 5$ mL per dose × 2 doses = 10 mL per day × 4 days = 40 mL total

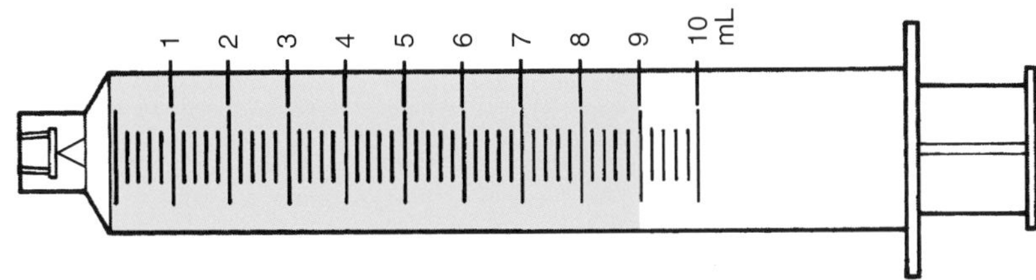

9. a. Add 26 mL of distilled water.

b.

KNOW	WANT TO KNOW	PROOF
10 mg : 1 mL = 50 mg : x mL		1 × 50 = 50
$10x = 1 \times 50 = 50$		10 × 5 = 50

$\frac{10 \text{ mg}}{1 \text{ mL}} \times \frac{50 \text{ mg}}{x \text{ mL}}$

$x = 5$ mL to administer

c.

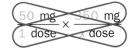

KNOW	WANT TO KNOW	PROOF
50 mg : 1 dose = 350 mg : x doses		1 × 350 = 350
$50x = 1 \times 350 = 350$		50 × 7 = 350

$\frac{50 \text{ mg}}{1 \text{ dose}} \times \frac{350 \text{ mg}}{x \text{ dose}}$

$x = 7$ doses in the bottle

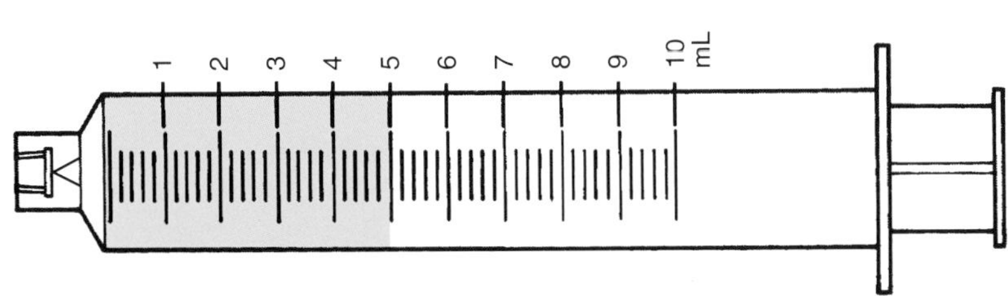

10. a. Add 55 mL of water.

b. KNOW　　　WANT TO KNOW　　　**PROOF**　　　**CROSS FRACTION**

125 mg : 5 mL = 200 mg : x mL　　　5 × 200 = 1000

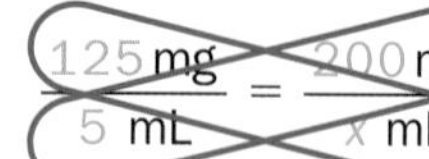

$125x = 5 \times 200 = 1000$　　　125 × 8 = 1000

x = 8 mL to administer

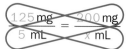

$125x = 5 \times 200 = 1000$

x = 8 mL

c. KNOW　　　WANT TO KNOW　　　**PROOF**

100 mL : x dose = 8 mL : 1 dose　　　1 × 100 = 100

$$\frac{100\text{ mg}}{x\text{ doses}} = \frac{8\text{ mL}}{1\text{ dose}}$$

$8x = 1 \times 100 = 100$　　　12.5 × 8 = 100

x = 12.5 doses in the bottle

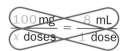

$8x = 100$

x = 12.5 doses

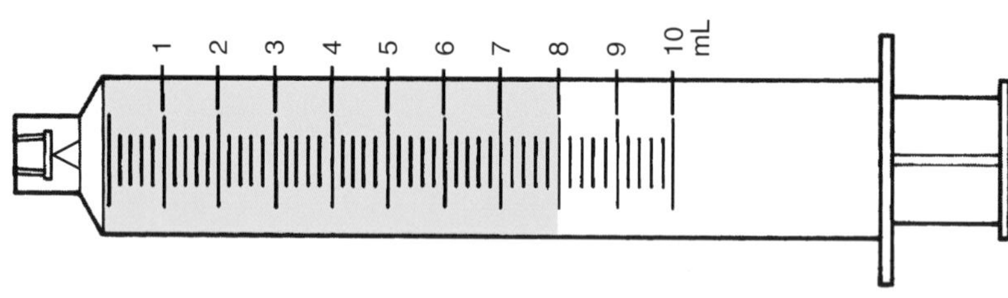

WORKSHEET **6B** (page 195)

1. a. Add 4.0 mL of diluent to yield 250,000 units/mL.

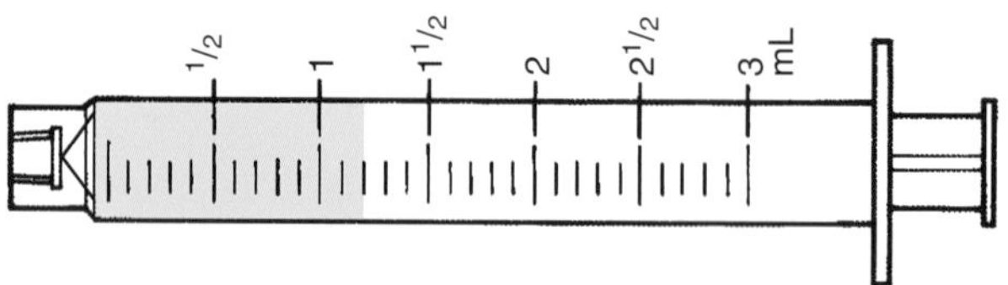

b. KNOW　　　WANT TO KNOW

25~~0,000~~ units : 1 mL = 30~~0,000~~ units : x mL

$25x = 30$

x = 1.2 mL

PROOF

25 × 1.2 = 30

1 × 30 = 30

CROSS FRACTION

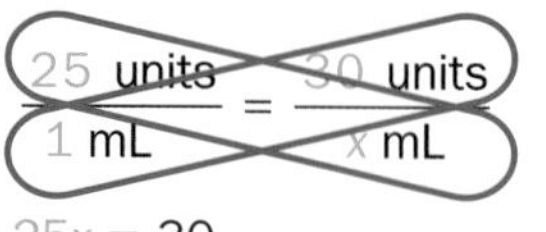

$25x = 30$

x = 1.2 mL

c. KNOW　　　WANT TO KNOW

3~~00,000~~ units : 1 dose = 1,0~~00,000~~ units : x dose

$3x = 10$

$3x = 10$

x = 3.3 = 3 full doses in the vial

PROOF

1 × 1,0~~00,000~~ = 1,0~~00,000~~

3.3 × 3~~00,000~~ = 9.9

If the 1.8 mL diluent were used, the resulting dosage would be 0.6 mL, which is concentrated and may create tissue inflammation.

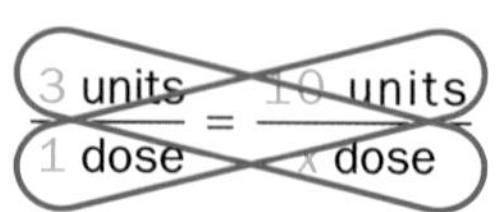

$3x = 10$

x = 3.3 doses

2. a. 4.2 mL 1% lidocaine
b. 350 mg per mL
c. 1.4 mL

KNOW	WANT TO KNOW	PROOF	CROSS FRACTION
350 mg : 1 mL =	500 mg : x mL	500 × 1 = 500	
350x = 500; x = 1.428 = 1.4 mL		350 × 1.428 = 499.8	350 x = 500; x = 1.4 mL

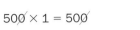

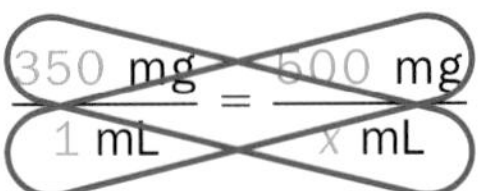

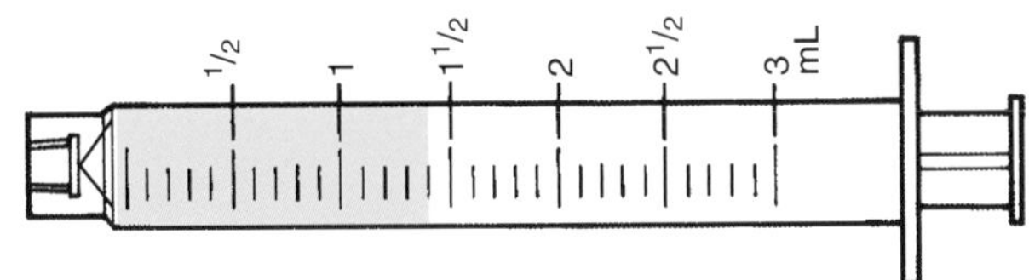

d. 5.7 doses

KNOW	WANT TO KNOW	PROOF
350 mg : 1 dose =	2000 mg : x dose	1 × 2000 = 2000
350x = 1 × 2000 = 200; x = 5.7 doses		5.71 × 350 = 1998.5 = 2000

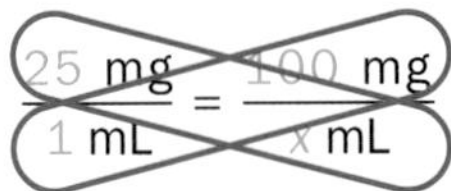

350 x = 2000
x = 5.7 doses

3. a. Administer 4 mL.

KNOW	WANT TO KNOW	PROOF	CROSS FRACTION
250 mg : 1 mL =	1000 mg : x mL	1 × 1000 = 1000	
250x = 1000; x = 4 mL		250 × 4 = 1000	25x = 100; x = 4 mL

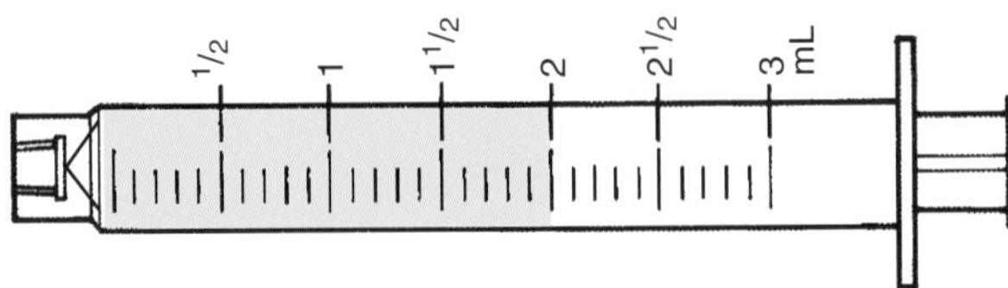

b. Give 2 mL in each site = 500 mg per injection.

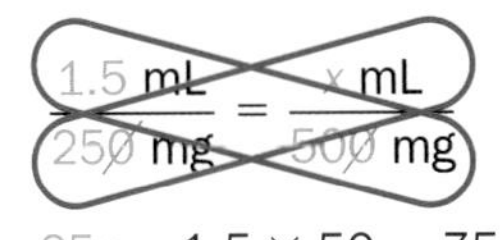

4. a. Add 5.7 mL sterile water for injection.
b. Administer: 3 mL.

KNOW	WANT TO KNOW	PROOF	CROSS FRACTION
1.5 mL : 250 mg =	x mL : 500 mg	25 × 3 = 75	
25x = 1.5 × 50 = 75; x = 3 mL		1.5 × 50 = 75	25x = 1.5 × 50 = 75; x = 3 mL

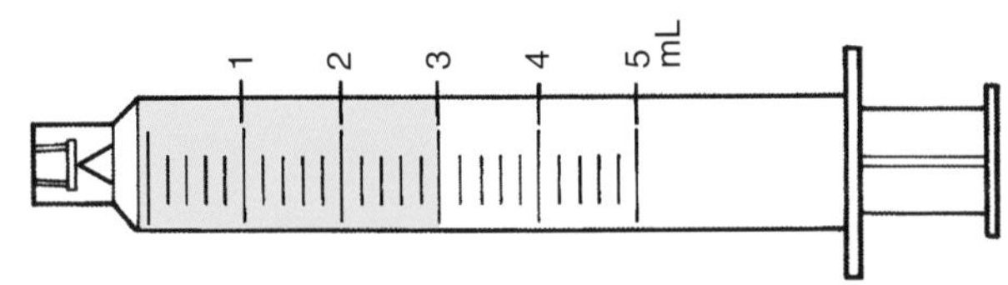

This can be given in divided doses.

5. Administer entire amount, 2.6 mL.

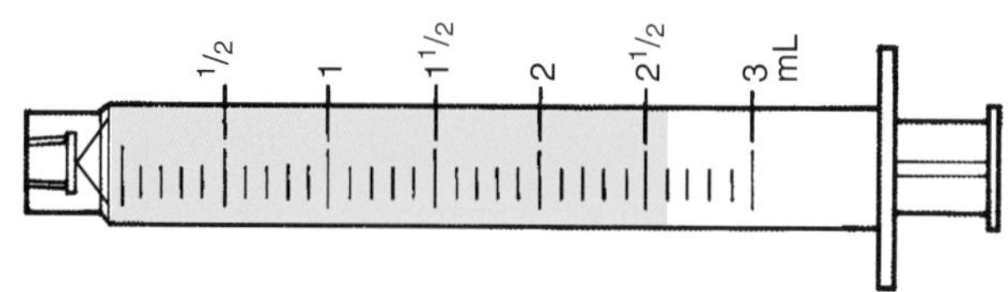

6. a. Add 1 mL of 1% lidocaine.

b. 1.3 mL

KNOW WANT TO KNOW

350 mg : 1 mL = 450 mg : x mL

$35x = 1 \times 45 = 45$

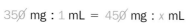

$x = 1.285 = 1.3$ mL

PROOF

$1 \times 45 = 45$

$35 \times 1.285 = 44.975$

CROSS FRACTION

$\frac{35 \text{ mg}}{1 \text{ mL}} = \frac{45 \text{ mg}}{x \text{ mL}}$

$35x = 45$

$x = 1.28 = 1.3$ mL

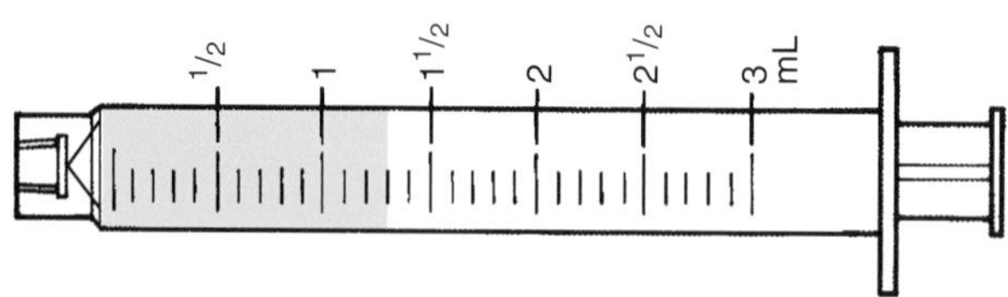

7. a. Add 3 mL of sterile water for injection as the diluent.

b. 280 mg/mL is the concentration.

c. KNOW WANT TO KNOW

280 mg : 1 mL = 250 mg : x mL

$280x = 250$

$x = 0.892 = 0.9$ mL

PROOF

$1 \times 250 = 250$

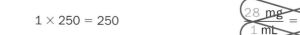

$0.892 \times 280 = 250$

CROSS FRACTION

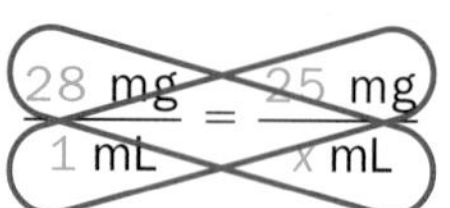

$28x = 25$

$x = 0.89$ mL $= 0.9$ mL

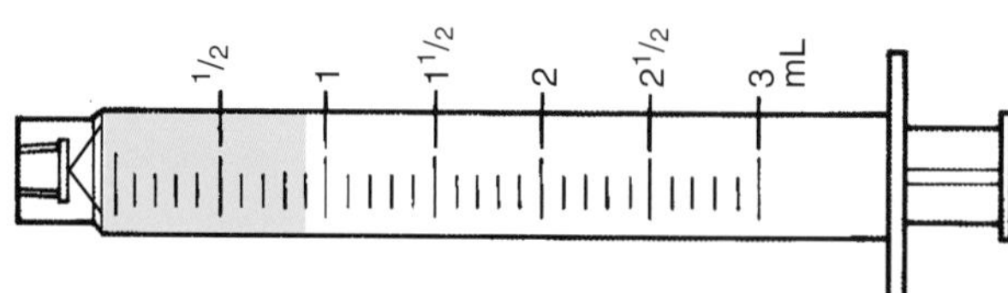

8. a. Add 3.5 mL of diluent.

b. 1 hour

c. 1 gram

d. KNOW WANT TO KNOW

250 mg : 1 mL = 100 mg : x mL

$250x = 100$

$x = 0.4$ mL

PROOF

$250 \times 0.4 = 100$

$100 \times 1 = 100$

CROSS FRACTION

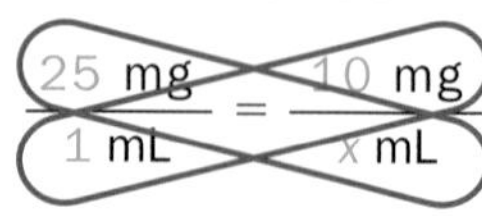

$250x = 100$

$x = 0.4$ mL

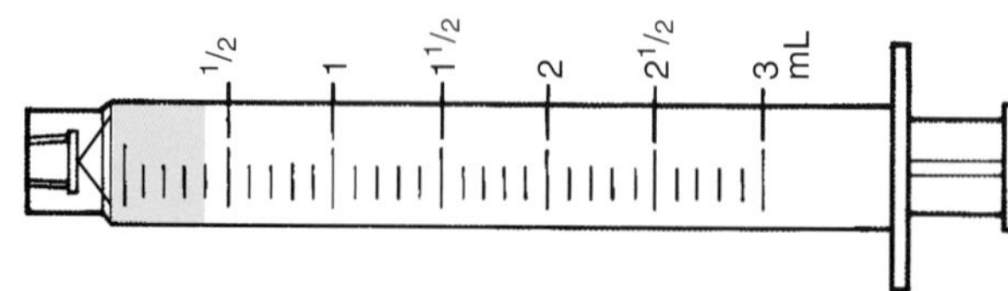

9. a. Administer 1.7 mL.

KNOW	WANT TO KNOW	**PROOF**	**CROSS FRACTION**
500 mg : 1.2 mL = 700 mg : x mL		5 × 1.68 = 8.4	$\frac{5\ \text{mg}}{1.2\ \text{mL}} = \frac{7\ \text{mg}}{x\ \text{mL}}$
5x = 1.2 × 7		1.2 × 7 = 8.4	5x = 7 × 1.2 = 8.4
5x = 8.4			x = 1.68 = 1.7 mL
x = 1.68 or 1.7 mL			

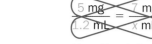

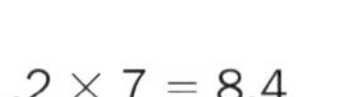
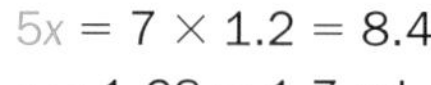
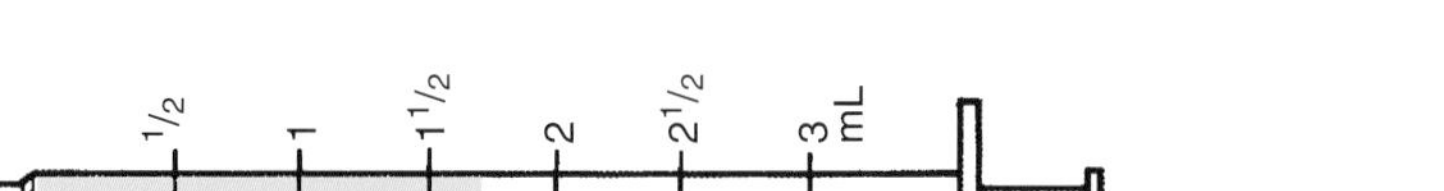
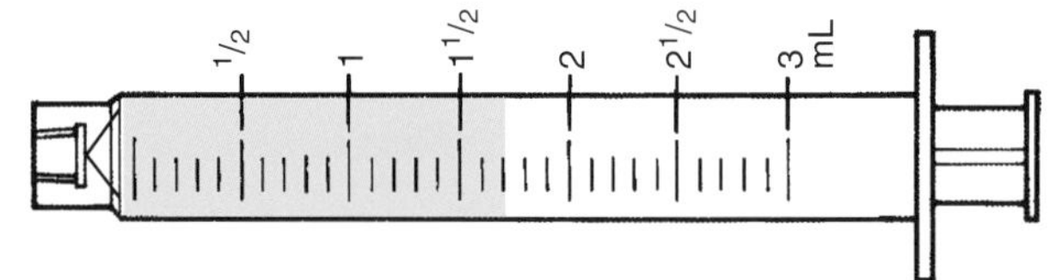

b. Patient will receive 2800 mg/day.

KNOW	WANT TO KNOW	**PROOF**	**CROSS FRACTION**
700 mg : 1 dose = x mg : 4 doses		700 × 4 = 2800	$\frac{700\ \text{mg}}{1\ \text{dose}} = \frac{x\ \text{mg}}{4\ \text{dose}}$
x = 4 × 700		1 × 2800 = 2800	x = 700 × 4 = 2800
x = 2800 mg/day			x = 2800 mg

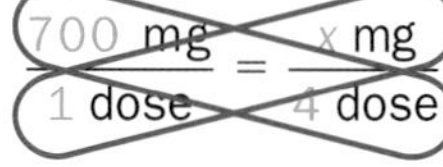

c. Need 2.8 or 3 vials per day.

KNOW	WANT TO KNOW	**PROOF**	**CROSS FRACTION**
1000 mg : 1 vial = 2800 mg : x vials		1 × 28 = 28	$\frac{10\ \text{mg}}{1\ \text{vial}} = \frac{28\ \text{mg}}{x\ \text{vials}}$
10x = 28 = 2.8 or 3 vials needed for a 24-hr period		10 × 2.8 = 28	10x = 28
			x = 2.8 vials

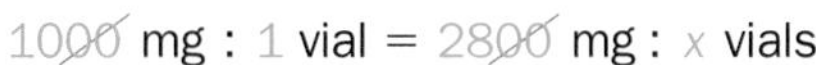
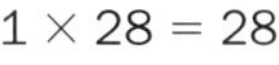
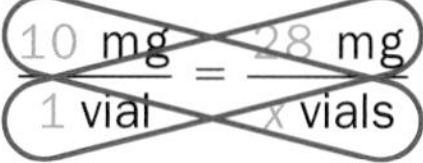

10. a. Administer 4 mL in first dose.
b. Divide into two equal injections.
c. Give deep intramuscularly in the right or left ventrogluteal area.

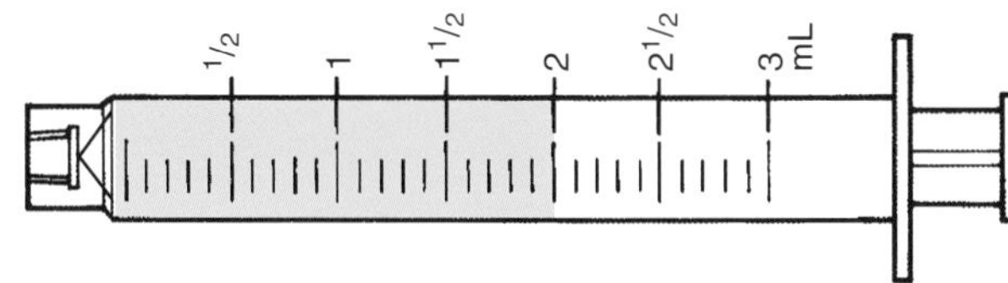

WORKSHEET **6C** (page 200)

1. a. 400 mg per mL.
b. 1.3 mL

KNOW	WANT TO KNOW	**PROOF**	**CROSS FRACTION**
400 mg : 1 mL = 500 mg : x mL		1 × 5 = 5	$\frac{4\ \text{mg}}{1\ \text{mL}} = \frac{5\ \text{mg}}{x\ \text{mL}}$
4x = 1 × 5 = 5		4 × 1.25 = 5	4x = 5
x = 1.25 = 1.3 mL			x = 1.25 = 1.3 mL

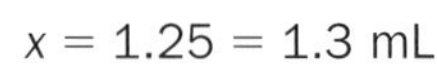
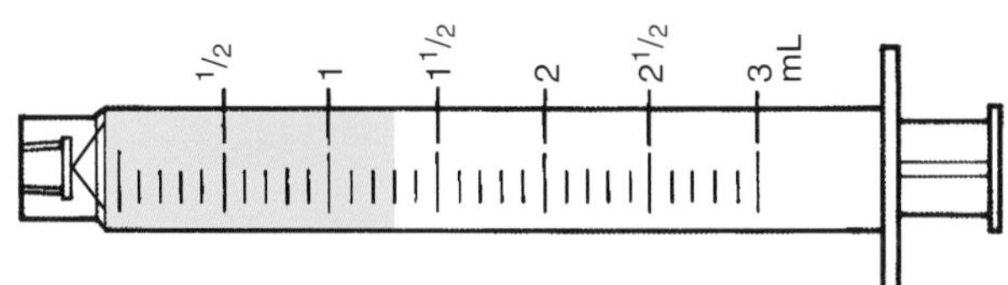

2. a. Add 2 mL of sterile water.

b. Have 500 mg/1.2 mL.

c. Administer 1.2 mL.

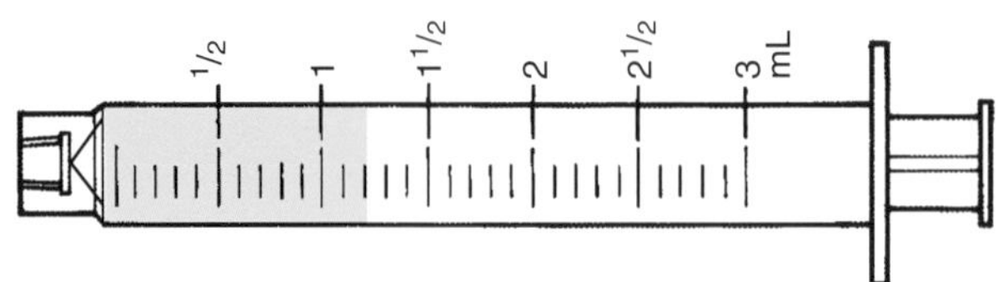

3. Choose the one next to the syringe that shows 1.4 mL.

KNOW WANT TO KNOW

250 mg : 1 mL = 500 mg : x mL

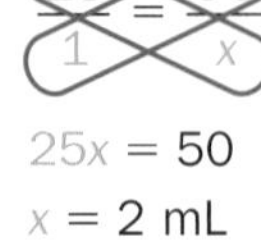

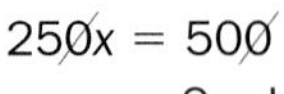

$250x = 500$

$x = 2$ mL

$25x = 50$

$x = 2$ mL

PROOF

$500 \times 1 = 500$

$250 \times 2 = 500$

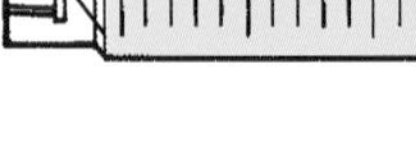

OR

KNOW	WANT TO KNOW	PROOF	CROSS FRACTION

→ 350 mg : x mL = 500 mg : x mL

$1 \times 500 = 500$

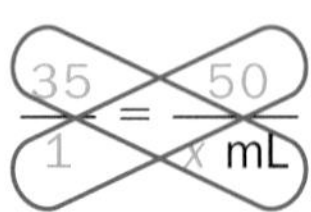

$350x = 1 \times 500 = 500$

$x = 1.428 = 1.4$ mL

$350 \times 1.428 = 500$

$35x = 50$

$x = 1.4$ mL

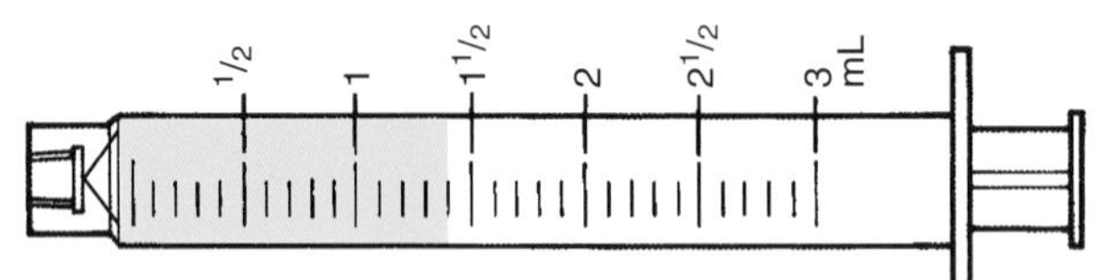

4. If you add 4 mL of diluent

KNOW WANT TO KNOW **PROOF**

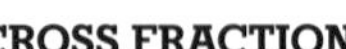

CROSS FRACTION

250,000 units : 1 mL = 400,000 units : x mL

$25 \times 1.6 = 40$

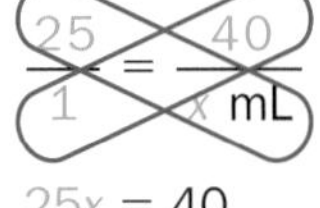

$25x = 40$

$x = 1.6$ mL would contain the dose 400,000 units

$1 \times 40 = 40$

$25x = 40$

$x = 1.6$ mL

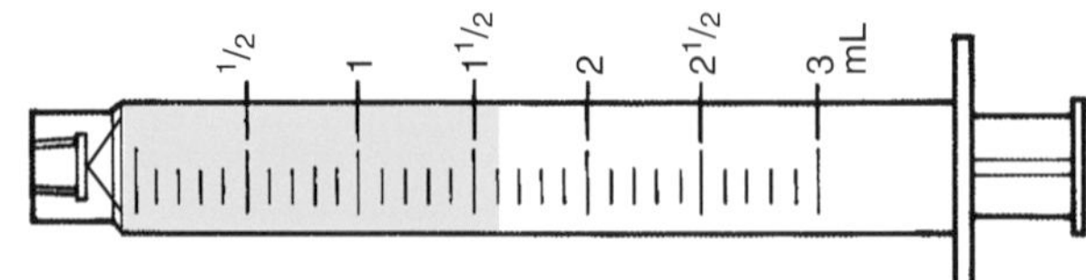

If you add 1.5 mL of diluent

KNOW WANT TO KNOW

500,000 units : 1 mL = 400,000 units : x mL

$5x = 4$

$x = 0.8$ mL would contain the dose 400,000 units

PROOF

$5 \times 0.8 = 4$

$1 \times 4 = 4$

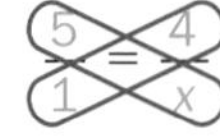

$5x = 4$

$x = 0.8$ mL

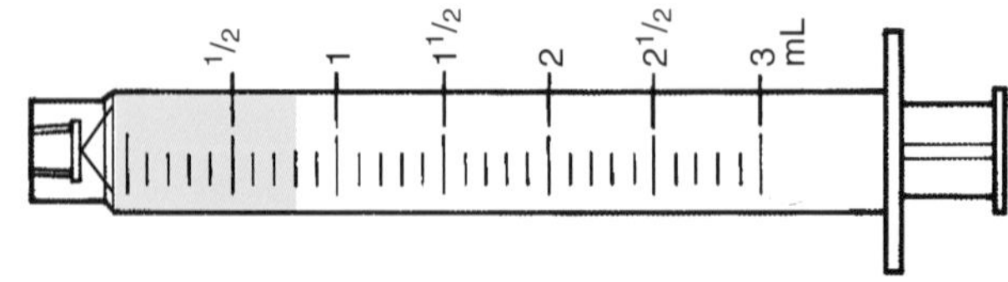

5. a. Add 16 mL of bacteriostatic water with benzyl alcohol.

b. 62.5 mg/mL

c.

KNOW	WANT TO KNOW	PROOF	CROSS FRACTION
62.5 mg : 1 mL = 125 mg : x mL		$1 \times 125 = 125$	$\frac{62.5}{1} = \frac{125}{x \text{ mL}}$
$62.5x = 1 \times 125 = 125$		$62.5 \times 2 = 125$	$62.5x = 125$
$x = 2$ mL/dose			$x = 2$ mL

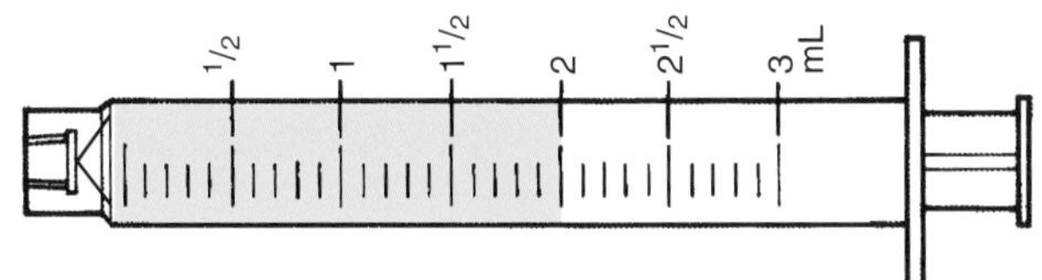

d.

KNOW	WANT TO KNOW	PROOF	
125 mg : 1 dose = 1000 mg : x doses		$1 \times 1000 = 1000$	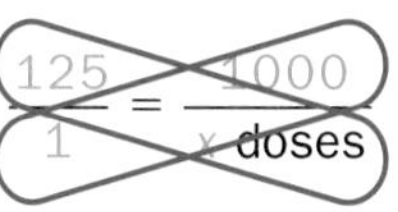
$125x = 1 \times 1000$		$125 \times 8 = 1000$	$125x = 1000$
$x = 8$ doses in the vial			$x = 8$ doses

e. The literature states the medication must be used within 48 hours.

f.

KNOW	WANT TO KNOW	PROOF	
500 mg : 1 day = 1000 mg : x days		$1 \times 1000 = 1000$	$\frac{5}{1} = \frac{10}{x \text{ days}}$
$500x = 1000$		$500 \times 2 = 1000$	$5x = 10$
$x = 2$ days to administer the vial.			$x = 2$ days

The allowed time is 48 hr, which is within the allotted time frame.

6. a. Choose the strength next to the syringe showing 0.8 mL.

KNOW	WANT TO KNOW	PROOF	CROSS FRACTION
250,000 units : 1 mL = 400,000 units : x mL		$1 \times 40 = 40$	$\frac{25}{1} = \frac{40}{x \text{ mL}}$
$25x = 1 \times 40 = 40$		$25 \times 1.6 = 40$	$25x = 40$
$x = 1.6$ mL twice a day			$x = 1.6$ mL

KNOW	WANT TO KNOW	PROOF	
500,000 units : 1 mL = 400,000 units : x mL		$5 \times 0.8 = 4$	$\frac{5}{1} = \frac{4}{x \text{ mL}}$
$5x = 1 \times 4 = 4$		$4 \times 1 = 4$	$5x = 4$
$x = 0.8$ mL twice a day			$x = 0.8$ mL

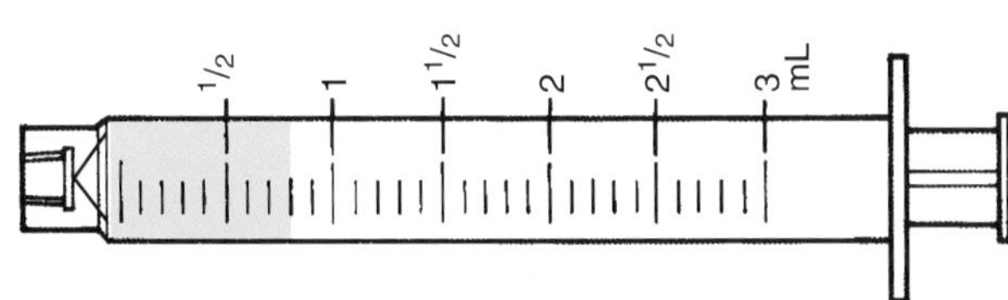

b. The muscle mass of your patient will help you decide which strength to use.

7. **a.** Add 2 mL of sterile water for injection.
b. The reconstituted medication will yield 1 g/2.6 mL.
c. Use medication promptly.
d. 1000 mg or 1 g
e. Administer 2 mL.

KNOW WANT TO KNOW

$100\not{0}\text{ mg} : 2.6\text{ mL} = 75\not{0}\text{ mg} : x\text{ mL}$

$1000x = 2.6 \times 750 = 1950$
$1000x = 1950$
$x = 1.95 = 2\text{ mL}$

PROOF

$1000 \times 1.95 = 1950$

$2.6 \times 750 = 1950$

CROSS FRACTION

$$\frac{100}{2.6} = \frac{75}{x\text{ mL}}$$

$100x = 2.6 \times 75 = 195$
$x = 1.95 = 2\text{ mL}$

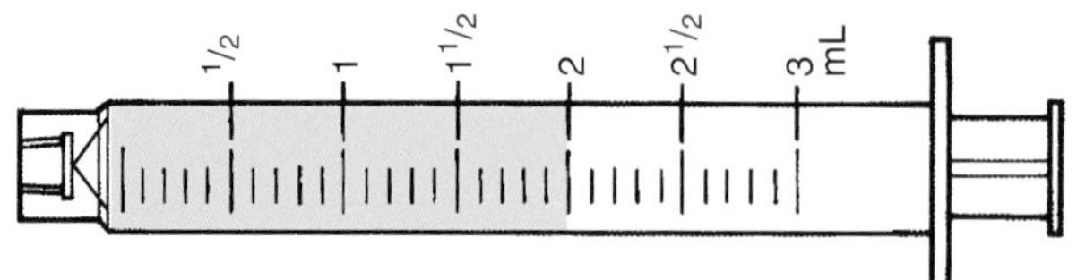

8. **a.** 3.5 mL of diluent
b. 250 mg per mL
c. 2 mL
d. Shelf life is 1 hour

KNOW WANT TO KNOW

$25\not{0}\text{ mg} : 1\text{ mL} = 50\not{0}\text{ mg} : x\text{ mL}$

$25x = 50$
$x = 2\text{ mL}$

PROOF

$1 \times 50 = 50$

$2 \times 25 = 50$

CROSS FRACTION

$$\frac{25}{1} = \frac{50}{x\text{ mL}}$$

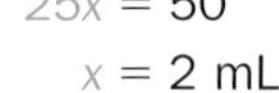

$25x = 50$
$x = 2\text{ mL}$

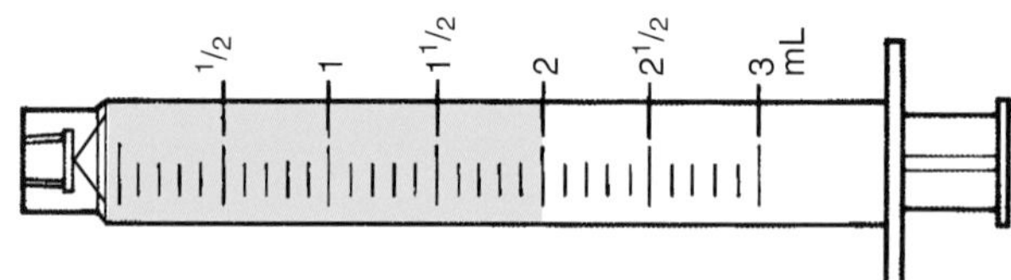

9. **a.** Add 3.5 mL diluent.
b. The reconstituted medication will yield 250 mg/mL.
c. Use within 1 hr, as this is a very unstable medication.
d. Administer 2 mL.

KNOW WANT TO KNOW

$25\not{0}\text{ mg} : 1\text{ mL} = 50\not{0}\text{ mg} : x\text{ mL}$

$25\not{0}\,x = 50\not{0}$
$x = 2\text{ mL}$

PROOF

$1 \times 500 = 500$

$250 \times 2 = 500$

CROSS FRACTION

$$\frac{25}{1} = \frac{50}{x\text{ mL}}$$

$25x = 50$
$x = 2\text{ mL}$

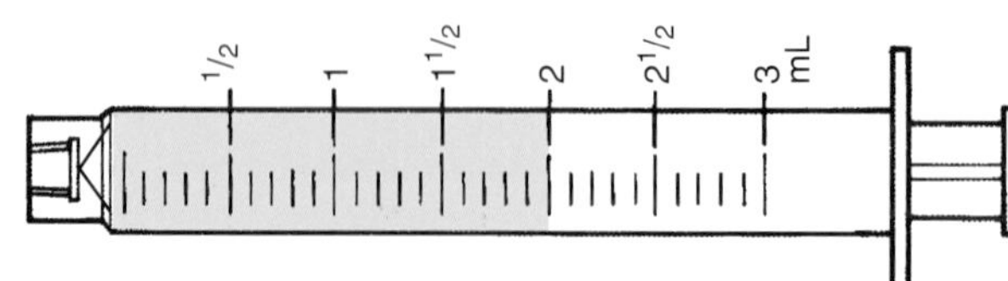

10. **a.** Add 2.7 mL of sterile water for injection.
b. 250 mg per 1.5 mL
c. Refrigerated, 7 days; room temperature, 3 days

d. 500 mg

b. Administer 2.7 mL.

KNOW	WANT TO KNOW	PROOF	CROSS FRACTION
25~~0~~ mg : 1.5 mL = 45~~0~~ mg : x mL		250 × 2.7 = 675	$\frac{25}{1.5} = \frac{45}{x\text{ mL}}$
25~~0~~x : 1.5 × 45~~0~~		1.5 × 450 = 675	25x = 1.5 × 45 = 67.5
25~~0~~ x = 67.5			x = 2.7 mL
x = 2.7 mL			

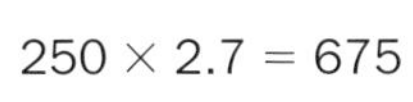
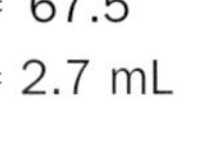
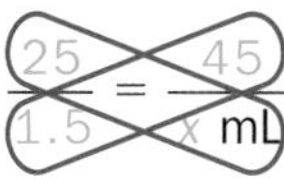

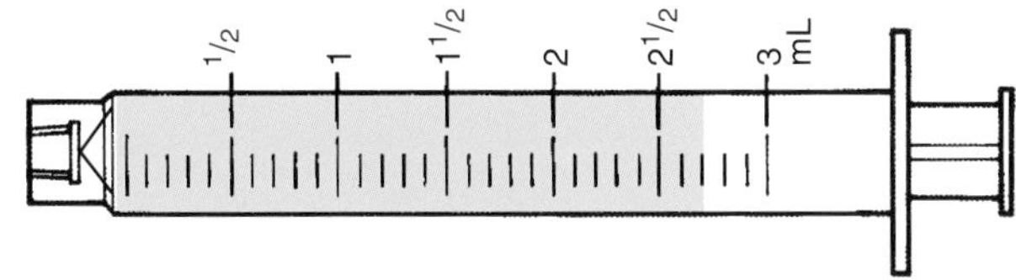

WORKSHEET **6D** (page 205)

1. b.

KNOW	WANT TO KNOW	PROOF	CROSS FRACTION
40 mcg : 1 mL = 60 mcg : x mL		1 × 60 = 60	$\frac{40}{1} = \frac{60}{x}$
40x = 1 × 60 = 60		40 × 1.5 = 60	40x = 60
x = 1.5 mL			x = 1.5 mL

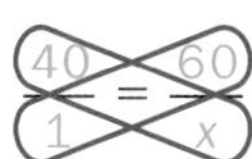

2. b. Directions read: Add 1.2 mL of diluent to yield 125 mg/mL.

d.

KNOW	WANT TO KNOW	PROOF	CROSS FRACTION
250 mg : 1 dose = x mg : 2 doses		1 × 500 = 500	$\frac{250}{1} = \frac{x}{2}$
x = 250 × 2 = 500		250 × 2 = 500	x = 500 mg
x = 500 mg for 2 doses			

KNOW	WANT TO KNOW	PROOF	
125 mg : 1 vial = 500 mg : x vials		1 × 500 = 500	$\frac{125}{1} = \frac{500}{x}$
125x = 1 × 500 = 500		125 × 4 = 500	125x = 500
x = 4 vials for 24 hr			x = 4 vials for 24 hr

3. d. Add 1.2 mL bacteriostatic water.

d. 0.9 mL.

KNOW	WANT TO KNOW	PROOF	CROSS FRACTION
40 mg : 1 mL = 35 mg : x mL		1 × 35 = 35	$\frac{40}{1} = \frac{35}{x}$
40x = 1 × 35 = 35		40 × 0.875 = 35	40x = 35
x = 0.875 = 0.9 mL			x = 0.87 = 0.9 mL

4. b.

KNOW	WANT TO KNOW	PROOF	CROSS FRACTION
2 mL : 1 g = x mL : 1.5 g		1 × 3 = 3	$\frac{2}{1} = \frac{x}{1.5}$
x = 2 × 1.5 = 3		2 × 1.5 = 3	x = 2 × 1.5 = 3
x = 3 mL divided into 2 injections depending on the assessment of the patient's muscle mass			x = 3 mL

d.

KNOW	WANT TO KNOW	PROOF	
1~~000~~ mg : 1 vial = 3~~000~~ mg : x vials		1000 × 3 = 3000	$\frac{1}{1} = \frac{3}{x}$
1000x = 3000		1 × 3000 = 3000	x = 3 vials
x = 3 vials needed			

5. c. KNOW — WANT TO KNOW

4 mL : 2000 mg = x mL : 1000 mg

$2000x = 4 \times 1000 = 4000$

$2x = 4$

$x = 2$ mL

PROOF

$2000 \times 2 = 4000$

$4 \times 1000 = 4000$

CROSS FRACTION

$\frac{4}{2} = \frac{x}{1}$

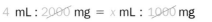

$2x = 4$

$x = 2$ mL

6. c. KNOW — WANT TO KNOW

2.6 mL : 1000 mg = x mL : 500 mg

$10x = 2.6 \times 5 = 13$

$x = 1.3$ mL

PROOF

$2.6 \times 500 = 1300$

$1000 \times 1.3 = 1300$

CROSS FRACTION

$\frac{2.6}{10} = \frac{x}{5}$

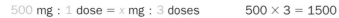

$10x = 5 \times 2.6 = 13$

$10x = 13$

$x = 1.3$ mL

7. c. KNOW — WANT TO KNOW

500 mg : 1 dose = x mg : 3 doses

$x = 500 \times 3 = 1500$

$x = 1500$ mg/24 hr

PROOF

$500 \times 3 = 1500$

$1500 \times 1 = 1500$

CROSS FRACTION

$\frac{500}{1} = \frac{x}{3}$

$x = 500 \times 3 = 1500$ mg

KNOW — WANT TO KNOW

1000 mg : 1 vial = 1500 mg : x vials

$1000x = 1500$

$x = 1.5$ vials

PROOF

$1 \times 1500 = 1500$

$1000 \times 1.5 = 1500$

You will need to have 2 vials on hand for 24 hr.

CROSS FRACTION

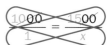

$\frac{1000}{1} = \frac{1500}{x}$

$10x = 15$

$x = 1.5$ vials

8. c. Directions read: Add 1.8 mL of diluent = 500,000 units/mL

d. KNOW — WANT TO KNOW

500,000 units : 1 mL = 400,000 units : x mL

$500{,}000x = 1 \times 400{,}000 = 400{,}000$

$5x = 4$

$x = 0.8$ mL

PROOF

$0.8 \times 500{,}000 = 400{,}000$

$1 \times 400{,}000 = 400{,}000$

CROSS FRACTION

$\frac{5}{1} = \frac{4}{x}$

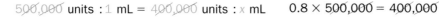

$5x = 4$

$x = 0.8$ mL

9. c. Add 9 mL of diluent = 400 mg/mL

a. KNOW — WANT TO KNOW

400 mg : 1 mL = 500 mg : x mL

$400x = 1 \times 500$

$4x = 5$

$x = 1.25 = 1.3$ mL

PROOF

$1 \times 500 = 500$

$400 \times 1.25 = 500$

CROSS FRACTION

$\frac{4}{1} = \frac{5}{x}$

$4x = 5$

$x = 1.25 = 1.3$ mL

10. c. 330 mg : 1 mL = 250 mg : x mL

$330x = 250$

$x = 0.757 = 0.8$ mL

PROOF

$1 \times 250 = 250$

$0.757 \times 330 = 249.8$

CROSS FRACTION

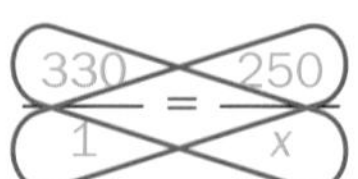

$330x = 250$

$x = 0.757 = 0.8$ mL

CHAPTER 6 FINAL: MEDICATIONS FROM POWDERS AND CRYSTALS: ORAL AND INTRAMUSCULAR (page 210)

1. **a.** Add 55 mL of water.
   b. 125 mg per 5 mL
   c. Give 6 mL.

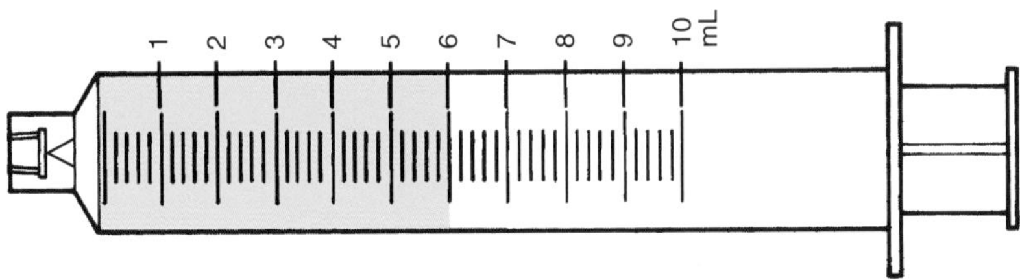

2. **a.** 700 mg
   b. doxycycline calcium
3. **a.** Add 3.5 mL diluent.
   b. Administer 1 mL.

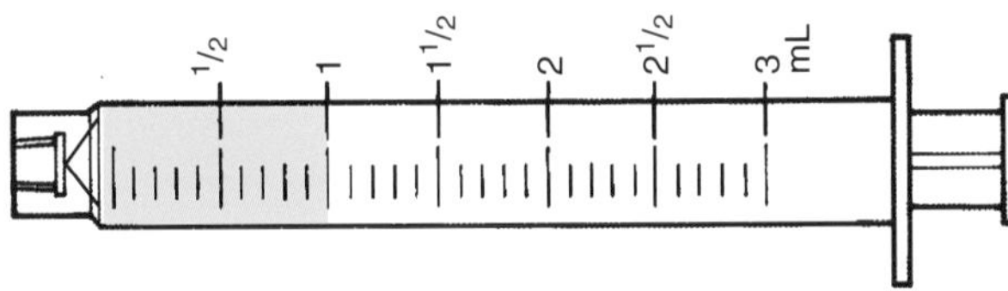

4. **a.** Add 2 mL of sterile water for injection.
   b. Administer 1.3 mL.

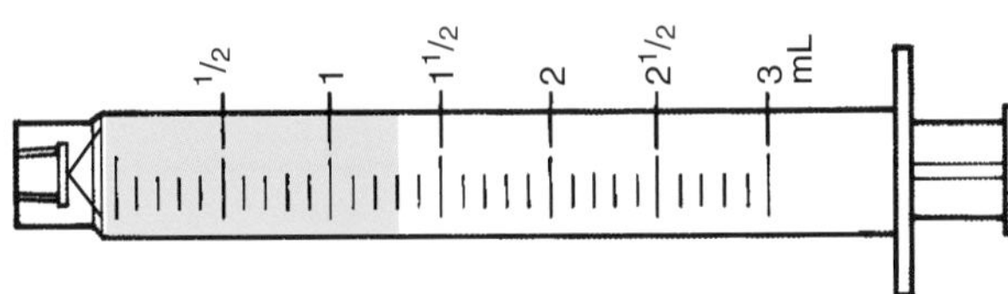

5. **a.** 250,000 units/mL
   b. 1.2 mL
   c. 16.6 doses in the vial

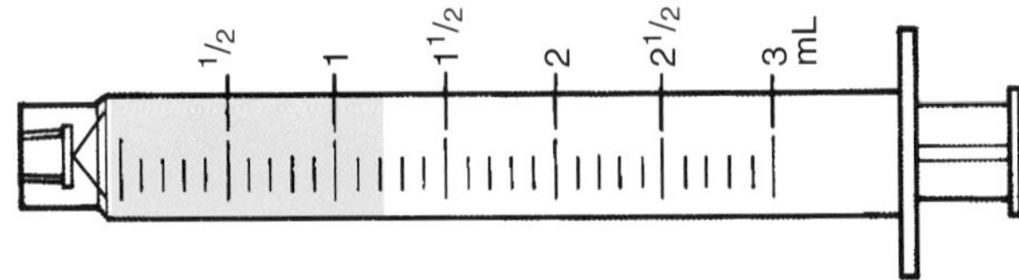

6. a. Add 9.5 mL of diluent.

b. Give 1.9 mL IM.

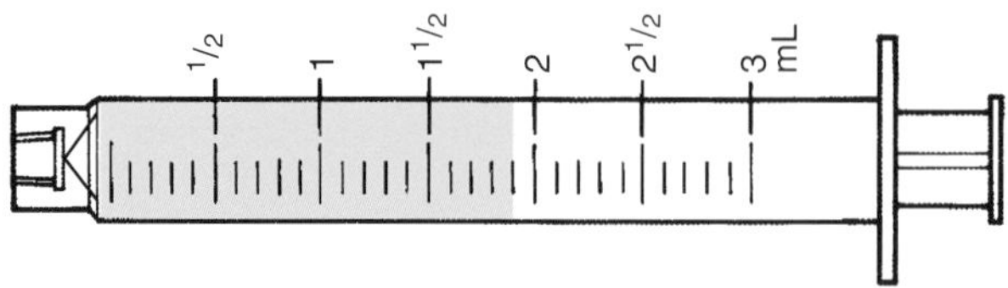

7. a. 3.0 mL of diluent

b. 280 mg per mL

c. 1.785 = 1.8 mL
Give 1.8 mL.

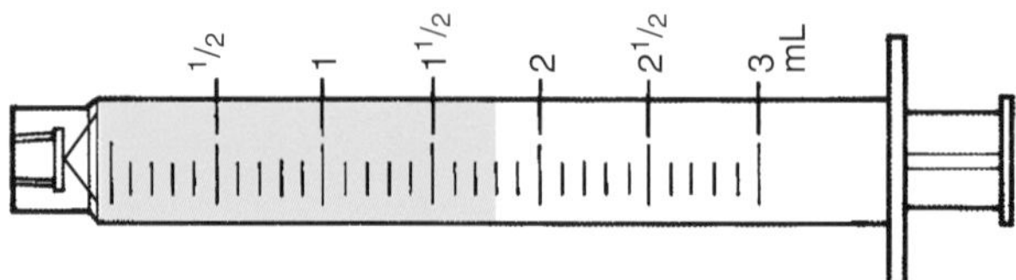

8. a. Add 9.6 mL of diluent to make 100,000 units/mL. A more concentrated solution may be caustic to the tissue.

b. Administer 1 mL.

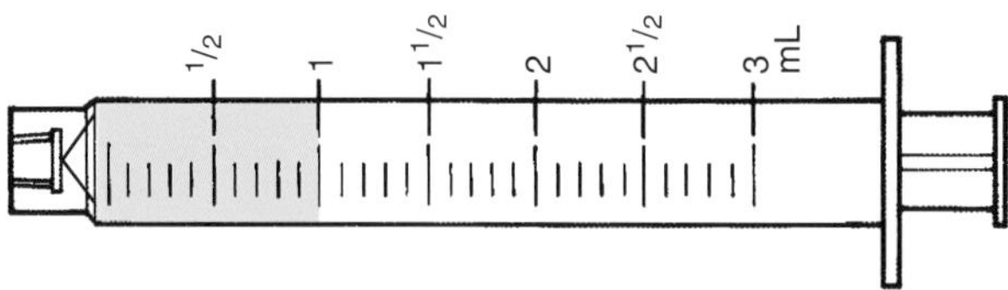

9. a. Add 2.7 mL sterile water for injection.

b. Administer 1.5 mL.

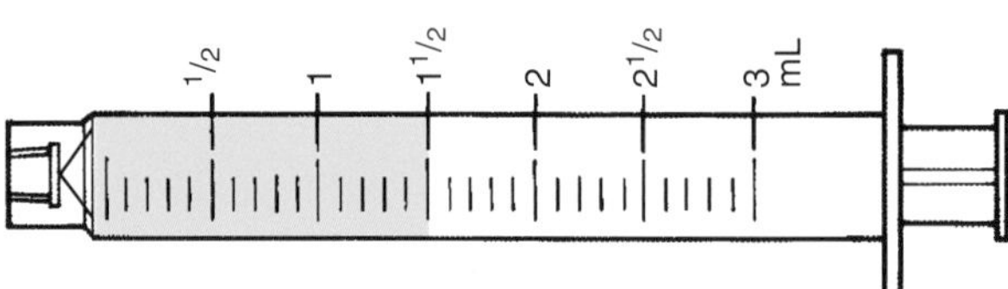

10. Administer 0.7 mL.

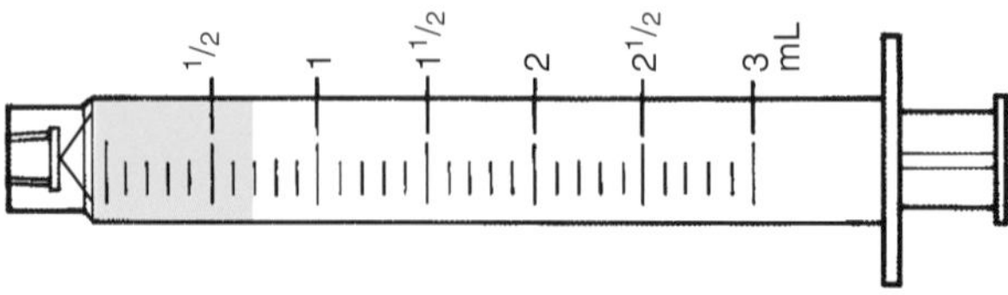

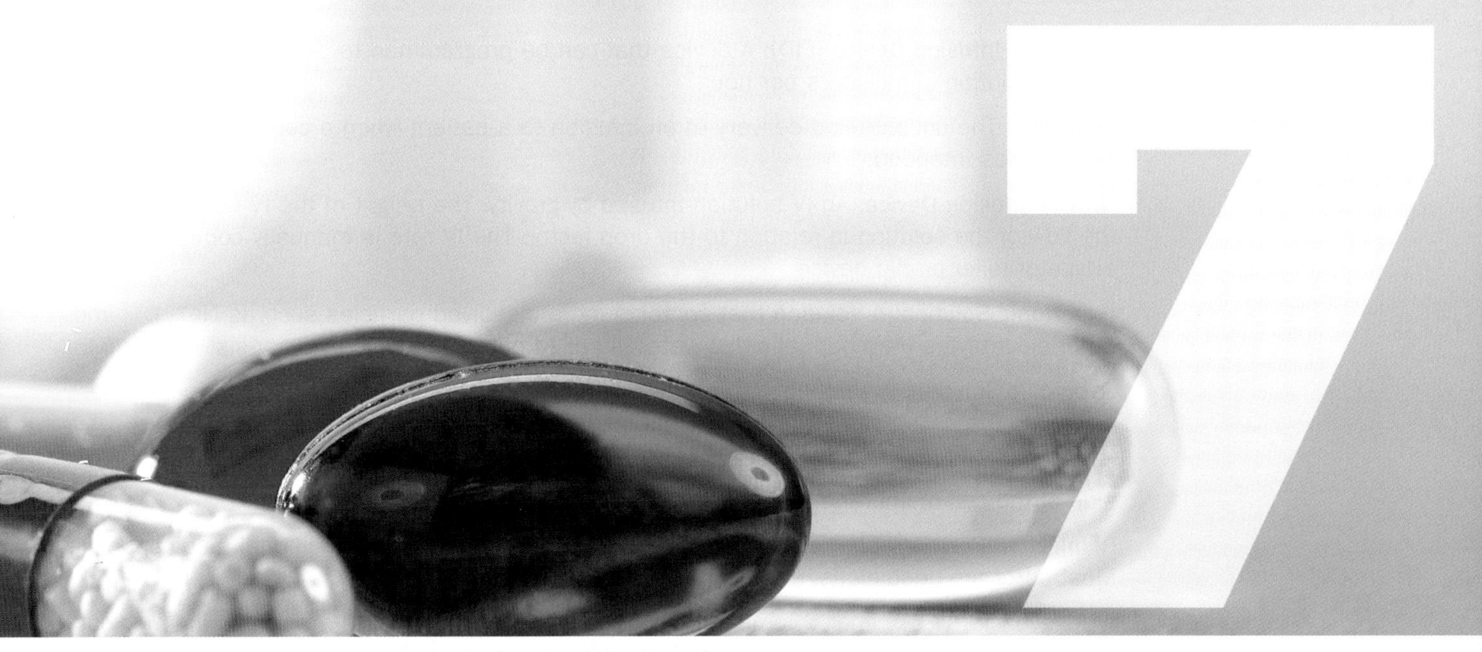

Basic Intravenous Therapy Calculations

Objectives

- State the rationale for administration of intravenous (IV) therapy.
- Check provider's IV order for type of solution, amount, additives, and rate of administration.
- Analyze IV orders for safe administration using critical thinking skills.
- Interpret IV labels.
- Calculate the grams of dextrose or sodium chloride in IV infusions.
- Identify osmolarity values for IV solutions.
- Identify IV sets: primary, primary with a port, IVPB extension tubing, transfusion sets, and venous access devices for intermittent use.
- Calculate IV flow rates for drops per min, mL per hr, mg per hr, g per hr, and infusion time.
- Identify various electronic IV infusion devices (EIDs).
- Explain the rationale for rate of infusion, initial and continuing, for blood and blood components.
- Understand PCA pumps using standard protocol.
- Identify a pressure-flow infusion device.
- Calculate the amount of saline or heparin for use in keeping venous access patent.
- Analyze medication errors using critical thinking skills.

Introduction

It is the nurse's responsibility to calculate the milliliters per hour or drops per minute to regulate an intravenous infusion. Knowledge of electronic infusion devices is required, as is knowledge of basic hand-regulated primary sets. The nurse is responsible for calculating the intravenous piggyback (IVPB) infusions that are timed for shorter periods.

Vocabulary

Bolus: A concentrated form of IV medication given in a short time period, usually given with a syringe into the IV port by a nurse or physician.

Continuous IV Infusion: An IV solution infused at a continuous, prescribed rate.

Drop Factor (DF): The number of drops per milliliter delivered through a given needle or dropper size into the drip chamber.

Electronic Infusion Device (EID): A device that can be programmed to deliver a prescribed rate of solution in milliliters per hour.

Free-Flow: The uncontrolled delivery of an infusion to a patient when a controlled or metered delivery was intended.

Gravity Infusion Device: An IV solution infused by gravity. The height of the IV solution affects the flow of the solution in relation to the drop factor. The IV rate is manually controlled with a type of roller or clip device.

Hypertonic Solution: A solution that contains more dissolved particles such as Na^+, C^-, and other electrolytes than normal cells; water is pulled out of the cells by osmosis.

Hypotonic Solution: A solution with a lower salt concentration than normal body cells; water flows into the cells across the cell membrane by osmosis.

Isotonic Solution: A solution that has the same concentration of dissolved solutes on each side of the cell membrane.

IV Injection Port: A rubber or latex port on IV infusion tubing to add additional medications. Most ports are needleless, ensuring safety from punctures.

IV Piggyback (IVPB): Small-volume infusions, usually 50, 100, or 250 mL containing medication, infused through a port on the existing primary line and delivered over 20 to 60 minutes.

Osmolarity: The total concentration of solutes, both penetrating and nonpenetrating. The milliosmole (mOsm) is in the cell and can also pass into the extracellular space. The exchange of milliosmoles (mOSm) from cellular to extracellular determines the isotonic, hypotonic, or hypertonic value of the solution.

Patient-Controlled Analgesia (PCA): An IV device/pump that is calibrated to deliver a prescribed amount of opioid medication operated by the patient and delivers the preset dose over a set period of time.

Tonicity: The concentration of extracellular, nonpenetrating solutes such as Cl^-, Na^+, and Ca^{++}.

Intravenous Therapy

Intravenous (IV) therapy is delivered through infusion into the venous system. IV therapy is used to correct or prevent fluid and electrolyte imbalances (IV solutions called crystalloids), provide parenteral nutrition (PN), administer blood and blood components (colloids), and/or deliver medication.

Intravenous Solutions

Administration of IV solutions requires a provider's order for the type of solutions, amount, additives, and rate of administration. Common IV solutions include saline solutions, dextrose in water solutions, balanced electrolyte solutions, and dextrose in saline solutions. The concentration of solutes in the solution determines if it is hypotonic, isotonic, or hypertonic.

Abbreviations for Common IV Solutions

Saline

NS	Normal saline; 0.9% sodium chloride solution (Figure 7.1)
½ NS	Normal saline; 0.45% saline or ½ strength sodium chloride (Figure 7.2)

Dextrose in Water

D5W or 5% D/W	Dextrose 5% in water (Figure 7.3)

Balanced Electrolyte

D5RL	Dextrose 5% in Ringer's lactate solution (Figure 7.4)
RL, LR, or RLS	Ringer's lactate solution (Figure 7.5)

Dextrose in Saline

D5NS Dextrose 5% in 0.9% normal saline (Figure 7.6)

D5 and ½ NS (0.45% NS) Dextrose 5% in ½ normal saline or Dextrose 5% in 0.45% sodium chloride (Figure 7.7)

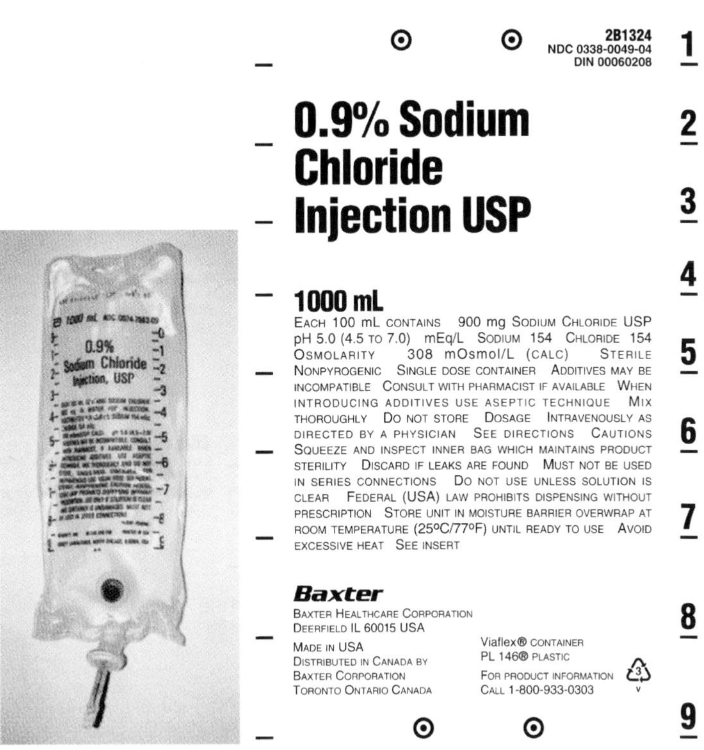

LOT
EXP
2B1324
NDC 0338-0049-04
DIN 00060208
0.9% Sodium Chloride Injection USP
1000 mL
EACH 100 mL CONTAINS 900 mg SODIUM CHLORIDE USP pH 5.0 (4.5 TO 7.0) mEq/L SODIUM 154 CHLORIDE 154 OSMOLARITY 308 mOsmol/L (CALC) STERILE NONPYROGENIC SINGLE DOSE CONTAINER ADDITIVES MAY BE INCOMPATIBLE CONSULT WITH PHARMACIST IF AVAILABLE WHEN INTRODUCING ADDITIVES USE ASEPTIC TECHNIQUE MIX THOROUGHLY DO NOT STORE DOSAGE INTRAVENOUSLY AS DIRECTED BY A PHYSICIAN SEE DIRECTIONS CAUTIONS SQUEEZE AND INSPECT INNER BAG WHICH MAINTAINS PRODUCT STERILITY DISCARD IF LEAKS ARE FOUND MUST NOT BE USED IN SERIES CONNECTIONS DO NOT USE UNLESS SOLUTION IS CLEAR FEDERAL (USA) LAW PROHIBITS DISPENSING WITHOUT PRESCRIPTION STORE UNIT IN MOISTURE BARRIER OVERWRAP AT ROOM TEMPERATURE (25°C/77°F) UNTIL READY TO USE AVOID EXCESSIVE HEAT SEE INSERT
Baxter
BAXTER HEALTHCARE CORPORATION
DEERFIELD IL 60015 USA
MADE IN USA
DISTRIBUTED IN CANADA BY
BAXTER CORPORATION
TORONTO ONTARIO CANADA
Viaflex® CONTAINER
PL 146® PLASTIC
FOR PRODUCT INFORMATION
CALL 1-800-933-0303
1
2
3
4
5
6
7
8
9

FIGURE 7.1 Normal saline 0.9%.

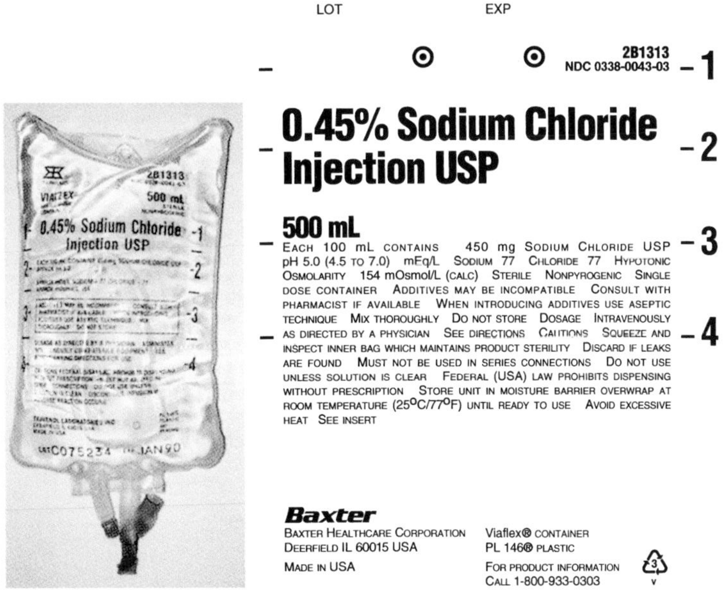

LOT
EXP
2B1313
NDC 0338-0043-03
0.45% Sodium Chloride Injection USP
500 mL
EACH 100 mL CONTAINS 450 mg SODIUM CHLORIDE USP pH 5.0 (4.5 TO 7.0) mEq/L SODIUM 77 CHLORIDE 77 HYPOTONIC OSMOLARITY 154 mOsmol/L (CALC) STERILE NONPYROGENIC SINGLE DOSE CONTAINER ADDITIVES MAY BE INCOMPATIBLE CONSULT WITH PHARMACIST IF AVAILABLE WHEN INTRODUCING ADDITIVES USE ASEPTIC TECHNIQUE MIX THOROUGHLY DO NOT STORE DOSAGE INTRAVENOUSLY AS DIRECTED BY A PHYSICIAN SEE DIRECTIONS CAUTIONS SQUEEZE AND INSPECT INNER BAG WHICH MAINTAINS PRODUCT STERILITY DISCARD IF LEAKS ARE FOUND MUST NOT BE USED IN SERIES CONNECTIONS DO NOT USE UNLESS SOLUTION IS CLEAR FEDERAL (USA) LAW PROHIBITS DISPENSING WITHOUT PRESCRIPTION STORE UNIT IN MOISTURE BARRIER OVERWRAP AT ROOM TEMPERATURE (25°C/77°F) UNTIL READY TO USE AVOID EXCESSIVE HEAT SEE INSERT
Baxter
BAXTER HEALTHCARE CORPORATION
DEERFIELD IL 60015 USA
MADE IN USA
Viaflex® CONTAINER
PL 146® PLASTIC
FOR PRODUCT INFORMATION
CALL 1-800-933-0303
1
2
3
4

FIGURE 7.2 0.45% normal saline.

LOT EXP

2B0064
NDC 0338-0017-04 1

5% Dextrose Injection USP 2

3

1000 mL

EACH 100 mL CONTAINS 5 g DEXTROSE HYDROUS USP pH 4.0 (3.2 TO 6.5) OSMOLARITY 252 mOsmol/L (CALC) STERILE NONPYROGENIC SINGLE DOSE CONTAINER ADDITIVES MAY BE INCOMPATIBLE CONSULT WITH PHARMACIST IF AVAILABLE WHEN INTRODUCING ADDITIVES USE ASEPTIC TECHNIQUE MIX THOROUGHLY DO NOT STORE DOSAGE INTRAVENOUSLY AS DIRECTED BY A PHYSICIAN SEE DIRECTIONS CAUTIONS SQUEEZE AND INSPECT INNER BAG WHICH MAINTAINS PRODUCT STERILITY DISCARD IF LEAKS ARE FOUND MUST NOT BE USED IN SERIES CONNECTIONS DO NOT ADMINISTER SIMULTANEOUSLY WITH BLOOD DO NOT USE UNLESS SOLUTION IS CLEAR FEDERAL (USA) LAW PROHIBITS DISPENSING WITHOUT PRESCRIPTION STORE UNIT IN MOISTURE BARRIER OVERWRAP AT ROOM TEMPERATURE (25°C/77°F) UNTIL READY TO USE AVOID EXCESSIVE HEAT SEE INSERT 4 5 6

7

Baxter

BAXTER HEALTHCARE CORPORATION DEERFIELD IL 60015 USA MADE IN USA

Viaflex® CONTAINER PL 146® PLASTIC FOR PRODUCT INFORMATION CALL 1-800-933-0303 8

9

FIGURE 7.3 5% dextrose in water.

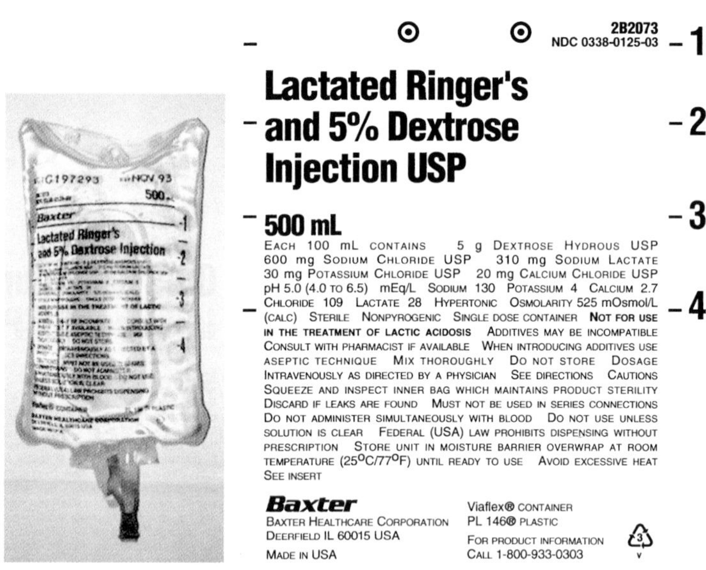
LOT EXP
2B2073
NDC 0338-0125-03 1
Lactated Ringer's and 5% Dextrose Injection USP 2
500 mL 3
EACH 100 mL CONTAINS 5 g DEXTROSE HYDROUS USP 600 mg SODIUM CHLORIDE USP 310 mg SODIUM LACTATE 30 mg POTASSIUM CHLORIDE USP 20 mg CALCIUM CHLORIDE USP pH 5.0 (4.0 TO 6.5) mEq/L SODIUM 130 POTASSIUM 4 CALCIUM 2.7 CHLORIDE 109 LACTATE 28 HYPERTONIC OSMOLARITY 525 mOsmol/L (CALC) STERILE NONPYROGENIC SINGLE DOSE CONTAINER NOT FOR USE IN THE TREATMENT OF LACTIC ACIDOSIS ADDITIVES MAY BE INCOMPATIBLE CONSULT WITH PHARMACIST IF AVAILABLE WHEN INTRODUCING ADDITIVES USE ASEPTIC TECHNIQUE MIX THOROUGHLY DO NOT STORE DOSAGE INTRAVENOUSLY AS DIRECTED BY A PHYSICIAN SEE DIRECTIONS CAUTIONS SQUEEZE AND INSPECT INNER BAG WHICH MAINTAINS PRODUCT STERILITY DISCARD IF LEAKS ARE FOUND MUST NOT BE USED IN SERIES CONNECTIONS DO NOT ADMINISTER SIMULTANEOUSLY WITH BLOOD DO NOT USE UNLESS SOLUTION IS CLEAR FEDERAL (USA) LAW PROHIBITS DISPENSING WITHOUT PRESCRIPTION STORE UNIT IN MOISTURE BARRIER OVERWRAP AT ROOM TEMPERATURE (25°C/77°F) UNTIL READY TO USE AVOID EXCESSIVE HEAT SEE INSERT 4
Baxter
BAXTER HEALTHCARE CORPORATION DEERFIELD IL 60015 USA MADE IN USA
Viaflex® CONTAINER PL 146® PLASTIC FOR PRODUCT INFORMATION CALL 1-800-933-0303

FIGURE 7.4 Ringer's lactate solution and 5% dextrose.

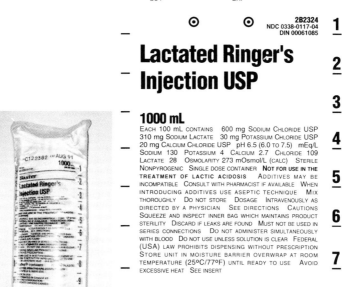

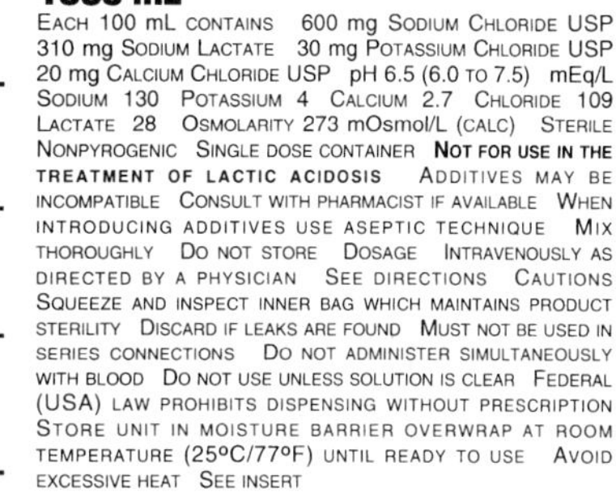

LOT
EXP
2B2324
NDC 0338-0117-04
DIN 00061085
Lactated Ringer's Injection USP
1000 mL
EACH 100 mL CONTAINS 600 mg SODIUM CHLORIDE USP 310 mg SODIUM LACTATE 30 mg POTASSIUM CHLORIDE USP 20 mg CALCIUM CHLORIDE USP pH 6.5 (6.0 TO 7.5) mEq/L SODIUM 130 POTASSIUM 4 CALCIUM 2.7 CHLORIDE 109 LACTATE 28 OSMOLARITY 273 mOsmol/L (CALC) STERILE NONPYROGENIC SINGLE DOSE CONTAINER NOT FOR USE IN THE TREATMENT OF LACTIC ACIDOSIS ADDITIVES MAY BE INCOMPATIBLE CONSULT WITH PHARMACIST IF AVAILABLE WHEN INTRODUCING ADDITIVES USE ASEPTIC TECHNIQUE MIX THOROUGHLY DO NOT STORE DOSAGE INTRAVENOUSLY AS DIRECTED BY A PHYSICIAN SEE DIRECTIONS CAUTIONS SQUEEZE AND INSPECT INNER BAG WHICH MAINTAINS PRODUCT STERILITY DISCARD IF LEAKS ARE FOUND MUST NOT BE USED IN SERIES CONNECTIONS DO NOT ADMINISTER SIMULTANEOUSLY WITH BLOOD DO NOT USE UNLESS SOLUTION IS CLEAR FEDERAL (USA) LAW PROHIBITS DISPENSING WITHOUT PRESCRIPTION STORE UNIT IN MOISTURE BARRIER OVERWRAP AT ROOM TEMPERATURE (25°C/77°F) UNTIL READY TO USE AVOID EXCESSIVE HEAT SEE INSERT
Baxter
BAXTER HEALTHCARE CORPORATION
DEERFIELD IL 60015 USA
MADE IN USA
DISTRIBUTED IN CANADA BY
BAXTER CORPORATION
TORONTO ONTARIO CANADA
Viaflex® CONTAINER
PL 146® PLASTIC
FOR PRODUCT INFORMATION
CALL 1-800-933-0303
1
2
3
4
5
6
7
8
9

FIGURE 7.5 Ringer's lactate solution.

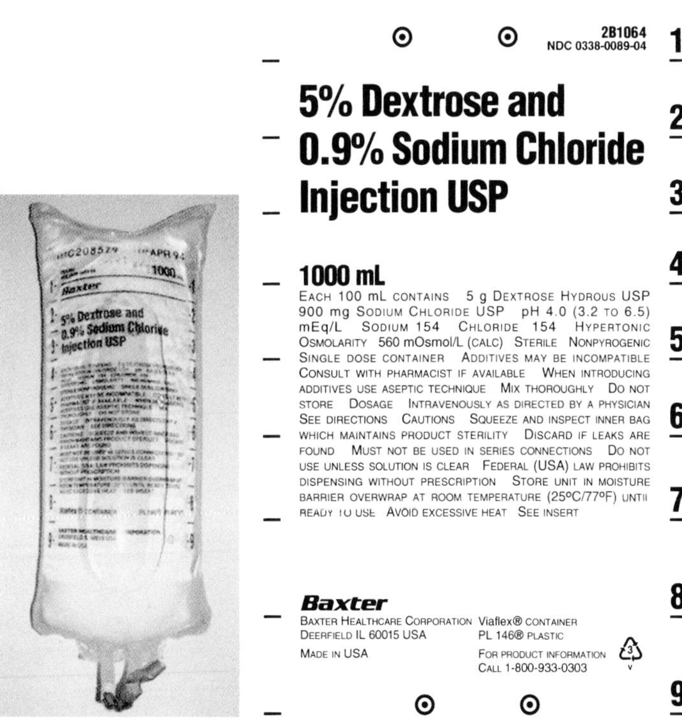

LOT
EXP
2B1064
NDC 0338-0089-04
5% Dextrose and 0.9% Sodium Chloride Injection USP
1000 mL
EACH 100 mL CONTAINS 5 g DEXTROSE HYDROUS USP 900 mg SODIUM CHLORIDE USP pH 4.0 (3.2 TO 6.5) mEq/L SODIUM 154 CHLORIDE 154 HYPERTONIC OSMOLARITY 560 mOsmol/L (CALC) STERILE NONPYROGENIC SINGLE DOSE CONTAINER ADDITIVES MAY BE INCOMPATIBLE CONSULT WITH PHARMACIST IF AVAILABLE WHEN INTRODUCING ADDITIVES USE ASEPTIC TECHNIQUE MIX THOROUGHLY DO NOT STORE DOSAGE INTRAVENOUSLY AS DIRECTED BY A PHYSICIAN SEE DIRECTIONS CAUTIONS SQUEEZE AND INSPECT INNER BAG WHICH MAINTAINS PRODUCT STERILITY DISCARD IF LEAKS ARE FOUND MUST NOT BE USED IN SERIES CONNECTIONS DO NOT USE UNLESS SOLUTION IS CLEAR FEDERAL (USA) LAW PROHIBITS DISPENSING WITHOUT PRESCRIPTION STORE UNIT IN MOISTURE BARRIER OVERWRAP AT ROOM TEMPERATURE (25°C/77°F) UNTIL READY TO USE AVOID EXCESSIVE HEAT SEE INSERT
Baxter
BAXTER HEALTHCARE CORPORATION
DEERFIELD IL 60015 USA
MADE IN USA
Viaflex® CONTAINER
PL 146® PLASTIC
FOR PRODUCT INFORMATION
CALL 1-800-933-0303
1
2
3
4
5
6
7
8
9

FIGURE 7.6 5% dextrose in normal saline 0.9%.

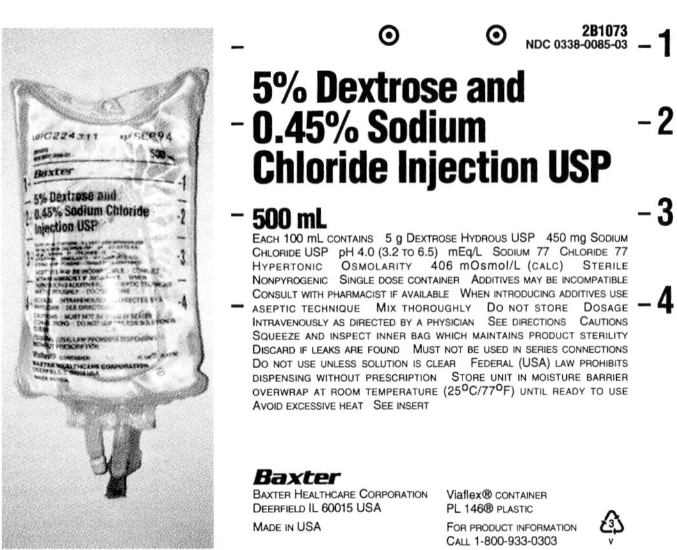

LOT
EXP
2B1073
NDC 0338-0085-03
1
5% Dextrose and
0.45% Sodium
Chloride Injection USP
2
500 mL
3
Each 100 mL contains 5 g Dextrose Hydrous USP 450 mg Sodium Chloride USP pH 4.0 (3.2 to 6.5) mEq/L Sodium 77 Chloride 77 Hypertonic Osmolarity 406 mOsmol/L (calc) Sterile Nonpyrogenic Single dose container Additives may be incompatible Consult with pharmacist if available When introducing additives use aseptic technique Mix thoroughly Do not store Dosage intravenously as directed by a physician See directions Cautions Squeeze and inspect inner bag which maintains product sterility Discard if leaks are found Must not be used in series connections Do not use unless solution is clear Federal (USA) law prohibits dispensing without prescription Store unit in moisture barrier overwrap at room temperature (25°C/77°F) until ready to use Avoid excessive heat See insert
4
Baxter
Baxter Healthcare Corporation
Deerfield IL 60015 USA
Made in USA
Viaflex® container
PL 146® Plastic
For product information
Call 1-800-933-0303

FIGURE 7.7 5% dextrose in ½ (0.45%) NS.

Percentage of Solutes in IV Solutions

The percentage indicated on the IV solution (5%, 0.9%, or 0.45%, for example) represents the amount of dextrose, sodium chloride, or other constituents in the infusion. The type of IV solution ordered is determined by the diagnosis. Patients with diabetes mellitus, kidney disease, hematologic disorders, or cardiac problems will need different types of solutions. The nurse must be aware of the diagnosis as it relates to the type of IV solution used. To determine the number of milliliters of dextrose or sodium chloride the percentage (%) represents, use the following formula. The dissolved substance or solute (dextrose, sodium chloride) is represented by a weight measurement (g). However, 1 mL of water weighs 1 g. Therefore the solute is weighed in grams per 100 mL of solution. The percentage = g solute per 100 mL solution.

remember **Percentage is based on 100.**

Example How many g of dextrose are in 1000 mL of D5W?

KNOW WANT TO KNOW

$$5 \text{ g (solute)} : 100 \text{ mL} = x \text{ g (solute)} : 1000 \text{ mL}$$

$$1x = 5 \times 1000 = 5000$$

$$1x = 5000$$

$$x = 50 \text{ g (solute)}$$

or mL of dextrose in 1000 mL

OR

FRACTION CROSS PRODUCT

$$\frac{5 \text{ g}}{100 \text{ mL}} = \frac{x \text{ g}}{1000}$$

$$x = 5 \times 10 = 50 \text{ g}$$

Therefore
50 g dextrose are in
1000 mL of D5W

LOT EXP

2B0064
NDC 0338-0017-04

5% Dextrose Injection USP

1000 mL

EACH 100 mL CONTAINS 5 g DEXTROSE HYDROUS USP pH 4.0 (3.2 TO 6.5) OSMOLARITY 252 mOsmol/L (CALC) STERILE NONPYROGENIC SINGLE DOSE CONTAINER ADDITIVES MAY BE INCOMPATIBLE CONSULT WITH PHARMACIST IF AVAILABLE WHEN INTRODUCING ADDITIVES USE ASEPTIC TECHNIQUE MIX THOROUGHLY DO NOT STORE DOSAGE INTRAVENOUSLY AS DIRECTED BY A PHYSICIAN SEE DIRECTIONS CAUTIONS SQUEEZE AND INSPECT INNER BAG WHICH MAINTAINS PRODUCT STERILITY DISCARD IF LEAKS ARE FOUND MUST NOT BE USED IN SERIES CONNECTIONS DO NOT ADMINISTER SIMULTANEOUSLY WITH BLOOD DO NOT USE UNLESS SOLUTION IS CLEAR FEDERAL (USA) LAW PROHIBITS DISPENSING WITHOUT PRESCRIPTION STORE UNIT IN MOISTURE BARRIER OVERWRAP AT ROOM TEMPERATURE (25°C/77°F) UNTIL READY TO USE AVOID EXCESSIVE HEAT SEE INSERT

Baxter

BAXTER HEALTHCARE CORPORATION
DEERFIELD IL 60015 USA
MADE IN USA

Viaflex® CONTAINER
PL 146® PLASTIC
FOR PRODUCT INFORMATION
CALL 1-800-933-0303

Osmolarity

Osmolarity is a measurement in osmols of *total* penetrating and non-penetrating solute concentration related to the *volume* of a solution. There are two abbreviations for milliosmoles per liter: mOsmol/L and the shorter abbreviation mOsm/L. IV labels contain the longer abbreviation—mOsmol/L.

Tonicity is a measurement of *estimated* osmolarity of *non*-penetrating solutes in extracellular solution. The shorter abbreviation, mOsm/L, is often used to measure tonicity and is seen on the headings of the tonicity chart, Page 237, Table 7.2. Both abbreviations are correct.

Table 7.2 Tonicity of Solutes

Hypotonic (less than 250 mOsm/L)	**Isotonic (250-375 mOsm/L)**	**Hypertonic (greater than 375 mOsm/L)**
Fluid shift out of intravascular compartment, hydrating cells	Osmolarity equal to that of serum	Fluid is drawn into the intravascular compartment from the cells
Examples: 0.45% normal saline (154 mOsm/L) 2.5% dextrose in water	Examples: 0.9% normal saline (308 mOsm/L) 5% dextrose in water (252 mOsm/L) lactated Ringer's solution (273 mOsm/L)	Examples: 5% dextrose and 0.9% NaCl (560 mOsm/L) 5% dextrose and lactated Ringer's solution (525 mOsm/L) 10% dextrose in water

Answers on page 265

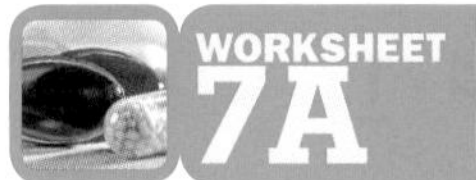

WORKSHEET 7A IV Solute Calculations

Calculate the grams of NaCl or dextrose in the following IV solutions and state the osmolarity and tonicity: hypotonic, hypertonic, or isotonic solution.

1.

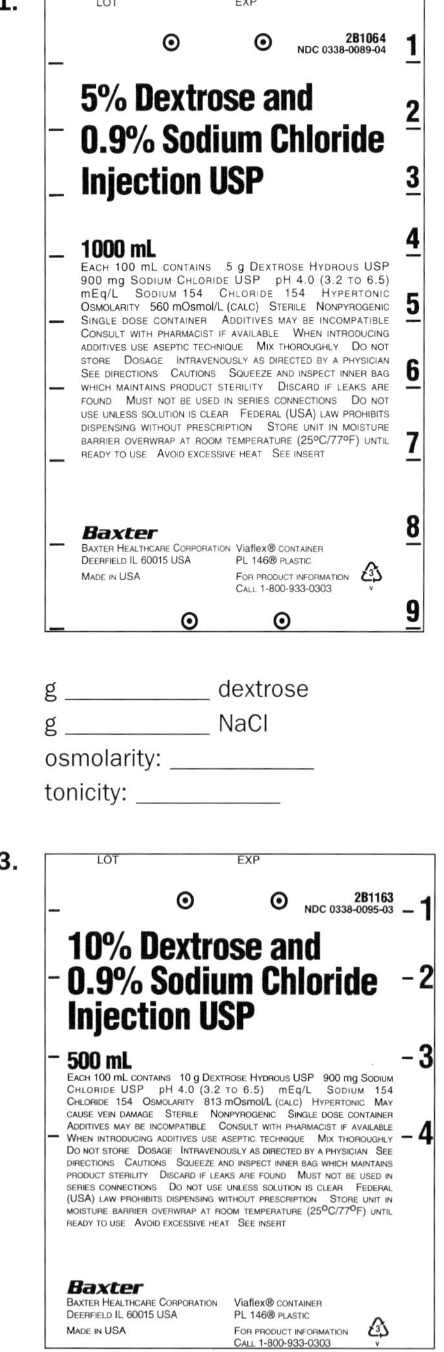
LOT
EXP
2B1064
NDC 0338-0089-04
1
5% Dextrose and
0.9% Sodium Chloride
Injection USP
2
3
1000 mL
4
Each 100 mL contains 5 g Dextrose Hydrous USP 900 mg Sodium Chloride USP pH 4.0 (3.2 to 6.5) mEq/L Sodium 154 Chloride 154 Hypertonic Osmolarity 560 mOsmol/L (calc) Sterile Nonpyrogenic Single dose container Additives may be incompatible Consult with pharmacist if available When introducing additives use aseptic technique Mix thoroughly Do not store Dosage Intravenously as directed by a physician See directions Cautions Squeeze and inspect inner bag which maintains product sterility Discard if leaks are found Must not be used in series connections Do not use unless solution is clear Federal (USA) law prohibits dispensing without prescription Store unit in moisture barrier overwrap at room temperature (25°C/77°F) until ready to use Avoid excessive heat See insert
5
6
7
8
Baxter
Baxter Healthcare Corporation
Deerfield IL 60015 USA
Made in USA
Viaflex® container
PL 146® Plastic
For product information
Call 1-800-933-0303
9
10% Dextrose and
0.9% Sodium Chloride
Injection USP
2B1163
NDC 0338-0095-03
500 mL
Each 100 mL contains 10 g Dextrose Hydrous USP 900 mg Sodium Chloride USP pH 4.0 (3.2 to 6.5) mEq/L Sodium 154 Chloride 154 Osmolarity 813 mOsmol/L (calc) Hypertonic May cause vein damage Sterile Nonpyrogenic Single dose container Additives may be incompatible Consult with pharmacist if available When introducing additives use aseptic technique Mix thoroughly Do not store Dosage Intravenously as directed by a physician See directions Cautions Squeeze and inspect inner bag which maintains product sterility Discard if leaks are found Must not be used in series connections Do not use unless solution is clear Federal (USA) law prohibits dispensing without prescription Store unit in moisture barrier overwrap at room temperature (25°C/77°F) until ready to use Avoid excessive heat See insert
Baxter
Baxter Healthcare Corporation
Deerfield IL 60015 USA
Made in USA
Viaflex® container
PL 146® Plastic
For product information
Call 1-800-933-0303

g ____________ dextrose
g ____________ NaCl
osmolarity: ____________
tonicity: ____________

2.

LOT EXP

2B1073
NDC 0338-0085-03

5% Dextrose and 0.45% Sodium Chloride Injection USP

500 mL

Each 100 mL contains 5 g Dextrose Hydrous USP 450 mg Sodium Chloride USP pH 4.0 (3.2 to 6.5) mEq/L Sodium 77 Chloride 77 Hypertonic Osmolarity 406 mOsmol/L (calc) Sterile Nonpyrogenic Single dose container Additives may be incompatible Consult with pharmacist if available When introducing additives use aseptic technique Mix thoroughly Do not store Dosage Intravenously as directed by a physician See directions Cautions Squeeze and inspect inner bag which maintains product sterility Discard if leaks are found Must not be used in series connections Do not use unless solution is clear Federal (USA) law prohibits dispensing without prescription Store unit in moisture barrier overwrap at room temperature (25°C/77°F) until ready to use Avoid excessive heat See insert

Baxter
Baxter Healthcare Corporation
Deerfield IL 60015 USA
Made in USA
Viaflex® container
PL 146® Plastic
For product information
Call 1-800-933-0303

g ____________ dextrose
g ____________ NaCl
osmolarity: ____________
tonicity: ____________

3.

g ____________ dextrose
g ____________ NaCl
osmolarity: ____________
tonicity: ____________

Calculate the g of NaCl in the following intravenous fluids. State the osmolarity.

4. Normal saline 0.9%

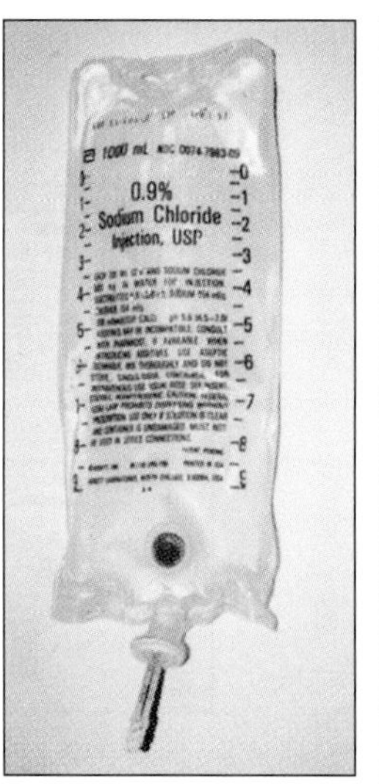

LOT EXP

2B1324
NDC 0338-0049-04
DIN 00060208

0.9% Sodium Chloride Injection USP

1000 mL

EACH 100 mL CONTAINS 900 mg SODIUM CHLORIDE USP pH 5.0 (4.5 TO 7.0) mEq/L SODIUM 154 CHLORIDE 154 OSMOLARITY 308 mOsmol/L (CALC) STERILE NONPYROGENIC SINGLE DOSE CONTAINER ADDITIVES MAY BE INCOMPATIBLE CONSULT WITH PHARMACIST IF AVAILABLE WHEN INTRODUCING ADDITIVES USE ASEPTIC TECHNIQUE MIX THOROUGHLY DO NOT STORE DOSAGE INTRAVENOUSLY AS DIRECTED BY A PHYSICIAN SEE DIRECTIONS CAUTIONS SQUEEZE AND INSPECT INNER BAG WHICH MAINTAINS PRODUCT STERILITY DISCARD IF LEAKS ARE FOUND MUST NOT BE USED IN SERIES CONNECTIONS DO NOT USE UNLESS SOLUTION IS CLEAR FEDERAL (USA) LAW PROHIBITS DISPENSING WITHOUT PRESCRIPTION STORE UNIT IN MOISTURE BARRIER OVERWRAP AT ROOM TEMPERATURE (25°C/77°F) UNTIL READY TO USE AVOID EXCESSIVE HEAT SEE INSERT

Baxter
BAXTER HEALTHCARE CORPORATION
DEERFIELD IL 60015 USA
MADE IN USA
DISTRIBUTED IN CANADA BY
BAXTER CORPORATION
TORONTO ONTARIO CANADA

Viaflex® CONTAINER
PL 146® PLASTIC
FOR PRODUCT INFORMATION
CALL 1-800-933-0303

1 2 3 4 5 6 7 8 9

g ____________ NaCl
osmolarity: ____________
tonicity: ____________

5. Normal saline 0.45%

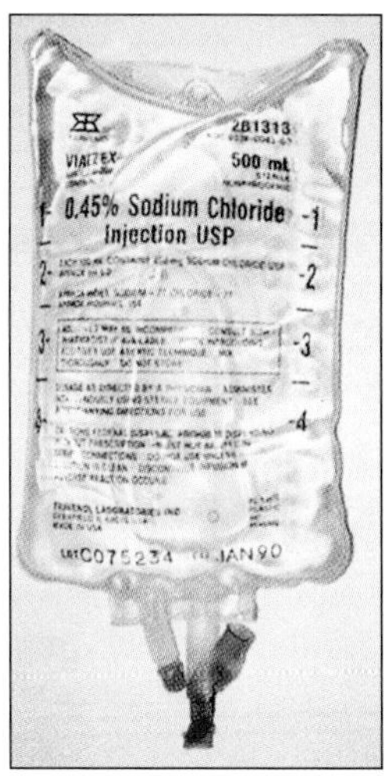

VIAFLEX
2B1313
500 mL
0.45% Sodium Chloride
Injection USP

LOT EXP

2B1313
NDC 0338-0043-03

0.45% Sodium Chloride Injection USP

500 mL

EACH 100 mL CONTAINS 450 mg SODIUM CHLORIDE USP pH 5.0 (4.5 TO 7.0) mEq/L SODIUM 77 CHLORIDE 77 HYPOTONIC OSMOLARITY 154 mOsmol/L (CALC) STERILE NONPYROGENIC SINGLE DOSE CONTAINER ADDITIVES MAY BE INCOMPATIBLE CONSULT WITH PHARMACIST IF AVAILABLE WHEN INTRODUCING ADDITIVES USE ASEPTIC TECHNIQUE MIX THOROUGHLY DO NOT STORE DOSAGE INTRAVENOUSLY AS DIRECTED BY A PHYSICIAN SEE DIRECTIONS CAUTIONS SQUEEZE AND INSPECT INNER BAG WHICH MAINTAINS PRODUCT STERILITY DISCARD IF LEAKS ARE FOUND MUST NOT BE USED IN SERIES CONNECTIONS DO NOT USE UNLESS SOLUTION IS CLEAR FEDERAL (USA) LAW PROHIBITS DISPENSING WITHOUT PRESCRIPTION STORE UNIT IN MOISTURE BARRIER OVERWRAP AT ROOM TEMPERATURE (25°C/77°F) UNTIL READY TO USE AVOID EXCESSIVE HEAT SEE INSERT

Baxter
BAXTER HEALTHCARE CORPORATION
DEERFIELD IL 60015 USA
MADE IN USA

Viaflex® CONTAINER
PL 146® PLASTIC
FOR PRODUCT INFORMATION
CALL 1-800-933-0303

1 2 3 4

g ____________ NaCl
osmolarity: ____________
tonicity: ____________

Calculate the g of dextrose and osmolarity in the following intravenous fluids.

6. Ringer's lactate solution and 5% dextrose

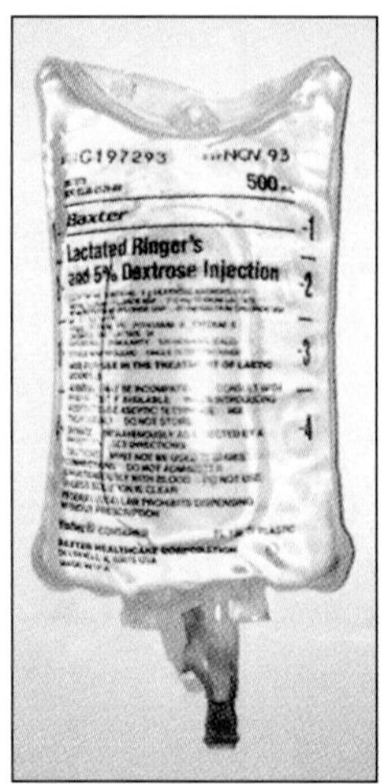

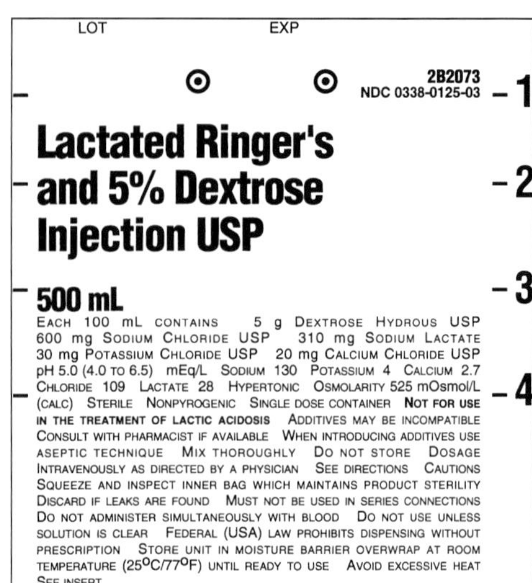

LOT
EXP
2B2073
NDC 0338-0125-03
1
Lactated Ringer's and 5% Dextrose Injection USP
2
3
500 mL
EACH 100 mL CONTAINS 5 g DEXTROSE HYDROUS USP 600 mg SODIUM CHLORIDE USP 310 mg SODIUM LACTATE 30 mg POTASSIUM CHLORIDE USP 20 mg CALCIUM CHLORIDE USP pH 5.0 (4.0 TO 6.5) mEq/L SODIUM 130 POTASSIUM 4 CALCIUM 2.7 CHLORIDE 109 LACTATE 28 HYPERTONIC OSMOLARITY 525 mOsmol/L (CALC) STERILE NONPYROGENIC SINGLE DOSE CONTAINER NOT FOR USE IN THE TREATMENT OF LACTIC ACIDOSIS ADDITIVES MAY BE INCOMPATIBLE CONSULT WITH PHARMACIST IF AVAILABLE WHEN INTRODUCING ADDITIVES USE ASEPTIC TECHNIQUE MIX THOROUGHLY DO NOT STORE DOSAGE INTRAVENOUSLY AS DIRECTED BY A PHYSICIAN SEE DIRECTIONS CAUTIONS SQUEEZE AND INSPECT INNER BAG WHICH MAINTAINS PRODUCT STERILITY DISCARD IF LEAKS ARE FOUND MUST NOT BE USED IN SERIES CONNECTIONS DO NOT ADMINISTER SIMULTANEOUSLY WITH BLOOD DO NOT USE UNLESS SOLUTION IS CLEAR FEDERAL (USA) LAW PROHIBITS DISPENSING WITHOUT PRESCRIPTION STORE UNIT IN MOISTURE BARRIER OVERWRAP AT ROOM TEMPERATURE (25°C/77°F) UNTIL READY TO USE AVOID EXCESSIVE HEAT SEE INSERT
4
Baxter
BAXTER HEALTHCARE CORPORATION
DEERFIELD IL 60015 USA
MADE IN USA
Viaflex® CONTAINER
PL 146® PLASTIC
FOR PRODUCT INFORMATION
CALL 1-800-933-0303

g ____________ dextrose
osmolarity: ____________
tonicity: ____________

Calculate the g of NaCl and the osmolarity in the following intravenous fluid.

7. Ringer's lactate solution

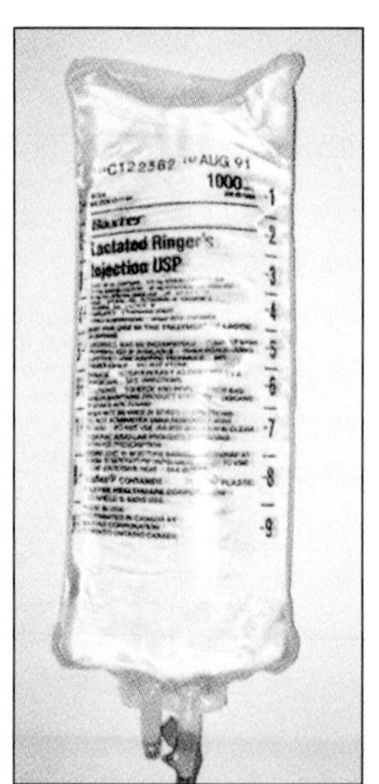

LOT EXP

2B2324
NDC 0338-0117-04
DIN 00061085

1

Lactated Ringer's Injection USP

2

3

1000 mL

EACH 100 mL CONTAINS 600 mg SODIUM CHLORIDE USP 310 mg SODIUM LACTATE 30 mg POTASSIUM CHLORIDE USP 20 mg CALCIUM CHLORIDE USP pH 6.5 (6.0 TO 7.5) mEq/L SODIUM 130 POTASSIUM 4 CALCIUM 2.7 CHLORIDE 109 LACTATE 28 OSMOLARITY 273 mOsmol/L (CALC) STERILE NONPYROGENIC SINGLE DOSE CONTAINER **NOT FOR USE IN THE TREATMENT OF LACTIC ACIDOSIS** ADDITIVES MAY BE INCOMPATIBLE CONSULT WITH PHARMACIST IF AVAILABLE WHEN INTRODUCING ADDITIVES USE ASEPTIC TECHNIQUE MIX THOROUGHLY DO NOT STORE DOSAGE INTRAVENOUSLY AS DIRECTED BY A PHYSICIAN SEE DIRECTIONS CAUTIONS SQUEEZE AND INSPECT INNER BAG WHICH MAINTAINS PRODUCT STERILITY DISCARD IF LEAKS ARE FOUND MUST NOT BE USED IN SERIES CONNECTIONS DO NOT ADMINISTER SIMULTANEOUSLY WITH BLOOD DO NOT USE UNLESS SOLUTION IS CLEAR FEDERAL (USA) LAW PROHIBITS DISPENSING WITHOUT PRESCRIPTION STORE UNIT IN MOISTURE BARRIER OVERWRAP AT ROOM TEMPERATURE (25°C/77°F) UNTIL READY TO USE AVOID EXCESSIVE HEAT SEE INSERT

4 5 6 7 8

Baxter
BAXTER HEALTHCARE CORPORATION
DEERFIELD IL 60015 USA
MADE IN USA
DISTRIBUTED IN CANADA BY
BAXTER CORPORATION
TORONTO ONTARIO CANADA

Viaflex® CONTAINER
PL 146® PLASTIC
FOR PRODUCT INFORMATION
CALL 1-800-933-0303

9

g ____________ sodium chloride
osmolarity: ____________
tonicity: ____________

Calculate the g of NaCl and dextrose and osmolarity in the following intravenous fluids.

8. 5% dextrose in 0.9% sodium chloride

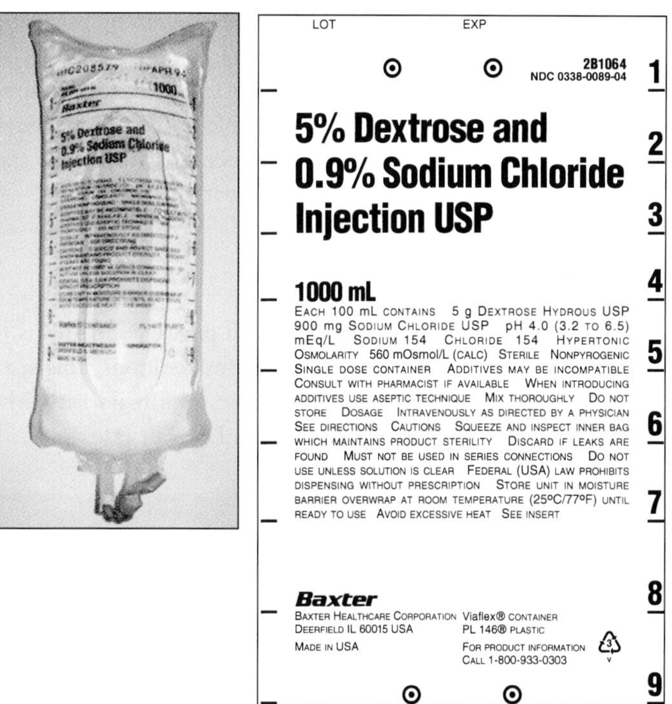
LOT
EXP
2B1064
NDC 0338-0089-04
5% Dextrose and
0.9% Sodium Chloride
Injection USP
1000 mL
EACH 100 mL CONTAINS 5 g DEXTROSE HYDROUS USP 900 mg SODIUM CHLORIDE USP pH 4.0 (3.2 TO 6.5) mEq/L SODIUM 154 CHLORIDE 154 HYPERTONIC OSMOLARITY 560 mOsmol/L (CALC) STERILE NONPYROGENIC SINGLE DOSE CONTAINER ADDITIVES MAY BE INCOMPATIBLE CONSULT WITH PHARMACIST IF AVAILABLE WHEN INTRODUCING ADDITIVES USE ASEPTIC TECHNIQUE MIX THOROUGHLY DO NOT STORE DOSAGE INTRAVENOUSLY AS DIRECTED BY A PHYSICIAN SEE DIRECTIONS CAUTIONS SQUEEZE AND INSPECT INNER BAG WHICH MAINTAINS PRODUCT STERILITY DISCARD IF LEAKS ARE FOUND MUST NOT BE USED IN SERIES CONNECTIONS DO NOT USE UNLESS SOLUTION IS CLEAR FEDERAL (USA) LAW PROHIBITS DISPENSING WITHOUT PRESCRIPTION STORE UNIT IN MOISTURE BARRIER OVERWRAP AT ROOM TEMPERATURE (25°C/77°F) UNTIL READY TO USE AVOID EXCESSIVE HEAT SEE INSERT
Baxter
BAXTER HEALTHCARE CORPORATION
DEERFIELD IL 60015 USA
MADE IN USA
Viaflex® CONTAINER
PL 146® PLASTIC
FOR PRODUCT INFORMATION
CALL 1-800-933-0303
1
2
3
4
5
6
7
8
9

g ____________ dextrose
g ____________ sodium chloride
osmolarity: ____________
tonicity: ____________

9. Calculate the dextrose, NaCl and osmolarity.

5% dextrose in ½ normal saline

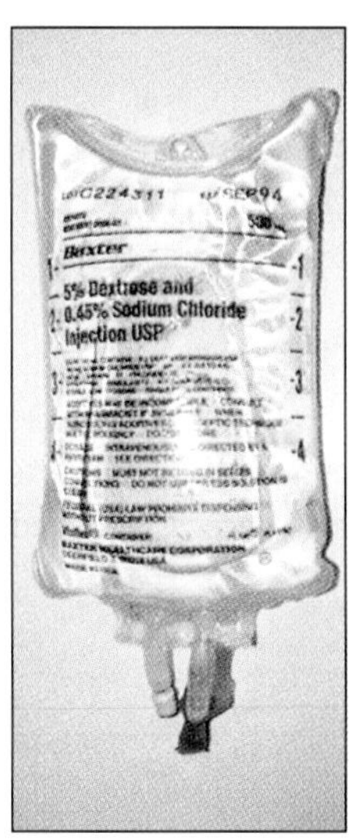

LOT EXP

2B1073
NDC 0338-0085-03

5% Dextrose and 0.45% Sodium Chloride Injection USP

500 mL

EACH 100 mL CONTAINS 5 g DEXTROSE HYDROUS USP 450 mg SODIUM CHLORIDE USP pH 4.0 (3.2 TO 6.5) mEq/L SODIUM 77 CHLORIDE 77 HYPERTONIC OSMOLARITY 406 mOsmol/L (CALC) STERILE NONPYROGENIC SINGLE DOSE CONTAINER ADDITIVES MAY BE INCOMPATIBLE CONSULT WITH PHARMACIST IF AVAILABLE WHEN INTRODUCING ADDITIVES USE ASEPTIC TECHNIQUE MIX THOROUGHLY DO NOT STORE DOSAGE INTRAVENOUSLY AS DIRECTED BY A PHYSICIAN SEE DIRECTIONS CAUTIONS SQUEEZE AND INSPECT INNER BAG WHICH MAINTAINS PRODUCT STERILITY DISCARD IF LEAKS ARE FOUND MUST NOT BE USED IN SERIES CONNECTIONS DO NOT USE UNLESS SOLUTION IS CLEAR FEDERAL (USA) LAW PROHIBITS DISPENSING WITHOUT PRESCRIPTION STORE UNIT IN MOISTURE BARRIER OVERWRAP AT ROOM TEMPERATURE (25°C/77°F) UNTIL READY TO USE AVOID EXCESSIVE HEAT SEE INSERT

Baxter
BAXTER HEALTHCARE CORPORATION
DEERFIELD IL 60015 USA
MADE IN USA

Viaflex® CONTAINER
PL 146® PLASTIC
FOR PRODUCT INFORMATION
CALL 1-800-933-0303

1 2 3 4

g ____________ dextrose
g: ____________ NaCl
osmolarity: ____________
tonicity: ____________

IV Calculations

Check IV orders before beginning calculations. There are two steps in IV calculations. The first step is to find out how many *milliliters per hour* (volume) the IV is ordered to infuse. The second step is to calculate the *drops per minute* needed to infuse the ordered volume.

Analyze your problem. If the order says to infuse the IV for 24 hours, calculate the mL per hr by beginning with Step 1. If the order states to infuse the IV at a specified rate per hour, such as 75 mL per hr, begin with Step 2.

IV Delivery Sets

Figure 7.8, *A* shows a primary set. This is the basic set that delivers IV fluids for a short duration. It does not have a port for additions. This is a needleless connector.

Figure 7.8, *B* shows a primary set with a port for adding piggyback medications. This set has a manual dial for the mL per hr rate.

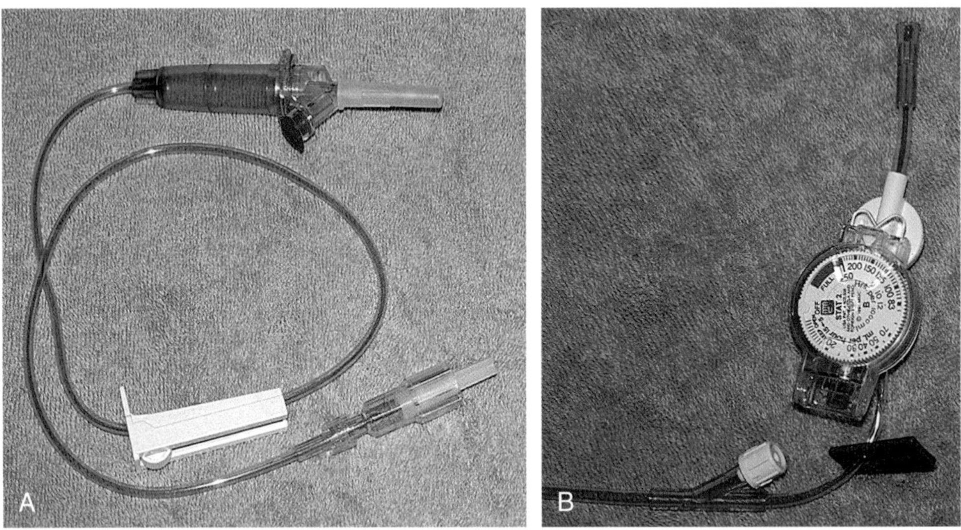

FIGURE 7.8 **A**, Primary set with a roller clamp (no port) to regulate the IV set. **B**, Primary set with a port.

Needleless IV systems are designed to protect caregivers from accidental punctures by contaminated needles. The BD SafetyGlide™ needle (see Figure 5.14, *D*, p. 155) used to inject medication into IV ports is another measure to avoid accidental punctures.

Drops per Minute by Manufacturer

A simple approach to calculate drops per min after you have determined the mL per hr is to memorize the reduced fraction numbers. Manufacturers have established rates for the products (Figure 7.9). Below is an example.

Product Drip Rates	Minutes	DF	=	Reduced Number
60 drops per mL	60	60	=	1
20 drops per mL	60	20	=	3
15 drops per mL	60	15	=	4
10 drops per mL	60	10	=	6

You may have to memorize only one number because most facilities purchase equipment from a single company.

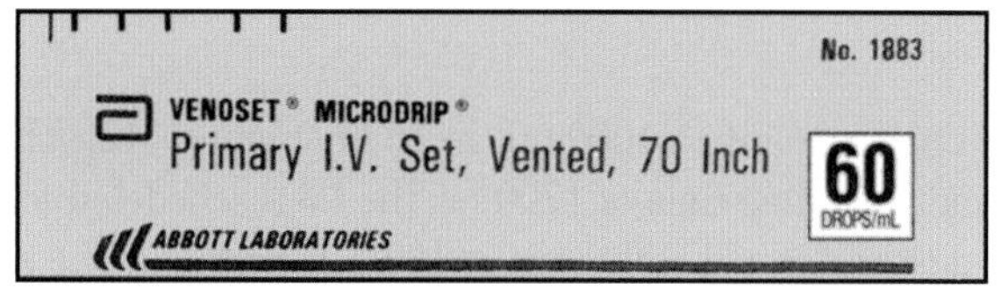

2C5419 s
Baxter-Travenol
Vented Basic Set
10 drops/mL
10

Catalog Number: ***IV3DO6***
Non-Vented Burette Set With Microbore Tubing And Luer-Lock ***Macrodrop Set: Approx. 20 drops/ml***

IVION CORPORATION
A wholly-owned subsidiary of Medex, Inc.

FIGURE 7.9 Various drop rates from different manufacturers.

Example If you know you are using a set that delivers 20 drops per mL, divide 3 into the mL per hr.

$$\frac{125}{3} = 41.6 = 42 \text{ drops per min}$$

As you already know, the formula for calculating drops per min is:

$$\frac{\text{DF}}{\text{Time in min}} \times \text{V per hr} \quad \text{or} \quad \frac{20}{60} \times 125 = \frac{1}{3} \times 125 = 41.6 = 42 \text{ drops per min}$$

Now you know two different methods for calculating drops per min.

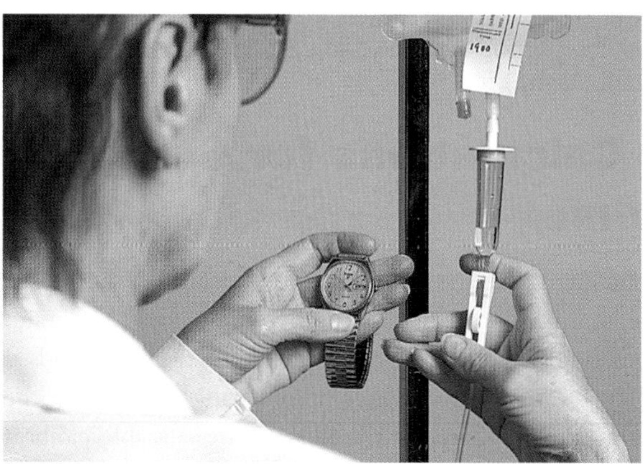

FIGURE 7.10 Count drops per minute by watching the drip chamber for 1 minute and adjusting the roller clamp as needed to deliver the desired number of drops per minute. (From Potter PA, Perry AG, Stockert P, Hall A: *Essentials for nursing practice,* ed. 8, St. Louis, 2014, Mosby.)

CLINICAL ALERT!

Check the IV every hour, even if an infusion device is used. Recheck drops per minute rate frequently because the IV rate can vary with position. Time taping the IV has become important, as electrical blackouts and brownouts can adversely affect the infusion accuracy (Figure 7.11).

Flo Meter Tape

The order is to infuse 1000 mL in 10 hr (Figure 7.12): The infusion label shows a starting time of 0700 hr and an ending time of 1700 hr. The IV is scheduled to infuse for 10 hr. Use the 10-hr rate per hr on the tape and initial each hour at 100 mL per hour. The ending time will be 1700 hr.

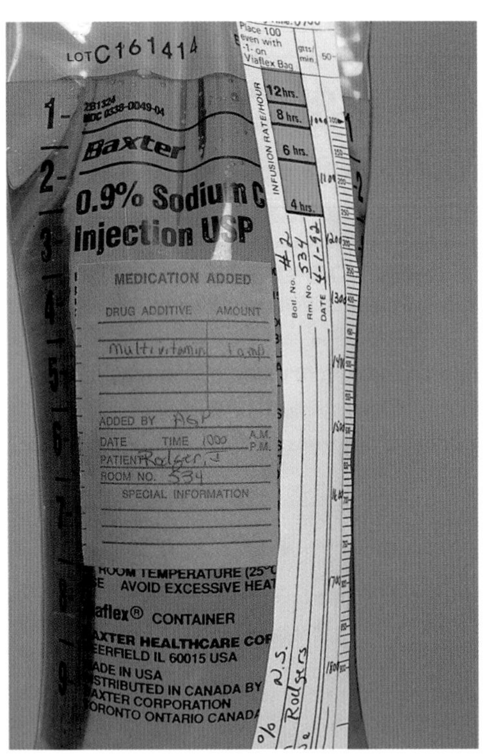

FIGURE 7.11 IV bag with timed tape. (From Potter PA, Perry AG, Stockert P, Hall A: *Essentials for nursing practice,* ed. 8, St. Louis, 2014, Mosby.)

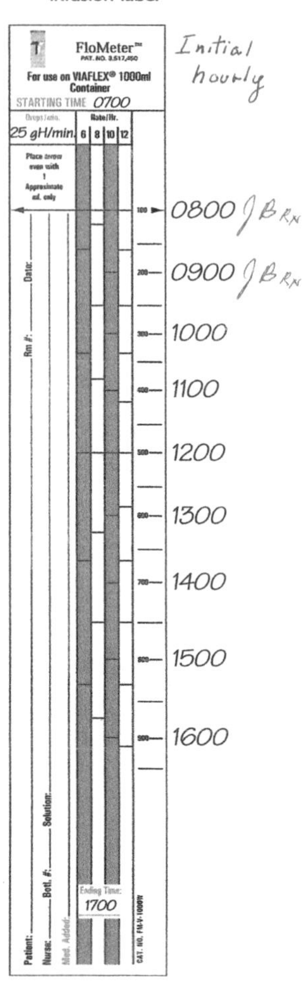

FIGURE 7.12 A FloMeter Tape on a 1000 mL IV bag indicating start time and the hourly rate at 100 mL per hour and initialed hourly.

Drop Factor Calculations for Gravity Infusions and Rounding IV mL

Rounding liquid medication doses depends on the nearest measurable amount on the equipment.

Round intravenous gravity doses to the nearest whole number of drops.

Rounding doses for electronic infusion devices depends upon the EID device. Round EID text problems to the nearest whole number unless directed otherwise.

Round syringe doses to the nearest measureable calibration on the syringe: whole numbers, tenths, hundredths or units.

Step 1 mL/hr

RULE **When the total volume is given, calculate the mL/hr.**

$$\frac{\text{Total volume (TV)}}{\text{Total time (TT) in hours}} = \text{mL per hr}$$

Example Ordered: 2000 mL D5W (dextrose 5% in water) to be infused for 24 hours. The problem is to find out how many mL per hour the patient must receive for the 2000 mL to be infused in 24 hours.

Formula

$$\frac{\text{Total volume (TV)}}{\text{Total time (TT) in hours}} = \text{mL per hr}$$

Calculation

$$\frac{TV}{TT} = \frac{2000}{24} = 83.33 = 83 \text{ mL per hr}$$

We now know that to infuse 2000 mL of fluid in 24 hours, the patient must receive 83 mL per hour. Infusion devices are calibrated for milliliters per hour (mL per hr).

Step 2 Drops per min

The drop factor is needed to calculate drops per minute. The drop factor is the number of drops in 1 mL. The diameter of the needle where the drop enters the drip chamber varies from one manufacturer to another. The bigger the needle, the fatter the drop (Figure 7.13, *A*); it takes only 10 macrodrops to make a milliliter. The smallest unit is the microdrop (60 drops per mL) (Figure 7.13, *B*). This is used

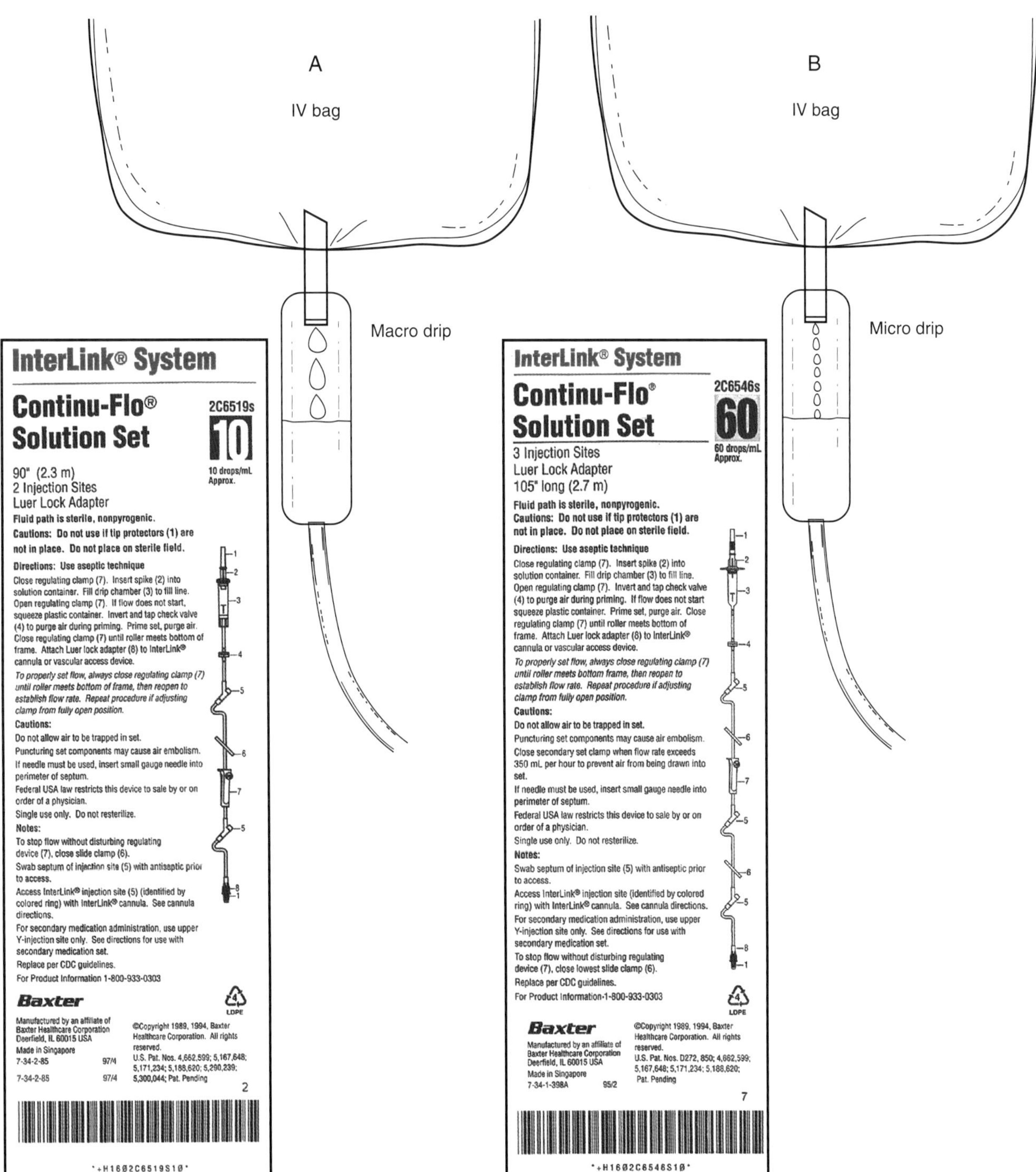

FIGURE 7.13 Drops per minute must be calibrated for gravity flow. **A,** InterLink System Continu-Flo Solution Set with drop factor of 10 (10 drops = 1 mL). **B,** InterLink System Continu-Flo Solution Set with drop factor of 60 (60 drops = 1 mL).

for people who can tolerate only small amounts of fluid, such as pediatric and geriatric patients and patients who require fluid restrictions. Drop factors of 10, 15, 20, and 60 (microdrip) are the most common. The drop factor is determined by the manufacturer and is found on the IV tubing package.

CLINICAL RELEVANCE

Gravity tubing is used by EMTs and in the emergency department, outpatient surgical centers, and long-term care facilities. The nurse will select the calibration of the IV set needed, based on the flow rate ordered. The drops per minute are printed on the IV tubing package (see Figure 7.13). The drops per minute are calculated by the nurse. When using a roller or slide pinch to regulate the IV, the nurse must check the IV rate every hour or more frequently because gravity rates are approximate and positional. The term *positional* means that the flow of the solution may vary depending on the position of the patient's extremity with the IV. For example, flow may be partially or fully obstructed as an extremity bends but becomes unobstructed when it extends, resulting in an inconsistent rate. The Dial-a-Flo tubing is calibrated in mL per hour (Figure 7.14).

RULE **When the mL per hour is given, calculate the drops per minute.**

$$\frac{\text{Drop factor or gtt/mL (from IV package)}}{\text{Time in minutes}} \times \text{Total hourly volume (V/hr)} = \text{drops per min}$$

Example Ordered: D5W to infuse at 83 mL per hour. The drop factor (DF) is 10.

$$\frac{\text{DF}}{\text{Time (min)}} \times \text{V/hr} = \frac{10\ (\text{DF})}{60\ (\text{min})} \times 83\ (\text{V/hr})$$

$$\frac{10}{60} \times \frac{83}{1} = \frac{1}{6} \times \frac{83}{1} = \frac{83}{6} = 13.8 \text{ or } 14 \text{ drops per min}$$

Drops cannot be timed in tenths, only in whole numbers. If the decimal is greater than or equal to 0.5, round to the next higher number.

Example Ordered: Antibiotic to infuse at 100 mL in 30 minutes. The drop factor is 15.

$$\frac{\text{DF}}{\text{Time (min)}} \times \text{V/hr} = \frac{15\ (\text{DF})}{30\ (\text{min})} \times 100\ (\text{V/hr})$$

$$\frac{15}{30} \times \frac{100}{1} = \frac{1}{2} \times \frac{100}{1} = \frac{100}{2} = 50 \text{ drops per min}$$

Summary Two-step IV flow rate calculations.

Step 1 $\frac{\text{TV}}{\text{TT in hr}} = \text{mL per hr}$

Step 2 $\frac{\text{DF}}{\text{Time in min}} \times \text{V per hr} = \text{drops per min}$

The reduced fraction is easier to calculate.

remember **Reduce the fraction DF per min *before* multiplying by the volume.**

Example Which would you rather calculate?

$$\frac{12}{60} \times 60 \text{ or } \frac{1}{5} \times 60$$

The reduced fraction is easier to calculate.

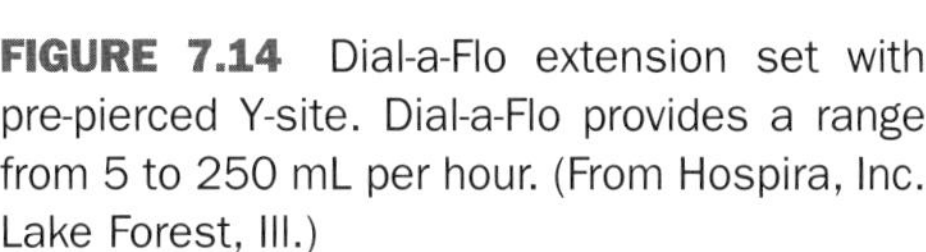

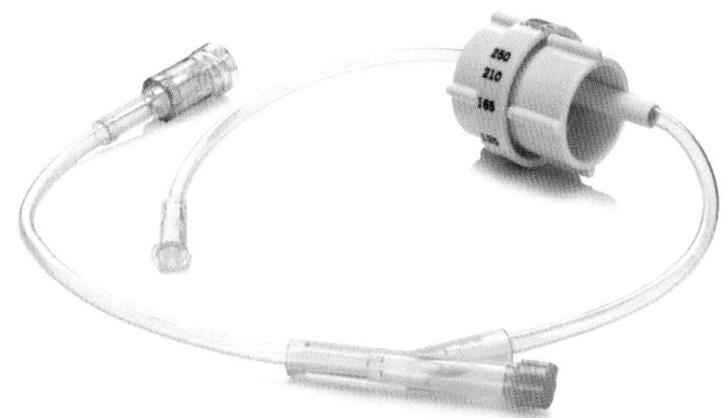

FIGURE 7.14 Dial-a-Flo extension set with pre-pierced Y-site. Dial-a-Flo provides a range from 5 to 250 mL per hour. (From Hospira, Inc. Lake Forest, Ill.)

remember **When the IV tubing is microdrip, 60 drops per mL, the drops per minute will be the same as the mL per hour.**

Example 1000 mL to infuse in 8 hours with a microdrip set.

Step 1 $\frac{\text{TV}}{\text{TT in hr}} = \frac{1000}{8} = 125 \text{ mL per hr}$

Step 2 $\frac{\text{DF}}{\text{Time in min}} \times \text{V per hr} = \frac{60}{60} \times 125 = 125 \text{ drops per min}$

Answers on page 267

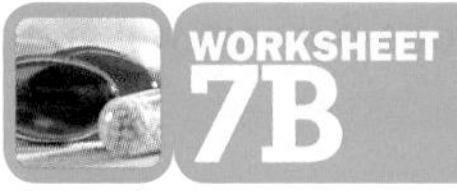

WORKSHEET 7B IV Calculations

Use either the Step 1 or the Step 2 formula to calculate mL per hr or drop per min to answer the following questions. Indicate STEP 2 if you only used it to solve the problem or indicate both STEP 1 and STEP 2 if both were needed.

Step 1 $\frac{\text{TV}}{\text{TT in hr}} = \text{mL per hr}$

Step 2 $\frac{\text{DF}}{\text{Time in min}} \times \text{V per hr} = \text{drops per min}$ or $\frac{\text{mL per hr}}{\text{reduced drop rate}}$

1. Ordered: 1000 mL to be infused for 8 hr. How many drops per min will be administered if the drop factor is 10?

2. Ordered: 50 mL to be infused for 1 hr. How many drops per min will be administered with microdrip?

3. Ordered: 100 mL to be infused for 30 min. How many drops per min is this if the drop factor is 10?

4. Ordered: 1500 mL to be infused for 12 hr. If the drop factor is 15, how many drops per min is this?

5. Ordered: 200 mL to be infused for 1 hr. If the drop factor is 15, how many drops per min will be administered?

6. Ordered: 1000 mL to be infused at 150 mL per hr. The drop factor is 20. How many drops per min will be infused?

7. Ordered: 75 mL to be infused for 45 min. The drop factor is 10. How many drops per min will be administered?

8. Ordered: 150 mL to be infused for 90 min. The drop factor is microdrip. How many drops per min will be administered?

9. Ordered: 150 mL to be infused for 40 min. The drop factor is 15 drops per mL. How many drops per min is this?

10. Ordered: 1500 mL to be infused for 8 hr. How many mL per hr will be administered?
    a. How many drops per min is this with a drop factor of 10?
    b. How many drops per min is this with a drop factor of 15?

Answers on page 268

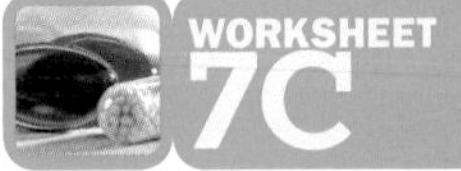

WORKSHEET 7C Additional Practice in IV Calculations

Use either the Step 1 or the Step 2 formula to calculate mL per hr or drops per min to answer the following questions. Indicate STEP 2 if you only used it to solve the problem or indicate both STEP 1 and STEP 2 if both were needed.

1. Ordered: 1000 mL to be infused for 12 hr on microdrip. At how many drops per min will you regulate the infusion?

2. You have 1500 mL normal saline (NS). The drop factor is 15. The solution is to be given for an 8-hr period.
   a. How many mL per hr will be infused?
   b. How many drops per min will be infused?

3. A solution of 3000 mL D5W with 1.5 g carbenicillin is being infused for 24 hr. The drop factor is 15 drops per minute.
   How many drops per min will be infused?

4. You have 500 mL 0.45% NS infusing for 4 hr. The drop factor is 15. How many drops per min will be infused?

5. Ordered: 2000 mL for 24 hr. The drop factor is 15. How many drops per min will be administered?

6. Ordered: 100 mL gentamicin to be infused for 30 min. The drop factor is 20. How many drops per min will be infused?

7. You have 2000 mL D5W being infused for 24 hr. How many mL per hr will be infused?

8. Ordered: 250 mL D5W is to be infused for 10 hr on a microdrip. How many drops per min will be administered?

9. Ordered: 1500 mL of Ringer's lactate solution to be infused for 12 hr.
   a. How many mL per hr will be infused?
   b. The drop factor is 15. How many drops per min will be infused?

10. Write your two-step formula again.
    Step 1 **Step 2**

Answers on page 269

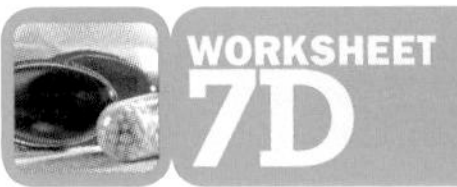

WORKSHEET 7D More Practice in IV Calculations

Use either the Step 1 or the Step 2 formula to calculate mL per hr or drops per min to answer the following questions.

1. Ordered: 500 mL for 8 hr by microdrip. How many drops per min is this?

2. Ordered: 50 mL to be infused for 30 min. At how many drops per min will you set the IV rate if the drop factor is 10?

3. Ordered: 1000 mL to be infused for 6 hr. How many drops per min will be administered if the drop factor is 15?

4. Ordered: 100 mL to be infused for 60 min. At how many drops per min will you set the IV rate if a microdrip is used? Is this the same as mL per hr?

5. Ordered: D5W continuous infusion at 85 mL per hr. The drop factor is 20. At how many drops per min will you set the IV rate?

6. Ordered: 100 mL per hr. At how many drops per min will you set the IV rate if the drop factor is 10?

7. Ordered: 1500 mL 0.45% NS for 24 hr. The drop factor is 10. At how many drops per min will you set the IV rate?

8. Ordered: 100 mL to be infused for 30 min. The drop factor is 15. At how many drops per min will you set the IV rate?

9. Ordered: 1000 mL Ringer's lactate solution at 75 mL per hr. The drop factor is 15. How many drops per min will be administered?

10. Ordered: 2000 mL to be infused for 12 hr. The drop factor is 20.
    a. At how many mL per hr will you set the IV rate?
    b. How many drops per min will this be?

IV Infusions

Intravenous (IV) infusions are used more frequently today than intramuscular (IM) injections. Continuous medication therapy can be delivered via an IV route, minimizing multiple injections via the IM route. Intermittent medication therapy can be delivered through a saline/heparin lock (Figure 7.15), which allows the patient free movement until the next scheduled dose. The saline lock is used for

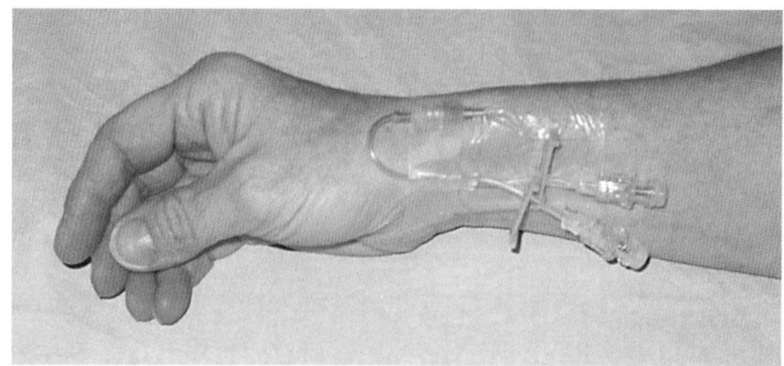

FIGURE 7.15 Intermittent lock covered with a transparent shield. (From Perry AG, Potter PA, Ostendorf WR: *Clinical nursing skills and techniques,* ed. 9, St. Louis, 2018, Mosby.)

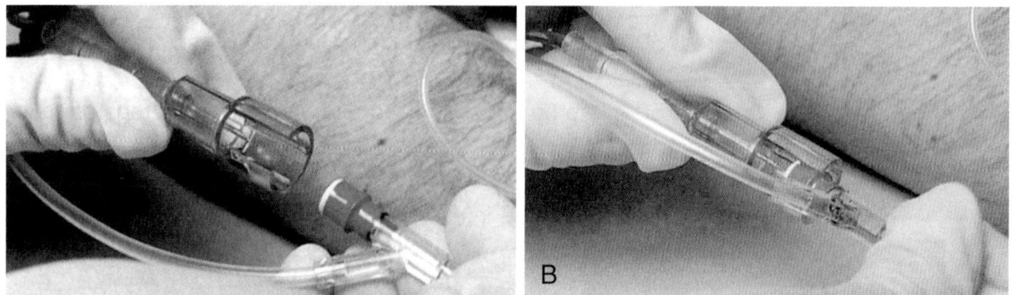

FIGURE 7.16 **A,** Needleless infusion system. **B,** Connection into an injection port. (From Perry AG, Potter PA, Ostendorf WR: *Clinical nursing skills and techniques,* ed. 8, St. Louis, 2014, Mosby.)

intermittent short-duration therapy in acute care, long-term care, and home care. Intermittent therapy can also be delivered as a piggyback with a continuous infusion. A heparin or saline flush can also be used to keep the port patent per manufacturer's guidelines or facility policy.

Medications can be added to the IV by the manufacturer, pharmacist, or nurse. The prescriber orders the medication, strength, and amount, and the manufacturer determines the type and amount of diluent. It is important that the person responsible for the IV understand the actions of the medication, flow rate, adverse reactions, and antidotes. IV fluids flow directly into the vein, resulting in immediate action, and cannot be retrieved. Therefore it is imperative that the nurse follows safe medication administration including correct calculations, medications, and accurate flow rate be administered.

An intermittent IV lock (see Figure 7.15) is known by many different terms. The terms most used are saline lock, hep/heparin lock, PRN cap, intermittent IV (INT), and intermittent peripheral infusion device (IPD). Most have needleless resealable valves (Figure 7.16).

CLINICAL ALERT!

For patient safety, before medication is added to any IV infusion, always verify compatibility with the existing IV solution. When the medication and solution are incompatible, precipitation (cloudiness) may result, which could harm the patient. If precipitation occurs, stop the IV administration immediately.

Gravity Piggyback Infusions

The acronym for intravenous piggyback is IVPB (Figure 7.17). When medications are ordered intermittently, the primary IV can be bypassed by introducing the medication through an entry or portal site. Piggyback (PB) medications are infused intermittently via the existing IV line. A secondary IV tube with a needleless attachment is inserted into the portal or entry site. The PB infusion amount is usually 50 to 250 mL of IV solution. Medication is then added. Calculations of patient's total input need to take the total milliliters into account.

Elevating the IVPB 12 inches above the existing IV allows the PB to infuse by **gravity** (Figure 7.18). When all of the medication has been infused, the existing IV will resume to the rate set for the PB infusion. The nurse must remember to regulate the primary IV to the previous rate. If an infusion device is used, the IV can be programmed to resume to the primary infusion rate at the completion of the PB.

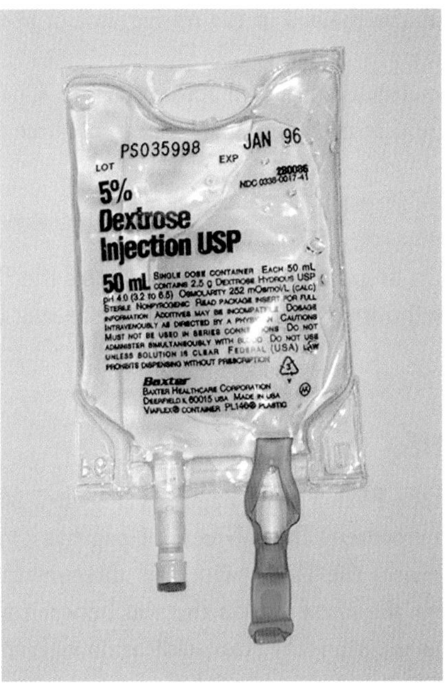

FIGURE 7.17 50 mL of solution for IV piggyback infusion.

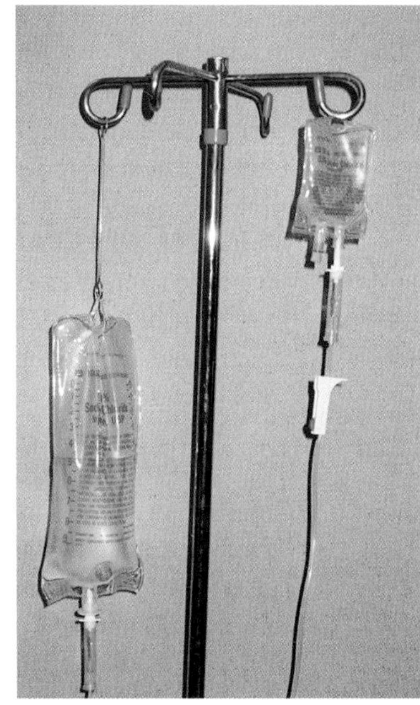

FIGURE 7.18 Gravity-flow IV piggyback. The IV piggyback is elevated above the existing IV, allowing it to infuse by gravity.

Piggyback medications are premixed by the pharmacy, drug manufacturer, or nurse. The manufacturer's insert provides recommended times for IVPBs to infuse if the provider does not state the rate in the order.

remember Gravity-flow sets are delivered in drops per minute.

Piggyback Premixed IVs

Piggyback IV additions are premixed by the pharmacy or the manufacturer. The medication is diluted in 50 to 250 mL of an iso-osmotic sterile solution. The amount of solution used depends on several factors. Factors include the type of medication, the presence of fluid restrictions, and the weight of the patient, as examples.

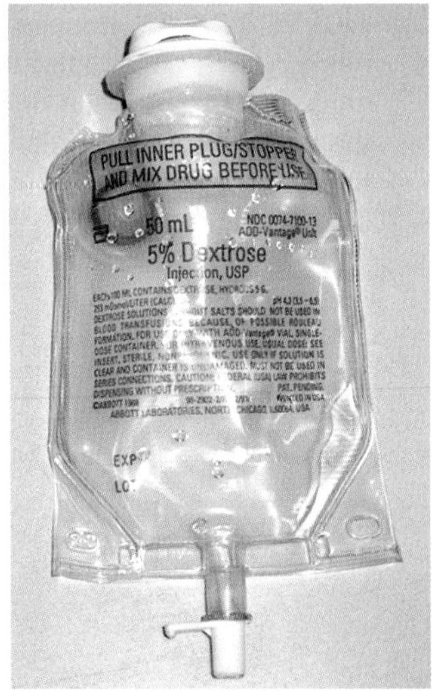

FIGURE 7.19 50 mL of dextrose. Medication can be added for infusion as an IV piggyback.

IVPB admixtures (Figure 7.19) are usually prepared in bulk by the pharmacist for more efficient use of time. If more than one day's supply is prepared, the IVPB can be frozen without altering its stability.

Premixed frozen IVPBs should be thawed in the refrigerator or at room temperature. Never thaw in a microwave oven or in hot or warm water.

All IVPB admixtures must be visually inspected before starting. Check the order, label, medication, strength, and quantity. Make sure that the admixture is clear and free from particles and that the expiration date has not passed.

CLINICAL RELEVANCE

Medication added to an IV bag in an upright position will cause the drug to be concentrated in the lower part of the bag. Disperse the medication by inverting the bag to avoid a concentrated dose, which could harm the patient.

Nurse-Activated Piggyback Systems

The Hospira ADD-Vantage and the Baxter Mini-Bag Plus (Figure 7.20) are used in home care as well as in hospitals and long-term care centers. The IVPB mini-bag has a vial of medication attached to a special port. The pharmacy dispenses the IVPB with the unreconstituted drug vial attached to the mini-bag. At the time of delivery, the nurse breaks the seal between the vial and the mini-bag. This allows the medication to flow into the mini-bag. The medication vial remains attached to the mini-bag, which is a safety feature created to decrease potential medication errors. Figure 7.21 shows the steps for assembling and using the ADD-Vantage system.

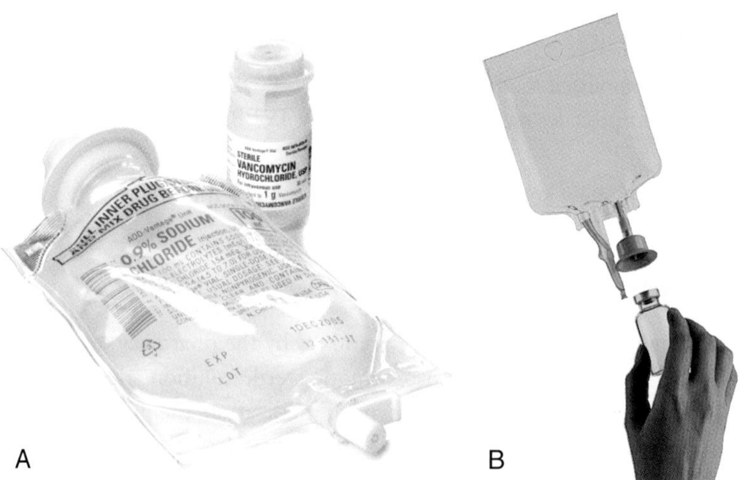

FIGURE 7.20 **A,** Hospira ADD-Vantage with a drug vial of vancomycin. **B,** The Mini-Bag Plus Container has a built-in vial adapter that fits standard powdered drug vials. The system can be assembled without immediately mixing the drug and diluent. The drug admixture is prepared by breaking the seal between the vial and the IV solution container. The vial remains attached to the Mini-Bag™ Plus Container, which reduces the potential for medication errors. (A, From Hospira, Inc., Lake Forest, IL. B, From Baxter Healthcare Corp., Deerfield, Ill.)

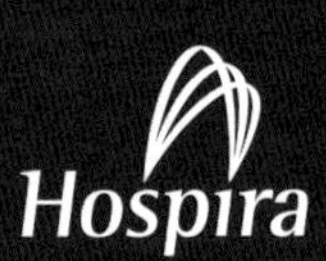
Hospira

ADD-Vantage® System

As Easy as 1, 2, 3

1 Assemble

Use Aseptic Technique

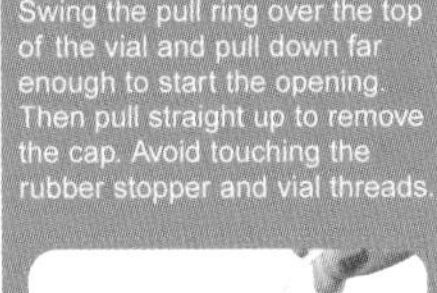
Swing the pull ring over the top of the vial and pull down far enough to start the opening. Then pull straight up to remove the cap. Avoid touching the rubber stopper and vial threads.

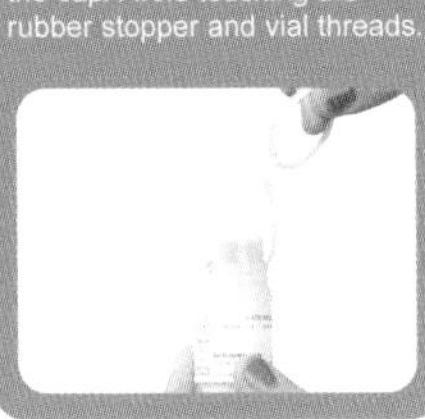

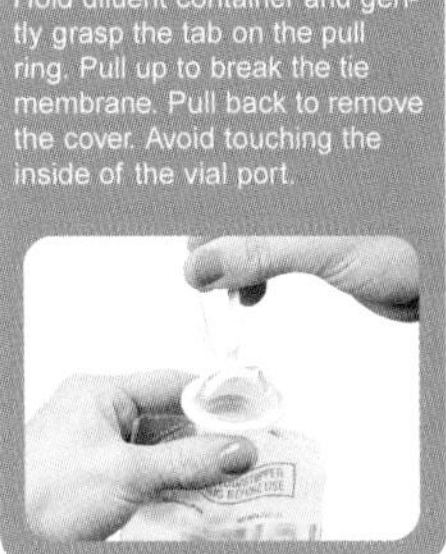
Hold diluent container and gently grasp the tab on the pull ring. Pull up to break the tie membrane. Pull back to remove the cover. Avoid touching the inside of the vial port.

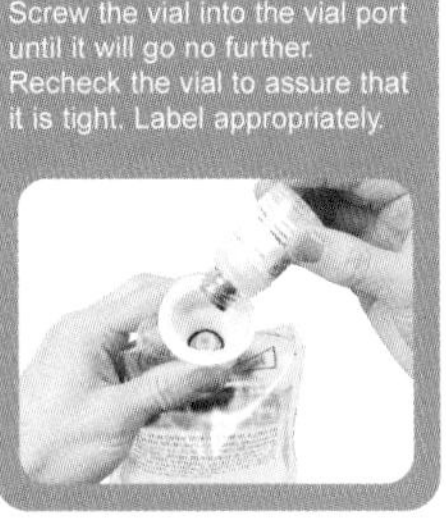
Screw the vial into the vial port until it will go no further. Recheck the vial to assure that it is tight. Label appropriately.

2 Activate

Pull Plug/Stopper to Mix Drug with Diluent

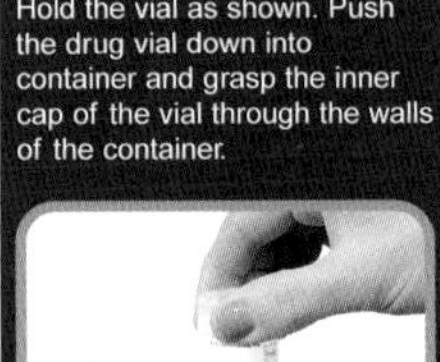
Hold the vial as shown. Push the drug vial down into container and grasp the inner cap of the vial through the walls of the container.

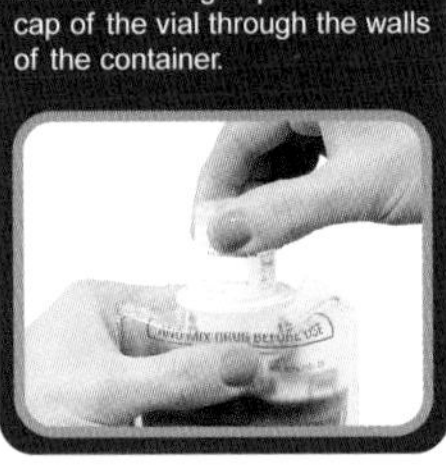

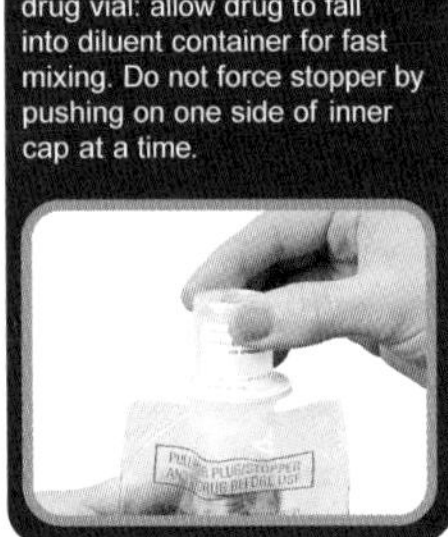
Pull the inner plug from the drug vial: allow drug to fall into diluent container for fast mixing. Do not force stopper by pushing on one side of inner cap at a time.

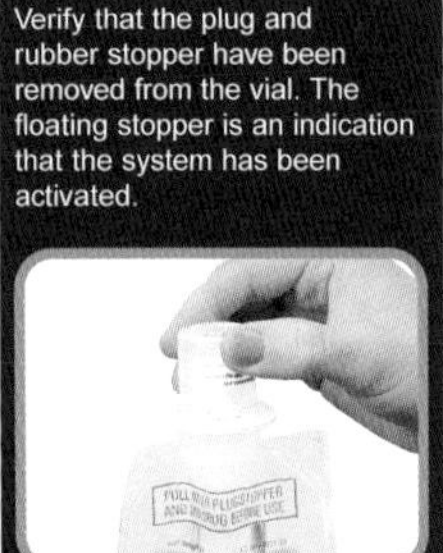
Verify that the plug and rubber stopper have been removed from the vial. The floating stopper is an indication that the system has been activated.

3 Mix and Administer

Within Specified Time

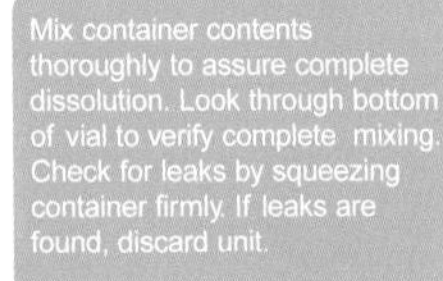
Mix container contents thoroughly to assure complete dissolution. Look through bottom of vial to verify complete mixing. Check for leaks by squeezing container firmly. If leaks are found, discard unit.

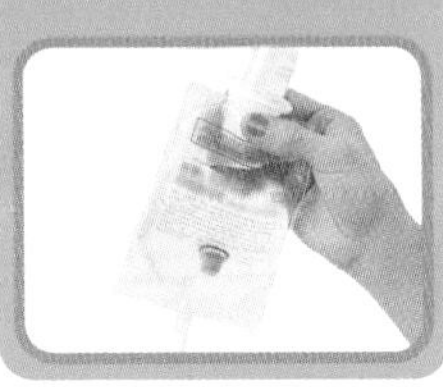

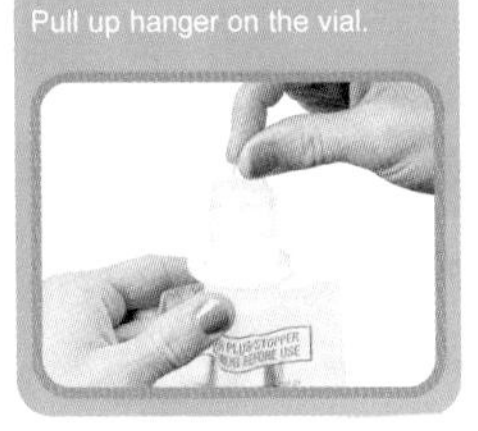
Pull up hanger on the vial.

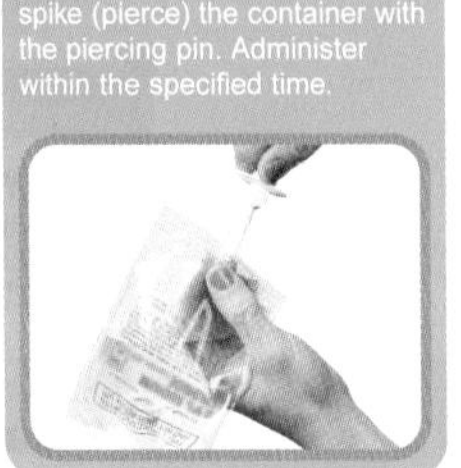
Remove the white administration port cover and spike (pierce) the container with the piercing pin. Administer within the specified time.

For more information on Advancing Wellness with ADD-Vantage® family of devices, contact your Hospira representative at 1-877-9467(1-877-9Hospira) or visit www.Hospira.com

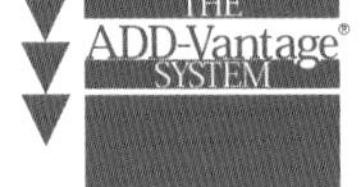
THE
ADD-Vantage®
SYSTEM

FIGURE 7.21 Hospira ADD-Vantage® System. From Hospira, Inc., Lake Forest, IL.

Electronic Infusion Devices (EIDs)

Electronic infusion devices are used in hospitals, extended-care facilities, home care, and ambulatory care settings. They deliver a set amount of intravenous solution per hour. Some examples of electronic infusion devices are shown in Figure 7.22. They are individually programmed to deliver a set amount of IV solution per hour.

CADD-Prizm (see Figure 7.22, *A*) is a battery-operated pump that provides IV medications to confined or ambulatory patients. There are four delivery modes:

- Patient-controlled analgesia (PCA)
- Continuous infusion
- Intermittent infusion
- Total parenteral nutrition

CLINICAL ALERT!

There is a wide variety of infusion devices/pumps. Make sure you understand how to program the pumps to avoid medication errors. Some institutions require another nurse to verify the setting. Adhere to the facility policy for IV device protocol.

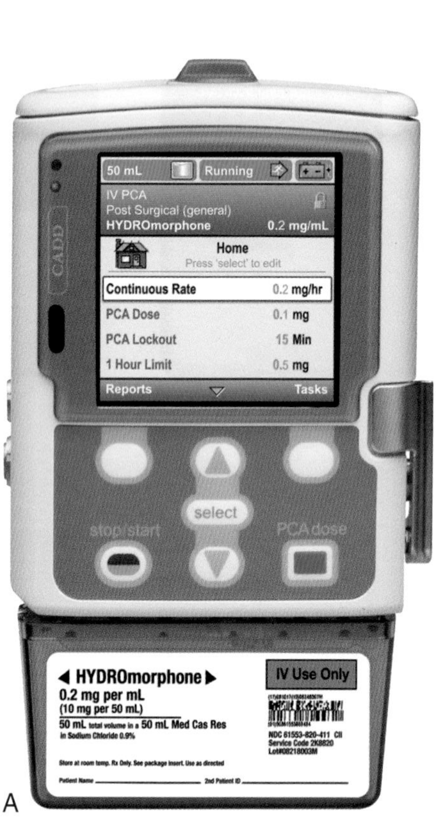

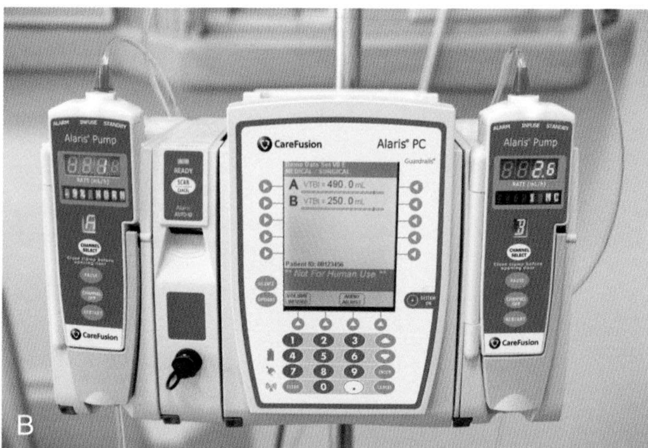

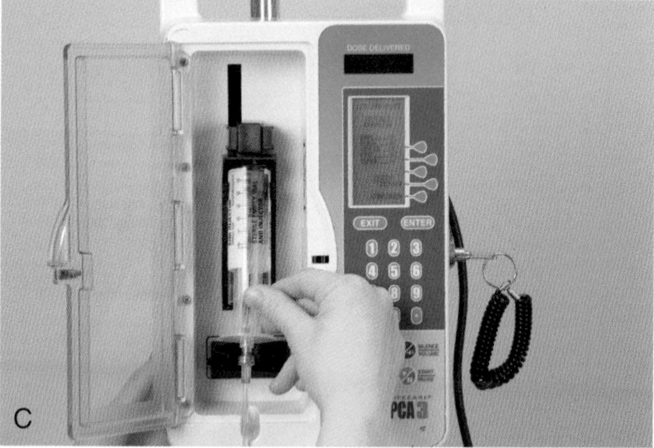

FIGURE 7.22 Electronic infusion devices. **A,** CADD® -Solls pain management pump. **B,** Alaris® PC System. **C,** Patient-controlled analgesia (PCA) ambulatory infusion pump. (**A,** From Smiths Medical ASD, Inc., St. Paul, Minn. **B,** From CareFusion, San Diego, Calif. **C,** From Perry AG, Potter PA, Ostendorf WR: *Clinical nursing skills and techniques,* ed. 9, St. Louis, 2018, Mosby.)

CLINICAL RELEVANCE

It is the nurses' responsibility to check the ordered IV rate for accuracy (mL per hr) and time or completion factor. If the IV is infusing too slowly, the rate can be adjusted, depending on the medication and the patient's condition. Check the facility protocol for discretionary adjustments. If the flow rate is too rapid, return to the ordered rate and notify the prescriber if deemed necessary.

Blood and Blood Components

Blood transfusions are the intravenous administration of blood or blood components. Packed red blood cells (RBCs) (250 to 300 mL) are derived from whole blood with two thirds of the plasma removed. Packed cells increase the oxygen-carrying capacity of the blood.

Whole blood (500 mL) is used to replace volume. It contains O_2-carrying cells as well as RBCs, plasma, proteins, and clotting factors that are needed for hypovolemic shock.

Frozen RBCs can be frozen for 3 years, but this product is infrequently used.

Fresh frozen plasma (FFP) (200 to 300 mL) improves the PT and PTT.

CLINICAL RELEVANCE

- Check the provider's order.
- Ensure that consent is signed.
- Check patient ID.
- Assess and record the patient's vital signs; alterations in baseline vital signs may indicate an adverse or transfusion reaction.
- For adults, ensure IV access with a large-bore catheter (18- to 20-gauge).
- Use a Y-tubing blood administration set with a filter.
- Start the IV with 0.9% normal saline solution and infusion pump.
- Two nurses must verify the numbers on the blood with the laboratory's type and cross-match.
- Blood should be completed within 3 to 4 hours after it is received from the blood bank or a chance of bacterial contamination may occur.

CLINICAL ALERT!

The rate for the first 15 minutes of blood administration should be set at 25 to 50 mL per hour. The nurse stays at the bedside during that time to monitor for an adverse or transfusion reaction (Figure 7.23). If no adverse reactions present, the EID flow rate is usually set at 100 to 120 mL per hour. Providers may order an antihistamine to be given to the patient before blood administration. Before initiating a transfusion, be familiar with the facility protocol for adverse or transfusion reactions as immediate intervention is required. If a reaction occurs, **stop** the transfusion and follow facility protocols.

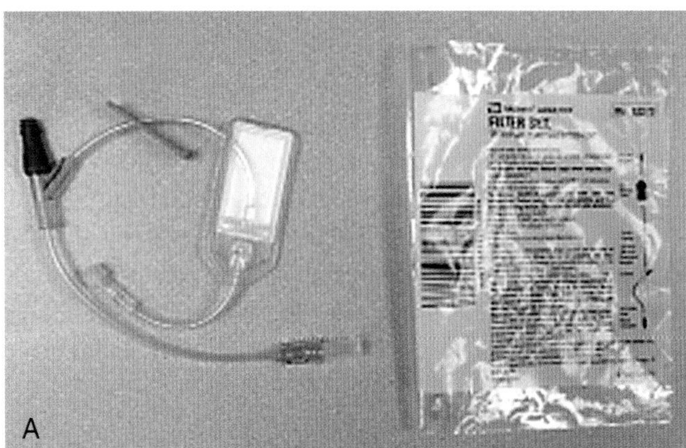

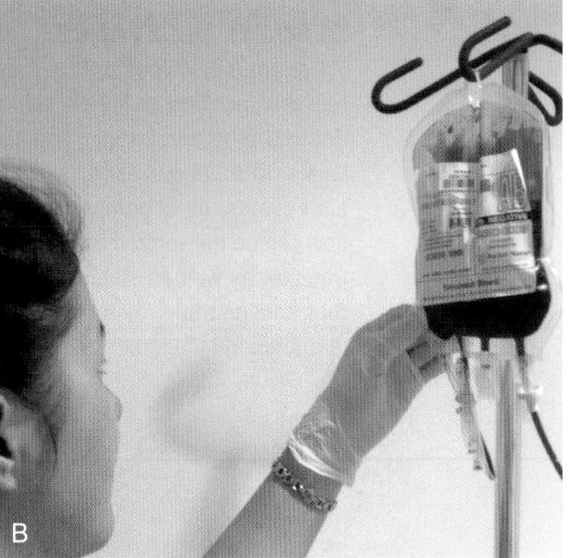

FIGURE 7.23 A, Filter used for blood administration. **B,** Blood administration with Y tubing and normal saline. (From Turner S: Mulholland's *The nurse, the math, the meds: Drug calculations using dimensional analysis,* ed. 4, St. Louis, 2019, Mosby.)

PCA Protocol

The patient-controlled analgesia (PCA) device allows a prespecified amount of narcotic to be available to the patient upon demand. This provides a more constant blood level of analgesia and better pain control (Figure 7.24, *A*). By pushing the button after the lockout phase, the patient can administer the medication to control pain level (Figure 7.24, *B*). An opioid such as morphine is usually the medication of choice. The nurse programs the amount and frequency of the ordered medication as well as the safety lockout time. The usual programmed amount is minimal effective analgesic concentration (MEAC), which can be *1 mg with a 6-minute lockout; 1.5 mg with a 9-minute lockout;* or *2 mg with a 12-minute lockout*. The device also stores information about how frequently the patient pushed the button during the lockout phase. This information allows the nurse to adjust the medication level or lockout time to achieve the MEAC after consulting with the physician. Evaluation of the patient's pain and respiratory status must be monitored every half hour when using opioid analgesia due to possible respiratory suppression.

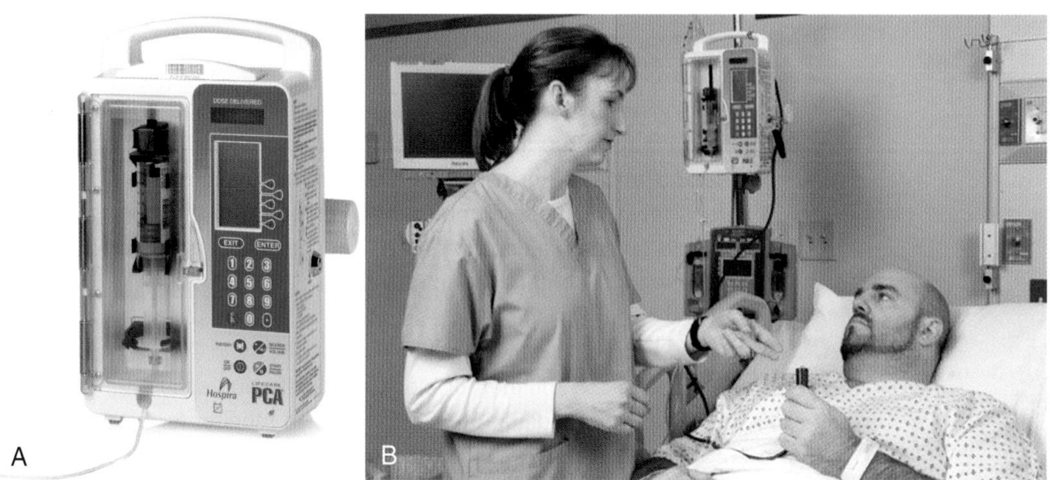

FIGURE 7.24 **A,** Lifecare® Patient-controlled analgesia 3 Infusion System. (From Hospira, Inc., Lake Forest, IL.) **B,** The nurse instructs the patient on the use of a PCA infusion pump for pain control. (**A,** From Hospira, Inc., Lake Forest, Ill. **B,** From Potter PA, Perry AG, Stockert PA: Essentials for nursing practice, ed. 9, St Louis, 2019, Mosby.)

CLINICAL RELEVANCE

There are many types of PCA pumps with different syringe calculations. Errors can result from incorrect programming. It is best to have another nurse check the ordered medication, the ordered dose, and the program setting. The Joint Commission (TJC) and a statement of National Patient Safety Goals (NPSG) have established goals to improve client safety when using PCA devices and IV infusion pumps. All IV pumps must have safety alerts when the IV is not infusing properly. Unregulated flow can be delivered if the pump tubing is improperly attached, disarming the mechanism to prevent free-flow as well as disarming the alarm. The institute for Safe Medication Practices (ISMP) reports that administration sets now have integral antisiphon valves to prevent a free-flow event if a pump is improperly loaded.

Pressure-Flow Infusion Device

The ambulatory infusion device system was developed for ambulatory use. It can be put in a pocket, inside a shirt, or in any other convenient place where it can be concealed. The flow rate is preset. Figure 7.25 shows an example of an ambulatory infusion device.

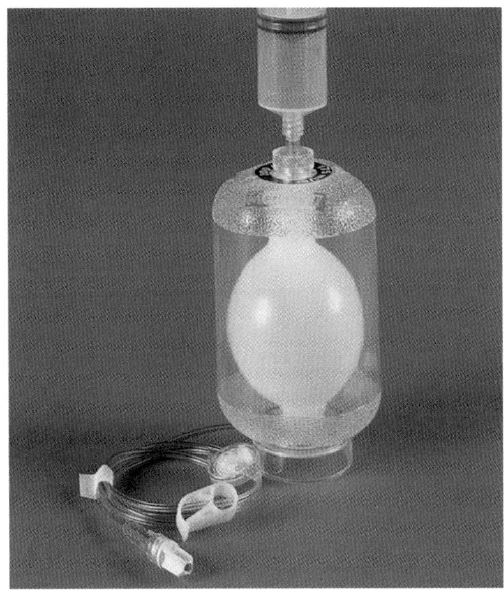

FIGURE 7.25 MedFlo postoperative pain management system, an ambulatory infusion device (Smith & Nephew Endoscopy, Andover, Mass.)

Piggyback Infusions

Examples

- Ordered: Cefazolin 1 g IV in 50 mL for 30 min. At how many mL per hr should the infusion pump be set?

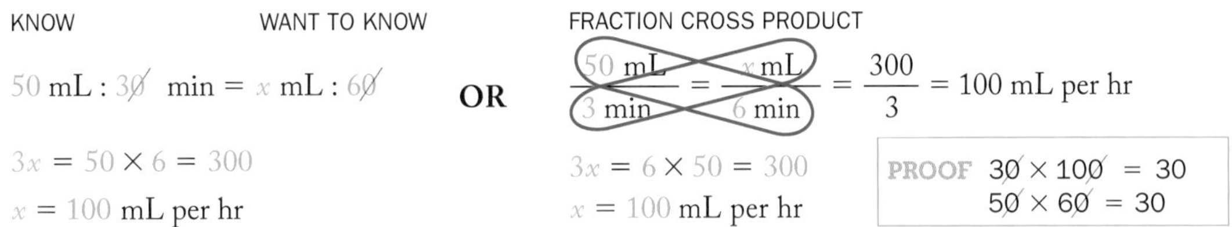

KNOW — WANT TO KNOW

$50 \text{ mL} : 3\cancel{0} \text{ min} = x \text{ mL} : 6\cancel{0}$

$3x = 50 \times 6 = 300$

$x = 100$ mL per hr

OR

FRACTION CROSS PRODUCT

$$\frac{50 \text{ mL}}{3 \text{ min}} = \frac{x \text{ mL}}{6 \text{ min}} = \frac{300}{3} = 100 \text{ mL per hr}$$

$3x = 6 \times 50 = 300$

$x = 100$ mL per hr

PROOF $3\cancel{0} \times 10\cancel{0} = 30$
$5\cancel{0} \times 6\cancel{0} = 30$

Set the infusion pump for 100 mL per hr.

- Ordered: Ampicillin 500 mg IV in 100 mL NS for 45 min. At how many mL per hr should the infusion pump be set?

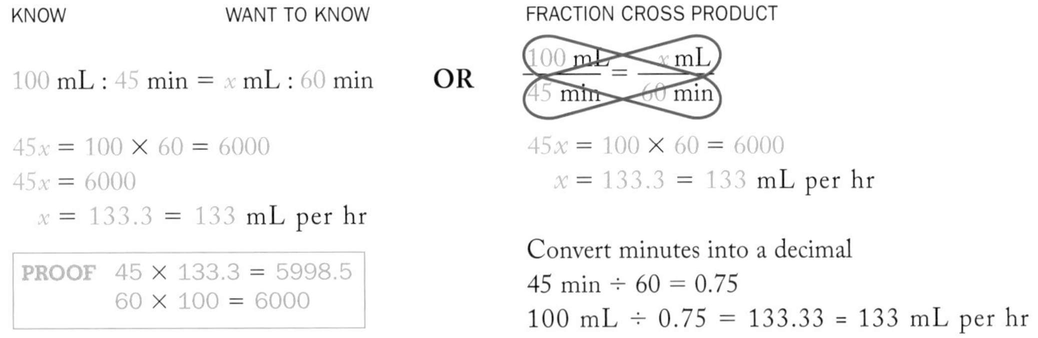

KNOW — WANT TO KNOW

$100 \text{ mL} : 45 \text{ min} = x \text{ mL} : 60 \text{ min}$

$45x = 100 \times 60 = 6000$

$45x = 6000$

$x = 133.3 = 133$ mL per hr

PROOF $45 \times 133.3 = 5998.5$
$60 \times 100 = 6000$

OR

FRACTION CROSS PRODUCT

$$\frac{100 \text{ mL}}{45 \text{ min}} = \frac{x \text{ mL}}{60 \text{ min}}$$

$45x = 100 \times 60 = 6000$

$x = 133.3 = 133$ mL per hr

Convert minutes into a decimal

$45 \text{ min} \div 60 = 0.75$

$100 \text{ mL} \div 0.75 = 133.33 = 133$ mL per hr

Set the infusion pump at 133 mL per hr.

CLINICAL ALERT!

Potassium chloride (KCL) as an additive to an IV can be dangerous. The IV solution must be clamped when the KCl is added. The IV bag must then be inverted or gently shaken for thorough mixing to avoid a bolus dose of potassium that could be lethal to the patient. Never administer KCL as a bolus.

CLINICAL ALERT!

When using an EID that infuses mL per hour, the device must be set at mL per hour when infusing an IVPB medication in less than 1 hour. Be aware that smart pumps can deliver different rates such as mL per hour, mg per kg, mg per kg per min, mg per min, mcg per min, and mcg per hour. It is the nurse's responsibility to be knowledgeable of the different types of EIDs and program the infusion depending on the device.

Answers on page 270

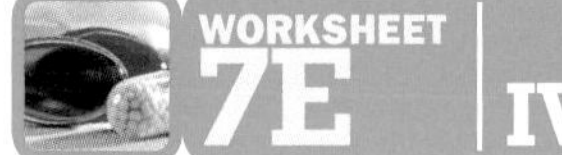

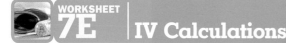

WORKSHEET 7E IV Calculations

Directions: Calculate mL per hr, hours to infuse, and completion time when indicated.

1. The patient is receiving an IV of D5W at 125 mL per hr. How many grams of dextrose per hour is the patient receiving?
2. Ordered: 1500 mL D5W to infuse in 4 hr. How many mL per hr should be delivered?
3. Ordered: Magnesium sulfate 2 g over 4 hr for hypomagnesium blood level.
   Available: 500 mL D5W with 2 g of magnesium sulfate.
   How many mL per hr should be infused?
4. Ordered: 5 g Rocephin IV for bronchitis to infuse in 6 hr.
   Available: 5 g Rocephin in 1000 mL of D5W.
   How many mL per hour should infuse?
5. Ordered: 1000 mL of lactated Ringer's solution to infuse at 125 mL per hour. The IV was started at 0900. When will the infusion be completed?
6. Ordered: 500 mg aminophylline in 250 mL normal saline IVPB for emphysema to infuse at 30 mL per hr. The IV started at 1330 hours. When will the infusion be complete?
7. Ordered: 1000 mL normal saline with 500 mg erythromycin for COPD lung infection to infuse in 8 hr. The infusion was started at 0715 hours. How many mL per hour will be infused? When will the infusion be complete?
8. Ordered: Aminophylline 1 g in 500 mL D5W for asthma to infuse at 40 mL per hr.
   Available: 1 g of aminophylline in 500 mL of D5W. The IV was started at 2100 hours.
   When will the infusion be complete?
9. Ordered: 2 g Keflin in 200 mL normal saline IVPB for infected sinus to infuse in 3 hr. How many mL per hour will the infusion device be set for?
10. Ordered: Rocephin 1 g in 500 mL of normal saline to infuse in 4 hr for endometriosis. At what rate will you set the IV pump?

IV medications must be charted on a flow sheet (Figure 7.26).

IV MEDICATION ADMINISTRATION RECORD

HOSPITAL

NURSING CARE RECORD

Medical/Surgical
Date 1-12-16

DATA FLOW RECORD

TIME	0600	1600																				
PULSE	84	80																				
RESPIRATION	20	22																				
BLOOD PRESSURE	150/92	152/90																				
COUGH/ DEEP BREATH	✓	✓																				
INITIALS	JG	CB																				

The IV flow sheet may record the vital signs prior to initiating IV therapy and again on every shift. The IV site and location is recorded along with the time and date it was started. The catheter type and needle size are recorded next to the type and rate of the IV solution. Additional IV solutions are recorded in the date/time inserted column. When the IV is discontinued, the reason is recorded under the comments column.

IV THERAPY

SITE	DATE/TIME INSERTED	SITE LOCATION	CATH TYPE/ SIZE	IV SOLUTION	RATE	DEVICE	TUBING CHANGE	APPEARANCE 7-3	APPEARANCE 3-11	APPEARANCE 11-7	SITE D/C'd	COMMENTS
R	1-12-16 0600	LPF	22 angio	1000 D5W	75°			1				
R	1-12-16 1900	LPF	22 angio	1000 D5W	75°		△		1			
R	1-12-16 2200	LPF	22 angio						2		✓	Slight redness noted at site pt
												denies pain or tenderness.

HEALTH DEVIATION NEEDS

DCP ASSESSED: In Progress ☐ Revise Plan ☐

DCP Conference ☐ ____________________

REFERRAL MADE: SS ☐ HHC ☐ Dietary ☐ Pharmacy ☐

Other ____________________

IV CODES

Site Location
L = Left
R = Right
S = Scalp
Ft = Foot
F = Femoral
H = Hand
W = Wrist
AC = Antecubital
UA = Upper Arm
UPF = Upper Posterior Forearm
LPF = Lower Posterior Forearm
UAF = Upper Anterior Forearm
LAF = Lower Anterior Forearm
IJ = Internal Jugular
SC = Subclavian

Catheter
S.G. = Swan Ganz
H.D. = Hemodialysis
Hick = Hickman
G = Groshong
Port = Port-A-Cath or other implanted port
I = Introducer
PP = Pace Port

Appearance
1 = Asymptomatic
2 = Red
3 = Swollen
4 = Ecchymotic
5 = Warm
6 = Cool
7 = Draining
8 = Leaking

Lumen
d = distal
m = middle
p = proximal

PATIENT/FAMILY TEACHING:

Pt/Other ____________________

PT/FAMILY TEACHING RESPONSE CODES
1 = Received Literature
2 = Communicates Understanding
3 = Requires Reinforcement
4 = Previous Experience
5 = Return Demonstration
6 = Objective Achieved
7 = Referral Initiated
8 = Refused
9 = Preprinted Teaching Protocol

EMOTIONAL SUPPORT CODES
1 = Active Listening
2 = Reassurance/Comfort
3 = Relaxation
  A = Breathing
  B = Visualization/Imagery
4 = Coping Skills Review

△ = Change

PROCEDURES

TIME	DEPT.	MODE	TRANSPORTER	RETURN

INITIAL	SIGNATURE/TITLE	INITIAL	SIGNATURE/TITLE
JG	J Gahle, RN		

FIGURE 7.26 Example of an IV therapy medication administration record (MAR).

CLINICAL RELEVANCE

When IVPBs are added to an existing IV solution, the nurse must ensure that the additive medication is compatible with both the IVPB solution and the primary IV solution of the existing IV line. When IVPBs are added to an existing IV line, the ports must be cleansed with antiseptic before puncturing.

Answers on page 271

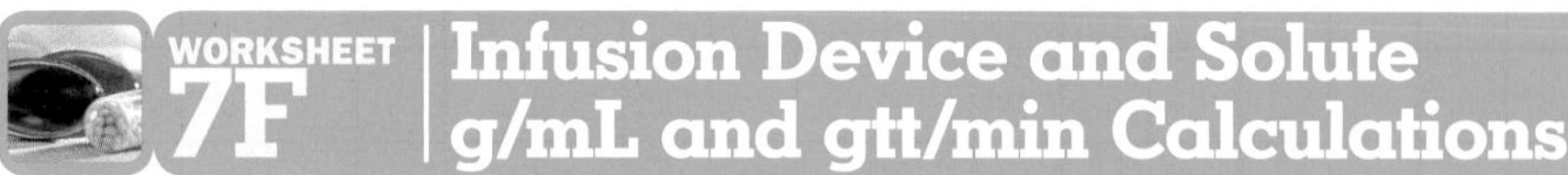

WORKSHEET 7F Infusion Device and Solute g/mL and gtt/min Calculations

Use the Step Two formula to answer the following questions.

1. **Ordered:** 100 mL IVPB to be infused for 1 hr. At how many mL per hr will you set the infusion device?

2. **Ordered:** 250 mL NS to be infused at 150 mL per hr. The drop factor is 15 drops per mL. How long will it take to infuse?

3. **Ordered:** 100 mL to be infused for 30 min by microdrip (microdrip = 60 drops per min).
   - **a.** How many drops per min will be infused on a gravity flow if the drop factor is used?
   - **b.** At how many mL per hr will you set the infusion device?

4. **Ordered:** 50 mL IVPB ADD-Vantage® System to be infused for 20 min.
   - **a.** At how many mL per hr would you set the infusion device?
   - **b.** How many drops per min will be administered on a gravity flow if the drop factor is 15?

5. **Ordered:** 100 mL IVPB to be infused for 1 hr. The drop factor is 15. How many drops per min is this? At how many mL per hr will you set the infusion device?

6. **Ordered:** 50 mL IVPB to be infused for 30 min.
   - **a.** At how many mL per hr will you set an infusion device?
   - **b.** How many drops per min will infuse for a gravity flow if the drop factor is 60?

7. **Ordered:** 200 mL to infuse for 90 min. The drop factor is microdrip.
   - **a.** How many drops per min will infuse?
   - **b.** At how many mL per hr will you set the infusion pump?

8. **Ordered:** 1000 mL 0.9% saline to infuse for 12 hr. The drop factor is 15 drops per mL.
   - **a.** How many drops per min will infuse?
   - **b.** At how many mL per hr will you set the infusion pump?
   - **c.** How many grams of sodium chloride will the patient receive?

9. **Ordered:** 2000 mL D5W to be infused for 8 hr. The drop factor is 15 drops per mL.
   - **a.** How many mL per hr will infuse?
   - **b.** How many drops per min will infuse?
   - **c.** How many grams of dextrose will the patient receive in 8 hours?

10. **Ordered:** 150 mL IVPB. Label reads to infuse for 40 to 60 min. The drop factor is microdrip.
    - **a.** What is the fastest rate for the IVPB to infuse? At what rate will you set the infusion device?
    - **b.** What is the slowest rate for the IVPB to infuse? At what rate will you set the device?

Answers on page 272

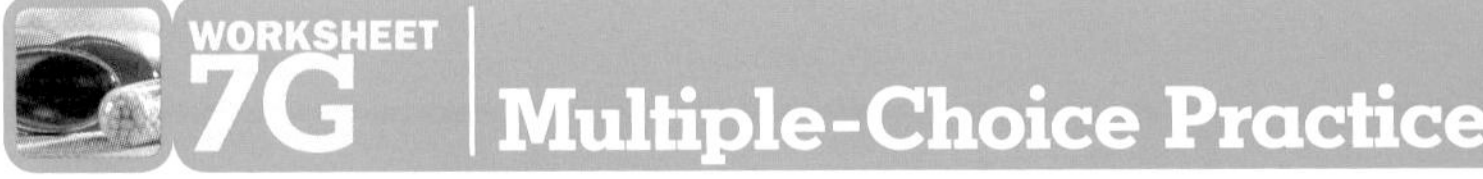

WORKSHEET 7G Multiple-Choice Practice

Circle the letter of the correct answer in the following problems. Remember: To convert tenths of an hour into minutes, multiply by 60. Example: 0.65 hr × 60 = 39 min

1. Calculate the infusion time for an IV of 1000 mL of D5W infusing at 25 drops per min with a drop factor of 10 drops per mL.

a. 6 hr, 40 min **b.** 6 hr, 10 min
c. 5 hr, 57 min **d.** 4 hr, 17 min

2. Administer 50 mL of an IV antibiotic for 15 min. The IV set is calibrated at 15 drops per mL. At how many drops per min will you set the rate?

a. 100 drops per min **b.** 50 drops per min
c. 25 drops per min **d.** 60 drops per min

3. Ordered: 50 mL piggyback to be infused for 30 min. The drop factor is 20. At how many drops per min will you set the rate?

a. 17 drops per min **b.** 100 drops per min
c. 20 drops per min **d.** 33 drops per min

4. Ordered: 300 mL of 0.9% NS for 6 hr. The IV set is microdrip. At how many drops per min will you set the rate?

a. 60 drops per min **b.** 50 drops per min
c. 30 drops per min **d.** 45 drops per min

5. Ordered: Dobutrex 150 mg in 150 mL Ringer's lactate (RL). The infusion device is set at 12 mL per hr. How long will it take to infuse?

a. 6 hr, 15 min **b.** 12 hr, 50 min
c. 8 hr, 15 min **d.** 12 hr, 30 min

6. The IV is infusing at 30 drops per min. The drop factor is 20 drops per mL. The IV bag label reads 500 mL of 0.45% NS. How many hours will it take to infuse?

a. 5 hr, 50 min **b.** 3 hr, 36 min
c. 4 hr, 40 min **d.** 5 hr, 30 min

7. Ordered: 2500 mL to be infused for 24 hr. Available: An IV tubing with 15 drops per mL. At what rate will you set the IV device?

a. 26 drops per min **b.** 35 drops per min
c. 52 drops per min **d.** 104 drops per min

8. A pint of blood (500 mL) is hung at 1100 hours. The flow rate is 42 drops per min. The drop factor on the administration set is 10 drops per mL. When will the infusion be complete?

a. 1733 hours **b.** 1920 hours
c. 1300 hours **d.** 1654 hours

9. Tridil is infusing at 30 mL per hr. The IV label reads: *500 mL D5W with Tridil 5 mcg per 3 mL.* How many hours will it take to infuse?

a. 15 hr, 10 min **b.** 18 hr, 45 min
c. 16 hr, 40 min **d.** 12 hr, 48 min

10. Ordered: Amicar 5 g in 250 mL for 2 hr. At how many mL per hr should the infusion device be set?

a. 150 mL per hr **b.** 100 mL per hr
c. 175 mL per hr **d.** 125 mL per hr

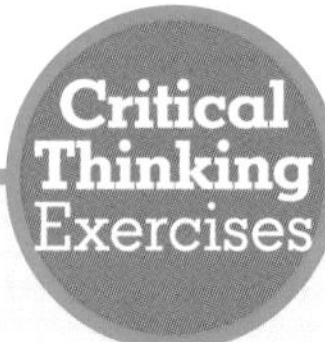

Critical Thinking Exercises provide math and medication-related patient safety issues for student discussion. Answers are not provided.

Analyze the following scenarios.

1. It is the change of shift. The patient with congestive heart failure (CHF) is being infused with an IV of 1000 mL D5W. The patient complains of being very short of breath. After checking the IV rate, you find that it is infusing at 175 mL per hr. Taking into consideration the patient's diagnosis, you check the IV order and it reads 500 mL D5W in 24 hr.

Ordered:

Given:

Error(s):

Potential adverse drug event:

Preventive measures:

Discussion

- What would be your first action?
- What are the serious effects that might jeopordize the patient's safety?
- At what rate should the IV be infusing?
- How can this type of error be reconciled to reduce potential risks?

2. Mr. K. has been transferred from the PACU to the surgical floor at 1400 hr after having a pneumonectomy. An IV with 1 gram of Rocephin in 500 mL of D5W is infusing at 42 mL per hr. The PACU nurse indicated on the chart that she had given Mr. K. 4 mg of morphine IV push about 10 minutes ago. Orders are to continue the Rocephin and start a PCA with 1 mg of morphine with a 6-minute lockout. At 1800 hr you notice that Mr. K. has pushed the lockout button three times, which indicated that the dose of 1 mg every 6 minutes was not adequate. The physician gave a verbal order to increase the dosage to 1.5 mg. You increase the morphine to 1.5 mg. At 2200 hr the evening nurse reports that Mr. K.'s respirations were 10 per min.

Discussion

- What will be your first action?
- What is the potential risk to the patient?
- Was the physician's order incomplete?
- How frequently should a patient on a PCA be checked?
- What is the protocol for a lockout time for 1.5 mg of morphine?
- To promote safety using a PCA, how would you reconcile this error?

3. A 75-year old patient, Mrs. J., has an IV of ampicillin 1 g in 500 mL D5W to be infused in 6 hours. The IV was started at 0730 hr. At 0830 hr when you check the IV, you notice that Mrs. J.'s face is flushed. You ask if she feels OK and she answers yes. You ask Mrs. J. if she has any allergies and she replies that a long time ago when she was little she had a rash when she was given what she thought was penicillin but never thought anything more about it because it was so long ago. You check Mrs. J.'s chart and find that penicillin was listed as an allergy. At 1030 hr Mrs. J. reports feeling frightened and that she was having a hard time breathing and feels as if her throat is closing. At this time, you stop the IV, notify the physican, and give the patient epinephrine, which is the protocol for allergy emergencies. You notice that the IV has 150 mL left to be infused.

Discussion

- Do you think you acted prudently?
- What was the correct rate for the IV? At what rate was it infusing?
- What was the potential risk to the patient?
- How can a situation like this be reconciled for patient safety?

CHAPTER 7

Final

1. **Ordered:** 250 mL to infuse for 90 min. How many mL per hr will infuse if the electronic infusion device is used? How many drops per min will infuse using a drop factor of 15?

2. **Ordered:** 3000 mL D5W to infuse for 24 hr with 0.5 g of penicillin in each 1000 mL. The drop factor is 20, by macrodrop. How many mL per hr will infuse? How many drops per min will be administered?

3. **Ordered:** 1000 mL to be infused for 12 hr IV. At how many mL per hr will you set the infusion device? How many drops per min will be administered via a gravity device if the drop factor is 20?

4. **Ordered:** 1200 mL to be infused for 8 hr. The drop factor is microdrip. How many drops per min will infuse using a gravity device?

5. **Ordered:** Infuse 2000 mL D5W for 24 hr. The drop factor is 10. At how many mL per hr will you set the infusion device? How many drops per min will be administered using a gravity device?

6. **Ordered:** 1500 mL NS to infuse for 12 hr. The drop factor is 15. How many mL per hr will be administered? How many drops per min will infuse?

7. **Ordered:** 75 mL to be infused for 45 min. The drop factor is 10. At how many mL per hr will you set the infusion device? How many drops per min will infuse via a gravity device if the drop factor is 10?

8. **Ordered:** 200 mL cefazolin to infuse for 45 min via the infusion device. At how many mL per hr will you set the infusion device?

9. **Ordered:** 1000 mL to run for 12 hr on microdrip. At how many drops per min will you regulate the flow?

10. **Ordered:** 3000 mL for 24 hr. The drop factor is 15. How many drops per min will infuse via a gravity device?

For additional practice problems, refer to the Intravenous Flow Rates section of the Elsevier's Interactive Drug Calculation Application, Version 1 on Evolve.

Answer Key

7 Basic Intravenous Therapy Calculations

WORKSHEET **7A** (page 238)

1. KNOW WANT TO KNOW

5 g : 100 mL = x g : 1000 mL

x = 5 × 10 = 50

x = 50 g or mL dextrose

PROOF

5 × 1000 = 5000

100 × 50 = 5000

CROSS FRACTION

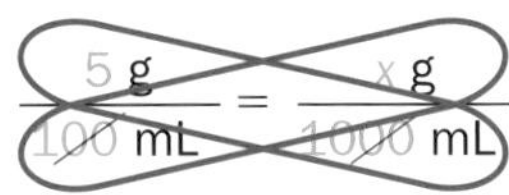

x = 5 × 10 = 50

x = 5 g

KNOW WANT TO KNOW

0.9 g : 100 mL = x g : 1000 mL

x = 0.9 × 10 = 9

x = 9 g of sodium chloride

PROOF

0.9 × 1000 = 900

100 × 9 = 900

Osmolarity: 560 mOsmol/L

Tonicity: Hypertonic

CROSS FRACTION

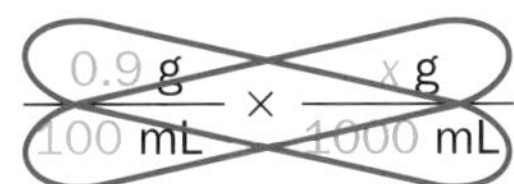

2. KNOW WANT TO KNOW

5 g : 100 mL = x g : 500 mL

x = 5 × 5 = 25

x = 25 g or mL of dextrose

PROOF

5 × 500 = 2500

100 × 25 = 2500

KNOW WANT TO KNOW

0.45 g : 100 mL = x g : 500 mL

x = 0.45 × 5 = 2.25

x = 2.25 g of sodium chloride

PROOF

0.45 × 500 = 225

100 × 2.25 = 225

Osmolarity: 406 mOsmol/L

Tonicity: Hypertonic

3. KNOW WANT TO KNOW

10 g : 100 mL = x g : 500 mL

x = 10 × 5 = 50

x = 50 g or mL of dextrose

PROOF

10 × 500 = 5000

100 × 50 = 5000

KNOW WANT TO KNOW

0.9 g : 100 mL = x g : 500 mL

x = 0.9 × 5

x = 4.5 g or mL of sodium chloride

PROOF

0.9 × 500 = 450

4.5 × 100 = 450

Osmolarity: 813 mOsmol/L

Tonicity: Hypertonic

4. KNOW WANT TO KNOW

$0.9\ \text{g} : 1\cancel{00}\ \text{mL} = x\ \text{g} : 10\cancel{00}\ \text{mL}$

$x = 0.9 \times 10 = 9$

$x = 9$ g or mL of sodium chloride

PROOF

$0.9 \times 1000 = 900$

$9 \times 100 = 900$

Osmolarity: 308 mOsmol/L

Tonicity: Isotonic

5. KNOW WANT TO KNOW

$0.45\ \text{g} : 1\cancel{00}\ \text{mL} = x\ \text{g} : 5\cancel{00}\ \text{mL}$

$x = 0.45 \times 5 = 2.25$

$x = 2.25$ g or mL of sodium chloride

PROOF

$0.45 \times 500 = 225$

$100 \times 2.25 = 225$

Osmolarity: 154 mOsmol/L

Tonicity: Hypotonic

6. KNOW WANT TO KNOW

$5\ \text{g} : 1\cancel{00}\ \text{mL} = x\ \text{g} : 5\cancel{00}\ \text{mL}$

$x = 5 \times 5 = 25$

$x = 25$ g or mL of dextrose

PROOF

$100 \times 25 = 2500$

$5 \times 500 = 2500$

Osmolarity: 525 mOsmol/L

Tonicity: Hypertonic

7. KNOW WANT TO KNOW

$600\ \text{mg} : 1\cancel{00}\ \text{mL} = x\ \text{mg} : 10\cancel{00}\ \text{mL}$

$x = 10 \times 600 = 6000$

$x = 6000$ mg of sodium chloride in 1000 mL

PROOF

$600 \times 1000 = 600{,}000$

$100 \times 6000 = 600{,}000$

KNOW WANT TO KNOW

$1\ \text{g} : 1\ \text{mg} = x\ \text{g} : 6\ \text{mg}$

$x = 6 \times 1 = 6$

$x = 6$ g of sodium chloride in 1000 mL

PROOF

$1 \times 6000 = 6000$

$6 \times 1000 = 6000$

Osmolarity: 273 mOsmol/L

Tonicity: Isotonic

8. KNOW WANT TO KNOW

$5\ \text{g} : 1\cancel{00}\ \text{mL} = x\ \text{g} : 10\cancel{00}\ \text{mL}$

$x = 5 \times 10 = 50$

$x = 50$ g or mL of dextrose

PROOF

$5 \times 1000 = 5000$

$100 \times 50 = 5000$

KNOW WANT TO KNOW

$0.9\ \text{g} : 1\cancel{00}\ \text{mL} = x\ \text{g} : 10\cancel{00}\ \text{mL}$

$x = 0.9 \times 10 = 9$

$x = 9$ g or mL of sodium chloride

PROOF

$100 \times 9 = 900$

$0.9 \times 1000 = 900$

Osmolarity: 560 mOsmol/L

Tonicity: Hypertonic

9. KNOW WANT TO KNOW

$5\ \text{g} : 1\cancel{00}\ \text{mL} = x\ \text{g} : 5\cancel{00}\ \text{mL}$

$x = 5 \times 5 = 25$

$x = 25$ g or mL of dextrose

PROOF

$5 \times 500 = 2500$

$100 \times 25 = 2500$

KNOW WANT TO KNOW

$0.45\ \text{g} : 1\cancel{00}\ \text{mL} = x\ \text{g} : 5\cancel{00}\ \text{mL}$

$x = 0.45 \times 5 = 2.25$

$x = 2.25$ g or mL of sodium chloride

PROOF

$0.45 \times 500 = 225$

$100 \times 2.25 = 225$

Osmolarity: 406 mOsmol/L

Tonicity: Hypertonic

remember

1 $\dfrac{\text{TV}}{\text{TT in hr}} = \text{mL per hr}$

2 $\dfrac{\text{DF}}{\text{Time in min}} \times \text{V per hr} = \text{drops per min}$

1. Step 1: $\dfrac{\text{TV}}{\text{TT}} = \dfrac{1000}{8} = 125$ mL per hr

Step 2: $\dfrac{1\not{0}}{6\not{0}} \times \dfrac{125\text{ mL}}{1} = \dfrac{1}{6} \times \dfrac{125}{1} = \dfrac{125}{6} = 20.8 = 21$ drops per min

2. Step 2: $\dfrac{\overset{1}{\cancel{60}}}{\underset{1}{\cancel{60}}} \times \dfrac{50}{1} = \dfrac{1}{1} \times \dfrac{50}{1} = \dfrac{50}{1} = 50$ drops per min

3. Step 2: $\dfrac{\overset{1}{\cancel{10}}}{\underset{3}{\cancel{30}}} \times \dfrac{100}{1} = \dfrac{1}{3} \times \dfrac{100}{1} = \dfrac{100}{3} = 33.3 = 33$ drops per min

4. Step 1: $\dfrac{1500}{12} = 125$ mL per hr

Step 2: $\dfrac{\overset{1}{\cancel{15}}}{\underset{4}{\cancel{60}}} \times \dfrac{125}{1} = \dfrac{1}{4} \times \dfrac{125}{1} = 31.25 = 31$ drops per min

5. Step 2: $\dfrac{\overset{1}{\cancel{15}}}{\underset{4}{\cancel{60}}} \times \dfrac{200}{1} = \dfrac{1}{4} \times \dfrac{200}{1} = \dfrac{200}{4} = 50$ drops per min

6. Step 2: $\dfrac{\overset{1}{\cancel{20}}}{\underset{3}{\cancel{60}}} \times 150 = \dfrac{1}{3} \times \dfrac{150}{1} = \dfrac{150}{3} = 50$ drops per min

7. Step 2: $\dfrac{10}{45} \times \dfrac{75}{1} = \dfrac{750}{45} = 16.6 = 17$ drops per min

8. Step 2: $\dfrac{\overset{2}{\cancel{60}}}{\underset{3}{\cancel{90}}} \times \dfrac{150}{1} = \dfrac{300}{3} = 100$ drops per min

9. Step 2: $\dfrac{\overset{3}{\cancel{15}}}{\underset{8}{\cancel{40}}} \times 150 = \dfrac{3}{8} \times \dfrac{150}{1} = \dfrac{450}{8} = 56.25 = 56$ drops per min

10. Step 1: $\dfrac{1500}{8} = 187.5 = 188$ mL per hr

Step 2: a. $\dfrac{1\not{0}}{6\not{0}} \times \dfrac{188}{1} = \dfrac{1}{6} \times \dfrac{188}{1} = \dfrac{188}{6} = 31.3 = 31$ drops per min

b. $\dfrac{\overset{1}{\cancel{15}}}{\underset{4}{\cancel{60}}} = \dfrac{1}{4} \times \dfrac{188}{1} = 47$ drops per min

WORKSHEET 7C (page 248)

remember 1 $\frac{\text{TV}}{\text{TT in hr}} = \text{mL per hr}$

2 $\frac{\text{DF}}{\text{Time in min}} \times \text{V per hr} = \text{drops per min}$

1. Step 1: $\frac{\text{TV}}{\text{TT}} = \frac{1000}{12} = 83.3 = 83 \text{ mL per hr}$

Step 2: $\frac{\overset{1}{\cancel{60}}}{\underset{1}{\cancel{60}}} \times \frac{83}{1} = \frac{83}{1} = 83 \text{ drops per min}$

2. Step 1: $\frac{\text{TV}}{\text{TT}} = \frac{1500}{8} = 187.5 = 188 \text{ mL per hr}$

Step 2: $\frac{\overset{1}{\cancel{15}}}{\underset{4}{\cancel{60}}} \times \frac{188}{1} = 47 \text{ drops per min}$

3. Step 1: $\frac{\text{TV}}{\text{TT}} = \frac{3000}{24} = 125 \text{ mL per hr}$

Step 2: $\frac{\overset{1}{\cancel{15}}}{\underset{4}{\cancel{60}}} \times \frac{125}{1} = \frac{125}{4} = 31.2 = 31 \text{ drops per min}$

4. Step 1: $\frac{\text{TV}}{\text{TT}} = \frac{500}{4} = 125 \text{ mL per hr}$

Step 2: $\frac{\overset{1}{\cancel{15}}}{\underset{4}{\cancel{60}}} \times \frac{125}{1} = \frac{125}{4} = 31.2 = 31 \text{ drops per min}$

5. Step 1: $\frac{\text{TV}}{\text{TT}} = \frac{2000}{24} = 83.3 = 83 \text{ mL per hr}$

Step 2: $\frac{\overset{1}{\cancel{15}}}{\underset{4}{\cancel{60}}} \times \frac{83}{1} = \frac{83}{4} = 20.75 = 21 \text{ drops per min}$

6. Start with Step 2 because we already know how many milliliters per 30 minutes.

Step 2: $\frac{\overset{2}{\cancel{20}}}{\underset{3}{\cancel{30}}} \times \frac{100}{1} = \frac{200}{3} = 66.66 = 67 \text{ drops per min}$

7. Step 1: $\frac{\text{TV}}{\text{TT}} = \frac{2000}{24} = 83.3 = 83 \text{ mL per hr}$

8. Step 1: $\frac{\text{TV}}{\text{TT}} = \frac{250}{10} = 25 \text{ mL per hr}$

Step 2: $\frac{\overset{1}{\cancel{60}}}{\underset{1}{\cancel{60}}} \times \frac{25}{1} = 25 \text{ drops per min}$

9. **Step 1:** $\frac{TV}{TT} = \frac{1500}{12} = 125$ mL per hr

Step 2: $\frac{\overset{1}{\cancel{15}}}{\underset{4}{\cancel{60}}} \times \frac{125}{1} = \frac{125}{4} = 31.25 = 31$ drops per min

10. **MEMORIZE** * **Step 1:** $\frac{TV}{TT \text{ in hr}} =$ mL per hr

Step 2: $\frac{DF}{\text{Time in min}} \times$ V per hr = drops per min

WORKSHEET 7D (page 249)

remember 1 $\frac{TV}{TT \text{ in hr}} =$ **mL per hr**

2 $\frac{DF}{\text{Time in min}} \times$ **V per hr = drops per min**

1. **Step 1:** $\frac{TV}{TT} = \frac{500}{8} = 62.5 = 63$ mL per hr

Step 2: $\frac{\overset{1}{\cancel{60}}}{\underset{1}{\cancel{60}}} \times \frac{63}{1} = 63$ drops per min

2. **Step 2:** $\frac{\cancel{10}}{\cancel{30}} \times \frac{50}{1} = \frac{50}{3} = 16.6 = 17$ drops per min

3. **Step 1:** $\frac{TV}{TT} = \frac{1000}{6} = 166.6 = 167$ mL per hr

Step 2: $\frac{\overset{1}{\cancel{15}}}{\underset{4}{\cancel{60}}} \times \frac{167}{1} = \frac{167}{4} = 41.75 = 42$ drops per min

4. **Step 2:** $\frac{\overset{1}{\cancel{60}}}{\underset{1}{\cancel{60}}} \times \frac{100}{1} = 100$ drops per min Yes, the mL per hr is the same as the drops per min rate.

5. **Step 2:** $\frac{\overset{1}{\cancel{20}}}{\underset{3}{\cancel{60}}} \times 85 = \frac{1}{3} \times \frac{85}{1} = \frac{85}{3} = 28.3 = 28$ drops per min

6. **Step 2:** $\frac{\cancel{10}}{\cancel{60}} \times 100 - \frac{100}{6} = 16.6 = 17$ drops per min

7. **Step 1:** $\frac{TV}{TT} = \frac{1500}{24} = 62.5 = 63$ mL per hr

Step 2: $\frac{\overset{1}{\cancel{10}}}{\underset{6}{\cancel{60}}} \times \frac{63}{1} = \frac{63}{6} = 10.5 = 11$ drops per min

8. **Step 2:** $\frac{\overset{1}{\cancel{15}}}{\underset{2}{\cancel{30}}} \times \frac{100}{1} = \frac{1}{2} \times \frac{100}{1} = \frac{100}{2} = 50$ drops per min

9. **Step 2:** $\frac{\overset{1}{\cancel{15}}}{\underset{4}{\cancel{60}}} \times \frac{75}{1} = \frac{75}{4} = 18.7 = 19$ drops per min

10. **Step 1:** $\frac{TV}{TT} = \frac{2000}{12} = 166.6 = 167$ mL per hr

Step 2: $\frac{\overset{1}{\cancel{20}}}{\underset{3}{\cancel{60}}} \times \frac{167}{1} = \frac{167}{3} = 55.6 = 56$ drops per min

WORKSHEET 7E (page 258)

1. KNOW WANT TO KNOW

   5 g : 100 = x g : 125 mL

   $100x = 5 \times 125 = 625$

   $x = 6.25$ g per hr

   PROOF

   $5 \times 125 = 625$

   $100 \times 6.25 = 625$

2. $\frac{\text{Total volume}}{\text{Total time}} = \text{mL per hr}$

   $\frac{1500 \text{ mL}}{4 \text{ hr}} = 375$ mL per hr

3. HAVE WANT TO HAVE

   500 mL : 4 hr = x mL : 1 hr

   $4x = 500 \times 1 = 500$

   $x = 125$ mL per hr

   PROOF

   $500 \times 1 = 500$

   $4 \times 125 = 500$

4. HAVE WANT TO HAVE

   1000 mL : 6 hr – x mL : 1 hr

   $6x = 1000$

   $x = 166.6 = 167$ mL per hr

   PROOF

   $1000 \times 1 = 1000$

   $6 \times 166.6 = 999$

5. KNOW WANT TO KNOW

   125 mL : 1 hr = 1000 mL : x hr

   $125x = 1000$

   $x = 8$ hr

   The IV will be completed by 1700 hours.

   PROOF

   $1 \times 1000 = 1000$

   $125 \times 8 = 1000$

6. HAVE WANT TO HAVE

   30 mL : 1 hr = 250 mL : x hr

   $30x = 250$

   $x = 8.33$ hr

   Convert 0.33×60 min $= 19.8 = 20$ min

   The IV will take 8 hr and 20 min to infuse.

   The IVPB was started at 1330 hr + 8 hr 20 min = 2150 for the hour of completion.

   PROOF

   $1 \times 250 = 250$

   $8.33 \times 30 = 249.9$

7. $\frac{\text{Total volume}}{\text{Total time}} = \text{mL per hr}$

   $\frac{1000 \text{ mL}}{8 \text{ hr}} = 125$ mL per hr

   The IV was started at 0715 + 8 = 1515 for the hour of completion.

8. HAVE WANT TO HAVE

   40 mL : 1 hr = 500 mL : x hr

   $40x = 500$

   $x = 12.5$ hr

   IV started at 2100 hr + 12.5 hr (12 hr 30 min) = 0930 for the hour of completion.

   PROOF

   $1 \times 500 = 500$

   $40 \times 12.5 = 500$

9. HAVE — WANT TO HAVE

200 mL : 3 hr = x mL : 1 hr

$3x = 200$

$x = 66.66 = 67$ mL per hr

OR

$$\frac{\text{Total volume}}{\text{Total time}} = \text{mL per hr}$$

$$\frac{200\text{ mL}}{3\text{ hr}} = 66.66 = 67\text{ mL per hr}$$

PROOF

$200 \times 1 = 200$

$3 \times 66.66 = 199.98$

10. $$\frac{\text{Total volume}}{\text{Total time}} = \text{vol per hr}$$

$$\frac{500\text{ mL}}{4\text{ hr}} = 125\text{ mL per hr}$$

WORKSHEET 7F (page 260)

1. KNOW — WANT TO KNOW

100 mL : 60 min = x mL : 60 min

$60x = 6000$

$x = 100$ mL per hr

PROOF

$100 \times 60 = 6000$

$60 \times 100 = 6000$

2. KNOW — WANT TO KNOW

150 mL : 60 min = 250 mL : x min

$150x = 250 \times 60 = 15{,}000$

$x = 100$ min $= 1.6$ hr $= 1$ hr 40 min

PROOF

$100 \times 150 = 15{,}000$

$250 \times 60 = 15{,}000$

3. a. $$\frac{\cancel{60}^{\,2}}{\cancel{30}_{\,1}} \times 100 = 200\text{ drops per min}$$

b. The infusion device will be set at 200 mL per hr.

KNOW — WANT TO KNOW

100 mL : 30 min = x mL : 60 min

$30x = 100 \times 60 = 6000$

$30x = 6000$

$x = 200$ mL per hr

4. a. KNOW — WANT TO KNOW

50 mL : 20 min = x mL : 60 min

$20x = 50 \times 60 = 3000$

$x = 150$ mL per hr

PROOF

$20 \times 150 = 3000$

$50 \times 60 = 3000$

b. $$\frac{15}{20} \times \frac{50}{1} = \frac{\cancel{15}^{\,3}}{\cancel{20}_{\,4}} \times \frac{50}{1} = \frac{150}{4}$$

$= 37.5 = 38$ drops per min

5. a. $$\frac{\cancel{15}^{\,1}}{\cancel{60}_{\,4}} \times \frac{100}{1} = \frac{1}{4} \times \frac{100}{1} = \frac{100}{4} = 25\text{ drops per min}$$

b. 100 mL : 60 min = x mL : 60 min

$60x = 100 \times 60 - 6000$

$60x = 6000$

$x = 100$ mL per hr

PROOF

$100 \times 60 = 6000$

$60 \times 100 = 6000$

6. a. KNOW — WANT TO KNOW

50 mL : 30 min = x mL : 60 min

$30x = 50 \times 60 = 3000$

$x = 100$ mL per hr

PROOF

$30 \times 100 = 3000$

$50 \times 60 = 3000$

b. $$\frac{60}{30} \times \frac{50}{1} = \frac{\cancel{60}^{\,2}}{\cancel{30}_{\,1}} \times \frac{50}{1} = 100\text{ drops per min}$$

7\. a. $\frac{\overset{2}{\cancel{60}}}{\underset{3}{\cancel{90}}} \times 200 = \frac{400}{3} = 133.33 = 133$ drops per min

OR

b. 200 mL : 90 min = x mL : 60 min

$90x = 200 \times 60 = 12{,}000$

$90x = 12{,}000$

$x = 133.33 = 133$ mL per hr

Set infusion device for 133 mL per hr.

8\. Step 1: $\frac{1000}{12} = 83.3 = 83$ mL per hr

a. Step 2: $\frac{\overset{1}{\cancel{15}}}{\underset{4}{\cancel{60}}} \times 83 = \frac{83}{4}$

$= 20.8 = 21$ drops per min

b. The infusion device will be set at 83 mL per hr.

KNOW WANT TO KNOW

c. 0.9 g : $1\cancel{00}$ mL = x g : $10\cancel{00}$ mL

$x = 0.9 \times 10 = 9$

$x = 9$ g of sodium chloride (solute)

PROOF

$0.9 \times 1000 = 900$

$100 \times 9 = 900$

9\. a. Step 1: $\frac{TV}{TT} = \frac{2000}{8} = 250$ mL per hr

b. Step 2: $\frac{\overset{1}{\cancel{15}}}{\underset{4}{\cancel{60}}} \times 250 = \frac{250}{4}$

$= 62.5$ or 63 drops per min

KNOW WANT TO KNOW

c. 5 g : $1\cancel{00}$ mL = x g : $20\cancel{00}$ mL

$x = 5 \times 20 = 100$

$x = 100$ g of dextrose

PROOF

$5 \times 2000 = 10{,}000$

$100 \times 100 = 10{,}000$

10\. a. $\frac{\overset{3}{\cancel{60}}}{\underset{2}{\cancel{40}}} \times 150 = \frac{450}{2}$

$= 225$ drops per min is the fastest rate. Set infusion device for 225 mL per hr using the microdrip formula.

b. $\frac{\overset{1}{\cancel{60}}}{\underset{1}{\cancel{60}}} \times 150 = 150$ drops per min is the slowest rate. Set infusion device for 150 mL per hr using the microdrip formula.

WORKSHEET 7G (page 261)

1\. a. KNOW WANT TO KNOW

25 drops : 1 min = 10 drops : x min

$25x = 10$

$x = 0.4$ min = 1 mL

PROOF

$25 \times 0.4 = 10$

$1 \times 10 = 10$

KNOW WANT TO KNOW

1 mL : 0.4 min = 1000 mL : x min

$x = 0.4 \times 1000 = 400$

$x = 400$ min divided by 60

$= 6.66$ hr = 6 hr 40 min

2\. b. $\frac{\overset{1}{\cancel{15}}}{\underset{1}{\cancel{15}}} \times 50 = 50$ drops per min

3. d. $\frac{\overset{2}{\cancel{20}}\text{ gtt}}{\underset{3}{\cancel{30}}\text{ min}} \times 50 = \frac{100}{3} = 33.33 = 33$ drops per min

4. b. KNOW WANT TO KNOW

300 mL : 6 hr = x mL : 1 hr

$6x = 300 \times 1 = 300$

$x = 50$ mL per hr. mL per hr and microdrip drops per min are the same, so 50 drops per min is correct

PROOF

$300 \times 1 = 300$

$6 \times 50 = 300$

OR

$\frac{\overset{1}{\cancel{60}}\text{ gtt}}{\underset{6}{\cancel{360}}\text{min}} \times 300\text{ mL} = \frac{300}{6} =$ 50 drops per min and 50 mL per hr

5. d. KNOW WANT TO KNOW

12 mL : 1 hr = 150 mL : x hr

$12x = 150$

$x = 12.5 = 12$ hr 30 min

PROOF

$1 \times 150 = 150$

$12.5 \times 12 = 150$

6. d. KNOW WANT TO KNOW

30 drops : 1 min = 20 drops : x min

$30x = 20$

$x = 0.66$ min

PROOF

$1 \times 20 = 20$

$30 \times 0.66 = 20$

KNOW WANT TO KNOW

1 mL : 0.66 min = 500 mL : x min

$x = 0.66 \times 500 = 330$

$x = 330$ min $\div 60 = 5.5$ hr = 5 hr 30 min

PROOF

$1 \times 330 = 330$

$0.66 \times 500 = 330$

7. a. KNOW WANT TO KNOW

2500 mL : 24 hr = x mL : 1 hr

$24x = 2500$

$x = 104.16 = 104$ mL per hr

PROOF

$2500 \times 1 = 2500$

$24 \times 104.16 = 2500 = 104$ mL per hr

KNOW WANT TO KNOW

15 gtt : 1 mL = x gtt : 104 mL

OR

$\frac{15}{60} \times 104 = \frac{1560}{60} = 26$ drops per min

$x = 15 \times 104 = 1560$

$x = 1560$ divided by 60 min = 26 drops per min

PROOF

$15 \times 104 = 1560$

$1 \times 1560 = 1560$

8. c. KNOW WANT TO KNOW

42 gtt : 1 min = 10 drops : x min

$42x = 1 \times 10 = 10$

$x = 0.238 = 0.24$ min per mL

PROOF

$1 \times 10 = 10$

$42 \times 0.24 = 10.08 = 10$

KNOW WANT TO KNOW

1 mL : 0.24 min = 500 mL : x min

$x = 0.24 \times 500 = 120$

$x = 120$ min divided by 60 = 2 hr

PROOF

$1 \times 120 = 120$

$0.24 \times 500 = 120$

The transfusion was started at 1100 hours. The completion time will be 1300 hours.

9. c. KNOW WANT TO KNOW

30 mL : 1 hr = 500 mL : x hr

$30x = 500$

$x = 16.66$ hr = 16 hr 40 min

PROOF

$30 \times 16.6 = 499.8 = 500$

$1 \times 500 = 500$

10. d. $\frac{250}{2}$ = 125 mL per hr

CHAPTER 7 FINAL: BASIC INTRAVENOUS THERAPY CALCULATIONS (page 264)

1. 42 drops per min if calculated with drop factor of 15. 167 mL per hr if infusion device is used

2. 125 mL per hr
42 drops per min

3. 83 mL per hr
28 drops per min

4. 150 drops per min

5. 83 mL per hr
14 drops per min

6. 125 mL per hr
31 drops per min

7. 100 mL per hr
17 drops per min

8. Set infusion device at 267 mL per hr.

9. 83 drops per min

10. 31 drops per min

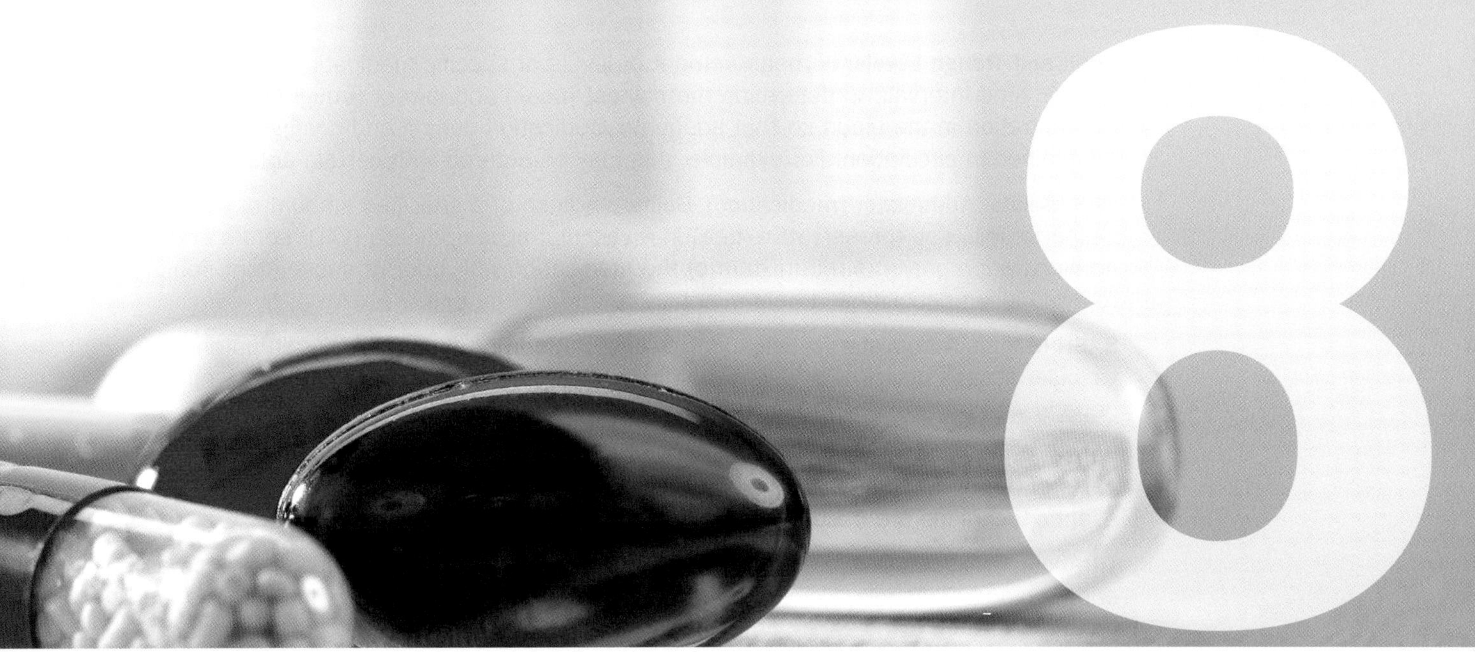

Advanced Intravenous Calculations

Objectives

- Calculate time and dose intervals for direct IV injection (bolus) medications administered by a syringe. Note: Often, the order may state "IV push." "IV injection" is used to emphasize safety.
- Calculate hourly drug dose and hourly flow rate for IV solutions.
- Calculate milligrams per kilogram and micrograms per kilogram per minute and per hour.
- Estimate and calculate infusion rates and drug doses using ratio and proportion.
- Evaluate existing infusions for correct flow rate and/or drug dose.
- Analyze IV medication errors using critical thinking to prevent future errors.

Introduction

This chapter builds on the basic IV calculations taught in Chapter 7. The problems cover single-dose intravenous medication administration and weight-based intravenous dosing in mcg per minute and per hour in solutions using ratio and proportion. The difference between basic IV calculations and more complex calculations is that there are more questions to be answered and sequenced to arrive at correct drug dosing, flow rates, and safe technique. Pharmacy, flow-rate charts, and IV pump equipment provide flow rates, but the nurse must be able to independently calculate and verify that they reflect the provider's order and that they will be diluted with compatible solutions. IV errors do occur, and because the medication is delivered directly into circulation, errors are more serious. Many of the problems involve ISMP-identified high-alert medications. Many practice problems to simplify the math as well as clinically relevant safety alerts are provided.

Vocabulary

Half-life ($t_{1/2}$): Amount of time for one half of a drug's concentration to be cleared from the plasma.

IV Flush: Injection of sterile normal saline for injection (preservative-free) into an existing vascular access device (VAD) to clear the line of existing medications or solutions that may be incompatible with subsequent products and to maintain patency of the device.*

---

*Always check compatibility of the medication to be administered with diluents, and any other IV medications the patient is receiving.

Peak and Trough Levels: IV measurement of levels of specific medications in the blood at *specific* time intervals to determine the highest (peak) and lowest (trough) levels of drug concentration in the blood so that adequate medication dosing and dosing intervals can be maintained in circulation. For example, this may be ordered with certain antibiotics.

SAS (Saline, Administer [medication], Saline): A flush of a *specified* amount of sterile normal saline for injection (preservative–free) in a vascular access device (VAD) before and after administration prevents the mixture of the medication with prior or subsequent substances to avoid incompatibility and help maintain patency of the line.

SASH (Saline, Administer [medication], Saline, Heparin): A flush to maintain patency of a vascular access device with a very small amount of heparin and to prevent the mixture of heparin with any existing incompatible substances in the line.

Sepsis: A grave complication of an infection that spreads into circulation and affects all parts of the body. This is why frequent handwashing, proper cleansing of injection ports, and aseptic technique are essential when administering IV medication.

Titration: The gradual adjustment of a drug dose to reach a *desired response,* such as lowering a blood pressure, raising a pulse, or easing respiratory difficulty. Intravenous medications are titrated by adjusting flow rate to increase or decrease a drug dose.

VAD (Vascular Access Device): An indwelling catheter, port, or other device in a vein or artery to give medications or monitor pressures.

Direct IV (Bolus) (IV Push)

IV injection medications are used to administer small amounts of a medication in a single administration to bring a drug level to a certain desired concentration. They may be prepared in relatively small amounts with a specific amount of compatible diluent to be administered over a specific limited amount of time. They usually deliver more concentrated drug mixtures and are smaller volumes than IV infusions.

CLINICAL ALERT!

Whenever the word "concentrate" is seen on any medication label, look for dilution directions.

CLINICAL ALERT!

Before administering any IV medication, including bolus injections, the following checks *must* be made to avoid an adverse drug event:

- Compare the provider's order with the supplied drug, dose, and solutions.
- Compatibility and interaction of the ordered drug with diluents, flushes, and with any other solutions with which the ordered drug may come in contact, for example, those infusing or recently infused in an existing line.
- Agency policies pertaining to flush volumes and safe syringe sizes for various sites and lines (see *Clinical Alert*).
- Recommended rates of flow—usually per minute—for the specific drug, dose, and purpose

Preservative-free solutions need to be used for intravenous flushes and bolus preparations. Because the appearance of the solutions is similar, check the labels carefully for the terms "preservative free" versus "bacteriostatic," which contains a preservative. Preferably the flush materials are single-use preparations to avoid the introduction of bacterial contaminants. If using multidose vials, check agency policy for discard dates—usually 24 hours—and examine for particulates and cloudiness before using. Multidose vials are needed for larger-volume diluents. Sterile technique is essential.

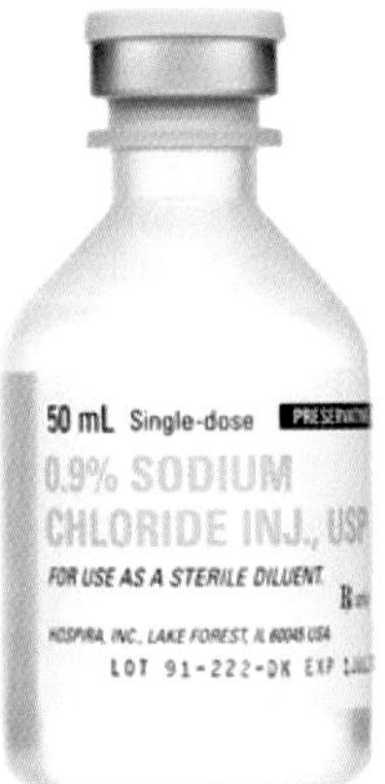

FIGURE 8.1 Hospira flush solutions. (From Hospira, Inc., Lake Forest, Ill.)

CLINICAL ALERT!

The words "direct" and "push" erroneously suggest push hard at a fast rate directly into a vein. Only a few emergency drugs are to be pushed quickly. Always check the recommended safe flow rate. Pushing any bolus injection (direct IV) (IV push) *hard and/or quickly,* particularly against resistance, increases the chance of damaging the line, vein, or port and/or having the syringe disengage from the connection, causing medication loss. Injecting faster than recommended can result in serious adverse drug events (ADE).

Check a current, reliable IV drug reference and/or pharmacist for the recommended rate limits and dilutions for all IV medications. It is also recommended to administer boluses via a VAD if available so that countermeasures can be taken promptly if complications arise.

Boluses may be delivered with a syringe, a syringe pump, or a volume-control device, or they may be connected to an IV as a piggyback (Figures 8.2, 8.3, and 8.4).

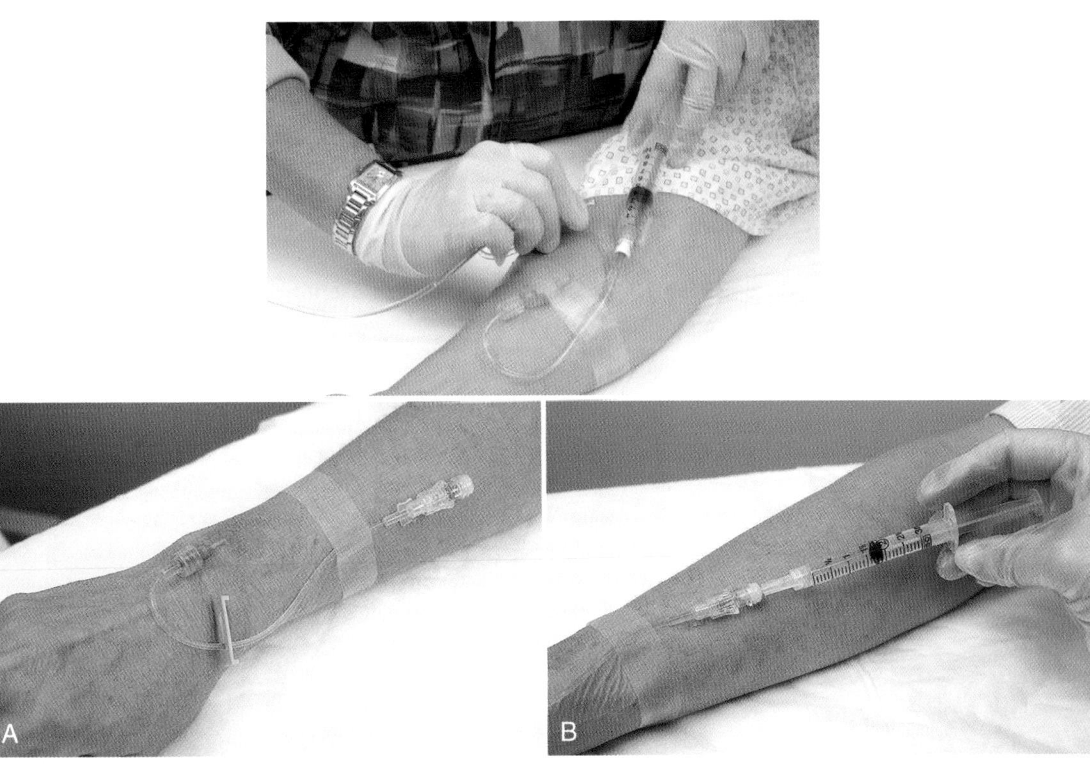

FIGURE 8.2 Using watch time to time an IV push medication. **A,** IV catheter with saline lock adapter. **B,** Syringe inserted into injection port. (From Potter PA, Perry AG, Ostendorf A: *Clinical nursing skills and Techniques*, ed. 9, St. Louis, 2018, Elsevier.)

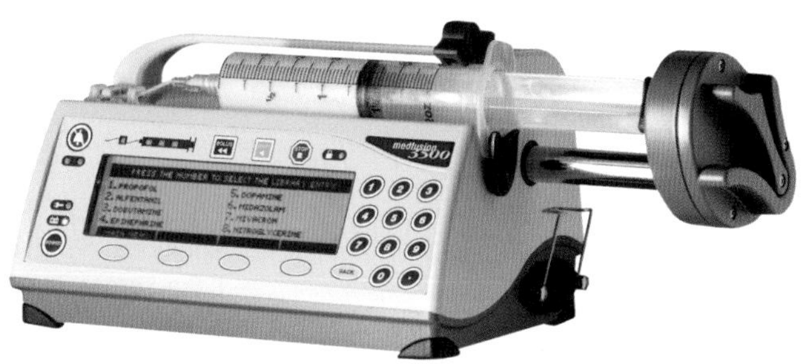

FIGURE 8.3 Syringe pump. (From Clayton BD, Willihnganz M: *Basic pharmacology for nurses,* ed. 16, St. Louis, 2013, Mosby.)

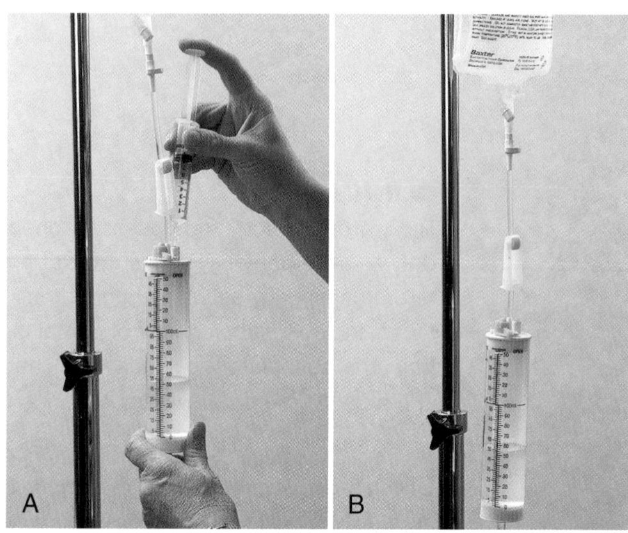

FIGURE 8.4 Volume-control device. **A,** Inject medication into device. **B,** Prepared dose. (From Potter PA, Perry AG, Stockert P, Hall A: *Essentials for nursing practice,* ed. 8, St. Louis, 2014, Mosby.)

CLINICAL ALERT!

There has been controversy about syringe size for bolus injections. A syringe with a wider barrel delivers less pressure and reduces the chance of damaging a vein or VAD. 10-mL syringes have been reported to cause less accurate doses and rates for small amounts because of their narrow calibrations. Smaller syringes deliver more accurate doses for small amounts because the calibrations are farther apart and easier to read, but they deliver more pressure because of their narrow diameter. Before selecting a syringe for IV bolus administrations, check agency policies and procedures.

CLINICAL ALERT!

Certain types of ports on central lines and most central lines require a wide-barreled 10-mL syringe.

To reduce needlestick injuries, the trend is to use infusion systems with safety features such as a needleless system (Figure 8.5).

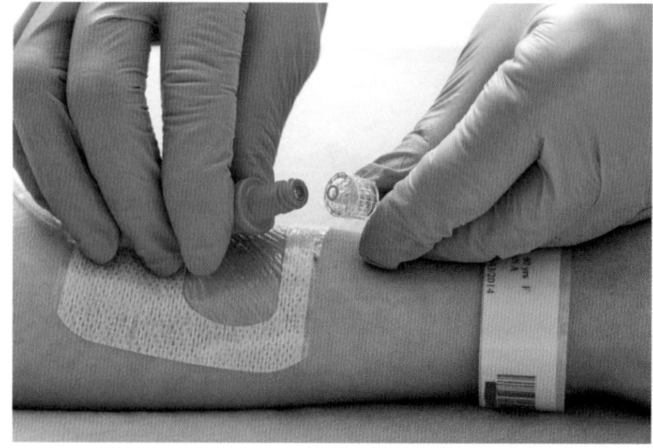

FIGURE 8.5 Needleless system. The syringe attaches without the use of a needle and therefore prevents needlesticks. (From Perry AG, Potter PA, Ostendorf WR: *Clinical nursing skills and techniques*, ed 9, St. Louis, 2018, Elsevier.)

There are two ways to time IV injection medications for direct administration of medication through a syringe. Regardless of the method you select, the first step is always to accurately calculate and prepare the correct volume.

Timing IV Injection Medications: Method 1 (mL per Minute)

This method calculates the amount in milliliters to be slowly and gradually injected over each minute.

Formula TV : TM = x mL : 1 minute
Total volume : Total minutes = x volume (mL) : 1 minute

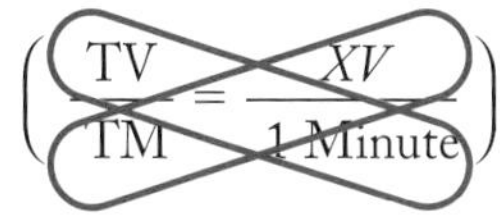

Example Ordered: Digoxin 0.5 mg IV over 5 min. Dilute to 4 mL with sterile water for injection.

TV : TM = x mL : 1 minute

4 mL : 5 min = x mL : 1 minute

$$\frac{4}{5} = \frac{x}{1}$$

x = 0.8 mL to be pushed slowly each minute

PROOF $4 \times 1 = 4$
$5 \times 0.8 = 4$

Schedule

1600 : 00	4 mL in syringe
1601	3.2 mL remaining
1602	2.4 mL remaining
1603	1.6 mL remaining
1604	0.8 mL remaining
1605	0 remaining

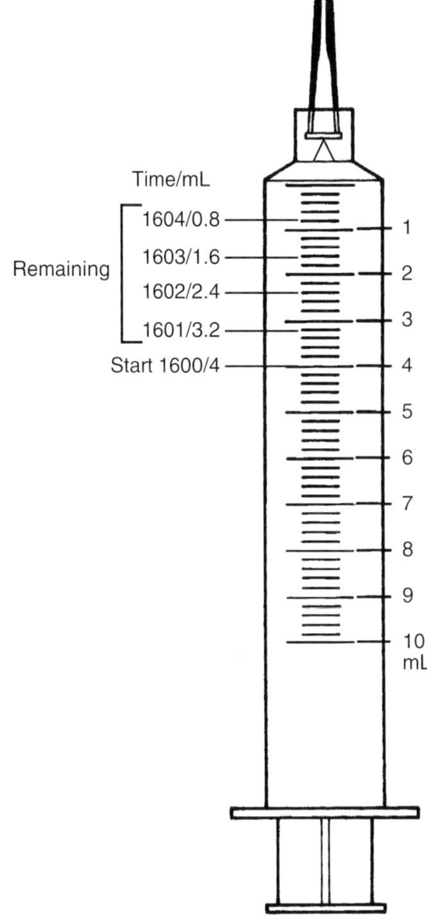

The schedule above reflects a start time of 1600 hours. It is helpful to write your start time and a schedule of "markers" (increments of time and volume) when you need to push over several minutes. Write this before beginning to inject and have it in front of you to avoid errors caused by distraction.

Timing IV Injection Medications: Method 2 (Seconds per Calibration)

Many IV injection medications have dilutions that permit 1 mL per minute so that the timing is easy to maintain. Occasionally, when the timing is to be very slow and is not 1 mL per minute, counting seconds per calibration permits more precise timing of the injection.

RULE **Divide the number of seconds of total time of administration by the number of calibrated increments in a syringe prepared with medication (lines on the syringe within each milliliter). This will yield the seconds per increment to be injected.**

Formula $\frac{\text{Total seconds}}{\text{Total increments}} = \text{Seconds to deliver each increment}$

Example Give 0.5 mg digoxin IV over 5 min. Directions say to dilute to 4 mL with sterile water for injection. There are 20 calibrations in 4 mL on this syringe.

$$\frac{300 \text{ seconds}}{20 \text{ calibrations (0.2 mL ea)}} = 1 \text{ calibration (0.2 mL) every 15 seconds}$$

PROOF $300 \times 1 = 300$
$15 \times 20 = 300$

Use the second hand on your watch and/or count each cycle (1 to 15) as you administer the medication, 1 calibration (0.2 mL) every 15 seconds.
Tip: start count when the second hand is on 12.
60 sec = 1 min
60 × 5 = 300 seconds

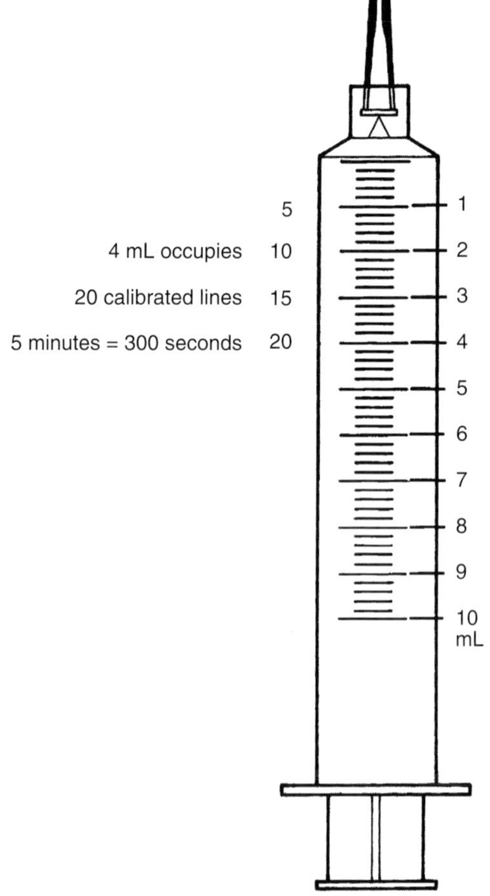

Answers on page 300

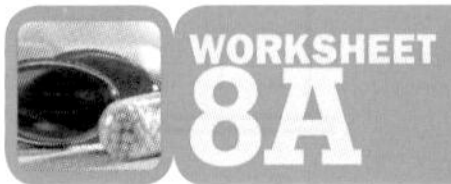

WORKSHEET 8A IV Injection Calculations

Solve the following problems using the syringes shown to calculate the seconds per calibration, if applicable, and mL/min to be administered.

1. Ordered: 10% calcium chloride (5 mL) over 5 min for a patient with hypocalcemia.
   a. For how many seconds will you administer each calibration?
   b. How many mL/min will be injected?
   c. Shade in amount on syringe.

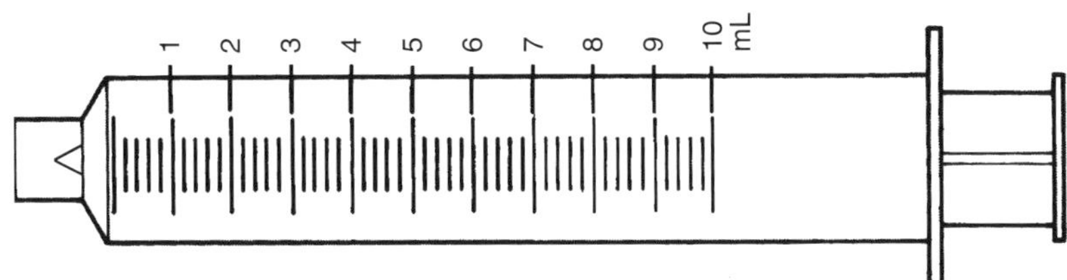

2. Ordered: Digoxin 0.5 mg IV over 10 min for a patient with heart failure. (The literature specifies a minimum of 5 min for administration.) Available: Digoxin 250 mcg per mL.
   a. Total mL you will inject:
   b. Total minutes for injection:
   c. mL per min to be injected:
   d. minutes per calibration:
   e. Shade in amount on syringe.

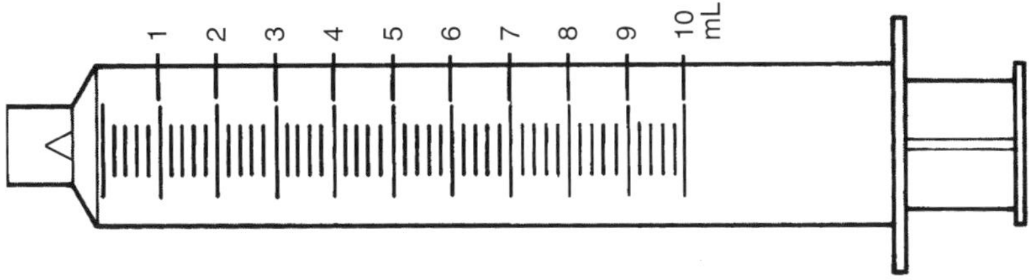

3. Ordered: Phenytoin sodium IV loading dose of 900 mg at 50 mg per min on an infusion device for a patient with seizures (Figure 8.6). Available: Phenytoin 100 mg per mL.
   a. Total mL to be injected:
   b. Total time for injection:
   c. mL per min to be administered:

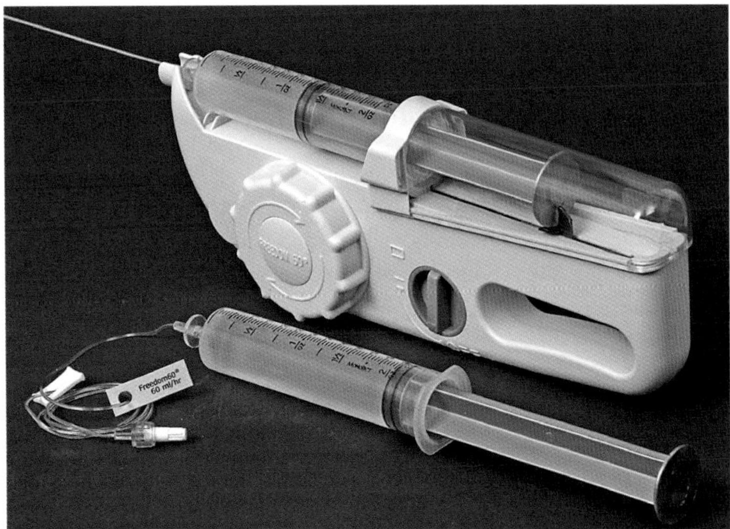

FIGURE 8.6 Freedom 60 infusion syringe pump. This portable reusable manual infusion uses standard 60 mL syringes and can be filled from 1 to 60 mL. It offers flow rates with rate-controlled tubing from 0.5 to 1200 mL per hr. It does not permit free flow. (From Repro-Med Systems, Inc., Chester, NY.)

4. Ordered: Furosemide 20 mg IV undiluted over 2 min for a patient with fluid retention. Available: Furosemide 10 mg per mL and a 10 mL syringe.
   a. Total mL to be injected:
   b. Total time in seconds:
   c. Seconds per calibration:
   d. mL per min to be administered:

5. Ordered: Morphine sulfate 4 mg IV injection for a patient with severe pain. The literature states that a single dose should be administered over 4 to 5 min and that the dose may be diluted in 4 to 5 mL with sterile water or normal saline for injection. The nurse dilutes it to 5 mL with NS.
   a. Total mL to be injected:
   b. Total time in minutes:
   c. mL per min to be administered:
   d. Shade in amount on syringe.

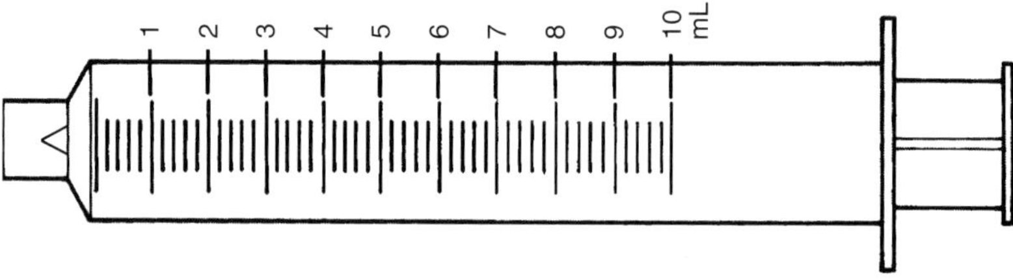

Calculating Intravenous Medicated Infusion Flow Rates and Drug Rates From the Order and Total Volume and Total Drug Supplied

Nursing responsibilities include independent calculation of flow rates of medication solutions in mg, mcg, g, or units per hour, and/or per minute and/or per kg of weight, depending on the provider order and the supplied solution and medication. Once the hourly volume and drug rates are known, variations such as the rate per minute and per kg are derived with simple arithmetic.

Steps for Calculating Hourly Volume Rate or Hourly Drug Rate

The first steps are always the same:

1. After checking the complete order with the supplied drug amount and solution volume, identify the on-hand total drug (TD) : total volume (TV) ratio (e.g., 250 mg : 1000 mL).
2. Reduce the ratio to lowest terms and place this on the *left* side of the equation (What you have) as in previous ratio and proportion problems.

Example

$$TD : TV = \left(\frac{250}{1000}\right)$$

250 mg : 1000 mL

TD : TV (Reduced ratio)

1 mg : 4 mL =

3. Place the hourly drug (HD) ordered or volume per hr (HV) on the right side of the equation, estimate the unknown (x) quantity, and solve the equation.

Check your answer with the estimate. Reducing the TD : TV ratio makes it easy to estimate a correct answer.

Example Hourly Drug and Flow Rate Formula for Medicated Infusions

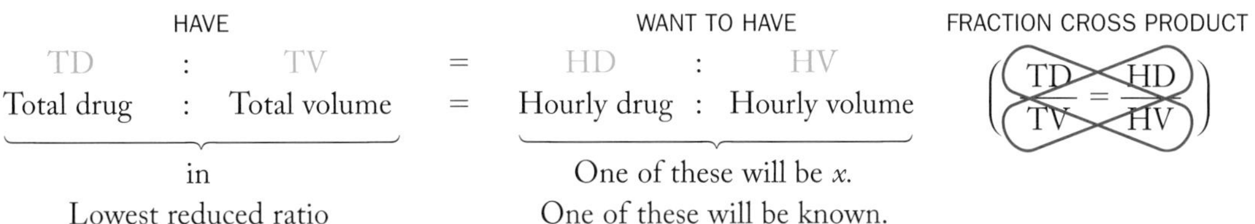

HAVE
WANT TO HAVE
FRACTION CROSS PRODUCT
TD : TV = HD : HV
Total drug : Total volume = Hourly drug : Hourly volume
in
Lowest reduced ratio
One of these will be x.
One of these will be known.
TD / TV = HD / HV

Example Ordered: A drug to infuse at 20 mg per hr IV
Available: An IV solution of 400 mg of a drug in 500 mL

Calculate an hourly flow rate (HV) after reducing the total drug/total volume ratio to lowest terms.

HAVE WANT TO HAVE

TD : TV = HD : HV

400 mg : 500 mL = 20 mg : x mL $\left(\frac{4}{5} = \frac{20}{x}\right) \rightarrow$ Make an estimate of x.

4 : 5 = 20 : x

x = 25 mL per hr

Set the flow rate on the IV infusion device to 25 mL/hr.

Example Existing IV infusing at 25 mL per hr

Calculate the hourly drug amount (HD) being infused.*

HAVE WANT TO HAVE

TD : TV = HD : HV

400 mg : 500 mL = x mg : 25 mL $\left(\frac{4}{5} = \frac{x}{25}\right) \rightarrow$ Make an estimate of x.

(reduced ratio) 4 : 5 = x : 25

$5x = 100$ x = 20 mg per hr of drug being infused

remember **When three quantities are known, the fourth can be obtained. The supply and the order provide three of the four quantities for the equation just as they did for basic calculations. The brief worksheets that follow provide sequential practice to increase your understanding and to help you master the calculations.**

Answers on page 300

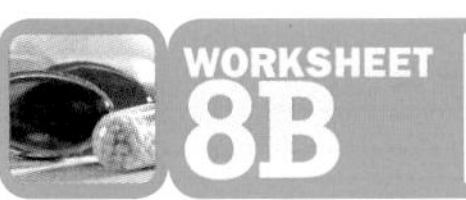

WORKSHEET 8B Medicated IV Calculations

1. Reduce the **T**otal **D**rug/**T**otal **V**olume ratio to lowest terms as shown in example 1a.

TD : TV	Lowest Ratio	
a. 250 mg : 1000 mL	1 : 4	$\left(\frac{1}{4}\right)$
b. 500 mg : 500 mL	______	
c. 100 mg : 1000 mL	______	
d. 250 mg : 500 mL	______	
e. 500 mg : 1000 mL	______	

RULE **To find the mL per hr for the order, reduce the ratio of total drug to total volume. Enter the known ordered mg per hour (HD). Enter x mL (HV) for the unknown. TD : TV = HD : x HV. Estimate the mL per hr.**

*This can be evaluated at the bedside to verify that it matches the order.

2. Estimate the value of x (hourly volume) after reducing the ratio of total drug to total volume. The ratio of hourly drug to hourly volume will be the same as total drug to total volume.

	TD : TV = HD : HV	ANSWER
Example	a. 250 mg : 1000 mL = 10 mg : x mL	1 : 4 = 10 : 40 mL per hr $\left(\frac{1}{4} = \frac{10}{40}\right)$
	b. 500 mg : 500 mL = 30 mg : x mL	______ mL per hr
	c. 100 mg : 1000 mL = 5 mg : x mL	______ mL per hr
	d. 250 mg : 500 mL = 3 mg : x mL	______ mL per hr
	e. 500 mg : 250 mL = 10 mg : x mL	______ mL per hr

RULE **To find the drug per hour being delivered in an existing infusion: Enter the existing IV solution concentration flow rate. Enter x for the drug per hr. Enter the existing flow rate to see if the rate is delivering the correct ordered amount of drug per hr.**

Note: x will either be the ordered drug rate or the flow rate. (TD : TV : x HD : HV)

3. Estimate the hourly drug (x).

	TD : TV = HD : HV	ANSWER
Example	a. 250 mg : 250 mL = x mg : 20 mL	1 : 1 = 20 : 20 20 mg per hr $\left(\frac{250}{250} = \frac{x}{20}\right)$
	b. 1000 mg : 500 mL = x mg : 6 mL	______ __ mg per hr
	c. 250 mg : 500 mL = x mg : 18 mL	______ __ mg per hr
	d. 400 mg : 1000 mL = x mg : 10 mL	______ __ mg per hr
	e. 500 mg : 250 mL = x mg : 18 mL	______ __ mg per hr

4. Calculate the IV drug order per hour based on the patient kg weight.

a. 2 mcg per kg per hr	Wt 60 kg	2 mcg × 60 kg = 120 mcg per hr
b. 10 mg per kg per hr	Wt 110 lb	______
c. 0.5 mcg per kg per hr	Wt 120 lb	______
d. 1.5 mg per kg per hr	Wt 68 kg	______
e. 6 mcg per kg per hr	Wt 60 kg	______

5. Change micrograms to milligrams by moving the decimal three places to the left. Reduce the total drug/total volume ratio to the lowest terms. Finally, estimate the hourly volume. (The hourly drug must always be calculated in the same terms as the total drug.)

	TD : TV = HD : HV	ANSWER
Example	a. 250 mg : 1000 mL = (4000 mcg) 4 mg : x mL	1 : 4 = 4 : 16 mL per hr
	b. 500 mg : 500 mL = (9000 mcg) __ mg : x mL	______ mL per hr
	c. 1000 mg : 500 mL = (20,000 mcg) __ mg : x mL	______ mL per hr
	d. 250 mg : 500 mL = (15,000 mcg) __ mg : x mL	______ mL per hr
	e. 400 mg : 250 mL = (8000 mcg) __ mg : x mL	______ mL per hr

Calculations for Various Types of IV Medication Orders

Once you understand the ratio of total drug to total volume and dose order per hour, variations on the calculations involve only metric conversions and basic arithmetic—multiplication or division. Medication orders based on weight are common and must be in terms of kg.

Medication orders based on mcg need to be changed to mg if the total drug available in the IV solution (Total Volume, or TV) is based in mg.

Answers on page 301

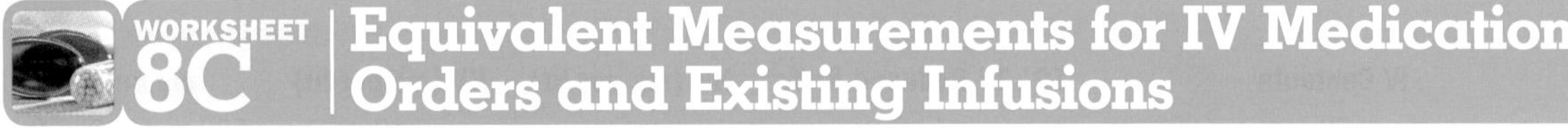

WORKSHEET 8C Equivalent Measurements for IV Medication Orders and Existing Infusions

Use a calculator where needed to solve the problems. Always enter calculator data twice for verification. Examine the relationships between minute and hour, and mg and mcg.

Formulas: 1000 mcg = 1 mg   60 minutes = 1 hr   1000 milliunits = 1 Unit   Patient wt: 80 kg

1. Ordered: 2 mg per minute. How many mcg per minute are ordered? mg per hr ordered?
2. Ordered: 300 mcg per minute. How many mg per minute would be needed? mg per hr?
3. Ordered: 0.2 mg per kg per minute. How many mg per minute would be needed? mg per hr?
4. Ordered: 5 mcg per kg per minute. How many mg per minute would be needed? mg per hr?
5. Ordered: 600 milliunits per hr. How many milliunits per minute?
6. *Infusing: 0.1 mg per hour. How many mcg are flowing per hr?
7. Infusing: 10 mg per hr. How many mg per minute are infusing?
8. Infusing: 100 mg per hr. How many mg per kg per hr are infusing?
9. Infusing: 2.5 mg per hr. How many mcg per minute are infusing?
10. Infusing: 3 units per hr. How many milliunits per minute are infusing?

*Note: Distinguish the need to multiply and the need to divide.

Answers on page 301

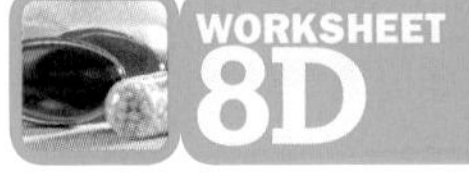

WORKSHEET 8D IV Drug/Flow Rates

Tip: Being able to convert drug, weight, time, and volume parameters within the metric system with ease facilitates advanced IV calculations.

1. Fill in the table by using a calculator and/or by moving decimals.

	mg per hr	mcg per hr	mg per min	mcg per min
Example	**a.** 0.050.	50	0.050 ÷ 60 = 0.0008	0.8
	b.		0.4	
	c. 30			
	d.			20
	e. 7.5			

2. Fill in the table using a calculator.

kg	mg per hr	mg per kg per min	mcg per kg per min
a. 85	25	25 ÷ 85 ÷ 60 = 0.005	5
b. 70		10	
c. 62			0.1
d. 55	75		
e. 48			50

3. Fill in the table for these IV drug/flow rate calculations using the TD : TV = HD : HV formula.

IV Contents	TD : TV Reduced Ratio	HD (mg per hr)	HV (mL per hr)	mg per mL
a. 500 mg per 1000 mL	1 : 2	5	10	500 ÷ 1000 = 0.5
b. 250 mg per 500 mL			30	
c. 400 mg per 250 mL		24		
d. 500 mg per 500 mL			75	
e. 500 mg per 250 mL		16		

CLINICAL ALERT!

Remember that the difference between a microgram (mcg) and a milligram (mg) is "× 1000." The difference between drug per minute and hourly drug is "× 60."

The difference between mcg per kg per minute and mcg per minute is based on "the weight in kilograms." Manipulating these differences is critical for safe medication administration.

Answers on page 302

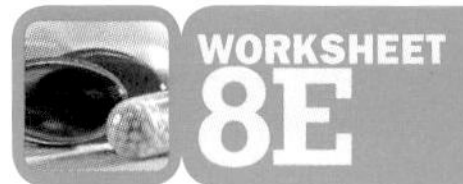

WORKSHEET 8E Medication Doses Infusing in Existing Solutions

It is often necessary to verify the amount of drug being delivered in an existing solution. The amount of drug in the IV solution is frequently a milligram dose, whereas the amount of drug the patient is receiving is a microgram dose or a microgram per kilogram dose.

Note the example in Problem 1 and do the following in the remaining problems:

- Set up the ratios and determine mg per hr. Prove your answer.
- Move decimals to change milligrams to micrograms (× 1000).
- Use a calculator to change hourly drug (HD) to drug per minute (divide by 60).
- Use a calculator to determine kilograms, and divide micrograms by kilogram weight to obtain mcg per kg per minute. Enter all calculator data *twice* for verification.

Example **1.** An IV drug 100 mg in 1000 mL is infusing at 20 mL per hr. The provider asks, "How many *mg per hr* is the patient receiving? How many *mcg per minute*? How many *mcg per kg per minute*? The patient weighs 143 lb (65 kg) today.

a. TD : TV reduced ratio: 100 : 1000 = 1 : 10 $\left(\frac{100}{1000} = \frac{1}{10}\right)$

b. TD : TV = HD : HV 1 mg : 10 mL = 2 mg : 20 mL

c. mg per hour infusing: 2 mg per hr

d. mcg per hour infusing: 2 × 1000 = 2000 mcg per hr

e. mcg per minute infusing: 2000 ÷ 60 = 33.3 mcg per minute

f. mcg per kg per minute infusing: 33.3 ÷ 65 kg = 0.5 mcg per kg per minute

PROOF 1 × 20 = 20
10 × 2 = 20

2. An IV drug 250 mg in 500 mL is infusing at 15 mL per hr. The patient weighs 110 lb today.

a. TD : TV = HD : HV reduced ratio:

b. mcg per hour infusing:

c. mcg per minute infusing:

d. mcg per kg per minute infusing:

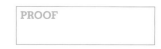

PROOF

3. An IV drug 400 mg in 1000 mL is infusing at 5 mL per hr. The patient weighs 121 lb today.

a. TD : TV = HD : HV reduced ratio:

b. mcg per hour infusing:

c. mcg per minute infusing:

d. mcg per kg per minute infusing:

PROOF

4. An IV drug 1000 mg in 250 mL is infusing at 10 mL per hr. The patient weighs 132 lb today.
   a. TD : TV = HD : HV reduced ratio:
   b. mcg per hour infusing:
   c. mcg per minute infusing:
   d. mcg per kg per minute infusing:

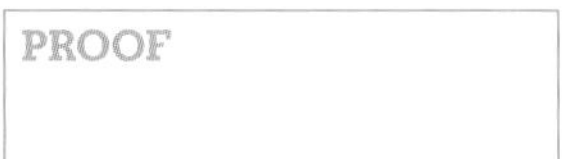

5. An IV drug 500 mg in 250 mL is infusing at 8 mL per hr. The patient weighs 175 lb today. (Calculate kilograms to nearest tenth.)
   a. TD : TV = HD : HV reduced ratio:
   b. mcg per hr infusing:
   c. mcg per minute infusing:
   d. mcg per kg per minute infusing:

PROOF

High-Tech Infusion Devices

A variety of sophisticated infusion pump devices have been developed to reduce IV medication errors. Known as "smart pumps," they may have capability to be connected to several different IV solutions and a mixture of IVs, syringes, and syringe pumps. Very small doses can be programmed in mcg per kg per minute up to very large doses in mL per hour (Figure 8.7). Flushes can be programmed, as can intermittent infusions. Alarms are programmed to warn of an overdose *(soft alert)* or to block the dose *(hard alert)*.

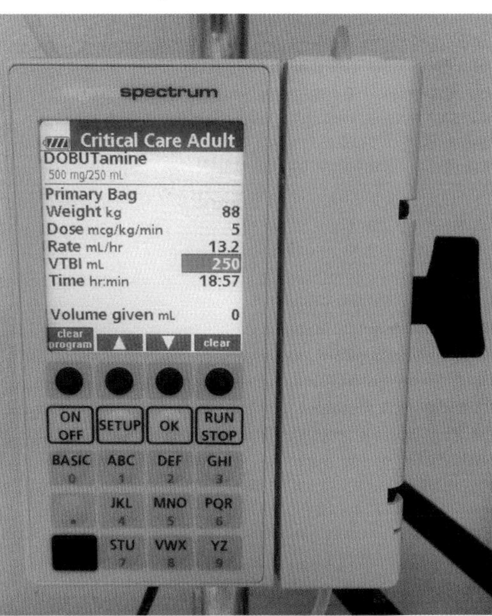

FIGURE 8.7 Sigma Spectrum Infusion Smart Pump has a master drug library that helps minimize the risk of pump-related programming mediction errors. (From Mulholland J, Turner S: *The nurse, the math, the meds: Drug calculations using dimensional analysis,* ed. 3, St. Louis, 2015, Mosby.)

CLINICAL ALERT!

Although these pumps can reduce errors, the nurse cannot be overly reliant on infusion alerts. The alerts depend upon the accuracy and scope of preprogrammed information as well as the function of the pump. Also, errors have been reported due to overrides of soft alerts. *Carefully research soft alerts and consult with pharmacy before overriding.

CLINICAL ALERT!

When entering data on an electronic IV device (EID), beware of decimal errors and of substituting mcg for mg or vice versa. Lack of familiarity with equipment function or equipment malfunction can cause medication errors. The nurse must confirm all the data with the order before initiating the flow of the drug and to ask for help if there is any question about the medication or the equipment.

CLINICAL ALERT!

Never override an IV alarm without rechecking the order. Consult a supervisor, pharmacist, or the provider before changing a program.

*The QSEN Institute (Quality and Safety Education for Nurses) Patient Goal No. 4 is: "Use Alarms Safely." www.jointcommission.org

APPENDIX A

Institute for Safe Medication Practices (ISMP)

ISMP List of *High-Alert Medications* in Acute Care Settings

High-alert medications are drugs that bear a heightened risk of causing significant patient harm when they are used in error. Although mistakes may or may not be more common with these drugs, the consequences of an error are clearly more devastating to patients. We hope you will use this list to determine which medications require special safeguards to reduce the risk of errors. This may include strategies such as standardizing the ordering, storage, preparation, and administration of these products; improving access to information about these drugs; limiting access to high-alert medications; using auxiliary labels and automated alerts; and employing redundancies such as automated or independent double-checks when necessary. (Note: manual independent double-checks are not always the optimal error-reduction strategy and may not be practical for all of the medications on the list.)

Classes/Categories of Medications
adrenergic agonists, IV (e.g., **EPINEPH**rine, phenylephrine, norepinephrine)
adrenergic antagonists, IV (e.g., propranolol, metoprolol, labetalol)
anesthetic agents, general, inhaled and IV (e.g., propofol, ketamine)
antiarrhythmics, IV (e.g., lidocaine, amiodarone)
antithrombotic agents, including: ■ anticoagulants (e.g., warfarin, low molecular weight heparin, IV unfractionated heparin) ■ Factor Xa inhibitors (e.g., fondaparinux, apixaban, rivaroxaban) ■ direct thrombin inhibitors (e.g., argatroban, bivalirudin, dabigatran etexilate) ■ thrombolytics (e.g., alteplase, reteplase, tenecteplase) ■ glycoprotein IIb/IIIa inhibitors (e.g., eptifibatide)
cardioplegic solutions
chemotherapeutic agents, parenteral and oral
dextrose, hypertonic, 20% or greater
dialysis solutions, peritoneal and hemodialysis
epidural or intrathecal medications
hypoglycemics, oral
inotropic medications, IV (e.g., digoxin, milrinone)
insulin, subcutaneous and IV
liposomal forms of drugs (e.g., liposomal amphotericin B) and conventional counterparts (e.g., amphotericin B desoxycholate)
moderate sedation agents, IV (e.g., dexmedetomidine, midazolam)
moderate sedation agents, oral, for children (e.g., chloral hydrate)
narcotics/opioids ■ IV ■ transdermal ■ oral (including liquid concentrates, immediate and sustained-release formulations)
neuromuscular blocking agents (e.g., succinylcholine, rocuronium, vecuronium)
parenteral nutrition preparations
radiocontrast agents, IV
sterile water for injection, inhalation, and irrigation (excluding pour bottles) in containers of 100 mL or more
sodium chloride for injection, hypertonic, greater than 0.9% concentration

Specific Medications
EPINEPHrine, subcutaneous
epoprostenol (Flolan), IV
insulin U-500 (special emphasis)*
magnesium sulfate injection
methotrexate, oral, non-oncologic use
opium tincture
oxytocin, IV
nitroprusside sodium for injection
potassium chloride for injection concentrate
potassium phosphates injection
promethazine, IV
vasopressin, IV or intraosseous

*All forms of insulin, subcutaneous and IV, are considered a class of high-alert medications. Insulin U-500 has been singled out for special emphasis to bring attention to the need for distinct strategies to prevent the types of errors that occur with this concentrated form of insulin.

Background
Based on error reports submitted to the ISMP National Medication Errors Reporting Program, reports of harmful errors in the literature, studies that identify the drugs most often involved in harmful errors, and input from practitioners and safety experts, ISMP created and periodically updates a list of potential high-alert medications. During May and June 2014, practitioners responded to an ISMP survey designed to identify which medications were most frequently considered high-alert drugs by individuals and organizations. Further, to assure relevance and completeness, the clinical staff at ISMP, members of the ISMP advisory board, and safety experts throughout the US were asked to review the potential list. This list of drugs and drug categories reflects the collective thinking of all who provided input.

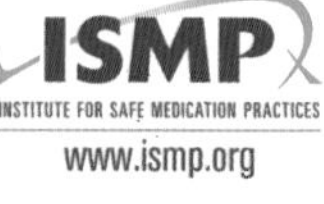

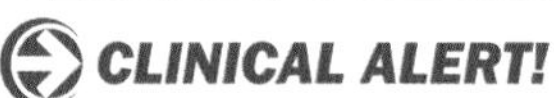

It has been recommended that all high-alert drug calculations and preparations be double-checked independently by a second, licensed person. **Check agency policy for additional required drugs.**

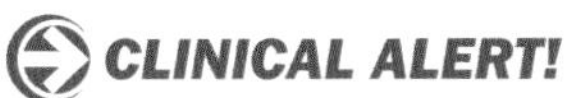

CLINICAL ALERT!

Most ISMP-identified high-alert medications must be administered on infusion pumps (Table 8.1). Check agency policies.

Hospital pharmacies often manage the multiple sources of preprogrammed software information, including drug libraries and types of safe dose parameters of specific medications for specific target populations. These parameters include doses based on age, weight, diagnosis, and other variables, with alerts if the data entered exceed the safe dose limits for the target population. Some smart pumps will alert if the same drug is being infused on another line. All infusions administered and alerts are logged to permit audits as needed.

Answers on page 302

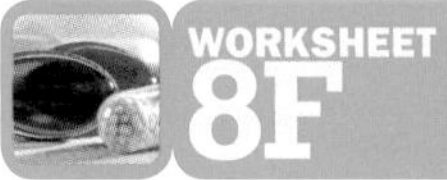

WORKSHEET 8F Advanced IV Flow Rate and Dose Evaluation

Perform the requested calculations. Use a calculator for long division or multiplication. Evaluate flow rates. Refer to ISMP's List of High-Alert Medications.

Example

1. Nitroprusside sodium infusion is ordered at 0.3 mcg per kg per minute IV and is being infused on a patient with hypertension in a pharmacy-prepared solution of 50 mg in 500 mL of D5W. Pharmacy directions instruct to set a flow rate of 12.6 mL an hr for this patient and administer on an IV pump. The patient's weight is 70 kg.

a. Hourly drug order in mcg:	**a.** 0.3 × 70 × 60 = 1260 mcg per hr
b. Hourly drug order in mg:	**b.** 1.26 mg per hr (decimal moved 3 places to left)
c. TD : TV reduced ratio:	**c.** 1:10 (50:500)
d. Hourly flow rate ordered to nearest tenth of a mL:	**d.** 12.6 mL per hr (1 mg:10 mL=1.26 mg:12.6 mL per hr)
e. Is the pharmacy direction correct?	**e.** Yes

2. Azithromycin 500 mg IV is ordered for a patient with pelvic inflammatory disease. Directions state that each 500 mg vial must be reconstituted first with 4.8 mL SW to give 100 mg per mL. Further dilute each 500 mg to 250 mL with D5W or other compatible solutions. Give over 1 hr. The nurse you are replacing on shift has set the flow at 500 mL per hour.
   - **a.** Mg per mL final dilution:
   - **b.** Is flow rate correct?
   - **c.** If not, what should it be?

3. Cefepime HCl 1 g is ordered IV q12h for a patient with severe pneumonia. Supplied is an ADD Vantage vial. 1 g vial to be diluted to 50 mL with NS in an ADD Vantage infusion container. Dose concentrations between 1 mg per mL and 40 mg per mL are acceptable. Current IV drug reference text for intermittent infusions states, "Infuse over 30 minutes."
   a. Mg per mL concentration after dilution:
   b. Is the concentration safe to administer?
   c. Flow rate to administer over 30 minutes:

4. Pantroprazole sodium 40 mg IV infusion once daily for 10 days is ordered for a patient with severe gastroesophageal reflux disease (GERD). A 40-mg dose is reconstituted first with 10 mL NS and further diluted to total volume of 100 mL with D5W and infused over at least 15 minutes, per label instructions. The IV is programmed when you come on duty for 6.7 mL per minute on a pump.
   a. Mg per mL after first dilution:
   b. Mg per mL after final dilution:
   c. Is the IV program approximately correct?
   d. IV flow rate per hr (to the nearest tenth of a mL):

5. Cytoxan* 5 mg per kg IV two times a week is ordered for an adult patient with malignant disease. The patient's weight is 50 kg. The pharmacy has sent a diluted solution of 250 mg in 250 mL NS. This order is to infuse over 90 minutes. When you arrive on duty, the IV is infusing at 100 mL per hr.
   a. Drug order in mg:
   b. TD : TV reduced ratio:
   c. Hr equivalent of 90 min:
   d. Flow rate on pump in tenth of a mL per hr:
   e. Is current infusion rate correct?

   *Nurses need certification to administer this drug.

CLINICAL ALERT!

Patient Safety Issue: Each nurse must refer to manufacturer instructions, current drug references, and personal calculations to protect the patient from prescriber, pharmacy, and prior caretaker IV drug dose errors and/or flow rate errors and ADE or sentinel events.

Beware of programming and mechanical errors with IV pumps.

Answers on page 303

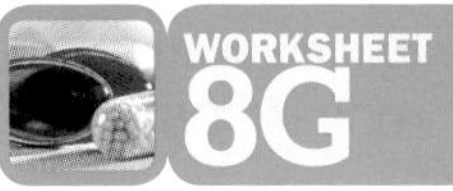

WORKSHEET 8G Critical Care IV Practice

Evaluate the following orders and infusions for safety. Use a calculator to determine kilogram weights to the nearest tenth. Change micrograms to milligrams, when applicable, by moving decimals. Use a calculator to determine the Safe Dose Range (SDR) when needed. Double-check and label all calculations. Prove the hourly flow-rate calculation. If requested, decide whether the order/infusion is:

1. Safe/Correct
2. Unsafe/Incorrect. Consult with provider.

Example **1.** Ordered: Dopamine HCl (Intropin) 4 mcg per kg per minute IV for a 110-lb patient with hypotension. The literature states that the usual dose is 2 to 5 mcg per kg per min. Available: Dopamine 200 mg in 250 mL D5W.

a. Patient's weight in kg: $110 \div 2.2 = 50$

b. SDR per minute: 100 – 250 mcg per minute (2 mcg × 50 kg : 5 mcg × 50 kg)

c. Is the order safe? Yes. 4 mcg × 50 = 200 mcg per minute. 200 mcg per minute is within the SDR

d. Hourly drug order in mcg: 12,000 (200 mcg × 60 minute)

e. Hourly drug order in mg*: 12 (decimal moved 3 places to left)

f. TD : TV reduced ratio: 4 : 5 (200 mg : 250 mL)

g. Hourly flow rate to be set on infusion device: 15 mL per hr (4 : 5 = 12 : x)

$$\frac{4}{5} \times \frac{12}{x}$$

$4x = 60$

$x = 15$ mL per hr

PROOF $4 \times 15 = 60$
$5 \times 12 = 60$

2. Ordered: Dobutamine HCl (Dobutrex) 5 mcg per kg per minute IV for a 132-lb patient in cardiogenic shock. Available: Dobutamine 250 mg in 250 mL D5W. The flow rate is currently infusing at 36 mL per hr.

a. Patient's weight in kg:
b. Hourly drug order in mcg:
c. Hourly drug order in mg*:
d. TD : TV reduced ratio:
e. Hourly flow rate to be set on infusion device:
f. Is current infusion correct?
g. Evaluation and decision:

PROOF

3. Ordered: Lidocaine 4 mg per minute to treat a patient with ventricular tachycardia. Available: 1 g of lidocaine in 500 mL of D5W.

a. TD : TV reduced ratio (mg : mL):
b. Hourly drug ordered:
c. Hourly flow rate to be set on infusion device:
d. Is it safe to give?

PROOF

4. Ordered: Isuprel (isoproterenol hydrochloride) 5 mcg per minute to treat a patient in shock. Available: Isoproterenol hydrochloride 1 mg in 250 mL D5W.

a. TD : TV reduced ratio:
b. Hourly drug ordered in mcg and in mg:
c. TD : TV = HD : HV ratio:
d. Hourly flow rate to be set on infusion device:
e. Is it safe to give?

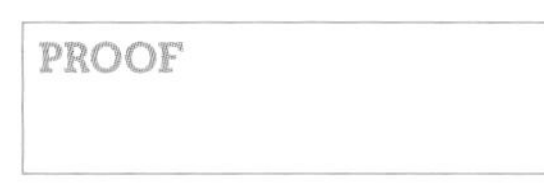

*Because the available drug (250 mg) is in mg, the hourly drug order must also be entered in mg.

5. Conversion: 1000 milliunits = 1 unit

Ordered: Initial dose: oxytocin, a uterine stimulant, 1 milliunit per minute to induce uterine contractions for a patient in labor. On hand: IV of 10 units of oxytocin in 1000 mL D5W. *Titrate* in 30 minutes by additional 1 milliunit per minute until there are two contractions every 10 minutes. Then call for orders and gradually decrease rate. Monitor fetal heart rate and uterine contractions continuously.

a. How many total milliunits of oxytocin are in the IV?
b. How many mL in the IV?
c. How many milliunits per mL?
d. What is ordered dose in milliunits per hr now that the terms are the same?
e. Flow rate in mL per hr on the pump? Is this order safe to give?

The patient needed to have the dose increased 30 minutes later:

f. What would the new dose be in milliunits per minute?
g. How many ordered milliunits per hr needed to infuse?
h. How many mL per hr should be set on the pump?

CLINICAL ALERT!

Document IVs carefully according to hospital policies. Consult the prescriber if the flow rate needs adjustment.

CLINICAL RELEVANCE

Titration orders do not require new methods of calculation. To get the desired response, the ordered dose starts low and the dose is gradually increased or lowered in a series of similar equations.

Example Initial: 0.1 mg per minute. Titrate every 15 minutes by additional 0.1 mg per minute until systolic BP is less than 160. Solution 10 mg in IV 5% DW 250 mL.

The total volume (TV) and the total drug supplied (TD) stay the same. A changed titrated drug order based on patient response is recalculated for a changed hourly dose (HD), which sets up the equation for the new hourly flow rate (HV). If the titrated dose is increased, the HV should increase. If the dose is decreased, the HV should decrease.

Note: If the blood pressure requires another dose, the only *entry* that needs to be recalculated is the hourly drug (HD), based on the increased new dose to be given.

CLINICAL ALERT!

If the supplied medicated IV solution is changed, the entire equation changes and must be recalculated. Assessment for expected responses, potential known side effects, and complications of the varying doses must be done frequently.

Answers on page 304

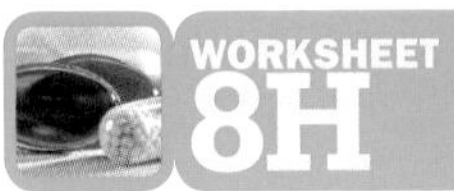

WORKSHEET 8H IV Calculations for Obstetrics

Calculate and evaluate the following orders. Remember that the terms must be the same in your TD : TV = HD : HV ratio and proportion.

Example **1.** Ordered: Magnesium sulfate 2 g to be infused over 60 minutes for a patient with eclampsia infusion IV. Available: Magnesium sulfate 4 g per 250 mL Ringer's lactate solution on an infusion device infusing at 125 mL per hr.

$\left(\frac{4}{250} = \frac{2}{x}\right)$

a. TD : TV = HD : HV — 4 g : 250 mL = 2 g : x mL
b. mL per hr ordered (HV): — $4x = 500$, $x = 125$ mL per hr
c. mL per hr infusing: — 125 mL per hr
d. Evaluation and decision: — Rate is correct.

PROOF $4 \times 125 = 500$
$250 \times 2 = 500$

2. Ordered: Stadol (butorphanol tartrate) 1 mg slow IV push to reduce pain in a patient with a full-term pregnancy in early labor. Available is a Stadol ampule 2 mg per mL. Directions state to deliver the medication over 3 to 5 minutes. It may be repeated every 4 hours prn pain but *not* within 4 hours of anticipated delivery. To give it slowly, the nurse adds 3.5 mL of sterile 0.9% NaCl solution preservative free in a 5- or 10-mL syringe and plans to deliver it in a vascular access device over 4 minutes. Monitor mental status, BP, and respirations.

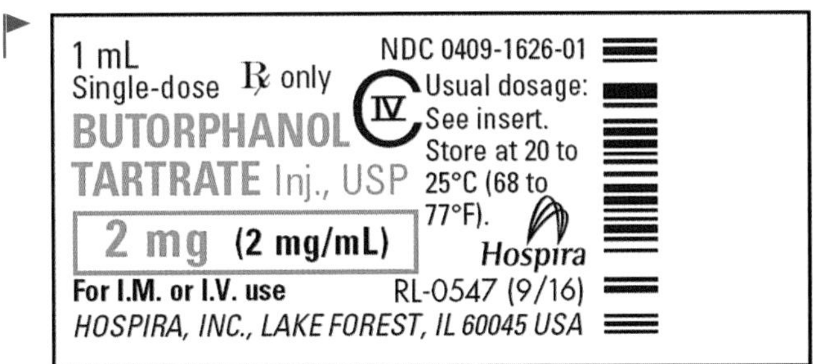

a. How many total mL will there be in the syringe? Mark total amount of mLs on syringe above.
b. At how many mL per minute will the medication be administered?
c. How many seconds per calibration should the nurse count in order to push each mL at a fairly even rate?

Note: It is difficult to give 1 mL evenly over 1 minute. It is better to count the seconds for each calibration.

3. Ordered: Magnesium sulfate 25 mL per hr for a patient with eclampsia. Call the doctor when 2 g have been infused. Available: 500 mL D5W with 20 g of magnesium sulfate on infusion device.
   a. TD (g) : TV reduced ratio:
   b. TD : TV = HD : HV (existing infusion):
   c. g per hr ordered at 25 mL per hr:
   d. Length of time 2 g to be infused:

PROOF

4. Ordered: Pitocin (oxytocin) 2 milliunits per minute. Available: 10 units Pitocin in 1000 mL of D5NS.
   a. milliunits per mL of Pitocin in IV container:
   b. TD : TV reduced ratio:
   c. Hourly drug ordered:
   d. TD : TV = HD : HV ratio:
   e. Flow rate on infusion device to be set:

PROOF

Answers on page 304

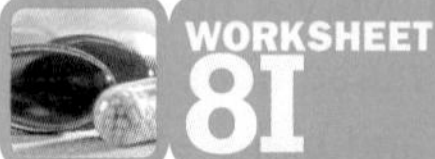

WORKSHEET 8I Multiple-Choice Practice

1. Ordered: Isoproterenol at 5 mcg per minute. How many mg per hr would be infused?
   a. 0.5 mg
   b. 50 mg
   c. 0.3 mg
   d. 300 mg

2. Available 2 g of lidocaine in 500 mL of D5W. What is the mg per mL ratio?
   a. 4 : 1
   b. 2 : 1
   c. 1 : 4
   d. 1 : 2

3. Why do the ISMP-identified High-Alert Medications need special attention?
   a. They can result in significant harm if given in error because they are powerful drugs.
   b. They are new drugs on the market and the manufacturers need feedback.
   c. They are expensive medications and must not be wasted.
   d. They are in clinical testing and can only be given to those patients who have signed up to be part of the study

4. Which diluent is isotonic and often (but not always) specified for intravenous medication IVP dilutions?
   a. 0.9% sodium chloride (NaCl) solution
   b. 0.9% bacteriostatic (NaCl) solution
   c. 10% NaCl solution
   d. Bacteriostatic sterile water for injection

5. Ordered: Levophed (norepinephrine bitartrate) IV infusion bolus for a patient with severe hypotension. Titrate every 10 to 15 minutes to maintain blood pressure of 90/60. Initial 0.1 mg per dose to 0.5 mg per dose. The patient's blood pressure is 70/30. Which diluted dose would you give this patient first?
   a. 0.5 mg
   b. 0.4 mg
   c. 0.3 mg
   d. 0.1 mg

CLINICAL ALERT!

Never leave the patient unattended. Monitor the BP continuously. Levophed bitartrate is for IV use. Norepinephrine base is for other routes. A dose of 2 mg of norepinephrine bitartrate is equal to 1 mg of norepinephrine base. They are *not* interchangeable. Recheck labels and orders. Contact the pharmacist if there is a question about the solution provided.

6. What size syringe is recommended for central lines?
   a. 1 mL because it is easier to manipulate
   b. 20 mL because it can deliver higher pressure to the line
   c. 10 mL because the wider barrel delivers lower pressure
   d. 3 mL because they are almost always available

7. What is the main reason for the recommendation to deliver a bolus medication into a vascular access device, such as a port or an existing infusion line?
   a. It avoids the trauma of a separate puncture for direct access to a vein.
   b. It reduces the risk of infection.
   c. It permits quick countermeasures if an adverse reaction occurs.
   d. It is easier to count the rate that is required for the medication IV push delivery.

8. Which statement about bolus, direct IV, and IV push is true?
   a. They are concentrated, and directions for rate vary and are specified.
   b. They need to be given very quickly directly into a vein.
   c. They are used only for emergencies.
   d. They are used to determine peak and trough levels.

9. Which sterile IV solution must be administered with blood?
   a. D5W
   b. Sterile water for injection
   c. Normal saline
   d. Lactated Ringer's solution

10. Ordered: An IV solution at 60 mg per hr on an infusion pump. Available 1 g in 1000 mL D5W. What flow rate should be programmed on the infusion pump?
   a. 30 mL per hr
   b. 60 mL per hr
   c. 100 mL per hr
   d. 120 mL per hr

Analyzing IV Medication Errors for Safe Nurse Practice

IV errors are not infrequent and have the potential to do serious damage because of immediate entry of drugs into circulation. As you review this list of errors, think about preventive methods.

1. Wrong patient
2. Wrong drug
3. Wrong dose
4. Wrong time
5. Wrong route
6. Incorrect reason for administration
7. Failure to conduct preadministration assessment
8. Failure to evaluate patient during or after administration of medication
9. Incompatible mixtures (medications and/or diluents)

10. Piggyback solutions' timing and compatibility errors
11. Infusion volume and rate errors
12. Bolus rate and dilution errors
13. Technique problems and site infections
14. Incorrect or lack of dilution of concentrated solutions
15. Delayed or omitted documentation
16. Lack of nursing experience with assignment
17. Unnoticed side effects
18. Subtle significant patient statements

Notes:

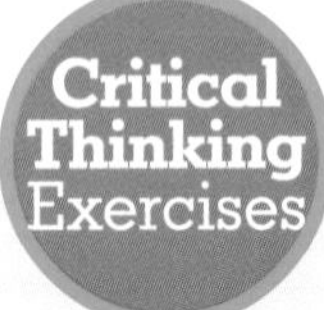

Critical Thinking Exercises provide math and medication-related patient safety issues for student discussion. Answers are not provided.

Analyze the following scenarios.

1. One night during a bedside emergency for a patient with ventricular fibrillation, a provider called for potassium chloride (KCl) 20 mEq to be added to an IV line of D5W and for Amiodarone to be given by direct injection into a second, separate IV line. Pharmacy prepared all KCl known ordered infusions but was closed for the night. The nurse obtained KCl 20 mEq concentrate from a locked cabinet. As the orders were called out, one nurse prepared the medications and handed them to the nurse who was assisting, who then administered the medications. At one point, the nurse was handed two syringes of medication. She was told that one was Amiodarone and that the other syringe contained KCl 20 mEq. The KCl was administered undiluted to the patient by direct IV injection, and the Amiodarone was placed in D5W. Refer to current drug reference for preparation of KCl IV and complications if given undiluted.

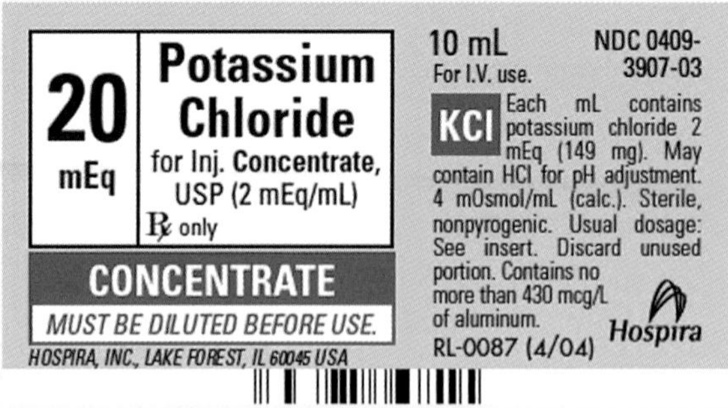

Error(s):

Causes of error(s):

Potential injuries:

Nursing actions:

Preventive measures:

2. A patient in the ICU weighing 60 kg was to receive an IV infusion of Dobutrex ordered to start at 3 mcg per kg per min. The nurse programmed the IV pump to infuse at 3 mg per kg per minute.

Error(s):

Amount of error:

Causes of error(s):

Potential injuries:

Nursing interventions:

Recommendations for the patient safety committee to prevent this type of error:

3. A patient was admitted with seizures. Phenobarbital 130 mg IV injection stat at 65 mg per minute was ordered. The nurse diluted the medication in 3 mL of sterile water for injection. It was administered over 1 minute.

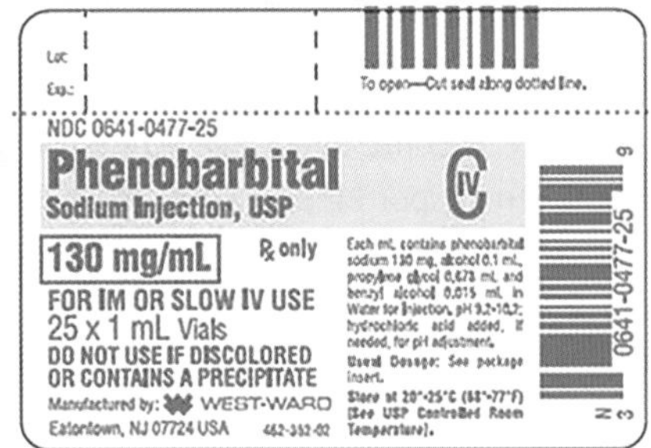

Error:

Cause(s) of error:

Potential adverse drug event(s) (ADE):
(Refer to side effects of phenobarbital IV in current IV drug reference)

Nursing interventions and antidotes needed:
(Refer to current IV drug reference)

Recommendations for the patient safety committee to prevent this type of error:

Answers on page 305

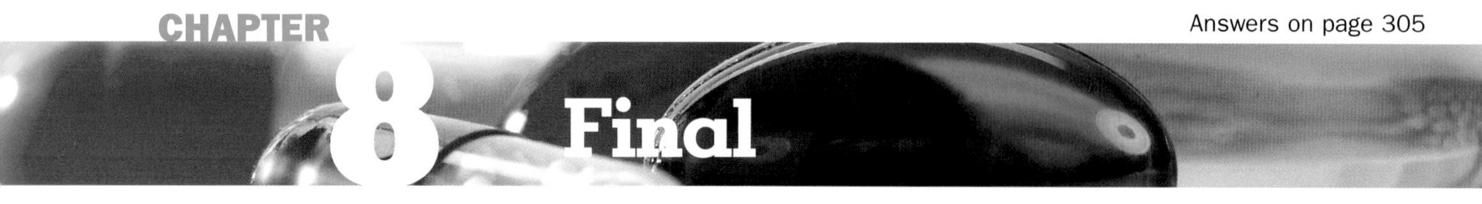

Solve the following problems by using a calculator, moving decimals, reducing ratios, and labeling your answers. Prove your work.

Make a decision:

A. Safe to give **B. Unsafe; consult with provider**

1. Ordered: Dobutamine HCl IV infusion 5 mcg per kg per min. Available: Dobutamine HCl 2000 mcg/mL in an infusion device. Patient's weight is 50 kg.
- **a.** mcg/hr needed:
- **b.** Flow rate to be set on IV infusion device: ________ hr
- **c.** Decision (Safe/Unsafe):

2. Ordered: Potassium chloride IV infusion 10 mEq to be administered to a 44-lb child with hypokalemia. Administer over 4 hr. Available: D5W 100 mL including 10 mEq KCl prepared by pharmacy. The literature states that the rate should not exceed 3 mEq per kg per 24 hr for a child.
- **a.** Patient's weight in kg:
- **b.** SDR for this child per 24 hr:
- **c.** Total drug ordered:
- **d.** Decision (Safe/Unsafe):
- **e.** Amount of drug in mL in IV (refer to label for mEq per mL):
- **f.** Hourly flow rate on infusion device in mL:

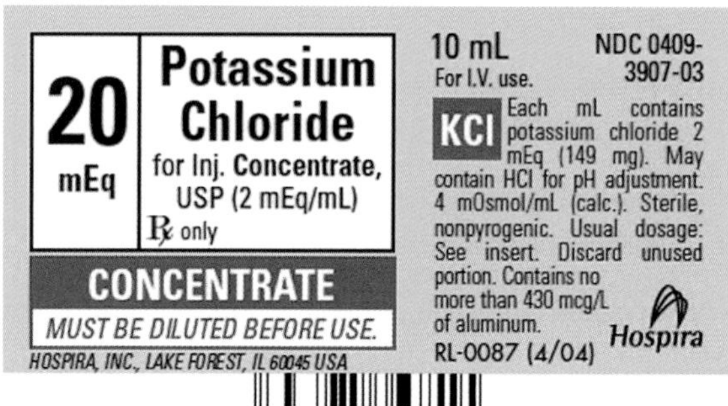

3. Ordered: An IV of Adrenalin (epinephrine) of 1 mg in 250 mL to be infused at 1 mcg per minute. The IV is infusing at 15 mL per hr for a patient in shock.
- **a.** Total drug amount in the solution in mcg (TD):
- **b.** Total volume of the solution (TV):
- **c.** TD : TV ratio:
- **d.** Hourly drug (HD) order in mcg:?:
- **e.** mL per hour needed for order?
- **f.** Is the existing hourly mL (HV) correct for the order?
- **g.** Decision (Safe/Unsafe):

4. Ordered: Dopamine IV at 4 mcg per kg per min for a patient in septic shock who weighs 110 lb today. The SDR is 2 to 10 mcg per kg per min. The IV is flowing at 15 mL per hr when you enter the room.
- **a.** Patient's weight in kg:
- **b.** SDR for this patient:
- **c.** Ordered drug rate per min:
- **d.** Decision (Safe/Unsafe):

e. TD : TV ratio:
f. mg per hr of drug ordered:
g. Hourly flow rate needed:
h. Decision (Safe/Unsafe):

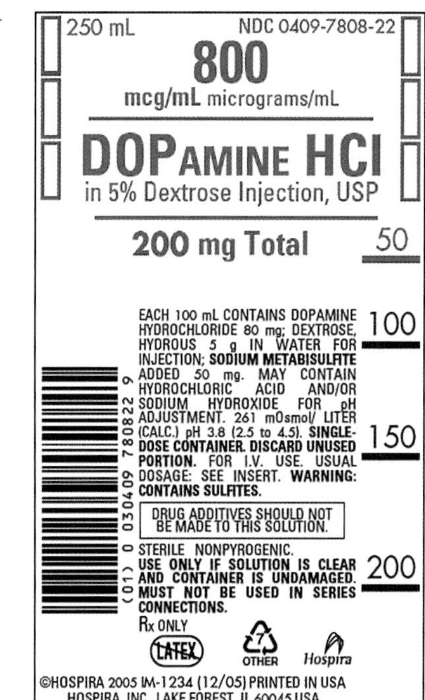

5. Ordered: Dilaudid (hydromorphone HCl) 3 mg IV injection for a patient with severe pain. Directions state it may be given undiluted slowly or diluted up to 5 mL with SW or NS to facilitate titration. It may be administered over 2 to 5 minutes slowly. The nurse dilutes it to 3 mL and plans to administer it over 3 minutes.*

a. Total amount of Dilaudid to be prepared (in mL, round to nearest tenth):
b. Total amount of diluted volume to be administered in mL:
c. Total number of minutes for injection:
d. Amount in mL per minute to be administered:
e. Shade amount on syringe.
f. Decision (Safe/Unsafe):

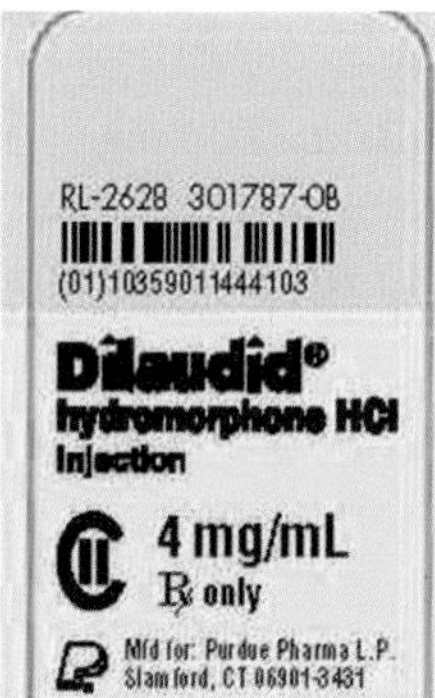

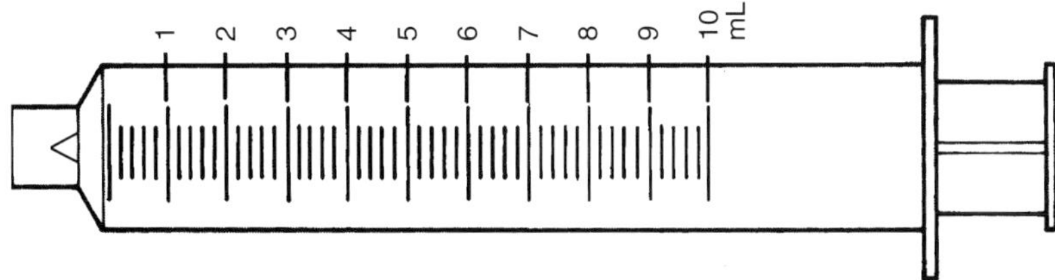

CLINICAL ALERT!

*When small amounts of medication are ordered, dilution makes it easier to control the rate of injection. This nurse wants to administer 1 mL per minute for ease of administration. There were other options. Always read the directions for dilution and rate of administration. If the patient begins to have side effects, the medication will be withdrawn. It is safer and always preferable to inject into an existing IV port or line so that side effects can be countered quickly when necessary.

Refer to the Advanced Calculation section of Drug Calculations Companion, version 5 on Evolve for additional practice problems.

Answer Key

8 Advanced Intravenous Calculations

WORKSHEET 8A (page 280)

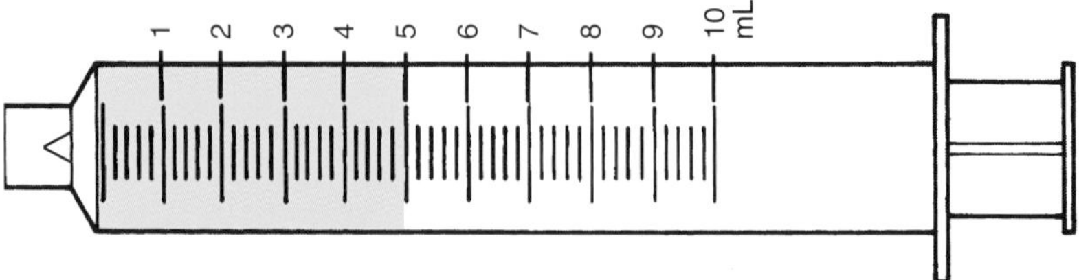

1. a. $5 \times 60 = 300$ sec
$300 \div 25$ lines $= 12$ sec per line
b. 5 mL : 5 min = x mL : 1 minute
$5x = 5$
$x = 1$ mL per minute

2. a. 250 mcg : 1 mL = 500 mcg : x mL
($x = 2$ mL)
b. 10 minutes
c. 2 mL : 10 minutes = x mL : 1 minute
$x = 0.2$ mL per minute
d. 1 minute per line ($10 \div 10$)

3. a. 100 mg : 1 mL = 900 mg : x mL
($x = 9$ mL)
b. 50 mg : 1 minute = 900 mg : x minute
$5\cancel{0}x = 90\cancel{0}$
$x = 18$ minutes
c. 9 mL : 18 minutes = x mL : 1 minute
$18x = 9$
$x = 0.5$ mL per minute

4. a. 10 mg : 1 mL = 20 mg : x mL
($x = 2$ mL)
b. $2 \times 60 = 120$ sec
c. $120 \div 10 = 12$ sec per line
d. 2 mL : 2 minute = x mL : 1 minute
$2x = 2$
$x = 1$ mL per minute

5. a. 5 mL
b. 5 minutes
c. 5 mL : 5 minutes = x mL : 1 minute
$5x = 5$
$x = 1$ mL per minute

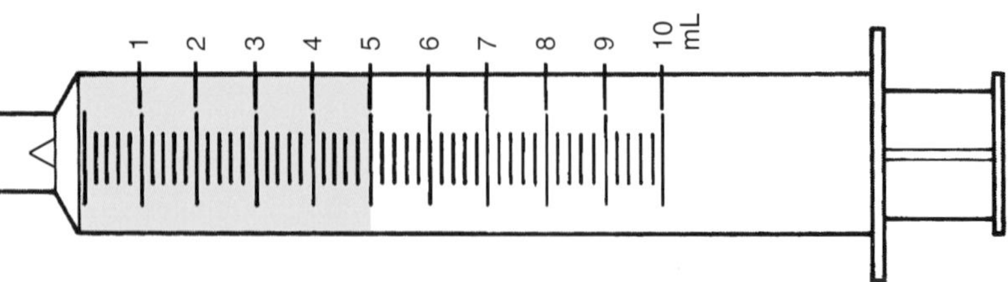

WORKSHEET 8B (page 283)

1. b. 1 : 1
c. 1 : 10
d. 1 : 2
e. 1 : 2

2. b. $x = 30$ mL per hr (1 : 1 = 30 : 30)
c. $x = 50$ mL per hr (1 : 10 = 5 : 50)
d. $x = 6$ mL per hr (1 : 2 = 3 : 6)
e. $x = 5$ mL per hr (2 : 1 = 10 : 5)

3. **b.** (2 : 1 = 12 : 6) 12 mg per hr
   c. (1 : 2 = 9 : 18) 9 mg per hr
   d. (4 : 10 = 4 : 10) 4 mg per hr
   e. (2 : 1 = 36 : 18) 36 mg per hr

4. **a.** 2 × 60 = 120 mcg per hr
   b. 10 × 50 = 500 mg per hr
   c. $\frac{120}{2.2} = 54.5$ kg
   0.5 × 54.5 = 27.3 mcg per hr
   d. 1.5 × 68 = 102 mg per hr
   e. 6 × 60 = 360 mcg per hr

5. **b.** (1 : 1 = 9 : 9) 9 mL per hr
   c. (2 : 1 = 20 : 10) 10 mL per hr
   d. (1 : 2 = 15 : 30) 30 mL per hr
   e. (8 : 5 = 8 : 5) 5 mL per hr

WORKSHEET **8C** (page 285)

1. 2000 mcg per minute (2 × 1000); 120,000 mcg per hr (2000 × 60); 120 mg per hr
2. 0.3 mg per minute (300 ÷ 1000); (0.3 × 60) 18 mg per hr
3. 16 mg per minute (0.2 × 80) 960 mg per hr (16 × 60)
4. 5 mcg × 80 kg ÷ 1000 = 0.4 mg per minute; 0.4 mg × 60 minutes = 24 mg per hr
5. 10 milliunits per minute (600 ÷ 60 = 10)
6. 100 mcg per hr (0.1 × 1000)
7. 0.167 mg rounded to 0.17 mg per minute (10 ÷ 60)
8. 1.25 mg per kg per hr (100 mg ÷ 80 kg = 1.25 mg per kg)
9. 41.66 rounded to 41.7 mcg per minute (2.5 × 1000 ÷ 60)
10. 50 milliunits per minute (3 × 1000 ÷ 60)

WORKSHEET **8D** (page 285)

		mg per hour	mcg per hr	mg per min	mcg per min
1.	**a.**	0.050	50	0.050 ÷ 60 = 0.0008	0.8
	b.	24	24,000	0.4	400
	c.	30	30,000	0.5	500
	d.	1.2	1200	0.02	20
	e.	7.5	7500	0.125	125

		kg	mg per hr	mg per kg per min	mcg per kg per min
2.	**a.**	85	25	25 ÷ 85 ÷ 60 = 0.005	5
	b.	70	10 × 70 × 60 = 42,000*	10	10,000
	c.	62	0.37	0.0001	0.1
	d.	55	75	0.02	20
	e.	48	144	0.05	50

*4.2 g per hour.

		IV Contents	TD : TV Reduced Ratio	HD (mg per hr)	HV (mL per hr)	mg per mL
3.	**a.**	500 mg/1000 mL	1 : 2	5	10	0.5
	b.	250 mg/500 mL	1 : 2	15	30	0.5
	c.	400 mg/250 mL	8 : 5	24	15	1.6
	d.	500 mg/500 mL	1 : 1	75	75	1
	e.	500 mg/250 mL	2 : 1	16	8	2

WORKSHEET **8E** (page 286)

2. a. 1 : 2 = x mg : 15 mL (x = 7.5 mg per hr)

PROOF

1 × 15 = 15

2 × 7.5 = 15

b. 7.5 mg × 1000 = 7500 mcg per hr

c. 7500 mcg ÷ 60 = 125 mcg per minute

d. 125 mcg per minute ÷ 50 kg = 2.5 mcg per kg per minute

3. a. 2 : 5 = x mg : 5 mL (x = 2 mg per hr)

PROOF

2 × 5 = 10

5 × 2 = 10

b. 2 mg per hr × 1000 = 2000 mcg per hr

c. 2000 mcg per hr ÷ 60 = 33.3 mcg per minute

d. 33.3 mcg per minute ÷ 55 kg = 0.605 or 0.6 mcg per kg per minute

4. a. 4 : 1 = x mg per hr : 10 mL per hr (x = 40 mg)

PROOF

4 × 10 = 40

1 × 40 = 40

b. 40 × 1000 = 40,000 mcg per hr

c. 40,000 mcg ÷ 60 = 667 mcg per minute

d. 667 mcg per minute ÷ 60 kg = 11.1 mcg per kg per minute

5. a. 2 : 1 = x mg : 8 mL per hr (x = 16 mg per hr)

PROOF

2 × 8 = 16

1 × 16 = 16

b. 16 mg × 1000 = 16,000 mcg per hr

c. 16,000 mcg per hr ÷ 60 = 266.7 mcg per minute

d. 266.7 mcg per minute ÷ 79.5 kg = 3.4 mcg per kg per minute

WORKSHEET **8F** (page 289)

2. a. 2 mg per mL (500 mg : 250 mL) = 2 : 1 ratio

b. No.

c. 250 mL per hr*

TD		TV		HD		HV
500 mg	:	250 mL	=	500 mg	:	250 mL
2	:	1	=	2	:	1

3. a. 20 mg per mL (1000 mg : 50 mL = 20 mg : 1 mL

PROOF: 1000 × 1 = 1000; 50 × 20 = 1000

b. Yes. Safe.

c. 100 mL per hr (50 mL : 30 minute = x mL : 60 minute)

PROOF: 50 × 60 = 3000

30 × 100 = 3000

4. a. 4 mg per mL (40 mg : 10 mL = x mg : 1 mL)

PROOF: 40 × 1 = 40; 10 × 4 = 40

b. 0.4 mg per mL (40 mg : 100 mL = x mg : 1 mL)

PROOF: 40 × 1 = 40; 100 × 0.4 = 40

c. Yes. (0.4 mg × 6.7 mL per minute × 15 minute = 40.2 mg total dose infused per label instructions)

d. 402 mL per hr (6.7 mg per minute × 60 min) or approximately 100.5 mL in 15 minutes

Recheck high-rate calculations and check with pharmacy if needed.

5. a. 250 mg (5 mg × 50 kg)

b. 1 : 1 (250 mg : 250 mL)

c. 1.5 hr (60 minute : 1 hr = 90 minute : 1.5 hr)

PROOF: 60 × 1.5 = 90; 1 × 90 = 90

d. 166.6 mL per hr (250 mL : 1.5 hr = x mL : 1 hr)

PROOF: 250 × 1 = 250; 166.6 × 1.5 = 249.9 rounded to approximately 250

e. Current rate is too slow. Assess patient; contact provider promptly for appropriate rate change if any. Report and document assessment, provider order and nurse action. Perform frequent follow-up assessments.

*Recheck the 250 mL per hr rate with current IV drug reference and pharmacist. It is very rapid but may be indicated for this patient.

Note: Doses are safe unless noted as UNSAFE in the answers for 8G

WORKSHEET **8G** (page 291)

2. a. 60 (132 ÷ 2.2)
b. 300 mcg per minute × 60 = 18,000 mcg per hr
c. 18 mg per hr (decimal moved 3 places to left)
d. 250 : 250 = 1 : 1
e. 18 mL per hr (1 : 1 = 18 : *x*)
PROOF
1 × 18 = 18
1 × 18 = 18
f. Incorrect flow rate. Should be 18 mL per hr, not 36 mL per hr.
g. Unsafe. Assess patient's vital signs, report per hospital policy, and contact provider for orders.

3. a. 1000 mg : 500 mL = 2 mg : 1 mL
b. 4 mg × 60 = 240 mg per hr
c. 2 : 1 = 240 : *x* = 120 mL per hr
PROOF
2 × 120 = 240
1 × 240 = 240
d. Safe/correct.

4. a. 1 mg : 250 mL
b. 5 mcg × 60 = 300 mcg per hr or 0.3 mg per hr
c. 1 : 250 mL = 0.3 mg : *x* mL
d. 0.3 × 250 = 75.0 mL per hr
PROOF
1 × 75 = 75
0.3 × 250 = 75
e. Safe/correct.

5. a. 10 units = 10,000 milliunits
1000 milliunits = 1 unit
b. 1000 mL
c. 10 milliunits per 1 mL (10,000 milliunits per 1000 mL)
d. 60 milliunits per hour (1 milliunit per minute × 60 minutes)
HAVE WANT TO HAVE
TD : TV = HD : HV
e. 6 mL per hour 10 milliunits : 1 mL = 60 milliunits : *x* mL
10*x* = 60
x = 6 mL per hour
f. 2 milliunits per minute
g. 120 milliunits per hour (2 milliunits per minute × 60 minutes)
TD : TV = HD : HV
h. 12 mL per hour 10 milliunits : 1 mL = 120 milliunits : *x* mL
10*x* = 120
x = 12 mL per hour

Note: The total drug, total volume did not change. The drug per hour changed. Total Drug : Total Volume is a "staple" of IV dose calculations and verification. When the ratio is reduced, the math becomes very simple. Titrated doses are a series of separate similar problems with a similar setup.

i. Safe/correct adjustment to correctly infusing medication.

WORKSHEET 8H (page 293)

2. a. 4 mL
b. 1 mL per minute (5 calibrations per minute)
c. 1 calibration every 12 seconds

3. a. $2\not{0} : 50\not{0} = 1 : 25$
b. 1 g : 25 mL = x g : 25 mL per hr
PROOF
$1 \times 25 = 25$
$25 \times 1 = 25$
c. $x = 1$ g per hr
d. 2 hr

4. a. 10,~~000~~ milliunits: 1~~000~~ mL
b. 10 milliunits : 1 mL
c. 2 milliunits $\times$ 60 = 120 milliunits per hr
d. $10 : 1 = 120 : x$
PROOF
$10 \times 12 = 120$
$1 \times 120 = 120$
e. $x = 12$ mL per hr

WORKSHEET 8I (page 294)

1. c. Finding mg per mL requires that mg is in the numerator and mL is in the denominator.

2. a. 2 g = 2000 mg to 500 mL. Ratio = 4 : 1

3. a.

4. a.

5. d. 0.1 mg; always start with the lowest dose unless otherwise ordered.

6. c. 10 mL. Smaller syringes need more pressure applied against resistance and can disengage and/or damage the line or blood vessel.

7. c. Side effects show up quickly with intravenous medications. Bolus medications are more concentrated (smaller volume, less dilution) and often are high-alert medications.

8. a. The three names convey speed. Many bolus medications are specified to be given *slowly. Serious ADE have resulted from giving them at the wrong rate.*

9. c. NS is administered with blood unless an order is received for another solution, which the nurse would check. Solutions with dextrose can cause hemolysis (breaking of the blood cells within or outside of the blood vessels). Blood should not be administered with IV products that contain calcium such as Lactated Ringer's. Checking any 2 or more IV mixtures for compatibility is critical for patient safety.

10. b. 60 mL per hr. The total drug, total volume is 1 g, or 1000 mg, and 1000 mL, a 1 : 1 ratio. Therefore the mL rate = mg amount.

CHAPTER 8 FINAL: ADVANCED INTRAVENOUS CALCULATIONS (page 298)

1. a. 15,000 mcg (5 mcg × 50 kg × 60 min)
b. 7.5 mL (2000 mcg : 1 mL = 15,000 mcg : *x* mL)
c. Safe

2. a. 20 kg
b. 60 mEq maximum per 24 hours
c. 10 mEq
d. Safe
e. 5 mL
f. 100 ÷ 4 = 25 mL per hr (95 mL D5W plus 5 mL KCl)

3. a. 1000 mcg
b. 250 mL
c. 4 : 1
d. 60 mcg per hour
e. 15 mL per hour $\frac{TD}{TV} = \frac{HD}{HV}$
f. Yes
Both drug measurements had to be in mcg or mg. The volume is always in mL.
g. Safe

4. a. 50 kg
b. 100 to 500 mcg per minute (2 to 10 mcg per kg per minute)
c. 200 mcg per minute (4 mcg per kg per minute)
d. Safe
e. 4 : 5 (200 mg : 250 mL)
f. 12 mg per hr (4 mcg × 50 kg × 60 minutes) ÷ 1000
g. TD TV HD HV
4 : 5 = 12 : *x* (*x* = 15 mL per hr)
h. Correct

5. a. 0.8 mL prepared in 1-mL syringe
b. 3 mL
c. 3 min
d. 1 mL per minute
e.

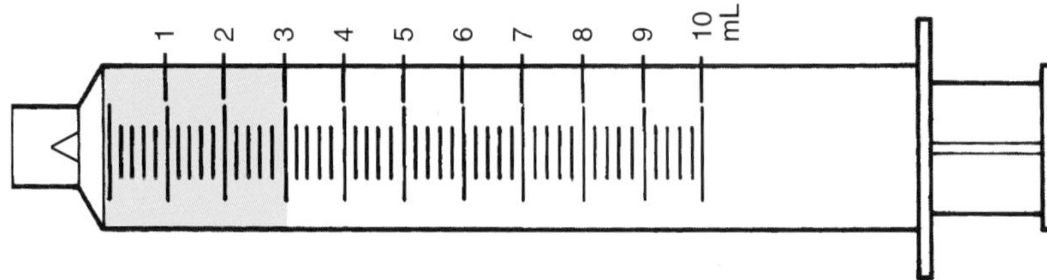

f. Safe

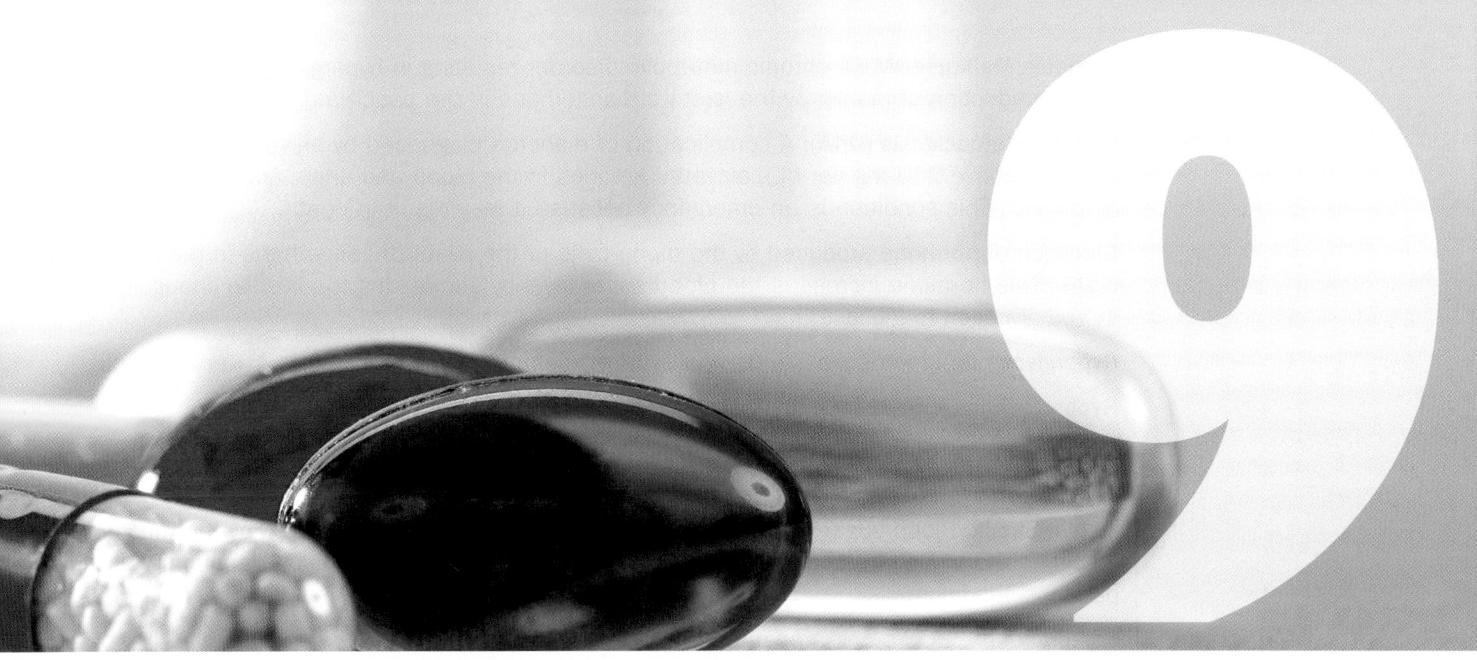

Insulin Administration and Type 2 Diabetes Medications

Objectives

- Identify appropriate sites for insulin injections.
- Identify the different types of insulin labels.
- Compare the actions of fast-, intermediate-, and long-acting insulins.
- Read calibrations on 30-, 50-, and 100-unit insulin syringes.
- Correctly prepare single- and mixed-dose insulin injections.
- Calculate units of insulin based on grams of carbohydrates or CHO.
- Interpret the sliding scale using the BMBS method.
- Use electronic intravenous devices to administer insulin dosages.
- Calculate insulin dosage as ordered for units per hr and mL per hr and duration.
- Analyze insulin and type 2 diabetes medication errors using critical thinking.

Introduction

According to the USP and the ISMP, insulin is the drug most commonly involved with medication errors. Insulin has been given as an overdose or confused with other unit-measured medications such as heparin. The importance of measuring the correct amount of insulin is vital. Different types of insulin syringes are shown for the practice of selecting the most appropriate syringe for the ordered dose. Mixing two types of insulin in one syringe is shown in drawings. The bedside monitor blood sugar (BMBS) flow sheet shows how to use the sliding scale to chart hourly insulin needs. IV infusions are calculated for units per hour based on the BS level.

Vocabulary

Basal Rate: Based on carbohydrate intake, weight, and exercise, A low continuous dose of insulin units needed to cover the glucose output of the liver.

BSL: Blood sugar level; measures the sugar level in blood.

Bolus Dose: A rapid-acting insulin injection to keep the blood sugar level under control following a meal or if the blood sugar level is too high.

Diabetes Mellitus (DM): A chronic metabolic disorder resulting in hyperglycemia due to inadequate production of insulin by the islets of Langerhans in the pancreas.

Diabetic Ketoacidosis (DKA): A complication of diabetes diagnosed by elevated blood sugar/glucose (above 250 mg per dL), elevated ketones in the blood and urine, and a blood pH below 7.3. This condition is an emergency because it may result in death.

Glucagon: A hormone produced by the alpha cells of the islets of Langerhans in the pancreas. This hormone increases the blood sugar level by stimulating the liver to change stored glycogen to glucose.

Hyperglycemia: Blood sugar levels above the basic normal values of 70 to 100 mg per dL.

Hypoglycemia: A decreased level of blood sugar (below 70 mg per dL).

Incretin Mimetics: A group of metabolic hormones that potentiate insulin release from the islets of Langerhans in the pancreas.

Insulin Shock: Blood sugar level below 60 mg per dL (hypoglycemia) caused by too much insulin in the blood. Treated by giving sugar orally or glucose intravenously, depending on the patient's condition.

Postprandial: Blood sugar measurement taken after a meal.

Preprandial: Blood sugar measurement taken before a meal.

Type 1 DM: Failure of the pancreas to produce insulin.

Type 2 DM: Insulin resistance or inadequate insulin secretion due to a decrease in sensitivity of muscle cells to uptake or recognize insulin.

Insulin

Insulin is an aqueous solution of the principal hormone of the pancreas. Insulin affects metabolism by allowing glucose to leave the blood and enter the body cells, preventing hyperglycemia or hypoglycemia.

Diabetes Mellitus

Diabetes mellitus (DM) is a deficiency of insulin and is classified according to its cause. Type 1 DM usually affects people before the age of 30 years. The pancreatic cells do not produce insulin. Insulin injections must be taken every day to control the blood glucose level.

The onset of type 2 diabetes usually occurs after 30 years of age; however, obesity has contributed to a rise in the diagnosis of type 2 diabetes in children and young adults. The pancreas produces some insulin but not enough to metabolize the glucose. In some cases, the insulin that is produced is not effective; this is known as insulin resistance. Of people with diabetes, 95% have type 2, and 40% of people with type 2 diabetes take insulin injections in conjunction with oral diabetes medications and the noninsulin incretin and amylin mimetic injections.

The most common complication of insulin therapy is hypoglycemia. This may be caused by injecting too much insulin (a risk in home care), by missing or delaying meals, or by being involved in more physical activity than usual. To treat hypoglycemia, a patient should always carry sugar in some form. The treatment of choice, if the patient can swallow, is glucose tablets (4 to 5 g carbohydrate [CHO] per tablet). Wait 15 minutes to retest the blood glucose. A glucose gel of 15 g is also available for the treatment of hypoglycemia. The glucose gel is to be used if the person cannot swallow but is still conscious. Put gel in the cheek along the gumline and rub vigorously. If the blood glucose level gets very low, unconsciousness may occur. At that point, the patient will need a glucagon injection. Emergency kits are available for home use (Figure 9.1). For patients weighing over 20 kg, use 1 mg. For patients weighing less than 20 kg, use 0.5 mg of glucagon. For unconscious patients, an IV of 50% dextrose solution should be administered.

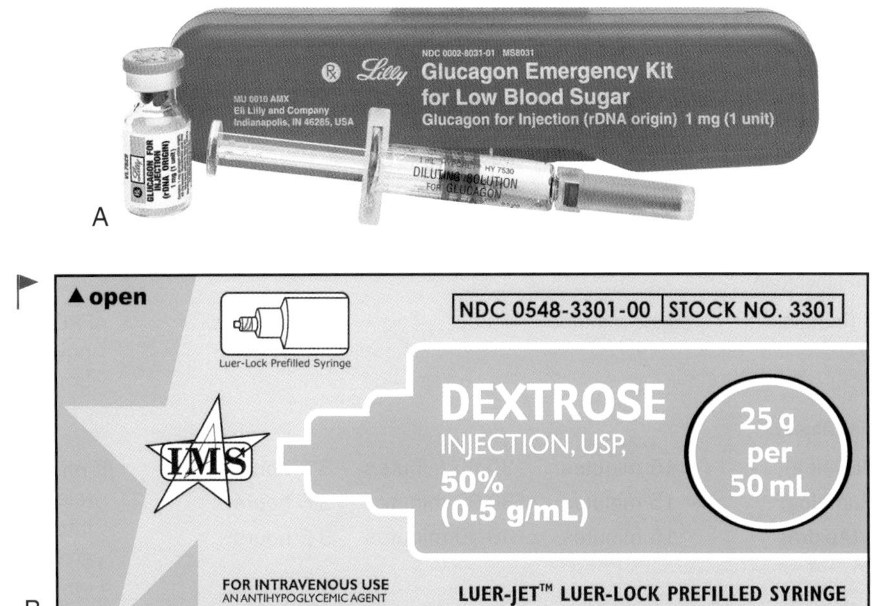

FIGURE 9.1 **A,** Glucagon emergency kit for home use. **B,** Dextrose 50% (**A,** Copyright Eli Lilly and Company. All rights reserved. Used with permission.)

Injection Sites

The abdomen is the preferred site for insulin injections. When insulin injections are required on a daily basis, it is important to rotate within that site to prevent lipodystrophy (Figure 9.2). The abdomen absorbs insulin more rapidly and is safer as an injection site than the upper arm, back, or thigh. If use of the abdomen is medically contraindicated, alternative sites may be used.

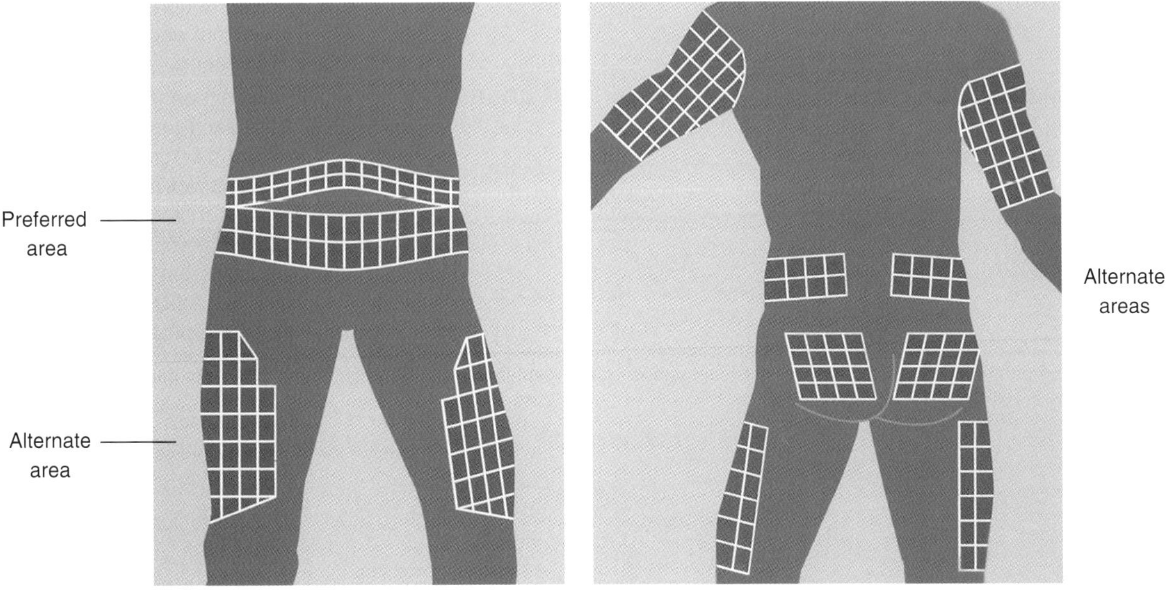

FIGURE 9.2 Insulin injection areas.

U-100 Insulins

Table 9.1 Insulin Comparison Chart

Insulin Name (Trade Name)	When Does It Start Working? (Onset)	When Will the Effect Be the Greatest? (Peak)	How Long Will It Lower Blood Glucose? (Duration)	Notes for Use
Ultra-Rapid Inhalation				
AFREZZA (insulin human)	10-12 minutes	1 hour	2.5-3 hours	AFREZZA® is a rapid-acting inhaled powder and can be taken at meal-time with long-acting insulin.
Rapid Acting Analogs				
Aspart (Novolog)	<15 minutes	30-90 minutes	3-5 hours	If mixing with NPH, rapid-acting insulin (clear formulation) should be drawn into syringe first. Mixture should be given immediately to avoid effects on peak action.
Lispro (Humalog)	<15 minutes	30-90 minutes	3-5 hours	
Glulisine (Apidra)	<15 minutes	30-90 minutes	3-5 hours	
Short Acting				
Regular (Novolin R or Humulin R)	0.5-1 hour	2-4 hours	4-8 hours	If mixing with NPH, short-acting insulin (clear formulation) should be drawn into syringe first. Mixture should be given immediately to avoid effects on peak action.
Intermediate Acting				
NPH (NovoLIN N or HumuLIN N)	1-2 hours	4-10 hours	10-18 hours	Cloudy formulation.
Long Acting Analogs				
Glargine (Lantus)	1-2 hours	No peak	20-24 hours	Do not mix with other insulin formulations. Both Glargine and Detemir are clear formulations.
Detemir (Levemir)	1-2 hours	Relatively flat	Up to 24 hours (dose-dependent)	
Combinations				
NovoLIN 70/30 or HumuLIN 70/30	0.5-1 hour	2-10 hours	10-18 hours	70% NPH +30% regular insulin. Insulin action includes two peaks (one from each formulation). Cloudy formulation.
Novolog Mix 70/30 or Humalog Mix 75/25 or 50/50	<15 minutes	1-2 hours	10-18 hours	Insulin action includes two peaks (one from each formulation). Novolog mix (cloudy formulation): 70% Aspart protamine + 30% Aspart Humalog mix (cloudy formulation): 75/25 = 75% Lispro protamine + 25% Lispro 50/50 = 50% Lispro protamine + 50% Lispro

*All insulin preparations are 100 units per mL except concentrated regular insulin U500 containing 500 units per mL. Onset, peak, and duration may vary considerably in different people.

Table 9.2 Non-Insulin Injectables for Diabetes Management

Generic Name (Brand Name)	Dosing	Action	When to Take
Amylin Mimetics			
Pramlintide acetate (Symlin)	Given subcutaneously. Prefilled pen.	Works with insulin to help maintain normal glucose concentrations. It has three actions: (1) helps control blood glucose levels by reducing the post-meal release of glucose from the liver; (2) slows the absorption of carbohydrate by slowing the rate of stomach emptying; (3) reduces appetite.	Taken with meals or snacks when more than 30 g of carbohydrates are eaten.

GLP-1 Agonist Medications Chart

Generic Name (Brand Name)	Dosing Schedule	Mixing Required	Preinjection Waiting Time	Dosing
Incretin Mimetics				
Exenatide (Byetta)	BID	No	None	5, 10 mcg
Exenatide extended release (Bydureon Kit)	QW	Yes	None	2 mg
Exenatide extended release (Bydureon Pen)	QW	Yes	None	2 mg
Albiglutide (Tanzeum)	QW	Yes	Yes, 15-30 minutes	30, 50 mg
Dulaglutide (Trulicity)	QW	No	None	0.75, 1.5 mg
Liraglutide (Victoza)	QD	No	None	0.6, 1.2, 1.8 mg

CLINICAL RELEVANCE

Humalog, Novolog, and Apidra may be taken 15 minutes before eating and can be mixed with NPH. Afrezza inhalation insulin can be taken 12 to 15 minutes before eating.

Incretin Mimetics for Type 2 Diabetes Mellitus

Incretin is a natural hormone the body makes to signal the release of insulin from the pancreas after eating to lower blood sugar. Incretin mimetics act like or mimic the action of the incretins the body creates to lower blood sugar after eating.

The Action of Incretin Mimetics

- Signals the pancreas to release insulin when blood sugar level rises
- Prevents the pancreas from releasing too much glucose, which would cause the liver to release stored sugar into the bloodstream
- Helps to slow the rate at which the stomach empties, which may reduce hunger and increase feeling satisfied after a meal
- Helps keep blood sugar level in target range without causing low blood sugar or weight gain
- Incretin mimetics may lower hemoglobin A1c by 0.5% to 1%

Insulin Syringes and Pens

Insulin is usually given in a 1-mL or 0.5-mL insulin syringe calibrated to U-100 insulin. The 0.5-mL insulin syringe is used for smaller doses because the calibrations are larger and easier to read.

Types of U-100 Insulin Syringes

Each calibration in the syringe shown in Figure 9.3 represents 1 unit. This syringe is used for small doses of 30 units or less and as a safety feature for people with diabetes who have vision problems (a Magni-Guide may also be useful for those people [Figure 9.4]) or for children who require small doses of insulin. This syringe is for use with U-100 insulin only.

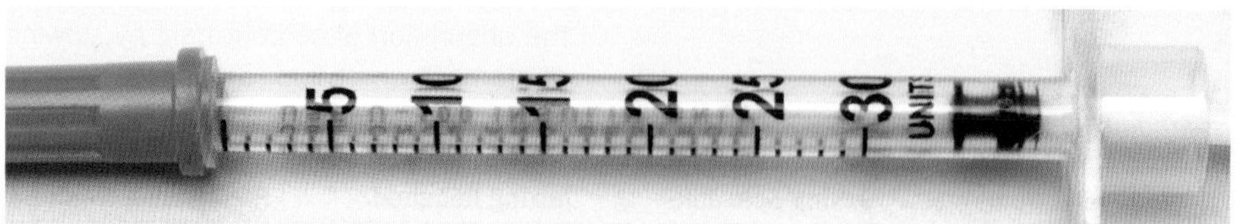

FIGURE 9.3 30-unit syringes.

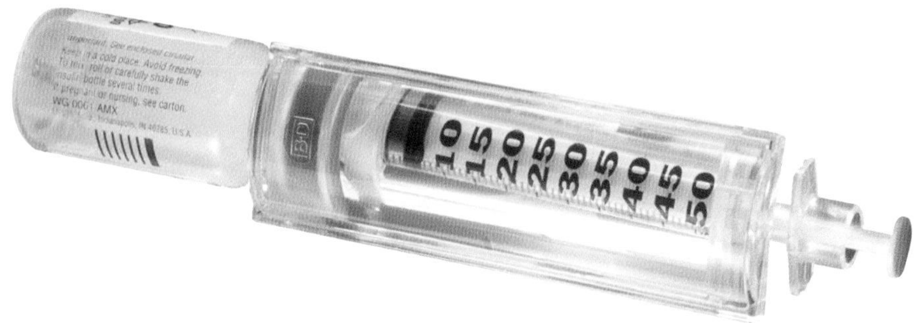

FIGURE 9.4 BD Magni-Guide. (From Becton, Dickinson, and Company, Franklin Lakes, N.J.)

CLINICAL ALERT!

Tuberculin syringes are calibrated in tenths and must never be substituted for insulin syringes, which are calibrated from 1 to 100 units.

CLINICAL RELEVANCE

Loss of vision is a complication of diabetes. U-30 and U-50 syringes have large numbers and are easier to read than the U-100 (1-mL) syringes. Tactile insulin measuring devices such as the Jordan Medical Count-a-Dose enable nonvisual insulin measurement and mixing.

Each calibration in the syringe shown in Figure 9.5 represents 1 unit. This syringe is used for small doses of 50 units or less and is used with U-100 insulin only. Needles are usually 24- to 26-gauge for subcutaneous injections. Clip-on magnifiers for syringes are available to enlarge the calibrations and numbers. The most commonly used insulin syringes are 30-, 50-, and 100-unit syringes.

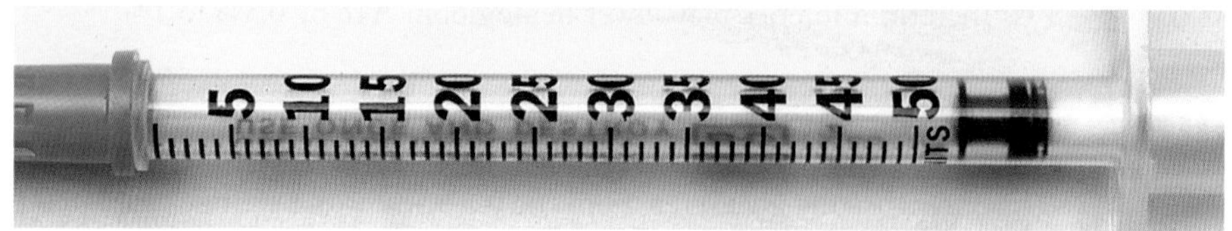

FIGURE 9.5 50-unit syringe.

Each calibration in the syringe shown in Figure 9.6 equals two units. This syringe is for use with U-100 insulin only.

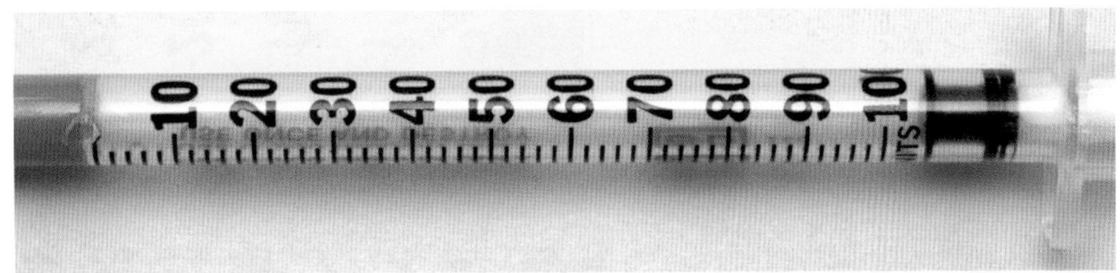

FIGURE 9.6 100-unit syringe.

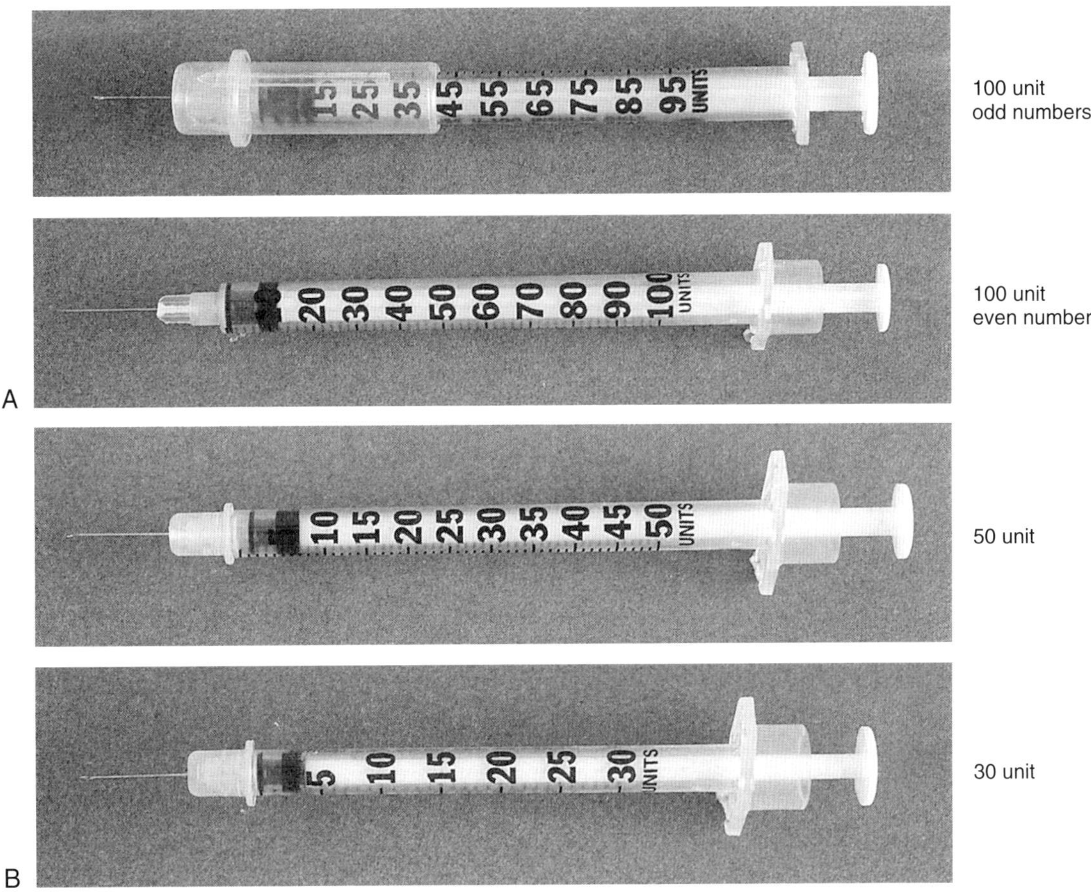

FIGURE 9.7 Insulin syringes. **A,** 100-unit syringes with odd and even numbers. **B,** 50- and 30-unit syringes. (From Becton, Dickinson and Company, Franklin Lakes, N.J.)

Insulin Orders

A typical order for insulin must include the following:

1. The *name* of the insulin: Humulin, Novolin, Lantus.
2. The *type* of the insulin: regular, lispro, aspart, N, detemir, or glargine.
3. The *number* of units or amount the patient will receive: 10 units.
4. The *time* to be given: AM, ½ hr before a meal.
5. The *route* is subcutaneous unless IV is specified.

Example Prepare 30 units of Humulin R insulin subcutaneously ½ hr before a meal. Using a 100-unit syringe, 50-unit syringe, or 30-unit syringe, fill the syringe to the 30 units calibration (Figure 9.8). (All insulins come in U-100, so orders no longer specify U-100.)

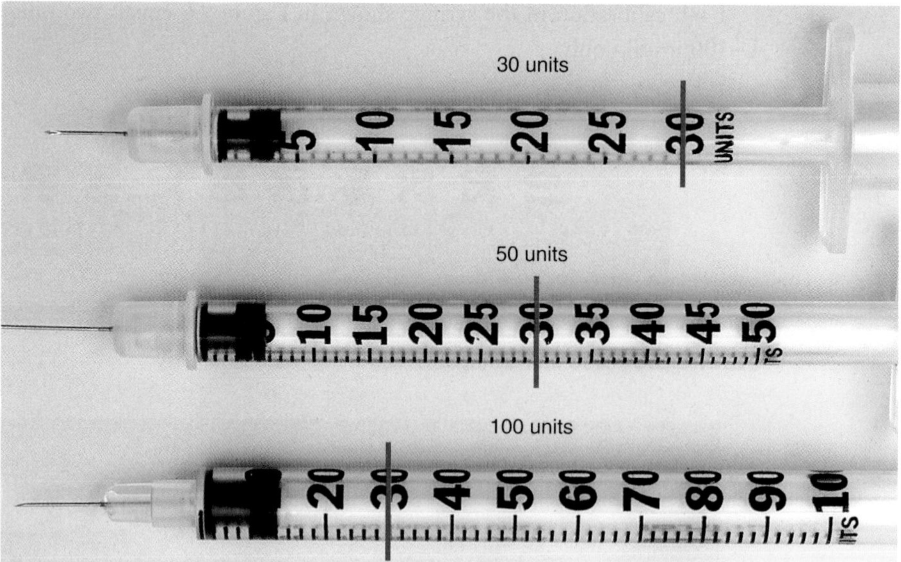

FIGURE 9.8 From left to right: 30 units measured on a 100-unit syringe (each calibration is 2 units), a 50-unit syringe (each calibration is 1 unit), and a 30-unit syringe (each calibration is 1 unit). (From Macklin D, Chernecky C, Infortuna H: *Math for clinical practice,* ed 2, St Louis, 2011, Mosby.)

CLINICAL RELEVANCE

Units must be spelled out (not abbreviated by a U) because abbreviating can be a source of medication errors (e.g., mistaking the U for a zero). Insulin dosages require two licensed nurses to double-check for accuracy.

Dial The prefilled, disposable Victoza pen can be dialed to the prescribed dose.

Dose Once a day, at any time, independent of meals, Victoza can be injected with a 32G Tip (6-mm) needle in the abdomen, thigh, or upper arm.

Types of Insulin

The source of insulin is either human or animal. This is known as the species of the insulin. It is essential to discuss with patients/families religious practices that may prohibit their receiving animal source medications such as porcine insulins. Human insulin is manufactured to be the same as insulin produced by the body. Human insulin is made in one of two ways:

- By recombinant DNA technology, a chemical process used to produce unlimited amounts of human insulin
- By a process that chemically changes animal insulin into human insulin

Humalog insulin (lispro) is recombinant DNA insulin with a rapid action of 5 to 15 minutes, allowing patients to dose and eat. Recombinant DNA insulins cause fewer allergies than those from animal sources.

All insulin is supplied in units denoting strength. Insulin is given via special insulin syringes (Figure 9.9) and pens. Byetta stimulates glucose-dependent insulin from pancreatic beta cells (GLP-1 and GIP) and decreases glucoagon production when glucose levels are elevated. Byetta is not insulin.

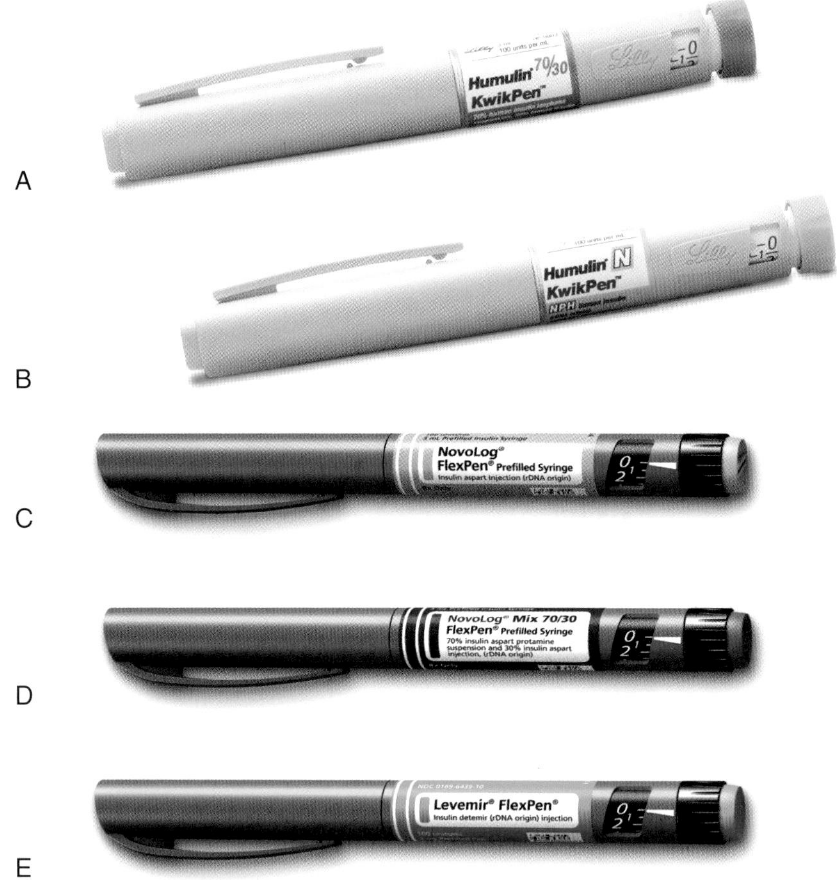

FIGURE 9.9 **A,** Humulin 70/30 short- and intermediate-acting insulins. **B,** Humulin N intermediate-acting insulin. Prefilled insulin pens. **C,** Novolog rapid-acting insulin. **D,** Novolog 70/30 short- and intermediate-acting insulin. **E,** Levemir long-acting insulin. (**A** and **B** Copyright Eli Lilly and Company. All rights reserved. Used with permission. **C-E,** from Novo Nordisk Inc., Princeton, N.J.)

Insulin is sometimes supplied in 10-mL vials labeled U-100, which means there are 100 units per mL (Figure 9.10). Insulin is also supplied in 10-mL vials of U-500, which means there are 500 units per mL. This strength is used for those whose blood glucose levels fluctuate to very high levels. This type of insulin is rarely used and rarely kept on the nursing unit. Table 9.1 lists the duration of activity of various types of insulins and other injectables. See examples of various U-100 insulins below and on the following pages.

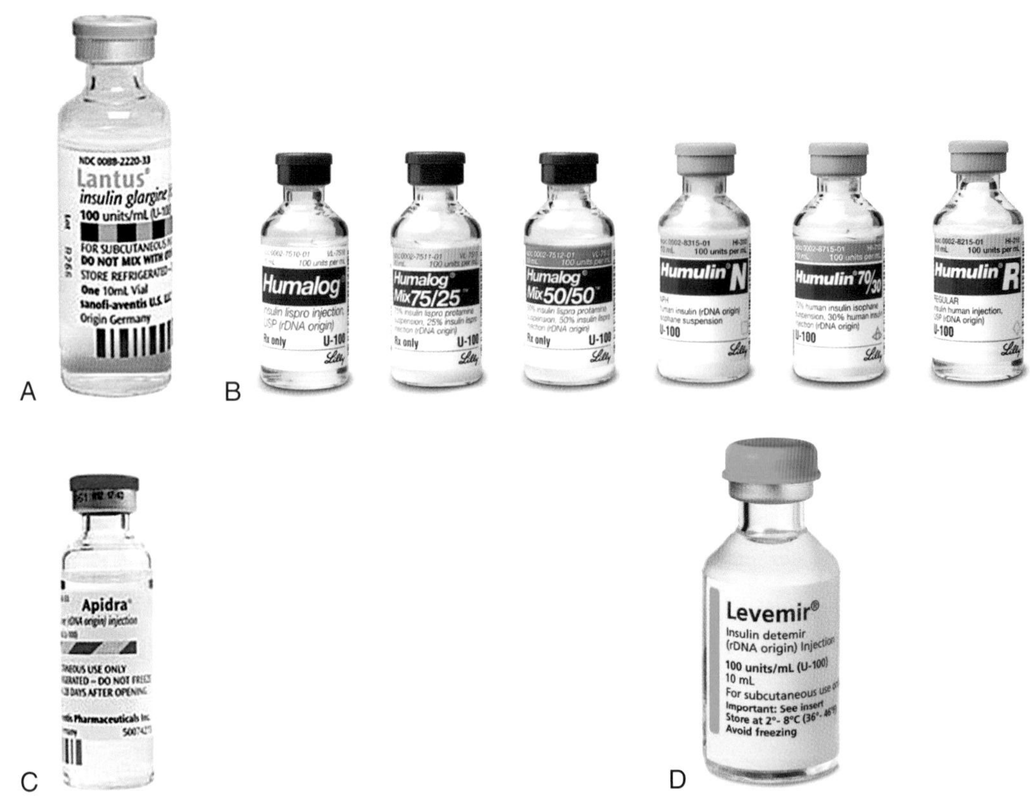

FIGURE 9.10 **A,** Lantus (insulin glargine). The Lantus vial is taller and narrower than the NPH, Regular, and Humalog vials. Lantus is written in purple letters. **B,** Various insulin vials. HUMULIN and HUMALOG are registered trademarks of Eli Lilly and Company. **C,** Rapid-acting Apidra. **D,** Long-acting Levemir. (**A** and **C,** Product images and trademarks are the property of and used with the permission of sanofi-aventis U.S. LLC, Bridgewater, N.J. **B,** Copyright Eli Lilly and Company. All rights reserved. Used with permission. **D** from Novo Nordisk Inc., Princeton, N.J.)

U-100 Insulin Labels

Short-Acting

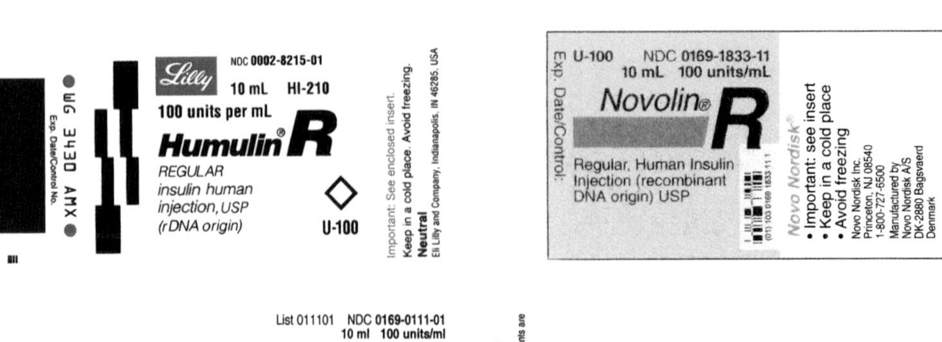

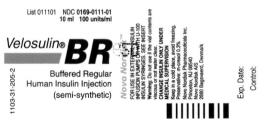

Rapid-Acting

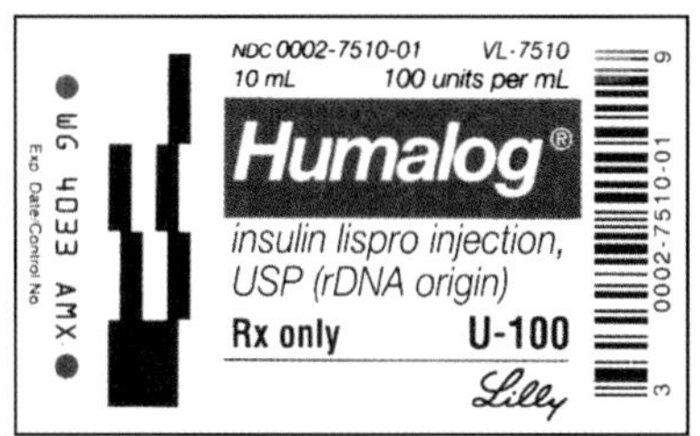

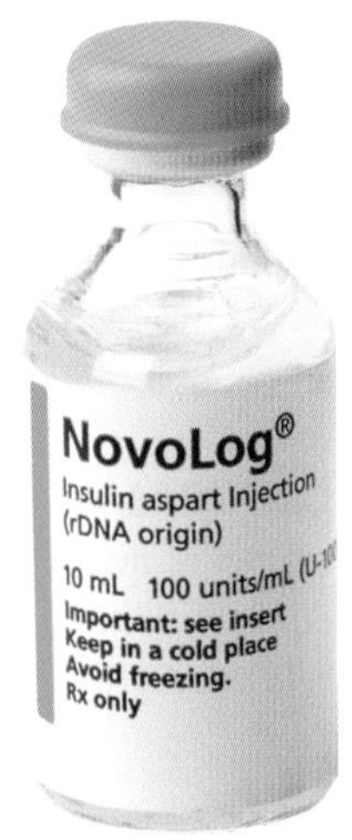

From Novo Nordisk Inc., Princeton, N.J.

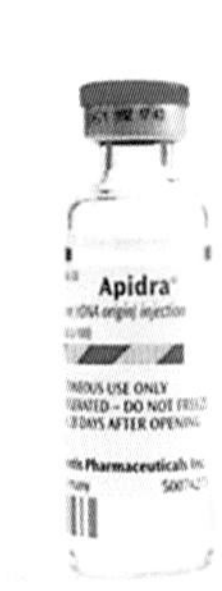

Product images and trademarks are the property of and used with the permission of sanofi-aventis U.S. LLC, Bridgewater, N.J.

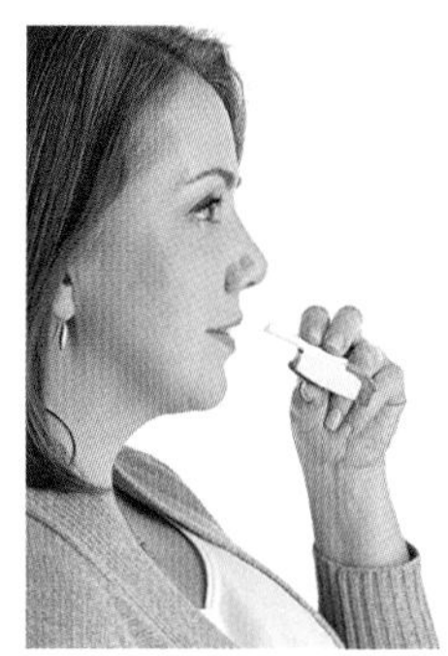

Afrezza® inhaled insulin. From sanofi-aventis U.S. LLC, Bridgewater, N.J.

CLINICAL ALERT!

Fast-acting and regular insulin should always be clear. Discard if unclear.

Mix insulins only with those of the **same name** because they may have differing amounts of preservatives. For example, Humulin R should be combined only with Humulin L or N. Humulin is a brand name.

Intermediate-Acting

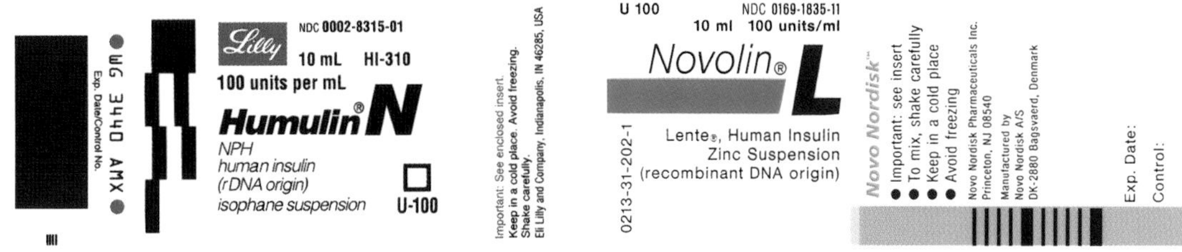

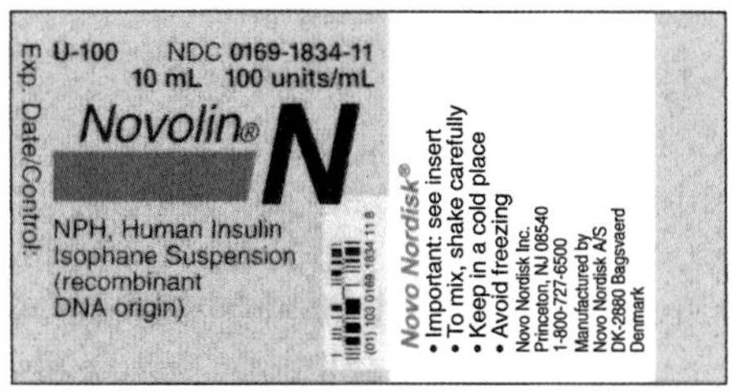

Intermediate- and Rapid-Acting Mixtures

The insulin combination of NPH and Regular is used to give a 24-hour effect.

In 1 mL of Humulin 70/30, there are 70 units of intermediate-acting insulin and 30 units of rapid-acting insulin. In 1 mL of Humulin 50/50, there are 50 units of intermediate-acting insulin and 50 units of rapid-acting insulin. The first number in the combination is always the intermediate-acting insulin. The second number and the smaller amount is rapid-acting insulin.

Note: Mix before administration by rolling *gently* between the palms. Never shake because this creates bubbles in the suspension, decreasing accuracy when withdrawing the insulin.

CLINICAL ALERT!
Insulin is available in various strengths: rapid-acting, regular, intermediate-acting, long-acting, and combinations of rapid- and intermediate-acting. READ LABELS CAREFULLY TO AVOID GIVING THE WRONG STRENGTH.

Long-Acting

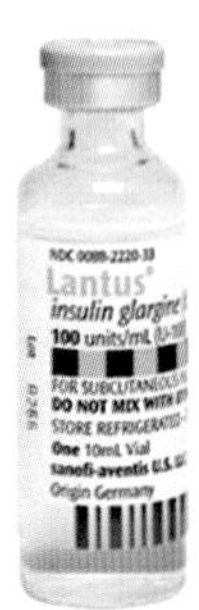

Product images and trademarks are the property of and used with the permission of sanofi-aventis U.S. LLC, Bridgewater, N.J.

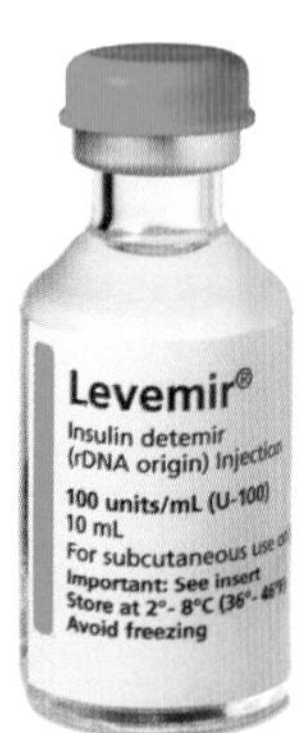

From Novo Nordisk Inc., Princeton, NJ.

CLINICAL ALERT!
Lantus must NOT be mixed in the same syringe with any other insulin or be diluted. It is NOT intended for IV administration. Caution: Lantus is clear like Regular Humalog. Lantus is given anytime for 24-hour coverage without a peak. Consistency in administration is necessary.

Answers on page 348

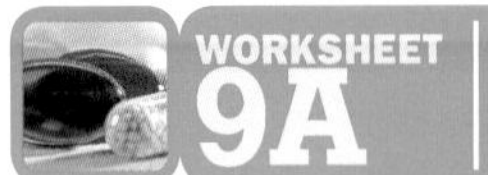

WORKSHEET 9A Single-Dose Measures

Read the syringes and write your answers in the spaces provided.

1. Units measured: __________

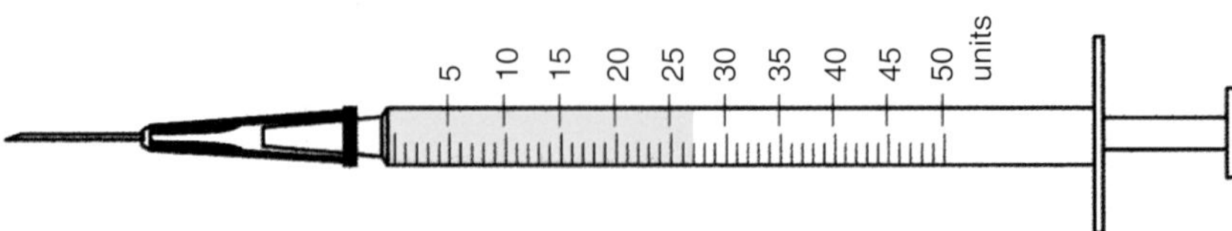

2. Units measured: __________

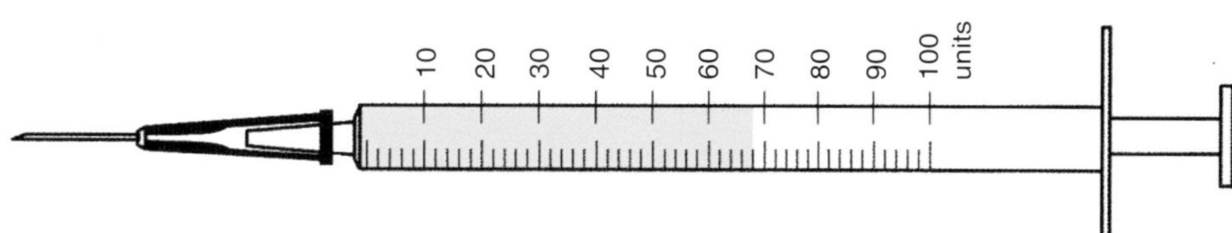

3. Units measured: __________

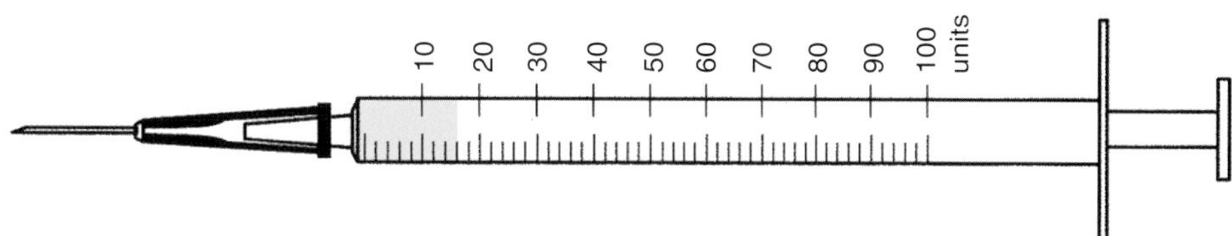

4. Units measured: __________

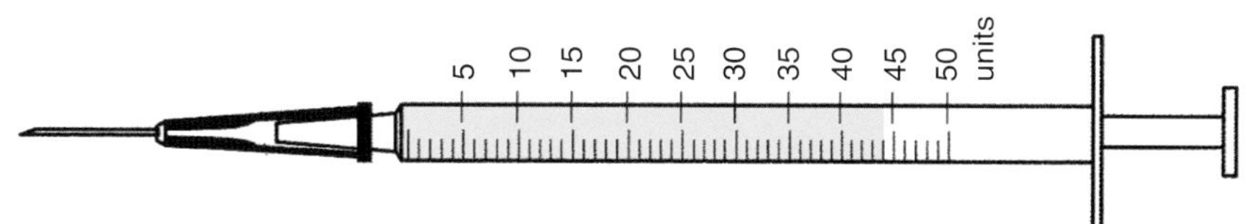

5. Units measured: __________

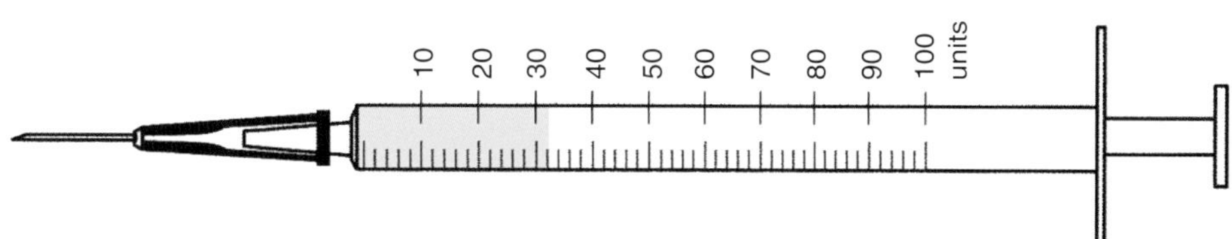

6. Units measured: __________

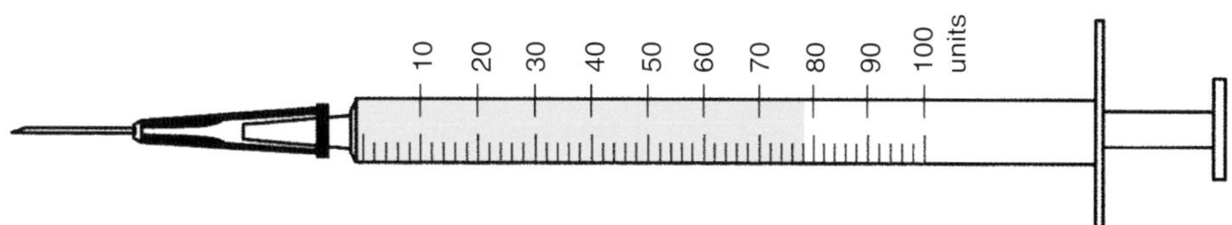

7. Units measured: __________

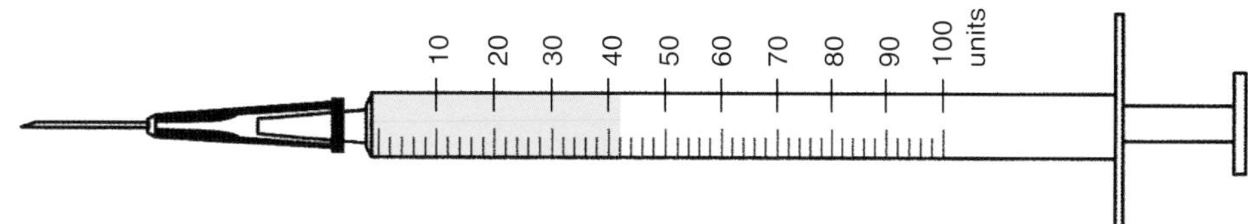

8. Units measured: __________

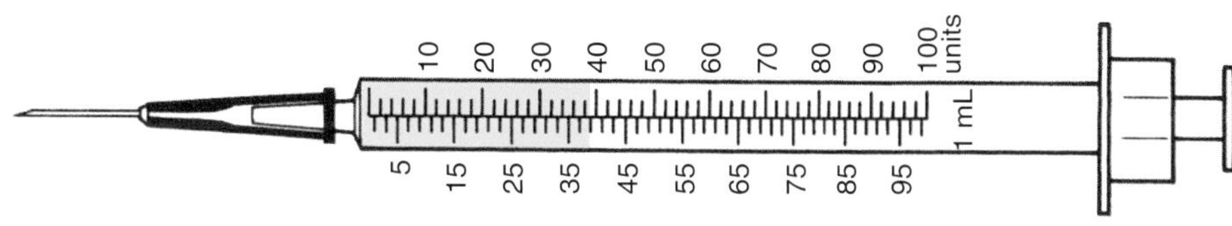

9. Units measured: ___________

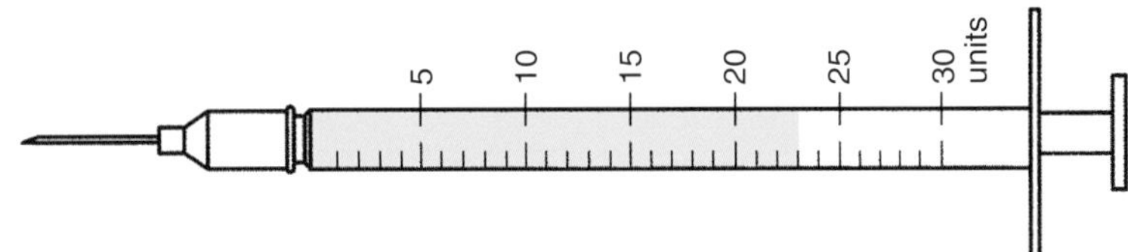

10. Units measured: ___________

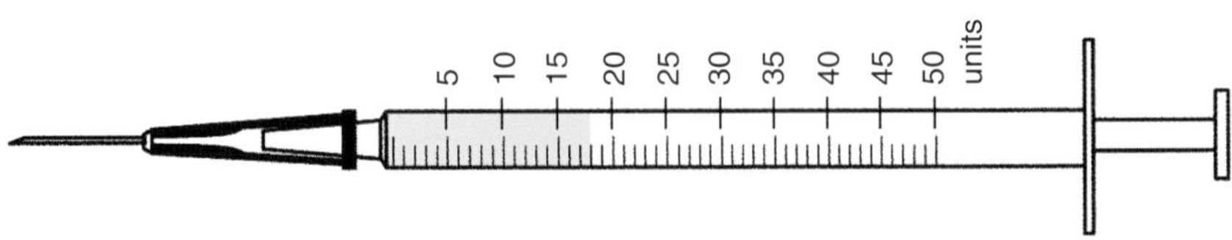

AM/PM INSULIN SHOT RECORD

NAME: JOHN DOE

Date		Time	Blood Sugar Level	Insulin Injected	Quantity	Site Where Injected
3/16	AM	0630	190 SMBG	Humulin R Humulin N	3 units 20 units	AB (R)
	PM	1530	150 SMBG	Humulin R Humulin N	1 units 20 units	AB (L)
Date		**Time**	**Blood Sugar Level**	**Insulin Injected**	**Quantity**	**Site Where Injected**
	AM					
	PM					
Date		**Time**	**Blood Sugar Level**	**Insulin Injected**	**Quantity**	**Site Where Injected**
	AM					
	PM					
Date		**Time**	**Blood Sugar Level**	**Insulin Injected**	**Quantity**	**Site Where Injected**
	AM					
	PM					
Date		**Time**	**Blood Sugar Level**	**Insulin Injected**	**Quantity**	**Site Where Injected**
	AM					
	PM					
Date		**Time**	**Blood Sugar Level**	**Insulin Injected**	**Quantity**	**Site Where Injected**
	AM					
	PM					
Date		**Time**	**Blood Sugar Level**	**Insulin Injected**	**Quantity**	**Site Where Injected**
	AM					
	PM					

BGM blood glucose monitor (capillary sample) performed by nurse
SMBG self blood glucose monitoring (by patient) (capillary sample)
Serum FBS fasting blood sugar (by lab or RN) (venous [serum] sample)

RA = Right Arm
LA = Left Arm
RT = Right Thigh
AB – Right abdomen
AB – Left abdomen

Answers on page 348

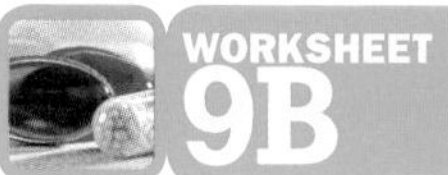

WORKSHEET 9B Additional Practice in Single-Dose Measures

Circle the letter of the syringe with the correct ordered amount.

1. Ordered: 13 units of Humulin NPH subcutaneous at 1100 hr.

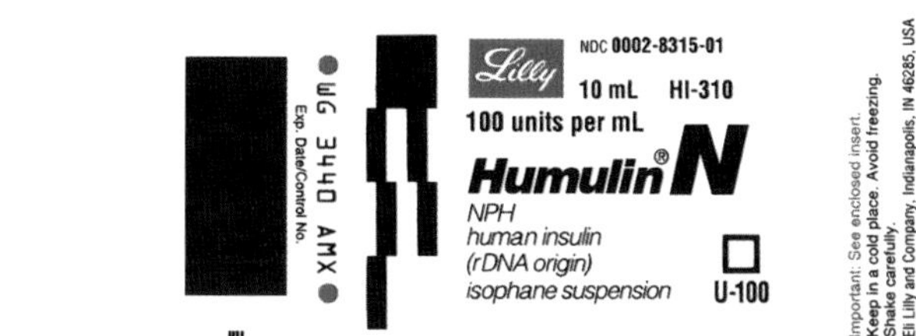

a.

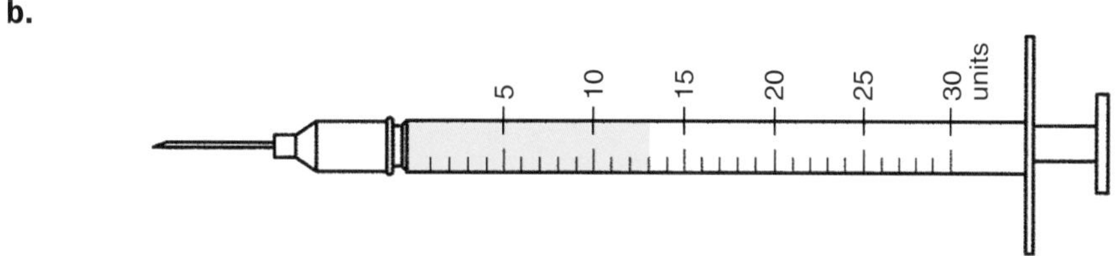

b.

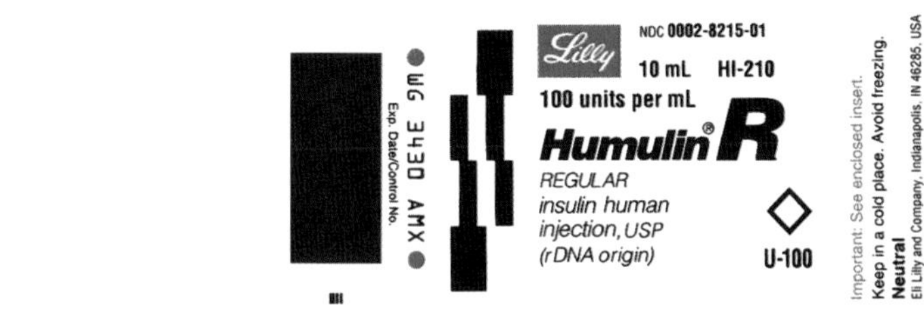

2. Ordered: 6 units of Humulin Regular subcutaneous ½ hr before a meal.

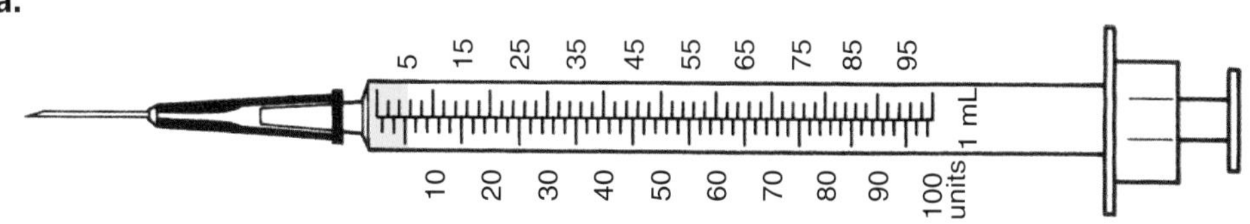

a.

b.

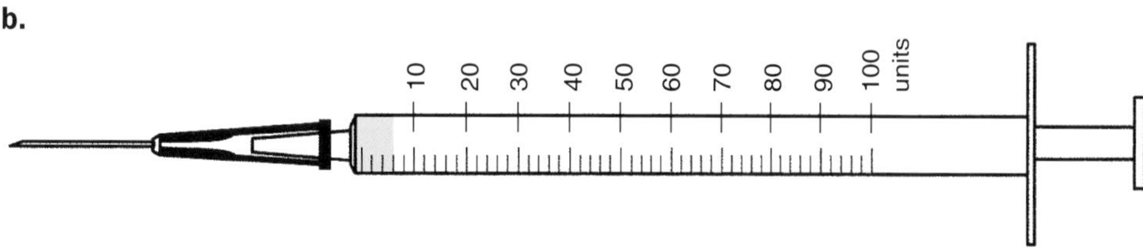

3. Ordered: 12 units of Novolin Regular subcutaneous 30 min before a meal.

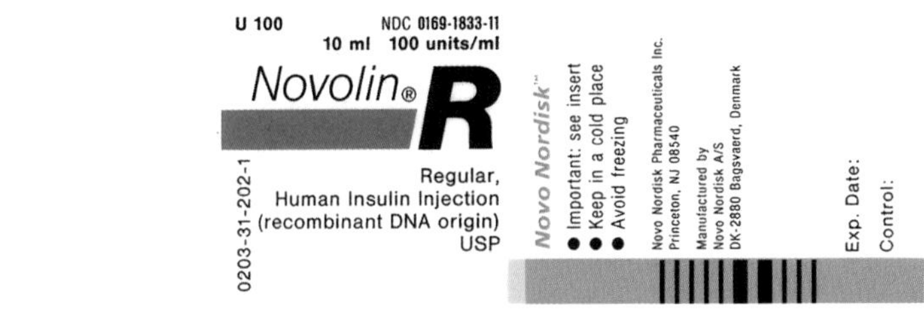

a.

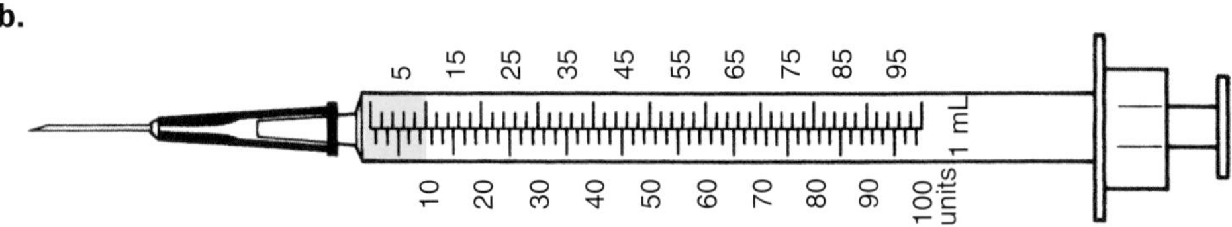

b.

4. Ordered: 12 units of Lantus subcutaneous at 2200 hr.

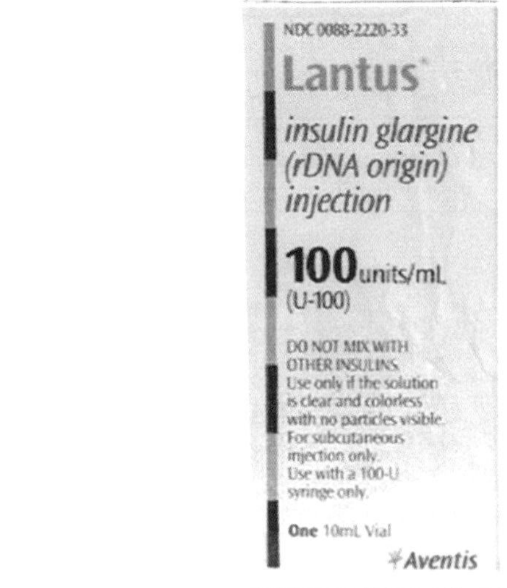

a.

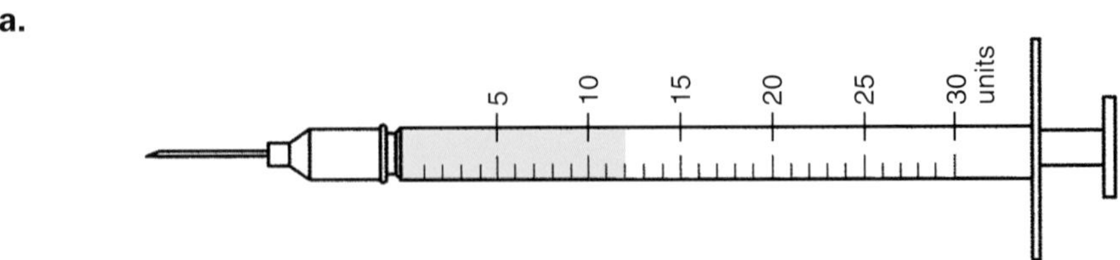

b.

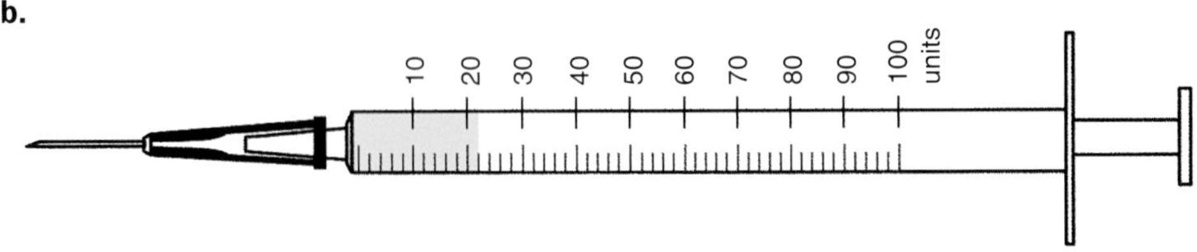

5. Ordered: 40 units of detemir subcutaneous at 0930.

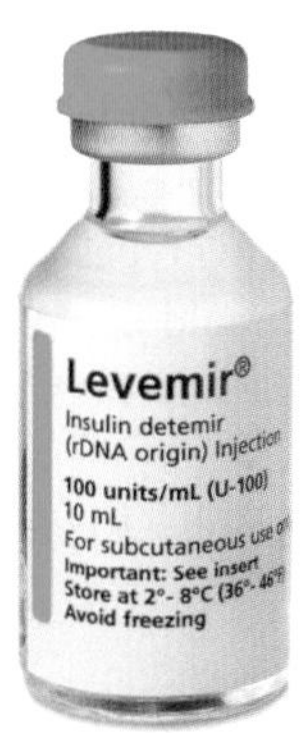

(From Novo Nordisk Inc., Princeton, N.J.)

a.

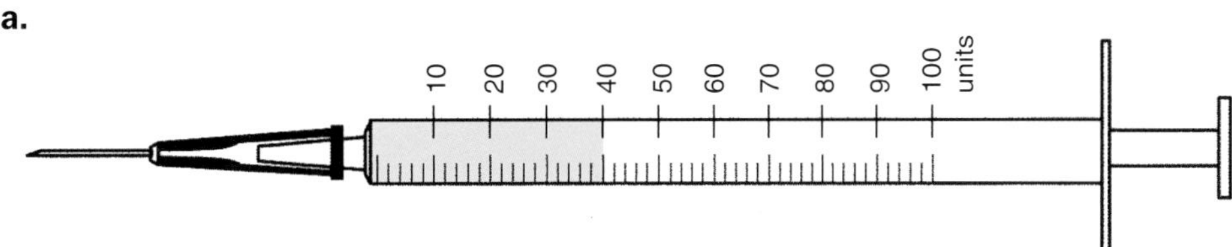

b.

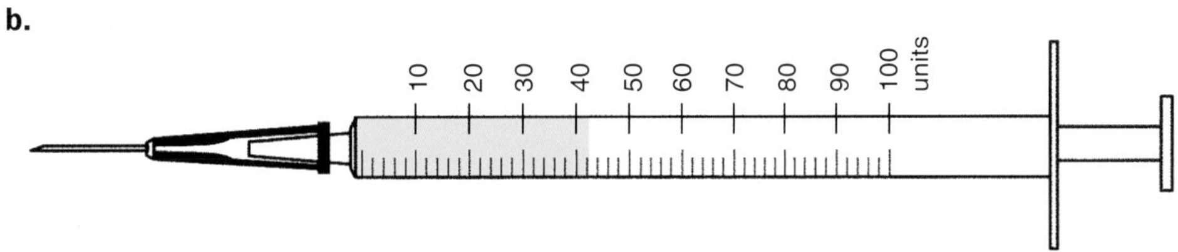

Mixing Insulin

Insulin dosages are drawn up *exactly* as ordered. An incorrect dosage could be devastating to the patient. Frequently, regular or rapid-acting insulin is combined with an intermediate-acting insulin. This gives insulin coverage (glucose control) within 15 to 60 minutes and lasts 10 to 16 hours. This technique of combining the two types of insulin is important for the nurse, patient, and family to master. The regular insulin vial should *not* be contaminated with the longer-acting insulin; therefore, the regular insulin should be drawn up first. The mixing procedure is illustrated in Figures 9.11 and 9.12.

Example

Ordered: 10 units of Humulin Regular and 40 units of Humulin N.
Total units: 50 units
Source: DNA and DNA
Which insulin will you draw up first? *Regular* (see Figure 9.11)

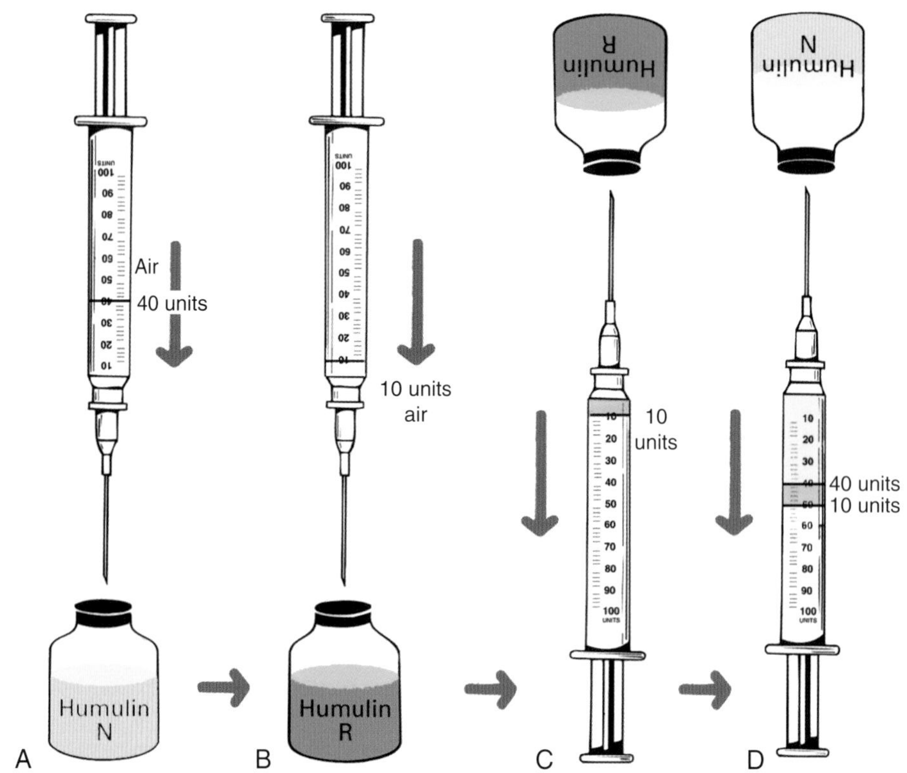

FIGURE 9.11 Order: Give 10 units of Humulin R and 40 units of Humulin N via subcutaneous injection. **A,** Inject 40 units of air into Humulin N first. Do **not** allow needle to touch insulin. Withdraw needle. **B,** Inject 10 units of air into Humulin R. **C,** With needle still in place, invert vial and withdraw 10 units of R. Withdraw needle. **D,** Insert needle into vial of Humulin N, invert vial and withdraw 40 units. Total amount in syringe equals 50 units.

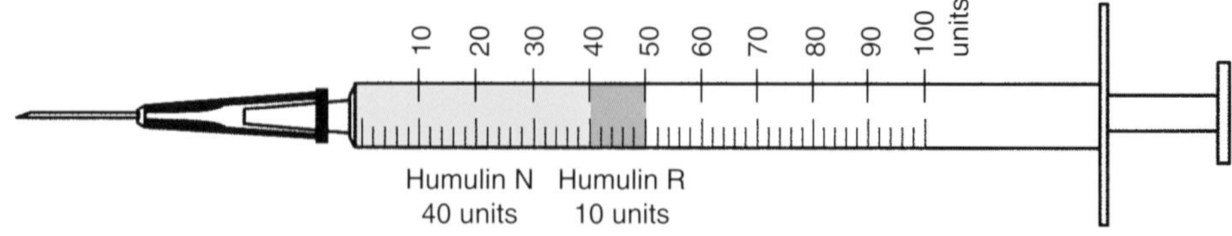

FIGURE 9.12 100-unit syringe showing the mixing of two insulins. Remember: **clear to cloudy when drawing up insulins.**

Example Ordered: 10 units of Novolin Regular and 20 units of Novolin N

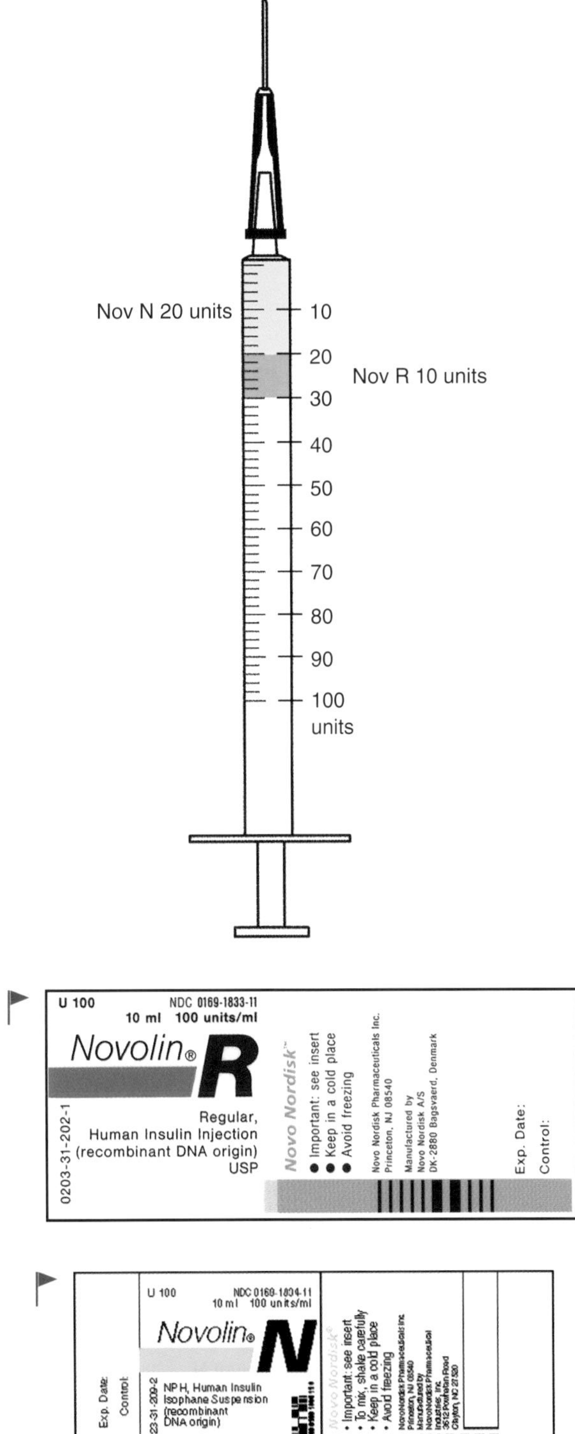

Insulin will not stay separated as pictured in the syringe.

CLINICAL ALERT!

Draw up regular (clear) insulin first before N (cloudy) is added (see Figure 9.11).

Regular insulin should not be contaminated with Humulin N or any N insulin. A multiple-dose vial of regular insulin can be used for IV infusion, and contamination with intermediate-acting insulin could be fatal. If the vial of regular insulin looks cloudy, do not use. It has been contaminated.

Answers on page 348

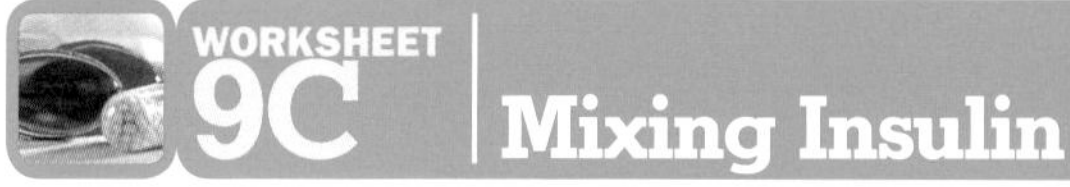

WORKSHEET 9C Mixing Insulin

Calculate the total number of units in the following problems. Circle the letter of the syringe with the correct amount.

1. Ordered: Lispro insulin 8 units and Humulin N 60 units ½ hr before breakfast.
Total units: ________

a.

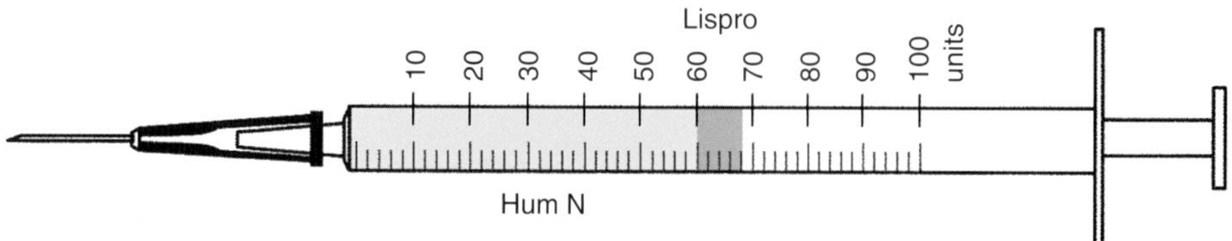

b.

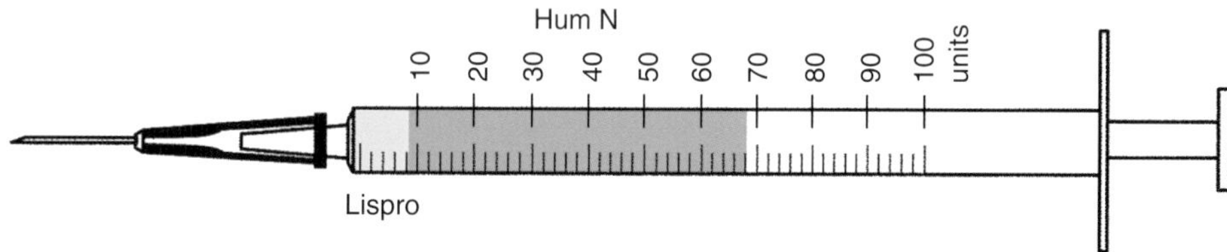

2. Ordered: Humalog R 14 units and Humulin N 25 units. Total units: ________

a.

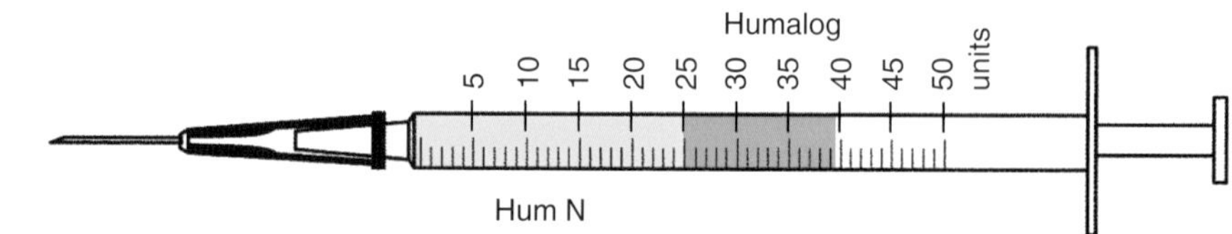

b.

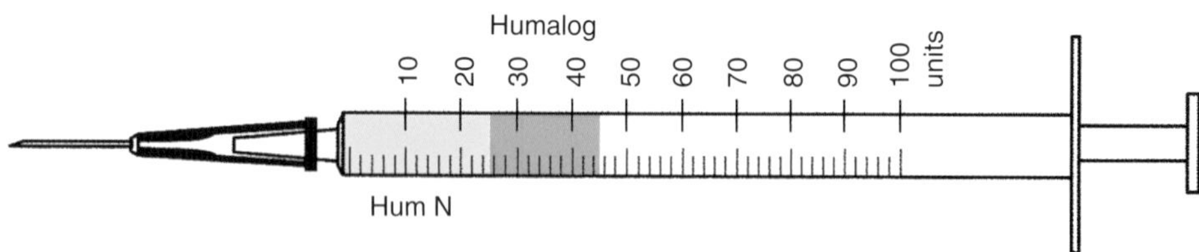

3. Ordered: Novolin R 8 units and Novolin N 15 units. Total units: ________

a.

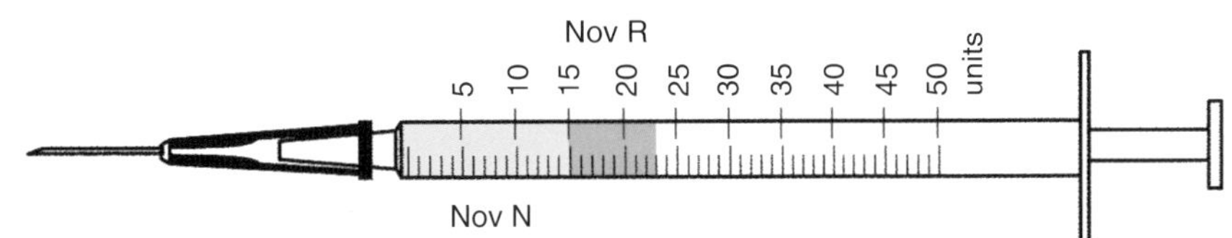

b.

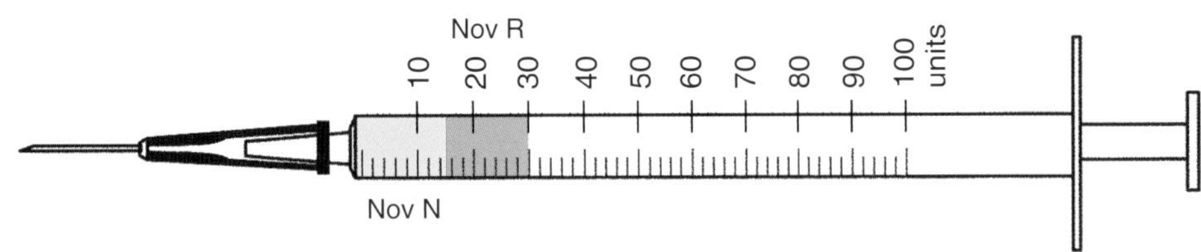

4. Ordered: Novolin 8 units and Novolin N 30 units. Total units: ________

a.

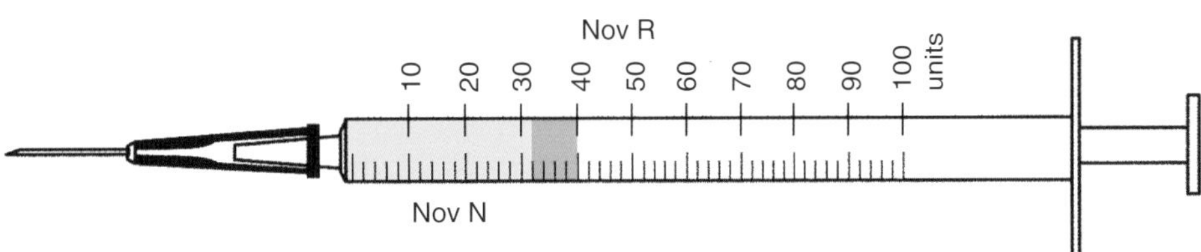

b.

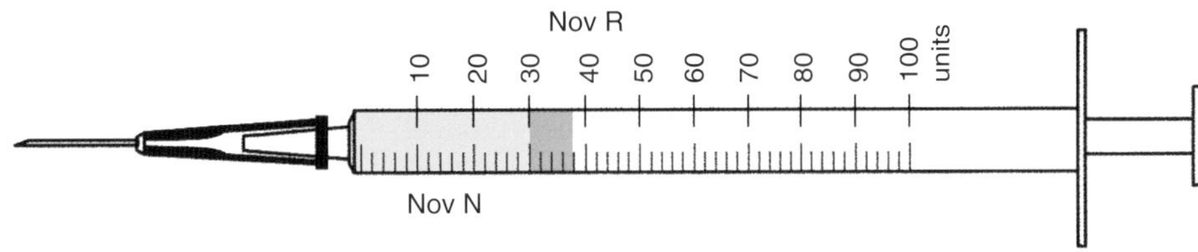

5. Ordered: 10 units of Humalog and 38 units Humulin N ½ hr before breakfast.
Total units: ________

a.

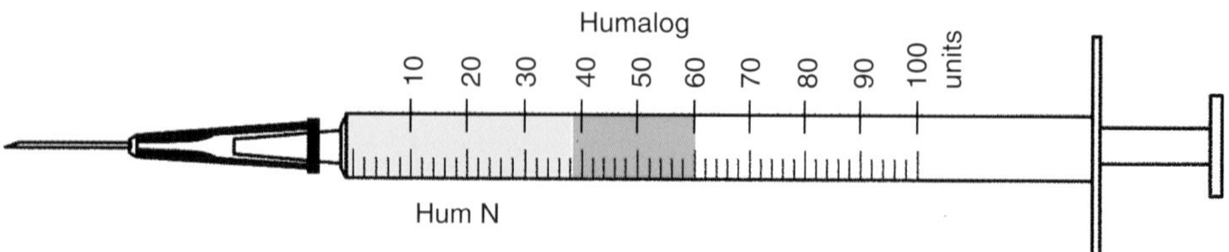

b.

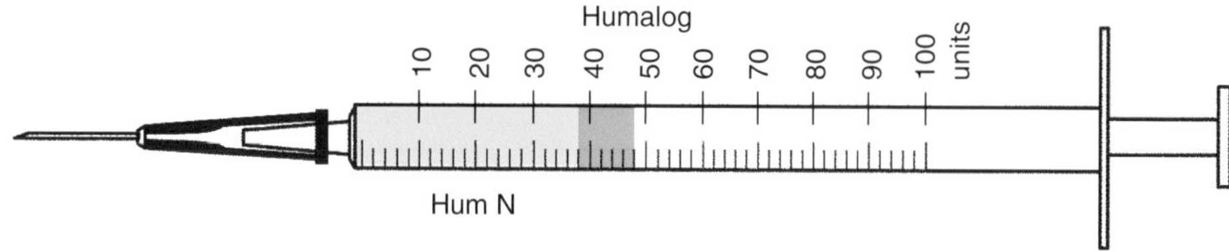

Shade in insulin dose on syringe. All orders are for U-100 insulin.

6. Ordered: Humulin R insulin 12 units and Humulin N 30 units every AM before breakfast. How many total units will you give? When will this peak? What is the duration?

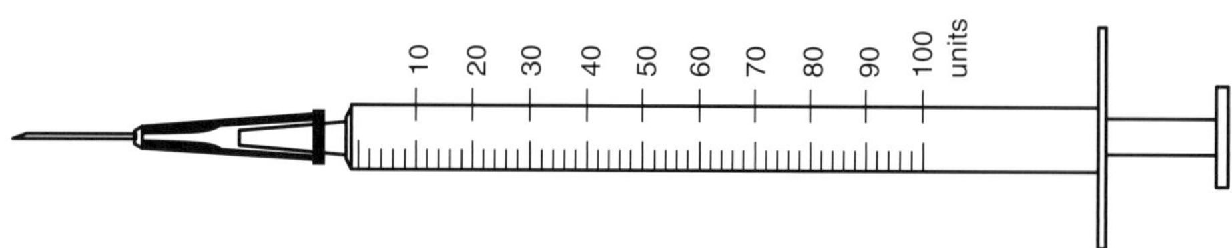

7. Ordered: 10 units of Apidra before meals. Available: Apidra U-100. How many units will you give? When will the action begin (onset)?

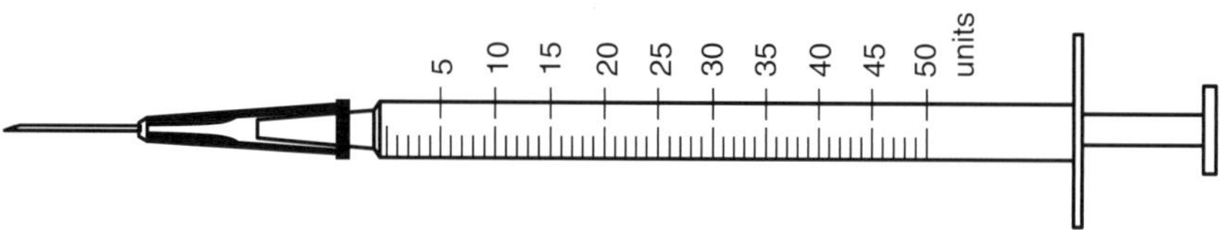

8. Ordered: Fixed combination of Humulin 70/30, 44 units daily. Available: Humulin Fixed 70/30. How many units will you give? When will it peak? What is the duration?

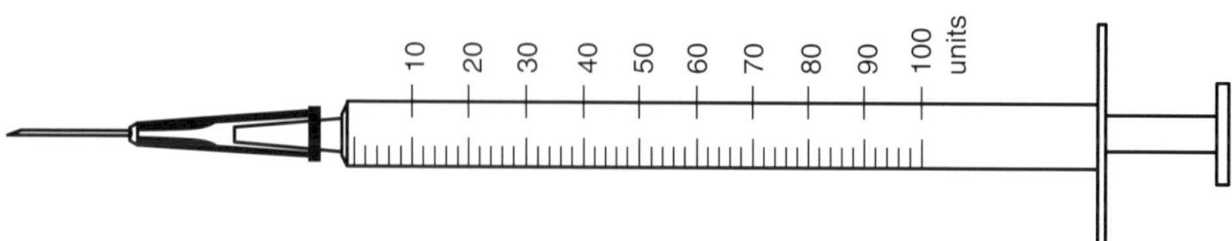

9. Ordered: Novolin R 10 units and Novolin N 40 units subcutaneous every AM ½ hr before meals. How many total units will you give? What is the duration?

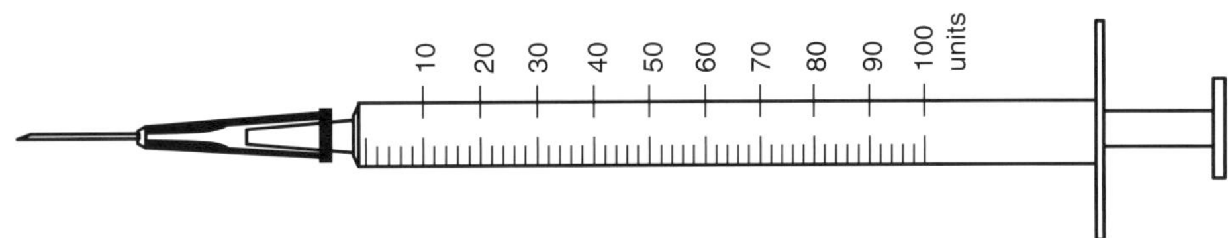

10. Ordered: 15 units of Novolog at 0830 before breakfast. Available: Novolog (aspart). How many units will you administer? When will it peak?

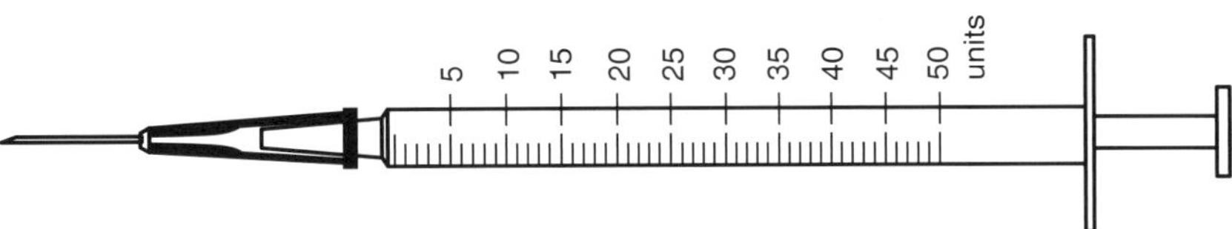

IV Insulin

During acute phases of illness, regular insulin is given by the IV route to ensure a controlled supply of medication that will vary depending on laboratory monitoring. A piggyback infusion is always administered with an IV-controlled infusion device. Discard the first 2 to 3 mL of combined infusion through IV tubing to prevent the insulin from binding to the tubing.

CLINICAL ALERT!

Only **clear regular** insulin can be used intravenously. Discard if cloudy (Figure 9.13).

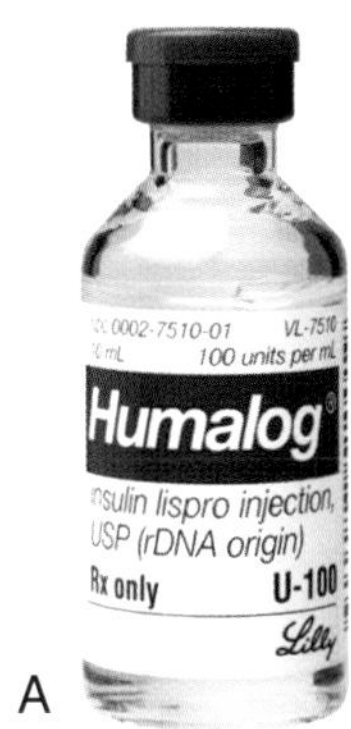

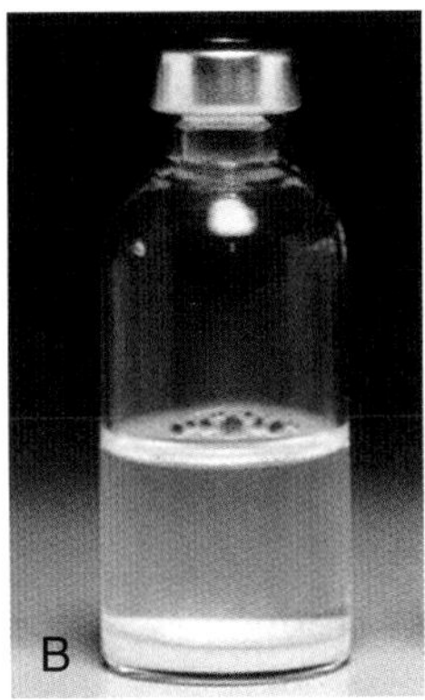

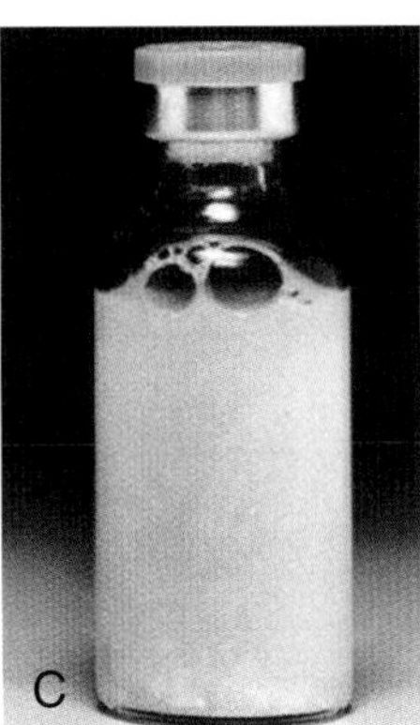

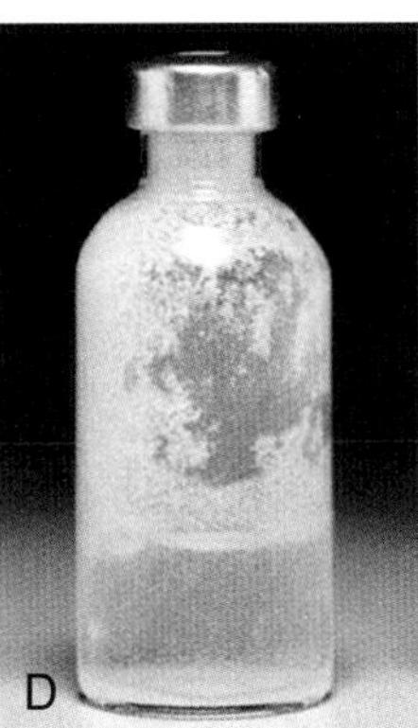

FIGURE 9.13 **A,** Regular and Humalog (lispro), Novolog (aspart), and Apidra (glulisine) should always look clear. **B,** Insulin at the bottom of the bottle; do not use if insulin stays on the bottom of the bottle after gentle rolling. **C,** Clumps of insulin; do not use if there are clumps of insulin in the liquid or on the bottom of the vial. **D,** Bottle appears frosted; do not use if particles of insulin are on the bottom or sides of the bottle and give it a frosty appearance. (Copyright Eli Lilly and Company. All rights reserved. Used with permission.)

Answers on page 349

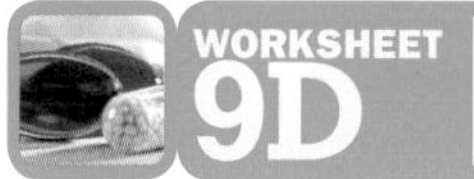

WORKSHEET 9D

IV Insulin Calculations

Answer questions 1 through 3 using Figure 9.14.

BG (mg/dL)	Std. Infusion Rate (units/hour)	☐ Stress Infusion Rate (units/hour)	☐ Customized (units/hour)
<80	0.2	0.2	______
80-100	0.5	1.0	______
101-140	1.0	2.0	______
141-180	1.5	3.0	______
181-220	2.0	4.0	______
221-260	2.5	5.0	______
261-300	3.0	6.0	______
301-340	4.0	8.0	______
>340	5.0	10.0	______

FIGURE 9.14 Standard insulin infusion chart. (Modified from Scottsdale Healthcare, Scottsdale, Ariz.)

RULE **Begin the problem with the known amount of medication in the total solution.**

The pharmacy standard insulin drip: 100 units Human Regular in 100 mL of NS.

Example Ordered: Regular human insulin 5 units per hr IV drip. Pharmacy has delivered 100 mL 0.9% NS with 100 units of regular human insulin.

- How many mL per hr will infuse 5 units per hr?
- For how many hours will the IV infuse?

Step 1 KNOW WANT TO KNOW FRACTION CROSS PRODUCT

$100 \text{ units} : 100 \text{ mL} = 5 \text{ units} : x \text{ mL}$

$\frac{100}{100} \times \frac{5}{x}$

$100x = 100 \times 5 = 500$

$100x = 500$

$x = 5 \text{ mL per hr} = 5 \text{ units of insulin}$

PROOF

$100 \times 5 = 500$

$100 \times 5 = 500$

Step 2 KNOW WANT TO KNOW FRACTION CROSS PRODUCT

$5 \text{ mL} : 1 \text{ hr} = 100 \text{ mL} : x \text{ hr}$

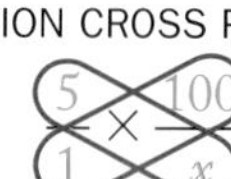

$5x = 100$

$x = 20 \text{ hr}$

PROOF

$20 \times 5 = 100$

$1 \times 100 = 100$

1. The patient's BS level is 310 mg per dL at 0820 hr.
   a. At what rate will you set the IV infusion device?
   b. At 0920 hr the BS level is 270 mg per dL. What will be the rate for the IV infusion device?

2. The patient's blood sugar level is 235 mg per dL at 0400 hr.
   a. At what rate will you set the infusion rate?
   b. In 1 hour, the BS level is 270 mg per dL. What will be the new IV rate?
   c. At 0600 hr the provider called and inquired about the BS level. He asked how many units of insulin the patient had received since the IV was started. What will you tell the provider?

3. Your patient is receiving insulin IV. The standard rate of 100 units in 100 mL of NS is sent from the pharmacy. The BS q1h is as follows: 350 mg per dL, 330, 270, 210, 190, 165, 145, 120 mg per dL. How many total units has the patient received?

4. The pharmacy has sent 50 mL of NS with 100 units of insulin. The order is for 5 units per hr until the BS level is stable at 130 mg per dL.
   a. At how many mL per hr will you set the IV infusion device?
   b. It took 16 hours for the BS level to stabilize at 130 mg per dL. How many total units of insulin did the patient receive during the 16 hours?

5. Ordered: 100 units Human Regular insulin in 50 mL of NS to be infused at 3 mL per hr until the blood sugar level is stable at 120 mg per dL.
   a. How many units per hr will be delivered?
   b. If it took 8 hours for the blood sugar level to stabilize at 120 mg per dL, how many total units of insulin did the patient receive?

For Problems 6 through 10, calculate the following:

- **mL per hr necessary to infuse the ordered amount via an infusion device**
- **length of time the IV is to infuse**

6. Ordered: Humulin R IV at 10 units per hr. Available: 150 mL of 0.9% NS with 100 units Humulin (lispro) R insulin.

7. Ordered: Humulin R in 50 mL to infuse at 8 units per hr. Available: 50 mL 0.9% NS with 50 units Humulin R insulin.

8. Ordered: Humulin R in 50 mL to infuse at 12 units per hr. Available: 50 mL 0.9% NS with 75 units Humulin R insulin.

9. Ordered: 120 units Humulin R insulin IV at 10 units per hr. Available: 100 mL of NS 0.9% with 120 units Humulin R insulin.

10. Ordered: 150 units Humulin R insulin IV at 12 units per hr. Available: 150 mL of NS 0.9% with 150 units Humulin R insulin.

Frequent Blood Sugar Monitoring/Insulin Drip Record

Normal Blood Sugar 70-100 mg/dL

DATE → 12/5/18					DATE →					DATE →				
Time ↓	Sugar (mg/dL)	Intervention Insulin (units/h) or other	Ketones S/M/L/Neg	Initial	Time ↓	Sugar (mg/dL)	Intervention Insulin (units/h) or other	Ketones S/M/L/Neg	Initial	Time ↓	Sugar (mg/dL)	Intervention Insulin (units/h) or other	Ketones S/M/L/Neg	Initial
00 __ __					00 __ __					00 __ __				
01 __ __					01 __ __					01 __ __				
02 __ __					02 __ __					02 __ __				
03 __ __	IV Insulin	Drip Started			03 __ __					03 __ __				
04 1 5	350	5.0		JB	04 __ __					04 __ __				
05 1 5	303	4.0		JB	05 __ __					05 __ __				
06 1 5	310	4.0		JB	06 __ __					06 __ __				
07 1 5	270	3.0		JB	07 __ __					07 __ __				
08 1 5	180	1.5		JB	08 __ __					08 __ __				
09 1 5	165	1.5		JB	09 __ __					09 __ __				
10 1 5	150	1.5		JB	10 __ __					10 __ __				
11 __ __					11 __ __					11 __ __				
12 1 5	140	1.0		JB	12 __ __					12 __ __				
13 1 5	130	1.0		JB	13 __ __					13 __ __				
14 __ __					14 __ __					14 __ __				
15 1 5	135	1.0		JB	15 __ __					15 __ __				
16 __ __					16 __ __					16 __ __				
17 1 5	140	1.0		JB	17 __ __					17 __ __				
18 __ __	Converted to	Subcutaneous Insulin			18 __ __					18 __ __				
19 __ __					19 __ __					19 __ __				
20 __ __					20 __ __					20 __ __				
21 __ __					21 __ __					21 __ __				
22 __ __					22 __ __					22 __ __				
23 __ __					23 __ __					23 __ __				
Insulin Total Daily Dose (TDD)					Insulin Total Daily Dose (TDD)					Insulin Total Daily Dose (TDD)				

Initial	Signature	Initial	Signature	Initial	Signature	Initial	Signature
JB	J Booth						

Original in Medical Chart **Copy to Pharmacy**

Diabetes flow sheet. Note: IV insulin should always be used with an infusion device, never via gravity flow. (Modified from Scottsdale Healthcare, Scottsdale, Ariz.)

Oral Diabetes Medications

Oral diabetes medications (ODMs) are used to treat type 2 DM. They are taken alone or in combination with insulin. Blood sugar levels determine the strength of oral medication needed. ODMs are *not* insulin. Many ODMs are combinations of two types of drugs. Examples include: Prandimet, Janumet, and Xigduo XR. Other type 2 ODMs have a specific action, as listed in the table below.

Class	Brand Name	Generic Name	Action
Biguanides	Glucophage, Glucophage XR	metformin	Decreases amount of glucose made by the liver.
Meglitinides	Prandin, Starlix	repaglinide nateglitinide	Stimulates the pancreas to produce a quick burst of insulin, plus it decreases glucose production in the liver.
	Prandimet	metformin and repaglinide	
Sulfonylurea	Diabeta	glyburide	Stimulates pancreas to increase insulin production. These are sometimes used in conjunction with insulin injections.
	Amaryl	glimepiride	
	Glucotrol	glipizide	
Alpha-glucosidase inhibitors	Precose	acarbose	Slows the absorption of starches
	Glyset	miglitol	
DPP-4 inhibitors	Nestina	alogliptin	Stimulates insulin production when blood sugar rises. Boosts incretin gut hormone to help lower blood glucose.
	Onglyza	sazagliptin	
	Tradjenta	linagliptin	
	Januvia	sitagliptin	
	Janumet	sitagliptin and metformin	
SGLT 2 inhibitors	Jardiance	empagliflozin	Causes excess blood glucose to be excreted in urine. Stops glucose from getting reabsorbed by the kidneys.
	Invokana	canagliflozin	
	Farxiga	dapagliflozin	
	Farxiga and Glucophage	dapagliflozin and metformin	
Thiazolidinedones	Actos Avandia	pioglitazone rosiglitazone	Makes body tissue more sensitive to insulin

Oral Antidiabetic Drug Labels

Example The following are some examples of providers' orders for oral antidiabetics, along with the drug labels:

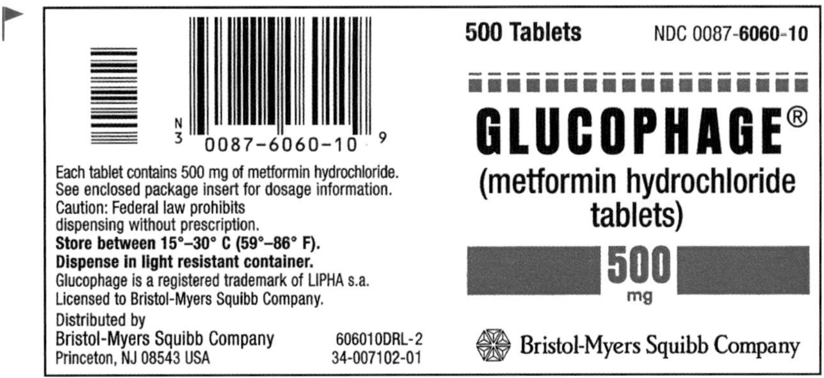

Glucophage 500 mg PO tid with meals.

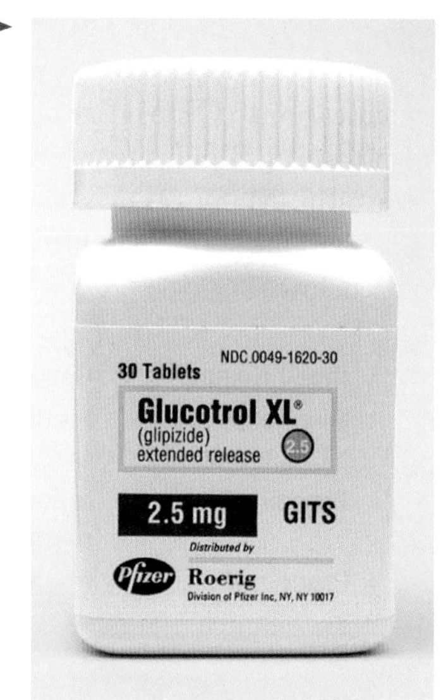

Glucotrol XL 2.5 mg daily with breakfast.

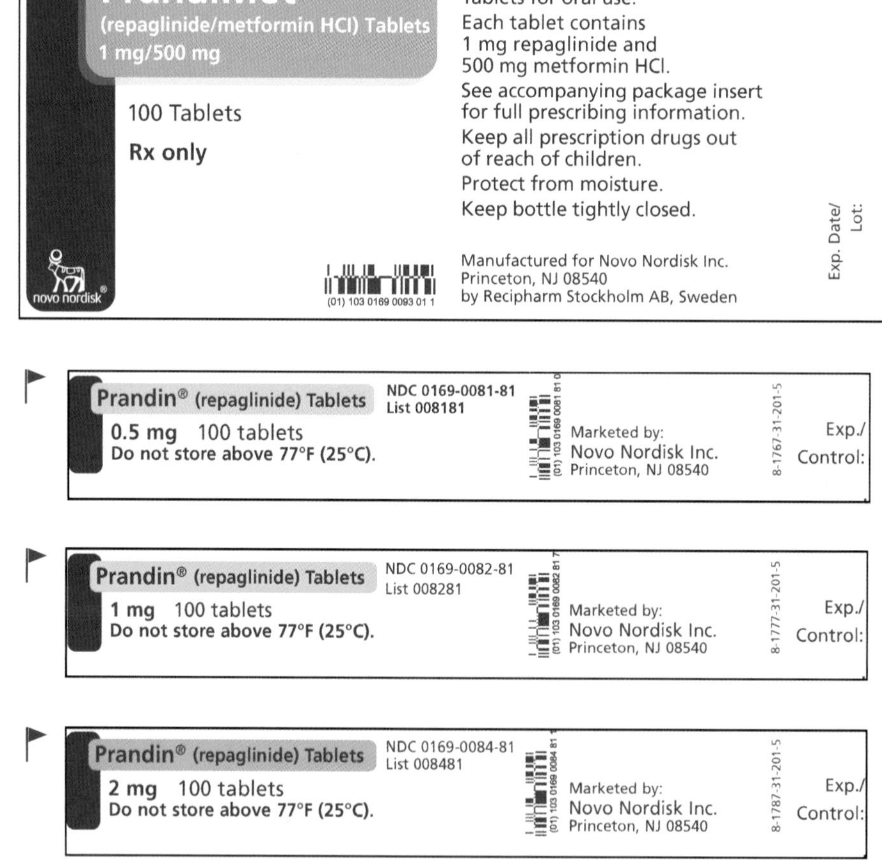

Prandin 1 mg PO tid 30 minutes ac.

Insulin Infusion Devices

Nurses must understand how to care for patients who are admitted with insulin pumps. It is the nurse's responsibility to ascertain the patient's knowledge of pump management. Patients must be able to manage their diabetes, monitor their blood sugar level four times a day, calculate carbohydrate intake (grams), and determine when a bolus dose is needed. Many times the patient is admitted because of a lack of knowledge or lack of compliance with the regimen. Most hospitals do not keep a supply of insulin pumps or batteries for the pump; therefore, determine if the patient has made arrangements for these supplies.

An insulin pump is a battery-powered pump that delivers a continuous subcutaneous insulin infusion (CSII) (Figure 9.15). The pump is attached to an infusion set (Figure 9.16) that has a very fine-gauge cannula inserted subcutaneously in the abdomen and is attached to the insulin reservoir via tubing. The reservoir can hold either 150 units, or, more commonly, 300 units of U-100 rapid-acting insulin. Insulin pumps generally take only rapid or short-acting insulin. Ketoacidosis can develop quickly if the insulin is interrupted. Because of this significant risk, *the device must not be stopped or disconnected without supplemental insulin coverage.* If the insulin pump has to be disconnected for computerized tomography scans and magnetic resonance imaging tests, the blood sugar level should be checked before disconnecting and after reconnecting the pump. An insulin IV may be needed during the tests.

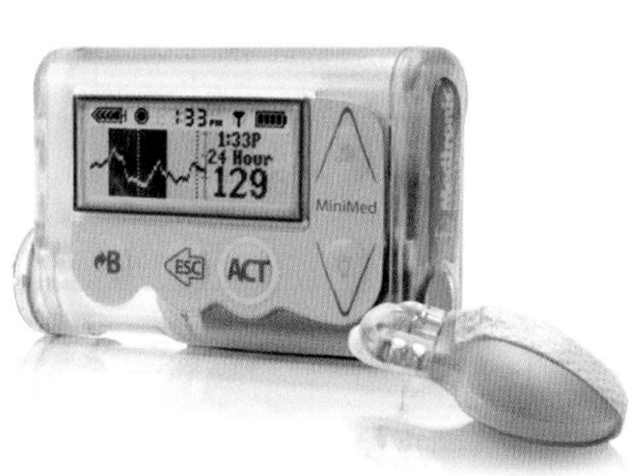

FIGURE 9.15 Paradigm Link blood glucose monitor and Paradigm 515 pump. (From Medtronic, Minneapolis, Minn.)

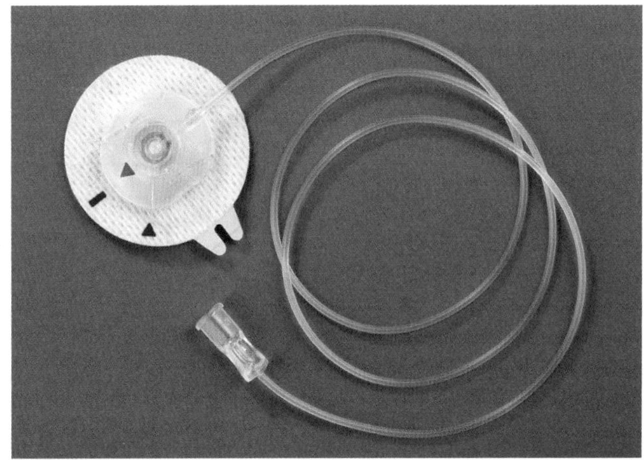

FIGURE 9.16 Quick-set infusion sets. (From Medtronic Diabetes, Northridge, Calif.)

When using insulin pumps, the blood sugar should be checked before meals and at bedtime. A continuous glucose monitoring (CGM) system device is a device worn by the patient to transmit glucose levels to the insulin pump. It is programmed to take blood sugar levels every 5 minutes. The blood sugar value is sent to the insulin pump, where the number is displayed.

Sensor glucose (SG) readings are taken from interstitial fluids. Fingersticks taken with the glucometer are taken from blood vessels. Therefore, the blood sugar (BS) level and the sensor level values are expected to be different. A big difference between the SG and the BS will most likely be after eating or exercising.

The patient will program the pump according to the basal rate set by the health care provider and the patient. If the basal rate is set correctly, the blood sugar should not fluctuate between meals. Basal rates are specific to each patient. They are set in units per hr. See Table 9.3, Basal Rates, Insulin Units Based on Required CHO Intake and Weight.

Insulin Dosage Based on Carbohydrate Intake

Because blood sugar levels fluctuate during the day (Figure 9.17), insulin doses should also fluctuate rather than being a constant dose every day. To keep the blood sugar level as close to the desired range as possible, carbohydrate intake must be calculated for each meal based on current blood sugar levels. This technique produces a more constant sugar level, which will help to minimize the detrimental effects of wide variations in blood sugar levels during the day. However, blood sugar levels must be measured before each meal and at bedtime. Usually, an insulin pump is used. If the carbohydrate ratio is high, the insulin pump can provide a bolus dose.

The health care provider will set a daily dose of long-acting insulin. For example, Lantus is used to cover blood sugar levels outside of meal times and is set for individualized parameters for each patient, depending on metabolic needs, such as exercise. The best type of diabetes management for some diabetics is the carbohydrate ratio technique, which is the closest way of replacing insulin made by the pancreas. A high level of compliance is needed for successful management. Rapid-acting insulin is used in the carbohydrate intake-to-weight ratio.

Week Starting / /	Sunday		Monday		Tuesday		Wednesday		Thursday		Friday		Saturday	
	Before	After	Before	After	Before	After	Before	After	Before	After	Before	After	Before	After
Breakfast	220	245												
Lunch	180	200												
Dinner	235	250												
Bed time	210													

Week Starting / /	Sunday		Monday		Tuesday		Wednesday		Thursday		Friday		Saturday	
	Before	After	Before	After	Before	After	Before	After	Before	After	Before	After	Before	After
Breakfast														
Lunch														
Dinner														
Bed time														

FIGURE 9.17 Preprandial and postprandial blood sugar level tracker.

remember **Blood sugar levels should be checked before meals and after meals for optimal diabetes control (see Figure 9.17).**

Example Based on blood sugar level (BS) and carbohydrate (CHO) intake.

- Desired blood sugar level is 130 mg per dL
- Order: Give 1 unit of insulin for every 15 mg per dL above 130 mg. Give 1 unit of insulin for every 10 g of CHO consumed.

Lunch	**CHO**
• ¾ cup of potato salad	21 g
• 2 slices of whole wheat bread	42 g
• 2 slices of Swiss cheese	2 g
• 2 slices of ham	2 g
• Mustard	1 g
• 1 12-oz. can of Pepsi	42 g
• Total	110 g CHO

Step 1 Desired BS is 130 mg per dL. The BS before lunch was 145 mg per dL. The difference between 130 and 145 is 15. The order states to give 1 unit of insulin for each 15 mg per dL above the desired 130 mg per dL. Therefore, 1 unit of insulin is required to treat the blood sugar level.

R & P Formula

15 mg : 1 unit = 15 mg : x units

$15x = 15$

$x = 1$ unit

Fraction Cross Product

$\frac{15 \text{ mg}}{1 \text{ unit}} \times \frac{15 \text{ mg}}{x \text{ unit}}$

Easy Method

Divide the BS difference by the order.

15 divided by 15 = 1 unit

Step 2 Total CHO for lunch is 110 g

Order: give 1 unit of insulin for each 10 g of CHO consumed.

R & P Formula

10 g : 1 unit = 110 g : x units

$10x = 110$

$x = 11$ units

Round to nearest whole number.

Fraction Cross Product

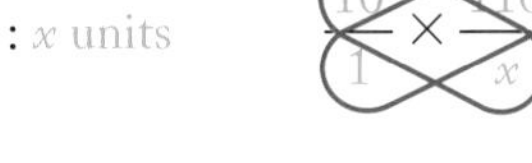

Easy Method

Divide the total grams of CHO by the order.

110 divided by 10 = 11 units

Give: 1 unit because the blood sugar level is above 15 g and give 11 units for the amount of CHO consumed. Give a total of 12 units of insulin.

Answers on page 350

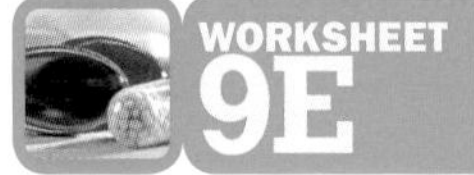

WORKSHEET 9E Insulin Dosage Based on CHO Intake

Use the following order to answer questions 1, 2, and 3. Round answers to the nearest whole number. Calculate the total number of insulin units required on the basis of the BS and the CHO intake.

Ordered: BS of 130 mg per dL is desired for this patient. Give 1 unit of insulin for each 10 mg above 130 mg. Give 1 unit of insulin for every 8 g of CHO consumed.

1. Breakfast — BS is 150 mg per dL

¾ cup Total cereal	CHO = 23 g
8 oz. low-carb milk	3 g
½ cup blueberries	1 g
1 slice wheat toast	21 g
1 pat butter	0 g
1 cup black coffee	0 g

Total units ______

2. Lunch — BS is 135 mg per dL

8 oz. yogurt	CHO = 25 g
⅓ cup dried cranberries	33 g
2 apple slices	1 g
5 grapes	1 g
5 saltines	11 g
Plain iced tea	0 g

Total units ______

3. Dinner — BS is 145 mg per dL

1 pork chop	CHO = 0 g
¾ cup mashed potatoes	34 g
¾ cup broccoli	0 g
8 oz. plain iced tea	0 g

Total units ______

Bedtime snack — BS is 145 mg per dL

¾ cup low-fat ice cream	CHO = 15 g

Total units ______

Use the following order to calculate the total insulin units in questions 4 and 5.

Ordered: The desired BS is 140 mg per dL. Give 1 unit of insulin for every 10 mg above 140 mg per dL. Give 1 unit of insulin for every 10 g of CHO consumed.

4. Breakfast — BS is 135 mg per dL

2 eggs	CHO = 1 g
2 slices wheat toast	42 g
2 slices bacon	0 g
2 cups black coffee	0 g

Total units ______

5. Lunch — BS is 160 mg per dL

4 oz. hamburger patty	CHO = 0 g
1 hamburger bun	28 g
½ cup cole slaw	20 g
1 small serving fries	45 g

Total units ______

SAMPLE

Logbook Based on CHO Intake, BS and Insulin																									
Name: John Doe										Start Date: 3 · 15 · 17										End Date:					
Date	RC	A.M. (Night/Morning)												P.M. (Afternoon/Evening)											
		24	1	2	3	4	5	6	7	8	9	10	11	12	13	14	15	16	17	18	19	20	21	22	23
Mon	Blood Sugar									240					250				245				245		
	Carbs									150					130				140				15		
	Insulin Bolus									2					2				3				2		
		Total Daily Dose:												Basal Dose:											
Tues	Blood Sugar																								
	Carbs																								
	Insulin Bolus																								
		Total Daily Dose:												Basal Dose:											
Wed	Blood Sugar																								
	Carbs																								
	Insulin Bolus																								
		Total Daily Dose:												Basal Dose:											
Thurs	Blood Sugar																								
	Carbs																								
	Insulin Bolus																								
		Total Daily Dose:												Basal Dose:											
Fri	Blood Sugar																								
	Carbs																								
	Insulin Bolus																								
		Total Daily Dose:												Basal Dose:											
Sat	Blood Sugar																								
	Carbs																								
	Insulin Bolus																								
		Total Daily Dose:												Basal Dose:											
Sun	Blood Sugar																								
	Carbs																								
	Insulin Bolus																								
		Total Daily Dose:												Basal Dose:											
Ave	Blood Sugar																								
	Carbs																								
	Insulin Bolus																								
		Total Daily Dose:												Basal Dose:											

FIGURE 9.18 Logbook based on CHO intake, BS and Insulin

Answers on page 351

WORKSHEET 9F Insulin Dosage Based on Blood Sugar and CHO Intake

Calculate the insulin requirements in questions 1, 2, and 3. The BS readings and CHO requirements are based on the following orders. **Mark each syringe** with the total dose required.

Ordered: Give 1 unit of insulin for every 20 mg BS above 160 mg per dL. Give 1 unit of insulin for every 15 g of CHO consumed.

1. BS is 190 mg per dL; 98 g of CHO were consumed.
How many total units of insulin are required?

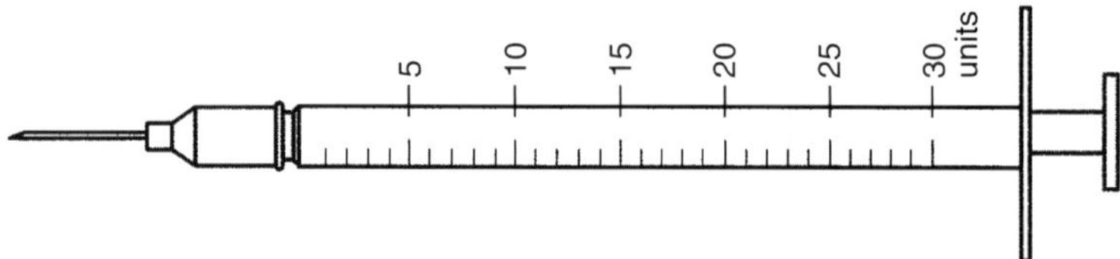

2. BS is 180 mg per dL; 40 g of CHO were consumed.
How many total units of insulin are required?

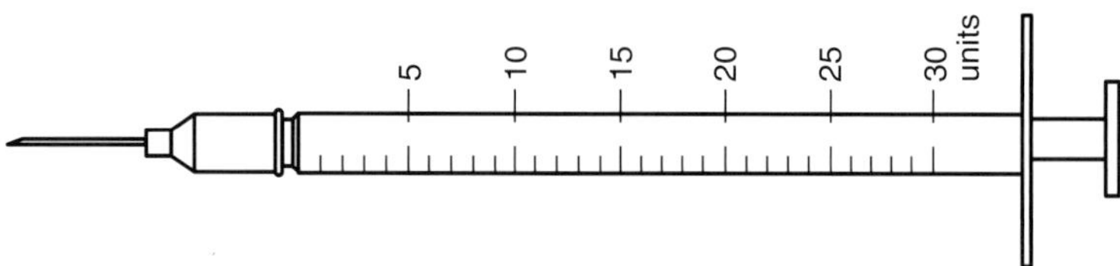

3. BS is 210 mg per dL; 118 g of CHO were consumed.
How many total units of insulin are required?

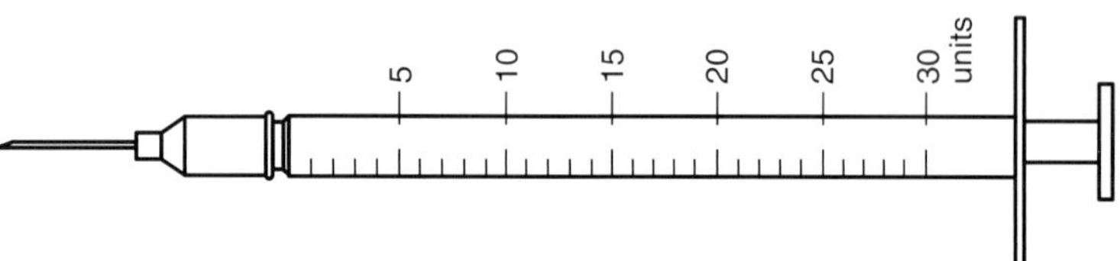

Calculate the total insulin requirements in questions 4 through 7. The BS reading and CHO requirements are based on the following orders. Mark each syringe with the total dose required.

Ordered: Give 1 unit of insulin for every 30 mg BS above 150 mg per dL. Give 1 unit of insulin for every 10 g of CHO consumed.

4. BS is 240 mg per dL; 58 g of CHO were consumed. How many total units of insulin are required?

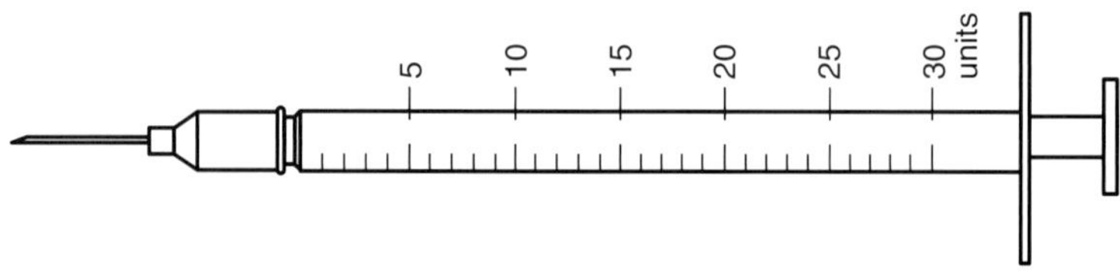

5. BS is 180 mg per dL; 120 g of CHO were consumed. How many total units of insulin are required?

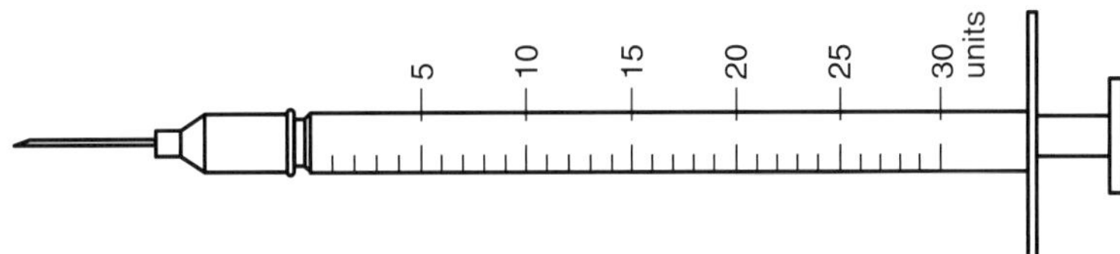

6. BS is 260 mg per dL; 58 g of CHO were consumed. How many total units of insulin are required?

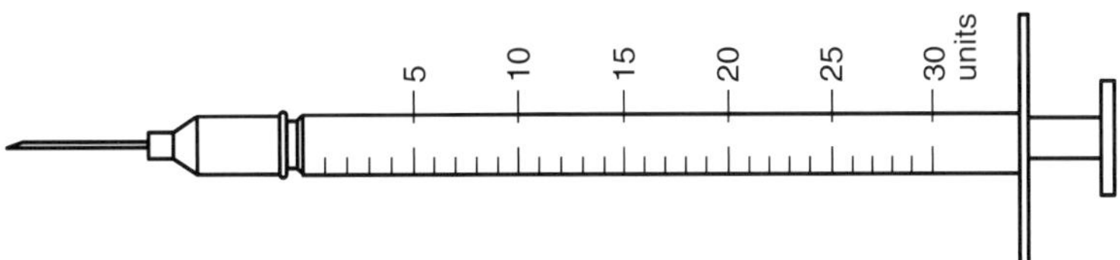

7. BS is 160 mg per dL; 28 g of CHO were consumed. How many total units of insulin are required?

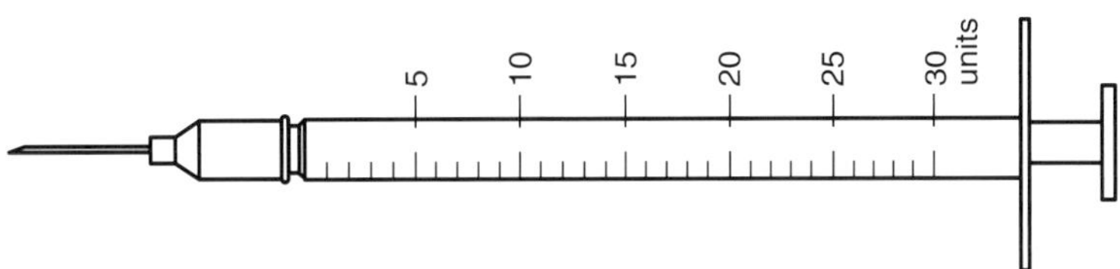

Sliding-Scale Calculations

Insulin administered according to a sliding scale is predicated on the blood sugar reading, the type of diabetes, insulin resistance, weight, age, renal status, and activity level. Blood sugar levels determine how much insulin to give. Blood sugar readings may be taken several times a day to determine daily insulin requirements. Sliding scales can vary greatly because they are individualized. Evidence-based computerized medical records information systems used in place of individualized sliding scales result in better glycemic control. The study was completed by the Department of Medicine, University of Washington, Seattle, WA, USA.

Example Ordered: Regular insulin q6h to follow the sliding scale.

Blood Sugar (mg per dL)	Low-Dose Scale
<70	Initiate Hypoglycemia Protocol
70-130	0 units
131-180	2 units
181-240	4 units
241-300	6 units
301-350	8 units
351-400	10 units
>400	12 units and call physician

Repeat blood sugar measurement 4 hr after it peaks.

At 1700 hr, the patient's blood sugar level was 168 mg per dL. How much regular insulin should be given? Shade the amount in the syringe.

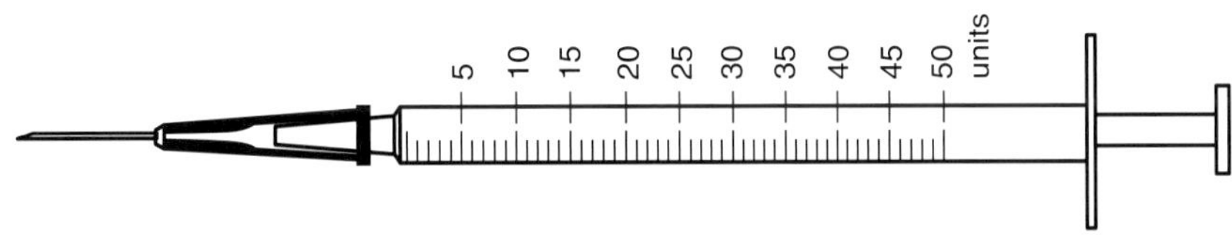

Estimating Insulin-to-Carbohydrate Ratio

This formula is based on estimates of insulin needs according to CHO intake and weight. It is a simple formula that gives estimates for categories of weight based on Table 9.3. Also given is the kilogram ratio for the same number of pounds.

Example Breakfast = 44 CHO. The patient's weight is 165 lb. Refer to Table 9.3. The ratio is 1 unit of insulin to 11 g of CHO consumed.

R & P Method	Fraction Cross Product	Total grams of CHO (Divided by) unit-to-CHO Ratio = Insulin Needs
1 unit : 11 CHO = x units : 44 CHO $11x = 44$ $x = 4$ units of R insulin	$\frac{1}{11} \times \frac{x}{44}$	44 (divided by) 11 = 4 units

Basal Rates

Table 9.3 Insulin Units Required Based on CHO Intake and Weight

Weight in Pounds	Weight in kg	Unit: grams of CHO
100-109	45.5-49.5	1:16
110-129	50-58.6	1:15
130-139	59-63.2	1:14
140-149	63.6-67.7	1:13
150-159	68.2-72.3	1:12
160-169	72.7-76.8	1:11
170-179	77.3-81.4	1:10
180-189	81.8-85.9	1:9
190-199	86.4-90	1:8
200-239	90.9-108.6	1:7
240+	109.1+	1:6

Answers on page 352

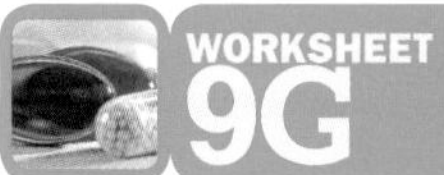

WORKSHEET 9G Insulin Dosage Based on CHO Intake and Weight

Calculate the insulin requirements for the following CHO intake related to the patient's weight. Refer to Table 9.3. Use either method shown in the example.

1. The patient ate 26 g CHO for breakfast. She weighs 142 lb. How many units of R are required?

2. The patient weighs 83 kg and ate 80 g CHO for lunch. How many units of R are required?

3. The patient ate 18 g CHO for lunch. She weighs 108 lb. How many units of R are required?

4. The patient consumed 90 g CHO for dinner and weighs 240 lb. How many units of R are required?

5. The patient weighs 162 lb. The total CHO intake during a 24-hour period was 160 g. How many units of R has the patient received in 24 hours?

6. The patient weighs 100 kg. The patient's total CHO intake during 24 hours was 145 g. How many units of R did she receive?

7. The provider calls at 1500 hours and wants to know how many total units of R his patient has received for the day. You calculate the following: breakfast included 45 g CHO, and he ate half of the CHO plus three quarters of his lunch, which had 72 g CHO. The patient weighs 190 lb. How many total units of R has the patient received?

8. You estimate that the patient ate half of his carbohydrates for lunch. The total CHO on his lunch menu was 50 g. His weight is 81 kg. How many units of R should he receive?

9. The patient weighs 70 kg. He has consumed 44 g CHO for breakfast, 72 g CHO for lunch, and 48 g CHO for dinner. His bedtime snack had 15 g CHO. What is the total amount of CHO the patient has consumed? What is the total amount of R he requires for the day?

10. Breakfast included 38 g CHO. The patient ate half of the CHO on the tray. Lunch included 50 g of CHO, and she ate one quarter of the CHO on the tray. Dinner included 48 g CHO, and she ate one third of the CHO. She weighs 112 lb. What is the total amount of CHO the patient has consumed? What is the total amount of R she requires for the three meals?

Answers on page 353

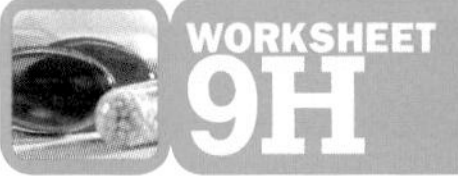

WORKSHEET 9H Multiple-Choice Practice

Calculate units per hr, mL per hr, and hours to infuse.

1. The IV is infusing at 10 mL per hr. You have NS 250 mL with 100 units of R insulin. How many units per hr of insulin is the patient receiving?
   a. 8 units **b.** 2 units **c.** 10 units **d.** 4 units

2. Using the units per hr in question 1, calculate how many hours it will take to infuse the 100 units of insulin.
   a. 50 hr **b.** 25 hr **c.** 15 hr **d.** 5 hr

3. Ordered: 15 units of Lantus (glargine) subcutaneous. What is the length of effectiveness of the insulin?
   a. 12 hr **b.** 4 hr **c.** 36 hr **d.** 24 hr

4. Ordered: 10 units of R insulin per hr IVPB. Available: 500 mL NS with 100 units of R insulin. At what rate will you set the IV infusion device?
   a. 50 mL per hr **b.** 25 mL per hr **c.** 100 mL per hr **d.** 5 mL per hr

5. Ordered: 30 units of R insulin to be infused over 12 hr. Available: 50 mL NS with 30 units of insulin. How many units per hr will be infused?
   a. 1.5 units **b.** 2.5 units **c.** 5 units **d.** 4 units

   At how many mL per hr will you set the infusion device?
   a. 4 mL per hr **b.** 12 mL per hr **c.** 41 mL per hr **d.** 8 mL per hr

6. The type of insulin that is used for infusions is
   a. Humulin N **b.** Levemir **c.** Humulin R **d.** Lantus

7. You have 100 mL of NS with 100 units of R insulin as an IVPB. The patient's BS level at 0600 is 300 mg per dL. Using the Standard Infusion Insulin Chart (see Figure 9.14), at what rate per hour will you start the IV?
   a. 5 mL per hr **b.** 4 mL per hr **c.** 3 mL per hr **d.** 2.5 mL per hr

8. Ordered: Humulin N 20 units subcutaneous at 0730.When will it peak?
   a. 4-5 hr **b.** 4-10 hr **c.** 1-3 hr **d.** 3-4 hr

9. Lantus (glargine) is the preferred insulin because it:
   a. peaks in 15 minutes
   b. has a duration of 16 hr
   c. is absorbed quickly
   d. is peakless

10. Lantus (glargine) is usually given subcutaneously:
   a. at breakfast **b.** at bedtime **c.** at midday **d.** anytime

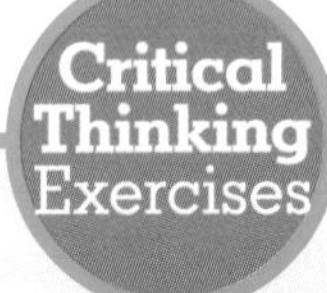

Critical Thinking Exercises provide math and medication-related patient safety issues for student discussion. Answers are not provided.

Analyze the following scenario.

1. Mr. Johnson's blood sugar level was 350 mg per dL. The orders on his chart read: Give 10 units of Humalog stat and check the bedside BS in 1 hour. The nurse gave the insulin at 1400 hr. After the change of shift, at 1430 hr, Mr. Johnson was incoherent. On checking the Diabetes Flow Sheet the nurse found that Mr. Johnson had been given 1 mL (100 units) of Humalog.

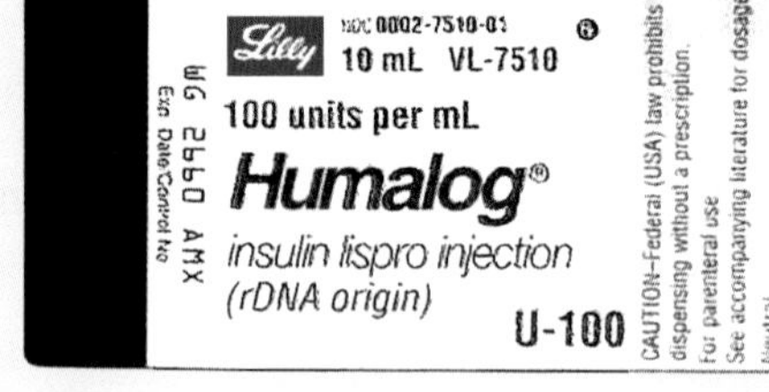

Ordered:

Given:

Error(s):

Discussion

What would be your immediate action?

How did this error occur?

How could this error have been prevented?

Do you think the nurse should have known the safe dosage range?

What were the potential injuries to the patient?

How can a safety issue like this be reconciled?

2. Mrs. B. was admitted to the surgical unit through the emergency department with a diagnosis of diabetic ulceration on right ankle. She has used an insulin pump for over 1 year and said it works well for her as she is able to be more ambulatory and free from giving herself multiple daily injections. At the time of admission, she did not have any diabetic supplies to care for the insulin pump. At 1100 hr, she asked the nurse to fill the reservoir on her insulin pump. The nurse checked the order, which read: Fill reservoir with 3 mL of U-100 insulin PRN. After filling the reservoir, the nurse then inserted the reservoir into Mrs. B.'s infusion device. After the change of shift at 1600 hr, the evening nurse noticed that Mrs. B. looked flushed. Her skin was warm and dry, and her reflexes were slow. The nurse took her vitals and found: BP 90/75, respirations 14, pulse 60 and weak. The nurse detected a fruity odor to her breath. The reservoir on the insulin device showed 2.5 mL left. The nurse then tested Mrs. B.'s blood sugar and found it to be 400 mg per dL.

Discussion:
What would be your immediate action?
What error occurred?
Was the order specific?
Should the nurse have known the type of insulin to put in the reservoir?
How can this type of error be remediated to ensure patient safety?

3. After shoulder replacement surgery, Mr. H., who is a type 1 diabetic, returned to the surgical unit in your care. He has an IV with 100 units of insulin in 100 mL of 0.9% normal saline infusing at 4 units per hr and heparin IV infusing with 1000 units of heparin in 250 mL infusing at 10 mL per hr. The PACU nurse transferred the MAR and stated that Mr. H. had been given a 5000-unit bolus dose of heparin and 10 mg morphine 10 minutes ago. When taking his vitals, the assigned nurse noticed Mr. H.'s blood sugar level had escalated to 300 mg per dL, probably due to the stress of surgery. When the nurse contacted the provider by phone, the provider ordered a bolus of 20 units of insulin and then a recheck of the blood glucose level in 1 hour. The nurse wrote the order and had it checked by the supervisor, who initialed it as being a correct order. The assigned nurse proceeded to give the 20 units into the IV port as a bolus dose.

After 1 hour, the nurse checked the blood glucose level and found it to be 380 mg per dL. The nurse contacted the supervisor and the provider. The two nurses analyzed the situation and realized that the assigned nurse had given a bolus dose of 20 units of heparin in place of the insulin.
What would be your first action?
Insulin is a high-alert drug; therefore, what preventative measures should have been followed?
What are the potential serious consequences for the patient?

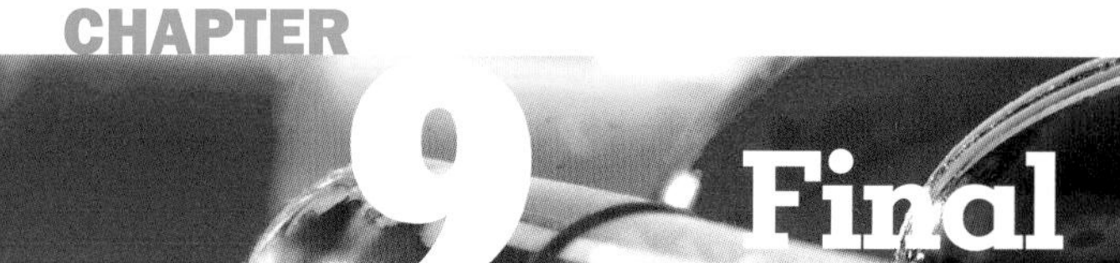

CHAPTER 9 Final

1. Ordered: Humalog insulin 15 units stat. Available: Humalog insulin.
   a. How many units will you give?

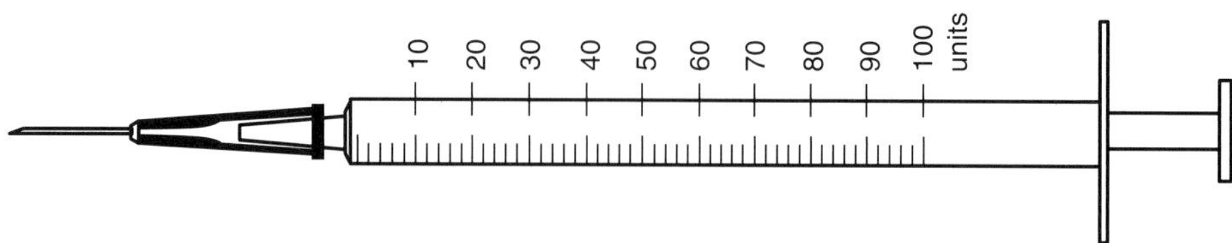

   b. Which syringe will give a precise measurement? Shade in correct amount.

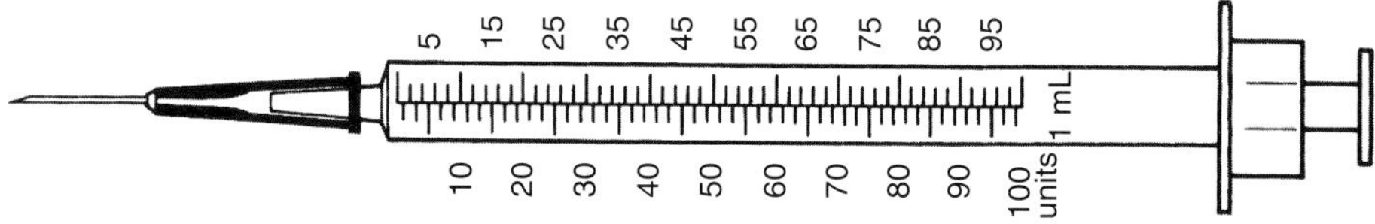

2. The blood sugar level is 280. How many units of Regular insulin will you give subcutaneously? Use the sliding scale on page 341.

3. Ordered: Novolin R 16 units with Novolin N insulin 30 units at 0700. Shade in the amount of regular insulin. Shade in the amount of N insulin and label.

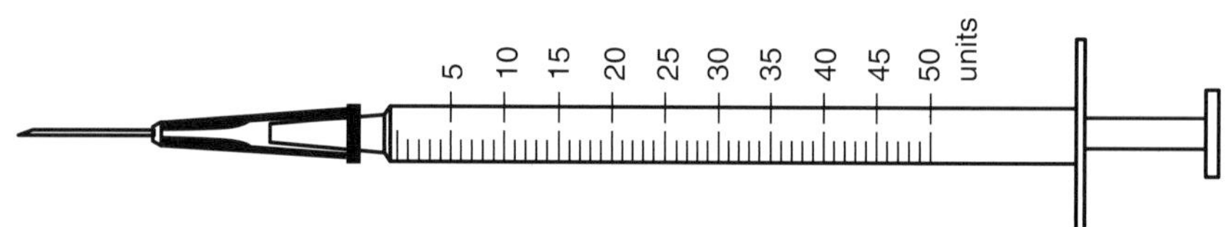

4. Ordered: Humalog 18 units before breakfast at 0930.
   a. How many units will you give?

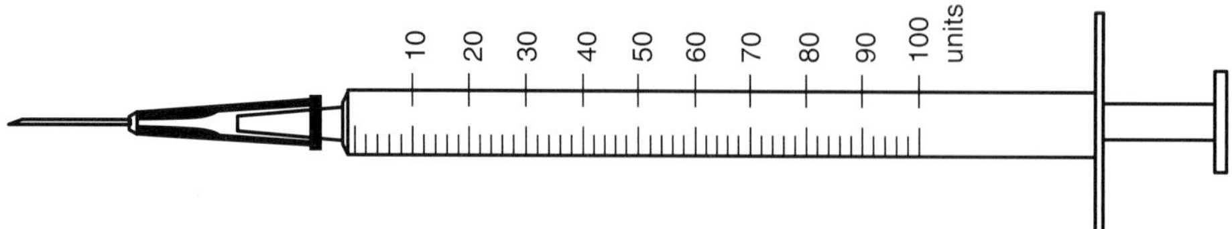

   b. Which syringe is easier to read?

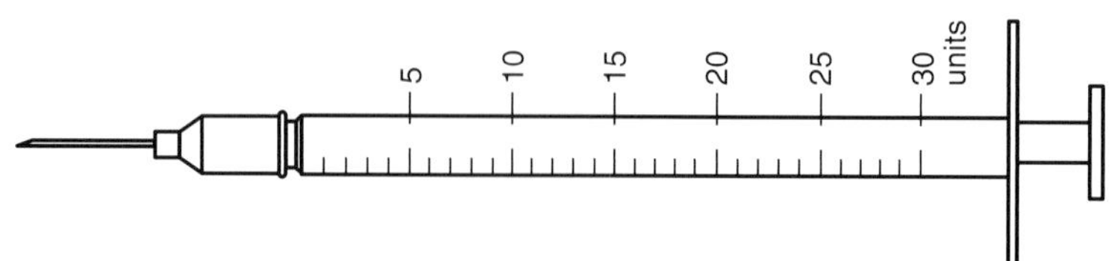

5. Ordered: Glucophage 850 mg tab and Novolin N 15 units before breakfast. How many total units will you give? Shade in the correct amount.

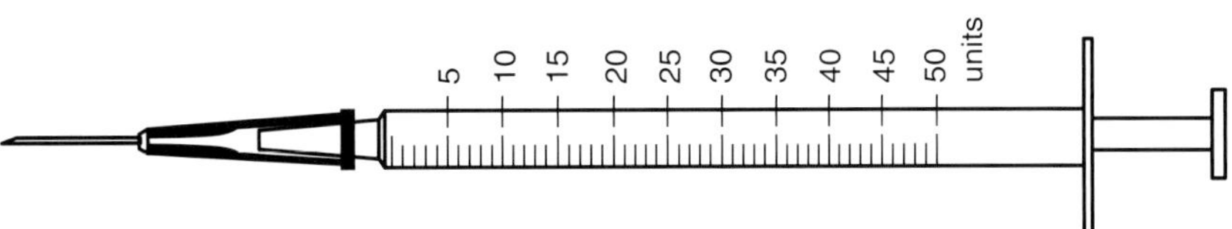

6. Ordered: 10 units per hr Novolin R insulin IV. Available: 500 mL 0.9% saline with 250 units Novolin R regular insulin.

a. How many mL per hr will deliver 10 units per hr?

b. How many hours will the IV infuse?

7. Ordered: 6 units per hr Novolin R IV. Available: 100 units Humulin R insulin in 250 mL of 0.9% saline.

a. How many mL per hr will infuse 6 units of insulin?

b. How many hours will the IV infuse?

8. Ordered: 8 units per hr Novolin R IV. Available: 250 mL NS with 100 units insulin.

a. How many mL per hr will infuse 8 units of insulin?

b. How many hours will the IV infuse?

9. Ordered: 7 units per hr Novolin R IV. Available: 200 mL NS with 100 units Novolin R.

a. How many mL per hr will infuse 7 units per hr?

b. How many hours will the IV infuse?

10. Ordered: Humulin R 9 units per hr IV. Available: 500 mL NS IV solution with 100 units Humulin R.

a. How many mL per hr will infuse 9 units per hr?

b. For how many hours will the IV infuse?

Refer to the Advanced Calculations section of Drug Calculations, version 5 on Evolve for additional practice problems.

Answer Key

9 Insulin Administration and Type 2 Diabetes Medications

WORKSHEET **9A** (page 318)

1. 27 units
2. 68 units
3. 16 units
4. 44 units
5. 32 units
6. 78 units
7. 42 units
8. 39 units
9. 23 units
10. 18 units

WORKSHEET **9B** (page 321)

1. b
2. b
3. a
4. a
5. a

WORKSHEET **9C** (page 326)

1. Total units: 68
a is correct
b insulins are reversed–drawn up incorrectly.

2. Total units: 39
a is correct

3. Total units: 23
a is correct

4. Total units: 38
b is correct

5. Total units: 48
b is correct

6. 42 units
Peak: 2 to 4 hr for R
Duration: 1 to 18 hr for N

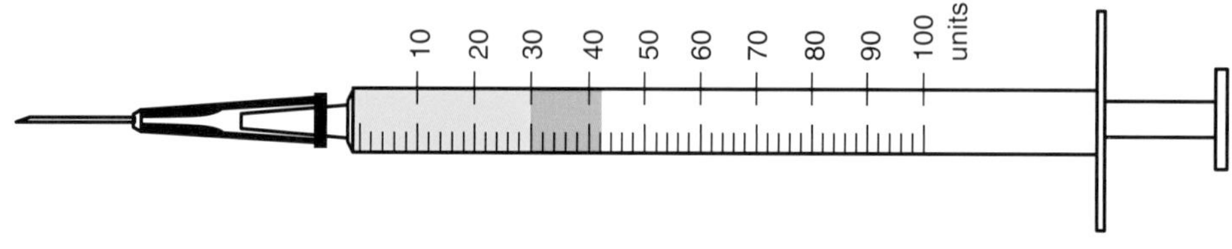

7. 10 units
Onset: 10 to 15 min

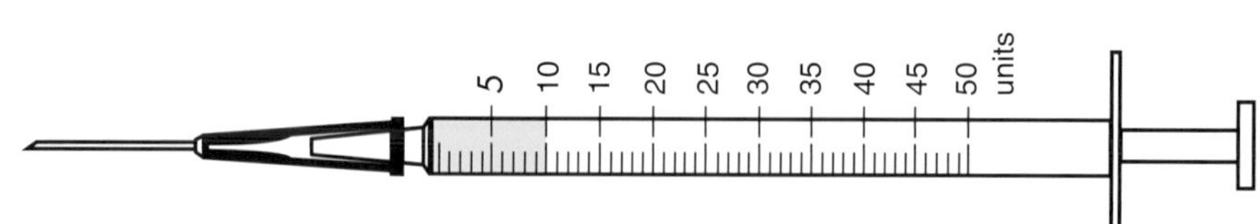

8. 44 units
Peak: 2-10 hr
Duration: 10 to 18 hr

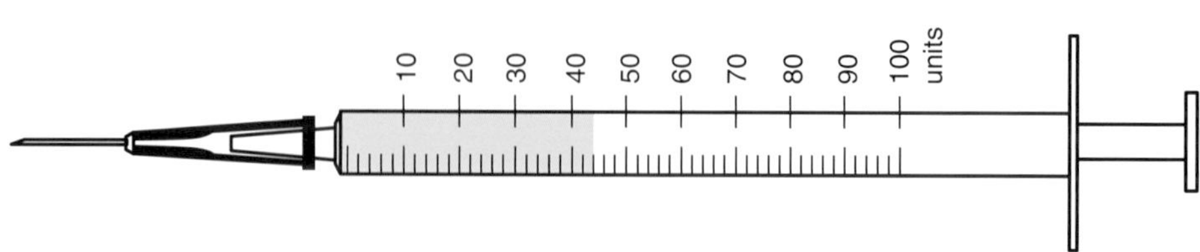

9. 50 units
Duration: 10 to 18 hr

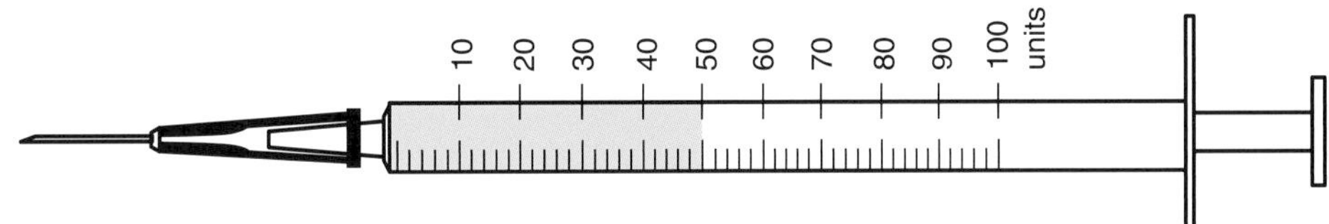

10. 15 units
Peak: 30-90 minutes

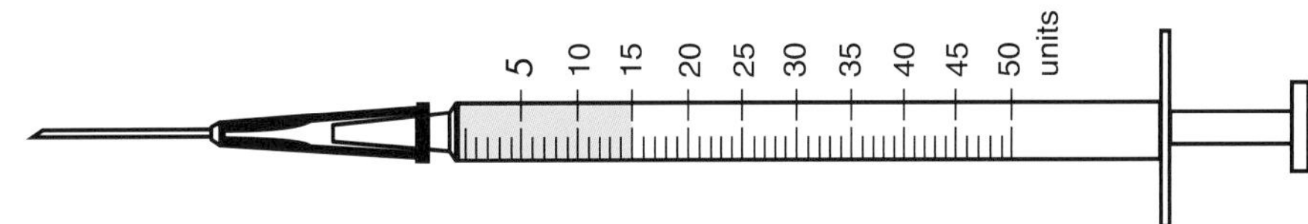

WORKSHEET 9D (page 330)

1. a. 4 units per hr or 4 mLs per hr
b. 3 units per hr or 3 mLs per hr

2. a. KNOW WANT TO KNOW
100 units : 100 mL = 2.5 units : x mL
$100x = 100 \times 2.5 = 250$
$x = 2.5$ mL/hr $\quad \frac{100}{100} \times \frac{2.5}{x}$
PROOF
$100 \times 2.5 = 250$
$100 \times 2.5 = 250$
b. Change IV rate to 3 mL/hr
c. 5.5 units

3. 20 total units
It would be prudent to check with the prescriber whether the patient should receive the insulin coverage if the BS goes below 120 mg per dL.

4. a. KNOW WANT TO KNOW
50 mL : 100 units = x mL : 5 units
$100x = 50 \times 5 = 250$
$x = 2.5$ mL/hr $\quad \frac{50}{100} \times \frac{x}{5}$
PROOF
$100 \times 2.5 = 250$
$50 \times 5 = 250$
b. 5 units per hour × 16 hours = 80 units of insulin

5. a. KNOW WANT TO KNOW
100 units : 50 mL = x units : 3 mL
$50x = 100 \times 3 = 300$
$x = 6$ units/hr $\quad \frac{100}{50} \times \frac{x}{3}$
PROOF
$100 \times 3 = 300$
$50 \times 6 = 300$
b. 8 hr × 6 units per hr = 48 units

6. KNOW WANT TO KNOW
100 units : 150 mL = 10 units : x mL
$100x = 150 \times 10 = 1500$
$100x = 1500$
$x = 15$ mL/hr = 10 units insulin $\quad \frac{100}{150} \times \frac{10}{x}$
PROOF
$100 \times 15 = 1500$
$150 \times 10 = 1500$
KNOW WANT TO KNOW
15 mL : 1 hr = 150 mL : x hr
$15x = 150$
$x = 10$ hr to infuse 100 units insulin $\quad \frac{15}{1} \times \frac{150}{x}$
PROOF
$15 \times 10 = 150$
$1 \times 150 = 150$

7. KNOW WANT TO KNOW

50 mL : 50 units = x mL : 8 units

$50x = 50 \times 8 = 400$ $\frac{50}{50} \times \frac{x}{8}$

$50x = 400$

$x = 8$ mL/hr = 8 units of insulin

PROOF

$50 \times 8 = 400$

$50 \times 8 = 400$

KNOW WANT TO KNOW

8 mL : 1 hr = 50 mL : x hr

$8x = 50$ $\frac{8}{1} \times \frac{50}{x}$

$x = 6.25$ hr to infuse 50 units insulin or 6 hr 15 min

PROOF

$8 \times 6.25 = 50$

$1 \times 50 = 50$

8. KNOW WANT TO KNOW

50 mL : 75 units = x mL : 12 units

$75x = 50 \times 12 = 600$ $\frac{50}{75} \times \frac{x}{12}$

$75x = 600$

$x = 8$ mL/hr = 12 units

PROOF

$50 \times 12 = 600$

$75 \times 8 = 600$

KNOW WANT TO KNOW

8 mL : 1 hr = 50 mL : x hr

$8x = 50$ $\frac{8}{1} \times \frac{50}{x}$

$x = 6.25$ hr = 6 hr 15 min to infuse

PROOF

$1 \times 50 = 50$

$8 \times 6.25 = 50$

9. KNOW WANT TO KNOW

100 mL : 120 units = x mL : 10 units

$120x = 100 \times 10 = 1000$ $\frac{100}{120} \times \frac{x}{10}$

$120x = 1000$

$x = 8.33$ mL/hr to deliver 10 units of insulin

PROOF

$120 \times 8.33 = 999.6$

$100 \times 10 = 1000$

KNOW WANT TO KNOW

8 mL : 1 hr = 100 mL : x hr

$8x = 1 \times 100 = 100$

$8x = 100$ $\frac{8}{1} \times \frac{100}{x}$

$x = 12.5$ hr to infuse 120 units of regular insulin

PROOF

$8 \times 12.5 = 100$

$1 \times 100 = 100$

10. KNOW WANT TO KNOW

150 mL : 150 units = x mL : 12 units

$150x = 150 \times 12$ $\frac{150}{150} \times \frac{x}{12}$

$150x = 1800$

$x = 12$ mL/hr to deliver 12 units of insulin

PROOF

$150 \times 12 = 1800$

$12 \times 150 = 1800$

KNOW WANT TO KNOW

12 mL : 1 hr = 150 mL : x hr

$12x = 150$ $\frac{12}{1} \times \frac{150}{x}$

$x = 12.5$ hr to infuse 150 units of regular insulin, or 12 hr 30 min

$12 \times 12.5 = 150$

$1 \times 150 = 150$

WORKSHEET **9E** (page 338)

1. BS difference is 20 divided by 10 = 2 units of R
   CHO is 48 g divided by 8 = 6 units R
   Total units = 8

2. BS difference is 5 divided by 10 = 0.5 = 1 unit R (rounded to nearest whole number)
   CHO is 71 g divided by 8 = 8.87 = 9 units R
   Total units = 10

3. BS difference is 15 divided by 10 = 1.5 = 2 units R
   CHO is 34 g divided by 8 = 4.25 = 4 units R
   Total units = 6

   Snack: BS difference is 15 divided by 10 = 1.5 = 2 units R
   CHO is 15 g divided by 8 = 1.87 = 2 units R
   Total insulin for the day = 28 units

4. BS difference is −5 = 0 units R
CHO is 43 g divided by 10 = 4.3 = 4 units R
Total units = 4

5. BS difference is 20 divided by 10 = 2 units
CHO is 93 g divided by 10 = 9.3 = 9 units R
Total units = 11

WORKSHEET **9F** (page 340)

1. BS difference is 30 divided by 20 = 1.5 = 2 units R
CHO is 98 g divided by 15 = 6.5 = 7 units R
Total = 9 units R

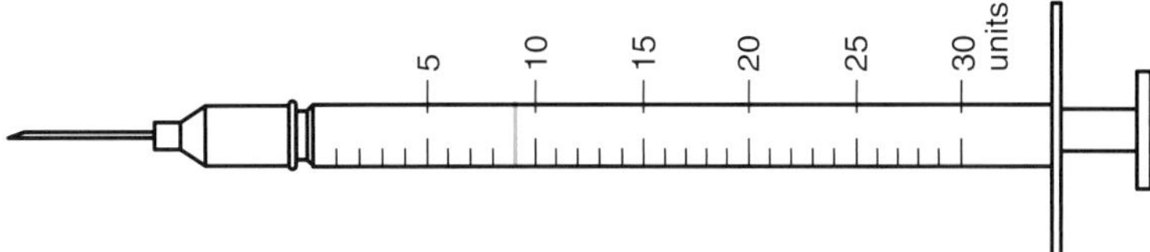

2. BS difference is 20 divided by 20 = 1 = 1 unit R
CHO is 40 g divided by 15 = 2.6 = 3 units R
Total = 4 units R

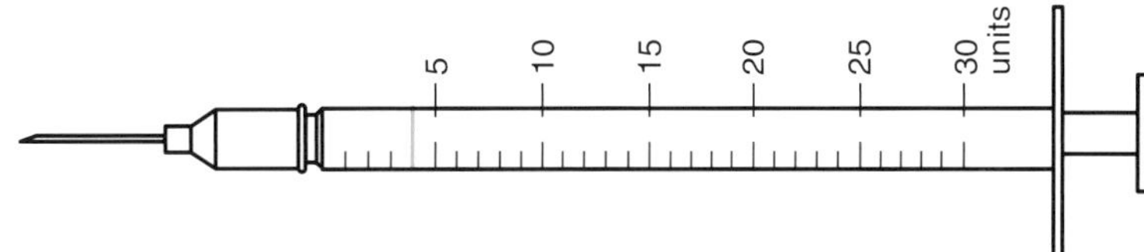

3. BS difference is 50 divided by 20 = 2.5 = 3 units R
CHO is 118 g divided by 15 = 7.8 = 8 units R
Total = 11 units R

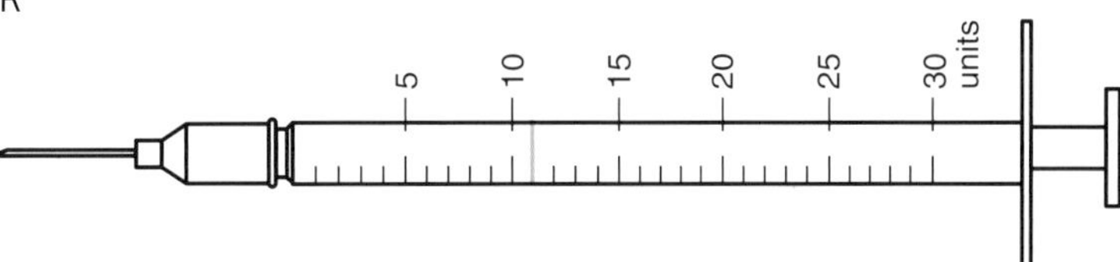

4. BS difference is 90 divided by 30 = 3 units R
CHO is 58 g divided by 10 = 5.8 = 6 units R
Total = 9 units R

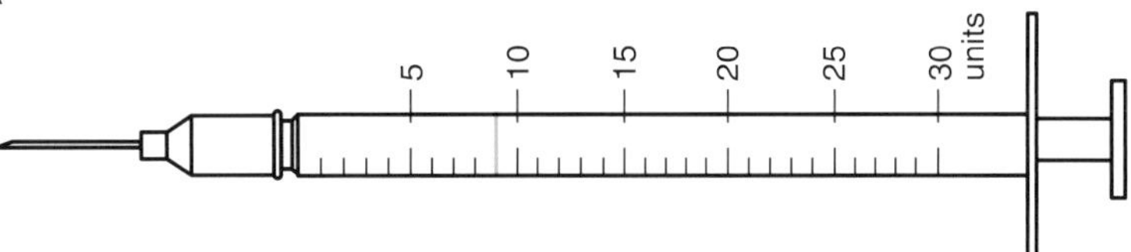

5. BS difference is 30 divided by 30 = 1 unit R
CHO is 120 g divided by 10 = 12 units R
Total = 13 units R

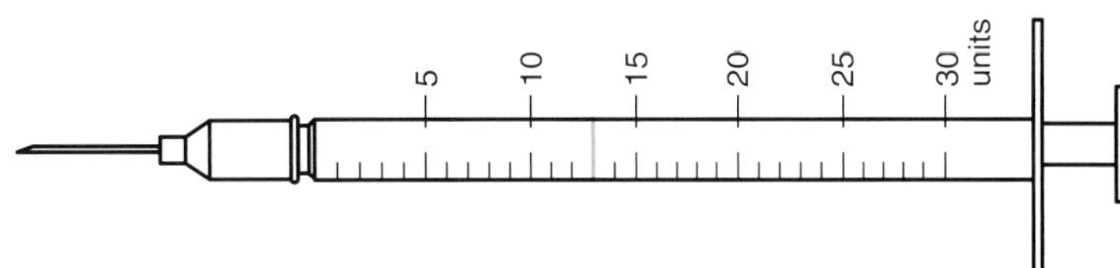

6. BS difference is 110 divided by 30 = 3.6 = 4 units R
CHO is 58 g divided by 10 = 5.8 = 6 units R
Total = 10 units R

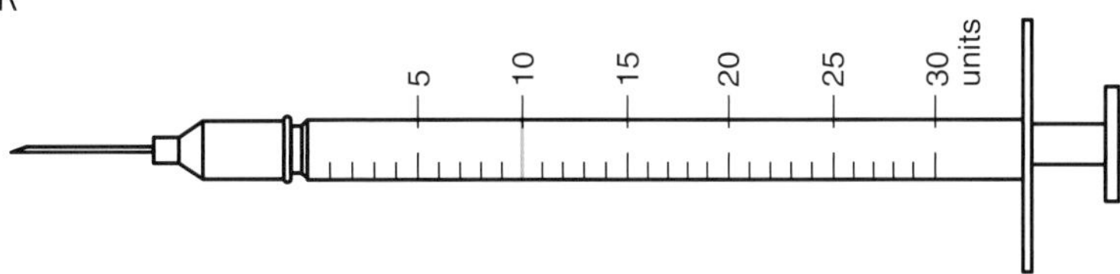

7. BS difference is 10 divided by 30 = 0.3 = 0 units R
CHO is 28 g divided by 10 = 2.8 = 3 units R
Total = 3 units R

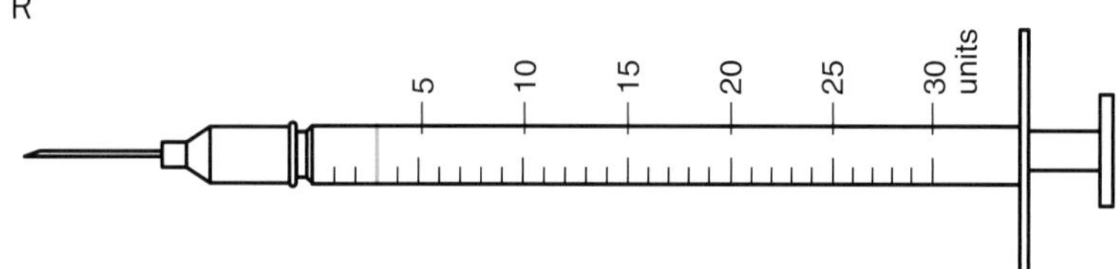

WORKSHEET **9G** (page 342)

1. $\frac{\text{total g}}{\text{units}} = \frac{26}{13}$ = 2 units R

2. $\frac{\text{total g}}{\text{units}} = \frac{80}{9}$ = 8.8 = 9 units R

3. $\frac{\text{total g}}{\text{units}} = \frac{18}{16}$ = 1.1 = 1 unit R

4. $\frac{\text{total g}}{\text{units}} = \frac{90}{6}$ = 15 units R

5. $\frac{\text{total g}}{\text{units}} = \frac{160}{11}$ = 14.5 units = 15 units R for 24 hr

6. $\frac{\text{total g}}{\text{units}} = \frac{145}{7}$ = 20.7 = 21 units R for 24 hr

7. $\frac{1}{2}$ of 45 = 22.5 + $\frac{3}{4}$ of 75 = 56.25 = 78.75; 78.75 ÷ 8 = 9.8 = 10 units R

8. 50 g divided by 2 = $\frac{25\text{ g}}{10}$ = 2.5 = 3 units R

9. Total amount of CHO = 179 g
   $\frac{179}{12}$ = 14.9 = 15 units for the day

10. $\frac{1}{2}$ of 38 = 19 g; $\frac{1}{4}$ of 50 = 12.5 g; $\frac{1}{3}$ of 48 = 16 g
    Total CHO grams = 47.5 = 3 units total for the 3 meals

WORKSHEET 9H (page 343)

1. d. 4 units

KNOW WANT TO KNOW

250 mL : 100 units = 10 mL : x units

$250x = 100 \times 10 = 1000$

$x = 4$ units/hr

$$\frac{250}{100} \times \frac{10}{x}$$

PROOF

$250 \times 4 = 1000$

$100 \times 10 = 1000$

2. b. 25 hr

KNOW WANT TO KNOW

4 units : 1 hr = 100 units : x hr

$4x = 100$

$x = 25$ hr

$$\frac{4}{1} \times \frac{100}{x}$$

PROOF

$1 \times 100 = 100$

$4 \times 25 = 100$

3. d. 24 hr

4. a. 50 mL/hr

KNOW WANT TO KNOW

500 mL : 100 units = x mL : 10 units

$100x = 500 \times 10 = 5000$

$x = 50$ mL/hr

$$\frac{500}{100} \times \frac{x}{10}$$

PROOF

$100 \times 50 = 5000$

$500 \times 10 = 5000$

5. b. 2.5 units/hr

KNOW WANT TO KNOW

30 units : 12 hr = x units : 1 hr

$12x = 30$

$x = 2.5$ units/hr

$$\frac{30}{12} \times \frac{x}{1}$$

PROOF

$30 \times 1 = 30$

$12 \times 2.5 = 30$

a. 4 mL/hr

50 mL : 12 hr = x mL : 1 hr

$12x = 50$

$x = 4.16 = 4$ mL/hr

$$\frac{50}{12} \times \frac{x}{1}$$

PROOF

$50 \times 1 = 50$

$12 \times 4.16 = 4.9$

6. c. Humulin R

7. c. 3 mL/hr

KNOW WANT TO KNOW

100 units : 100 mL = 3 units : x mL

$100x = 100 \times 3 = 300$

$x = 3$ mL/hr

$$\frac{100}{100} \times \frac{3}{x}$$

PROOF

$100 \times 3 = 300$

$100 \times 3 = 300$

8. b. 4 to 10 hr

9. d. is peakless

10. b. at bedtime

CHAPTER 9 FINAL: INSULIN ADMINISTRATION AND TYPE 2 DIABETES MEDICATIONS (page 346)

1. 15 units
b

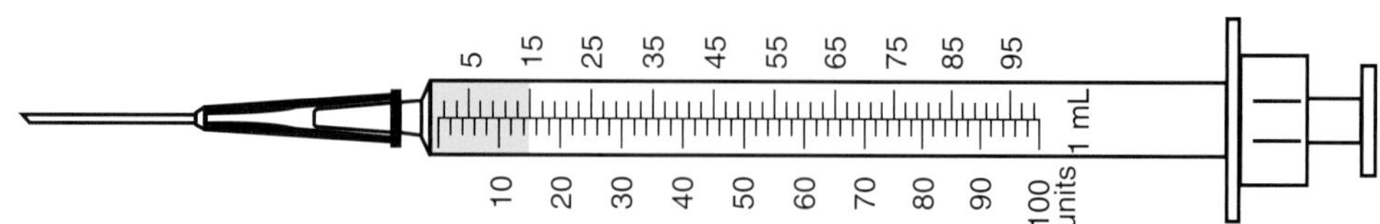

2. Sliding scale
Give 6 units.

3. 16 units Humulin R
30 units Humulin N
Total amount is 46 units.

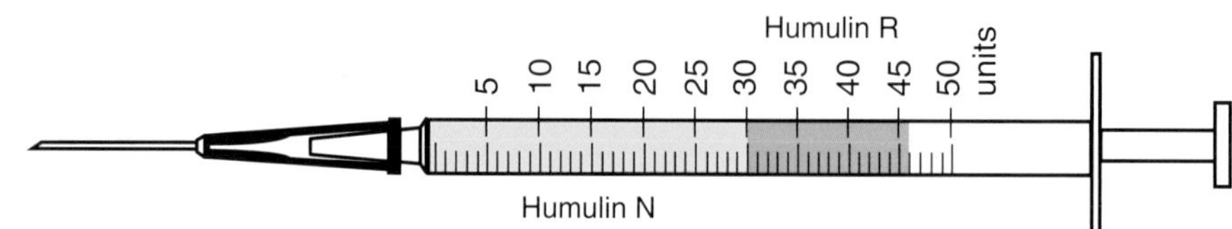

4. 18 units Humalog
b is easier to read

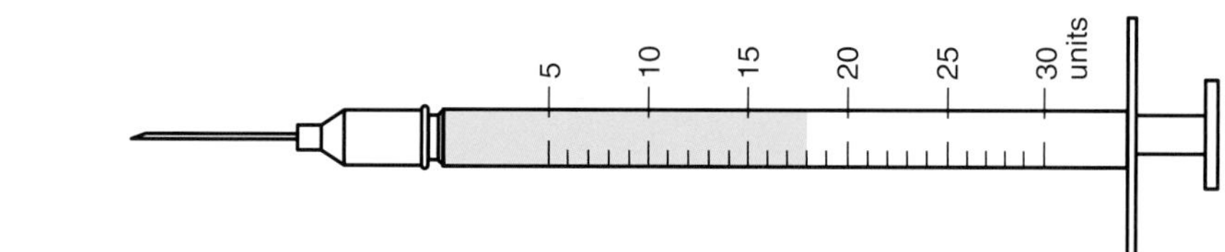

5. 15 units Novolin N

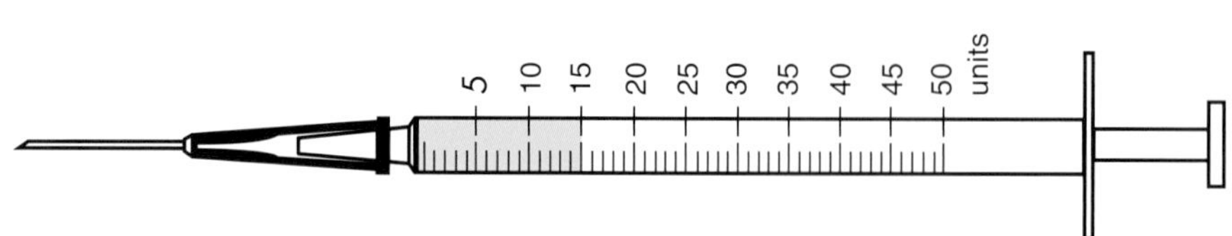

6. 20 mL per hr = 10 units
25 hr to infuse. An IV solution can hang for only 24 hr (CDC guidelines).

7. 15 mL per hr to infuse 6 units insulin
16.6 hr to infuse = 16 hr 36 min

8. 20 mL per hr to infuse 8 units insulin
12.5 hr to infuse = 12 hr 30 min

9. 14 mL per hr to infuse 7 units insulin
14.28 hr to infuse = 14 hr 17 min

10. 45 mL per hr to infuse 9 units insulin
11.1 hr to infuse = 11 hr 6 min

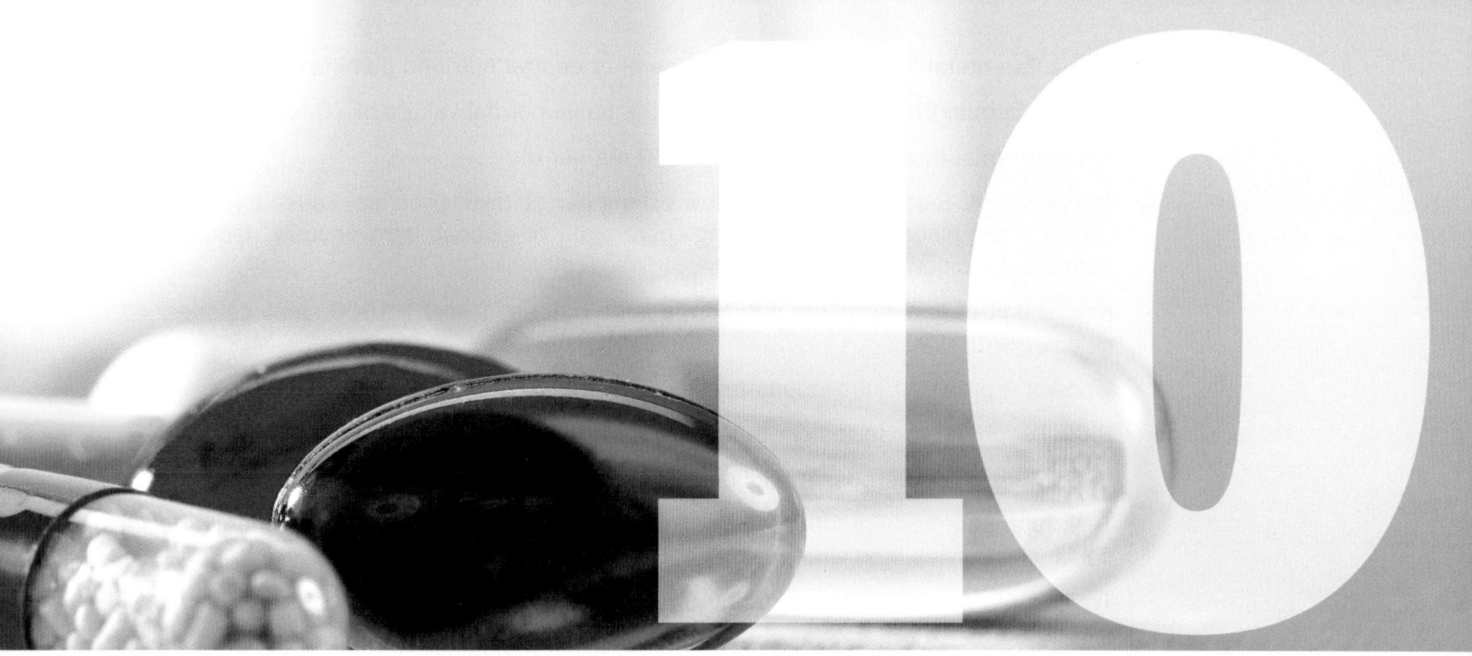

Parenteral Nutrition

Objectives

- Calculate grams of protein, carbohydrate, and lipids per order.
- Calculate the percentage of protein, carbohydrate, and lipids per infusion.
- Discuss the reasons different concentrations of additives are used in peripheral and central lines.
- Calculate the kilocalories for protein, carbohydrate, and lipids per infusion.
- Calculate the total kilocalorie per infusion.
- Compare the provider's order for parenteral nutrition with the infusion label for each unit (bottle/bag) supplied from the pharmacy.
- Analyze medication errors using critical thinking.

Introduction

The IV requirements for patients who are unable to ingest food and fluid are calculated on a daily basis. Concentrations of nutrients are calculated to show the differing strengths and percentages of additives for peripheral and central lines. The percentage of additives is calculated to ensure that the electrolyte and mineral requirements are being met. Standard orders for peripheral and central lines are compared. The importance of parenteral orders and of verification of the labels on the bag is stressed.

Vocabulary

AA: Amino acids or protein.

CHO: Carbohydrates. In parenteral nutrition, the carbohydrate is a specific concentration of dextrose, a sugar.

CPN: Nutrition delivered by central (venous) parenteral infusion.

Diabetes Mellitus (DM): A chronic metabolic disorder resulting in hyperglycemia caused by inadequate or no production of insulin by the islets of Langerhans in the pancreas or the inability of the body to use the available insulin that is produced.

Diabetic Ketoacidosis (DKA): A complication of diabetes diagnosed by elevated blood sugar (above 250 mg per dL), elevated ketones in the blood and urine (from the partial breakdown of body fat) and a blood pH below 7.3; this condition is an emergency for the patient because death may result if the pH is not corrected quickly.

Glucagon: A hormone produced by the alpha cells of the islets of Langerhans in the pancreas that increases the blood glucose level by stimulating the liver to convert stored glycogen to glucose. Used to reverse hypoglycemia and insulin shock by opposing the action of insulin.

Home Parenteral Nutrition (HPN): Peripheral or central nutrition administered in the home.

Hyperglycemia: Blood sugar level above the basic normal values of 70 to 100 mg per dL.

Hypoglycemia: Blood sugar level below 70 mg per dL.

Insulin Shock: Blood sugar level below 60 mg per dL (hypoglycemia) caused by too much insulin in the blood. Treated by giving sugar orally or glucose intravenously, depending on the patient's condition.

Kcal: A unit of energy, and in nutrition, a large Calorie; 1 kcal = 1000 small calories = 1 calorie USA.

Liposyn: A prepared intravenous fat emulsion.

PICC: Peripherally inserted central (venous) catheter.

PPN: Nutrition delivered by peripheral (venous) parenteral infusion.

TPN: Total parenteral nutrition; the non-GI administration of CHO (dextrose), amino acids, lipids, electrolytes, and vitamins.

Type 1 DM: Metabolic disorder related to a failure of the pancreas to produce insulin.

Type 2 DM: Inadequate insulin secretion or insulin resistance due to decreased sensitivity or recognition of muscle cells to uptake insulin.

Total Parenteral Nutrition

Nutritional support of the sick patient in various care agencies as well as in the home has become increasingly important. More people are being treated with total parenteral nutrition (TPN) in the home, and it is the nurse's responsibility to teach the patient and the family to care for the catheter insertion site and the infusion pump, and to educate them about possible side effects of the infusion. Survival of the patient with a gastrointestinal problem has been made possible by advances in the field of parenteral nutrition.

TPN permits the venous administration of dextrose, amino acids, lipids, electrolytes, and vitamins to sustain life when the gastrointestinal system must be bypassed or during serious illness or injury (e.g., burns). A TPN bag is shown in Figure 10.1.

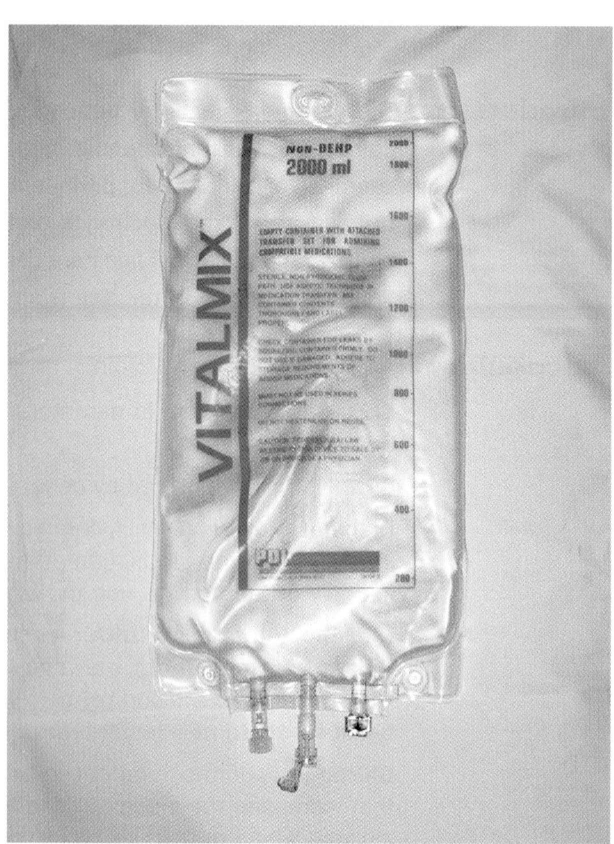

FIGURE 10.1 TPN bag. The content label will be put on the bag by the pharmacist.

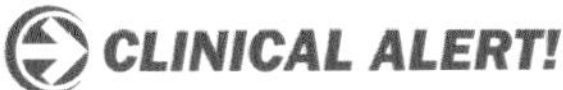

CLINICAL ALERT!

Medication incompatibility can occur when IV drugs are delivered along with TPN administration. A pharmacist with special training in intravenous TPN should be consulted to determine compatibility. A dedicated PICC line, Groshong catheter, Hickman/Broviac port should be established.

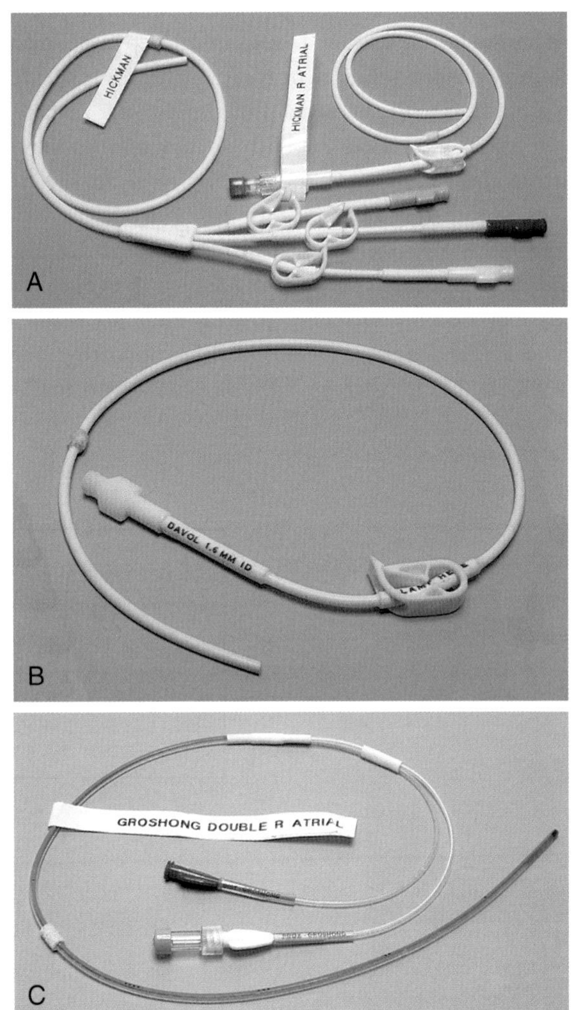

A, Hickman catheter. **B,** Broviac catheter. **C,** Groshong catheter. (From Clayton BD, Willihnganz MJ: *Basic pharmacology for nurses,* ed. 16, St. Louis, 2013, Elsevier.)

A routine maintenance IV solution of 1000 mL with 5% dextrose delivered over an 8-hour period provides approximately 200 calories derived from dextrose. If a patient is restricted from ingesting anything by mouth (NPO, npo) and receives 3 liters of D5W a day, the 600 total calories received would not be enough to promote or maintain health for a sustained period. In contrast, TPN may deliver as much as 1 calorie per mL, depending on the concentration of nutrients.

TPN administered via a central vein such as the subclavian or internal jugular is known as *central parenteral nutrition (CPN).* Peripheral administration, known as *peripheral parenteral nutrition (PPN),* is delivered via peripheral veins. The choice depends on the patient, vein condition, and how long the patient will need the therapy. The larger central veins are selected for longer-term therapy and higher concentration of nutrients. The contents of TPN are customized according to the patient's condition and need, the venous route, relevant laboratory values, and the patient's weight. Orders for the contents may be changed daily. TPN formulas are specific to the patient and are determined by the individual's energy, protein, fluid, and caloric requirements. Special formulas are created for patients with diabetes, renal or hepatic problems, bowel obstruction, or pancreatitis. This list is not all inclusive.

PPN is used for nutritional therapy lasting 2 weeks or less. A PPN solution must be kept at the following concentration levels to prevent vein irritation: amino acids, 5.5%; dextrose, 10%; lipids, 10%. CPN permits higher levels of concentration because it is infused into larger veins. CPN solutions are hypertonic and have higher osmolarity. CPN is used when nutritional therapy is needed for more than 2 weeks. CPN concentrations usually are as follows: amino acids, 8.5%; dextrose, 20% to 70%; lipids, 20%. Dextrose administered with amino acids spares the protein for tissue repair. Parenteral nutrition must always be administered by an infusion pump—**never** by gravity.

A three-in-one solution, or total nutrition admixture, combines lipids, amino acids, and dextrose. The solution is white because of the lipids, which make precipitation difficult to observe. The three-in-one solution is used for both agency and home therapy. When lipids are administered with dextrose and amino acids, the osmolarity of the solution will improve the tolerance for peripheral venous administration. Lipids are isotonic because of added glycerol and can therefore be administered either peripherally or centrally. Lipids can also be administered separately (Figure 10.2). Lipids help control hyperglycemia, which is a complication of parenteral nutrition. After 12 hours, lipids may become unstable. If a fat embolus could be a problem, monitor the patient closely. Amino acids, vitamins, and other life-supporting additives are easily denigrated when exposed to sunlight. Home therapy TPN is usually run for 12 hours to give the patient some infusion-free time.

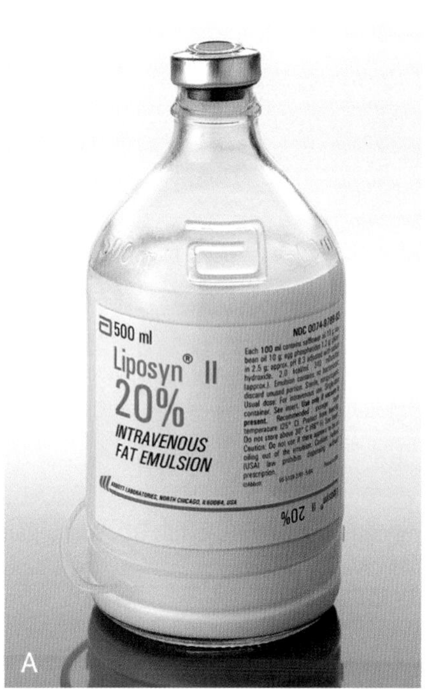

B

```
                A                              RM#:          (N ED )
RX# NO1922945   DUE:07/13/18          BAG#:1   @: 16. ml/hr
FAT EMULSIONS 20%                200ML

* CHANGE TUBING/BOTTLE EVERY 12 HOURS.
* INFUSE AT 17CC/HR X 12 HOURS DAILY.

PREP BY:____ RPH:____ 07/13/18 at: ____  RX.MSALAR
 *** RETURN IV TO PHARMACY IF NOT USED IN 24 HOURS***
```

FIGURE 10.2 **A,** Liposyn II (fat emulsion) 20% for parenteral nutrition. Notice the opaque contents contrasted with the parenteral infusion without lipids (fat emulsion). **B,** Fat emulsion (lipid) order. (**A,** From Abbott Laboratories, Abbott Park, Ill.)

Types of IV Lines

There are many types of IV tubing used for temporary and long-term access to veins and arteries (Figure 10.3).

- **Peripheral** A peripheral line is usually used for fluid replacement and temporary intermittent medication administration. The IV line is inserted in the hand, arm, or possibly leg if the hand or arm cannot be accessed. Foot and scalp sites are used for infants.
- **Peripherally inserted central catheter (PICC)** A PICC line (Figure 10.4) is longer than a central catheterline (approximately 22 inches in length). The insertion point is usually the vein in the antecubital region of the arm, where the line is then advanced into the superior vena cava. It is inserted by a PICC-certified RN or provider. Only solutions with an osmolarity of less than 10% should be administered via peripheral lines.

A Subclavian Catheter Site

Peripherally Inserted Central Catheter (PICC) B

C Femoral Catheter Site

Hickman Catheter Site D

Skin line

Self-sealing septum

Suture

Fluid flow

Catheter

E Subclavian Catheter with Implantable Vascular Access Port

Implantable Vascular Access Port F

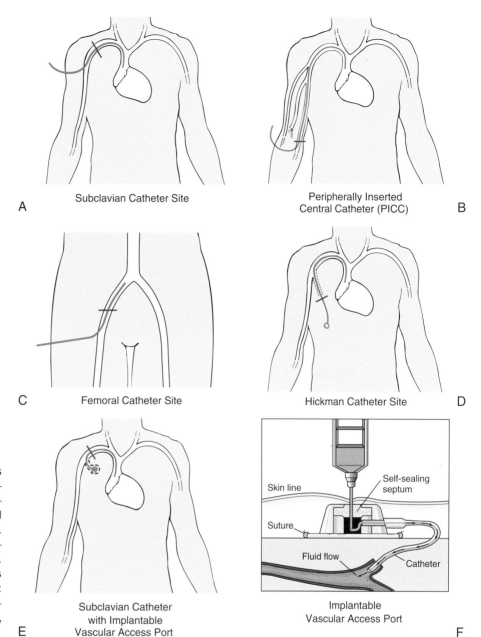

FIGURE 10.3 Central venous access sites. **A,** Subclavian catheter. **B,** Peripherally inserted central catheter (PICC). **C,** Femoral catheter. **D.** Hickman catheter. **E,** Subclavian catheter with implantable vascular access port. **F,** Implantable vascular access port. (**F,** from Perry AG, Potter PA: *Clinical nursing skills and techniques,* ed. 6, St. Louis, 2006, Mosby.)

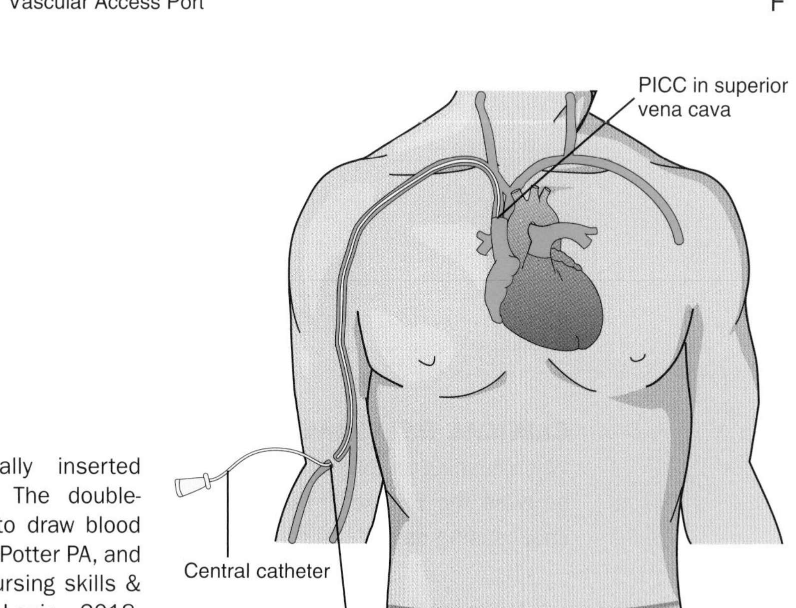

FIGURE 10.4 Peripherally inserted central catheter (PICC). The double-lumen catheter is used to draw blood samples. (From Perry AG, Potter PA, and Ostendort WR: Clinical nursing skills & techniques, ed. 9, St. Louis, 2018, Elsevier.)

- **Central line** A central line (Figure 10.5) is inserted directly into the jugular or subclavian vein and then into the superior vena cava. This type of line is for therapy requiring a longer period of time or when a peripheral line is not possible. The femoral vein may also be used as a central line site.

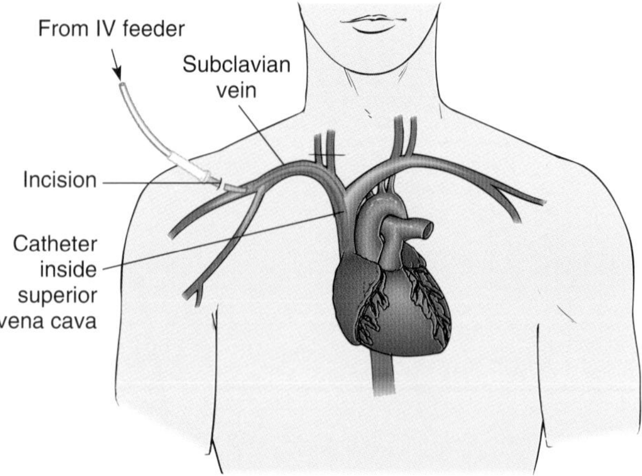

FIGURE 10.5 Placement of central venous catheter inserted into subclavian vein. [(Courtesy Rolin Graphics) From Perry AG, Potter PA, and Ostendort WR: *Clinical nursing skills & techniques*, ed. 9, St. Louis, 2018, Elsevier.]

CLINICAL ALERT!

Only solutions with an osmolarity of less than 10% should be administered via peripheral lines.

Table 10.1 is a guide that can be used to maintain patency by flushing intermittent-access locks. Always refer to manufacturer's insert or agency protocol for type of solution, volume, and frequency.

Table 10.1 Intermittent Flushing Ranges

Catheter	Flush Solution	Volume
Peripheral	Normal saline	1-3 mL
Peripherally inserted central catheter (PICC)	Normal saline	3-5 mL
Central venous	Heparinized saline	5-10 mL of saline followed with 3 mL heparin 1:100 units per mL

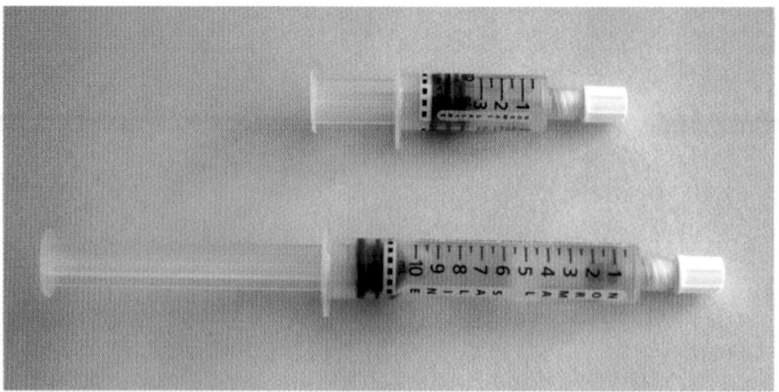

CLINICAL RELEVANCE

When flushing peripheral IV lines, prefilled sterile normal saline should be used. The syringe should be twice the volume of the solution. Smaller syringes may create greater pressure within the IV line, causing damage to the vein.

Automatic dose calculators (Figure 10.6) or electronic infusion devices (EIDs) are programmed by the patient's caregiver to deliver lipids and parenteral nutrition at the accurate mL per hour ordered. Gravity infusion tubing should ***never*** be used because the rate could fluctuate and harm the patient.

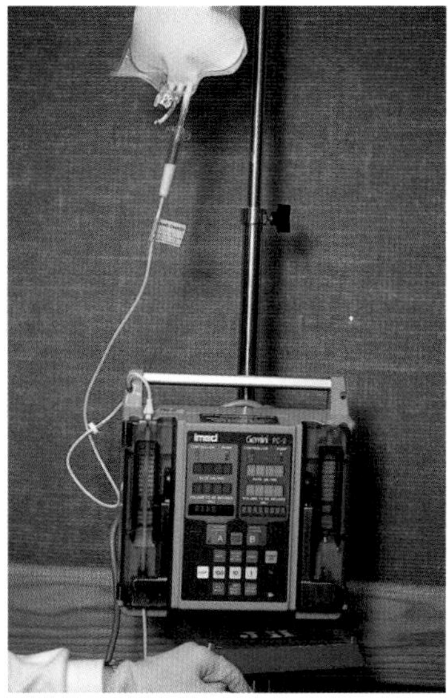

FIGURE 10.6 Automatic dose calculation device showing lipid infusing. (From Perry AG, Potter PA, Ostendorf WR: *Clinical nursing skills and techniques,* ed. 9, St. Louis, 2018, Elseveir.)

A tunneled catheter is surgically inserted into a vein in the neck or chest and passes under the skin (Figure 10.7). This type of catheter allows freedom of movement for the patient during long-term parenteral nutrition.

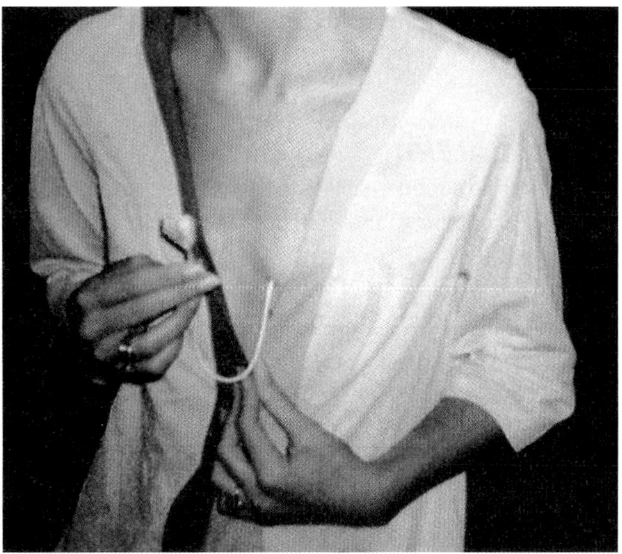

FIGURE 10.7 Tunneled catheter used for central parenteral nutrition given at home. (From Morgan SL, Weinsier RL: *Fundamentals of clinical nutrition*, ed. 2, St. Louis, 1998, Mosby) as presented in Perry AG, Potter PA, and Ostendort WR: *Clinical nursing skills & techniques*, ed. 9, St. Louis, 2018, Elsevier.]

Validation of TPN Label With the Provider's Order

Validate the contents listed on the TPN bag label (Figure 10.8) with the provider's order (Figure 10.9).

The 341 mL of quantity sufficient additive sterile water includes the volume for the additives of calcium gluconate, magnesium sulfate, potassium phosphate, sodium chloride, and multivitamins. In this order, the pharmacist included all of the additives except for the 10 units of insulin, which the nurse will add immediately before administering the bag of TPN.

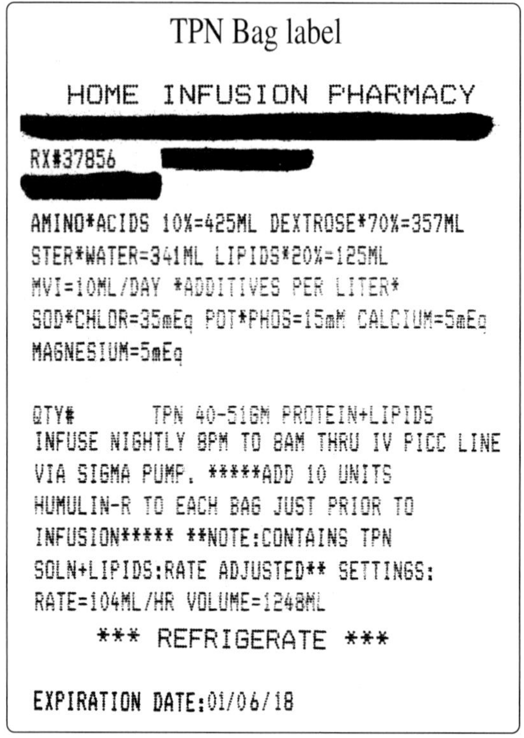

TPN Bag label

HOME INFUSION PHARMACY

RX#37856

AMINO*ACIDS 10%=425ML DEXTROSE*70%=357ML
STER*WATER=341ML LIPIDS*20%=125ML
MVI=10ML/DAY *ADDITIVES PER LITER*
SOD*CHLOR=35mEq POT*PHOS=15mM CALCIUM=5mEq
MAGNESIUM=5mEq

QTY# TPN 40-51GM PROTEIN+LIPIDS
INFUSE NIGHTLY 8PM TO 8AM THRU IV PICC LINE
VIA SIGMA PUMP. *****ADD 10 UNITS
HUMULIN-R TO EACH BAG JUST PRIOR TO
INFUSION***** **NOTE:CONTAINS TPN
SOLN+LIPIDS:RATE ADJUSTED** SETTINGS:
RATE=104ML/HR VOLUME=1248ML

*** REFRIGERATE ***

EXPIRATION DATE:01/06/18

FIGURE 10.8 TPN bag label. It is the nurse's responsibility to check the label on the TPN bag with the provider's order. Quantities of nutrients and additives are calculated based on 1 liter. The total volume (TV) is calculated by adding the amount over 1 liter as a decimal (e.g., 1248 mL = 1.248 L).

CLINICAL ALERT!

It is the nurse's responsibility to check the provider's order to determine if the pharmacy has filled the order according to the directions. Compare the order shown in Figure 10.9 with the label shown in Figure 10.8.

Example Refer to Figure 10.9, a sample provider's order form.

Calculate grams, percentage of concentration, and kilocalories per bag of TPN.

TPN ORDER SHEET

HOME HEALTH | DATE

PATIENT | ADDRESS

TPN FORMULA:

AMINO ACIDS: ☐ 5.5% ☐ 8.5% ☑ 10% ☐ WITH STANDARD ELECTROLYTES	425 mL
DEXTROSE: ☐ 10% ☐ 20% ☐ 40% ☐ 50% ☑ 70% (check one)	357 mL
LIPIDS: ☐ 10% ☑ 20% FOR ALL-IN-ONE FORMULA	125 mL

FINAL VOLUME qsad STERILE WATER FOR INJECTION 341 mL	1248 mL

Calcium Gluconate	0.465 mEq/mL	5 mEq
Magnesium Sulfate	4 mEq/mL	5 mEq
Potassium Acetate	2 mEq/mL	mEq
Potassium Chloride	2 mEq/mL	mEq
Potassium Phosphate	3 mM/mL	15 mM
Sodium Acetate	2 mEq/mL	mEq
Sodium Chloride	4 mEq/mL	35 mEq
Sodium Phosphate	3 mM/mL	mM
TRACE ELEMENTS CONCENTRATE	☐ 4 ☐ 5 ☐ 6	mL

Patient Additives:

☐ MVC 9 + 3 10 mL Daily

☐ HUMULIN-R 10 units DAILY

☐ FOLIC ACID ________ mg
______ times weekly

☐ VITAMIN K ________ mg
______ times weekly

☐ OTHER: MVI 10 mL/daily

☐ OTHER: ____________

Directions:

INFUSE: ☐ DAILY

☐ _____ TIMES WEEKLY

OTHER DIRECTIONS:

____

Rate: ☐ CYCLIC INFUSION:
OVER _____ HOURS
(TAPER UP AND DOWN)

☐ CONTINUOUS INFUSION:
AT _____ mL PER HOUR

☑ STANDARD RATE:
AT 104 mL PER HOUR
FOR 12 HOURS

LAB ORDERS:

☐ STANDARD LAB ORDERS
SMAC-20, CO2, Mg+2 TWICE WEEKLY
CBC WITH AUTO DIFF WEEKLY
UNTIL STABLE, THEN:
SMAC-20, CO2, Mg+2 WEEKLY
CBC WITH AUTO DIFF MONTHLY

☐ OTHER: ____________

VALIDATION:

____
PROVIDER'S SIGNATURE

Print Name: ____________

Office Address: ____________

Phone: ____________

WHITE: Home Health CANARY: Provider

FIGURE 10.9 Sample provider's order form.

Total Grams per Bag

Formula: % × mL = g/L

Step 1
Amino acids (AA) 10% in 425 mL
0.10 × 425 = 42.5 g/L

Formula g/L × TV*/L = g/bag

Step 2
42.5 g/L × 1.248 TV/L = 53 g/bag
There are 53 g of AA in 1248 mL of TPN

Shortcut method: % × mL = g/L × TV/L = g/bag
AA 10% in 425 mL
0.10 × 425 = 42.5 g/L × 1.248 TV/L = 53 g of AA in the bag

Shortcut method: % × mL = g/L × TV/L = g/bag

Dextrose 70% in 357 mL
0.70 × 357 = 250 g/L × 1.248 TV/L = 312 g of dextrose per bag

Shortcut method: % × mL = g/L × TV/L = g/bag

Lipids 20% in 125 mL

Step 1 **Step 2**
0.20 × 125 = 25 g/L × TV/L 1.248 ml = 31.2 g/bag
There are 31.2 g of lipids in 1248 mL per bag

Percentage of Amino Acids, Dextrose, and Lipids per Bag

Formula: $\frac{\textbf{g/bag}}{\textbf{TV}} = \textbf{\%/bag}$

AA $\frac{53}{1248}$ = 0.042 = 4.2% of bag is AA (PRO)

Dextrose $\frac{312}{1248}$ = 0.250 = 25% of bag is dextrose (CHO)

Lipids $\frac{31.2}{1248}$ = 0.0250 = 2.5% of bag is lipids (FAT)

Percentage of Additives

Formula:	**Step 1**	**mEq/L × TV/L = mEq/bag**
	Step 2	**mEq/bag ÷ TV = % in bag**
Shortcut method:		**mEq/L × TV/L ÷ TV = % in bag**
Calcium gluconate		5 mEq × 1.248 TV = 6.24 mEq/bag
		6.24 ÷ 1248 TV = 0.5% in bag
Magnesium sulfate		5 mEq × 1.248 TV = 6.24 ÷ 1248 = 0.5% in bag
Potassium phosphate		15 mEq × 1.248 TV = 18.72 ÷ 1248 = 1.5% in bag
Sodium chloride		35 mEq × 1.248 TV = 43.68 ÷ 1248 = 3.5% in bag

A milliequivalent (mEq) is a measurement of weight that represents 1000th of a gram.

mL per Hour to Set the Pump

$\frac{\text{TV}}{\text{Total Time (hr)}}$ = mL per hr $\frac{1248}{12}$ = 104 mL per hr

*TV, Total volume.

Kilocalories (kcal) per Bag

Formula:	kcal/g × g/bag = kcal/bag		
	1 g CHO = 4 kcal	312 g × 4 kcal =	1248 kcal of CHO
	1 g PRO = 4 kcal	53 g × 4 kcal =	212 of PRO
	1 g FAT = 9 kcal	31.2 g × 9 kcal =	281 kcal of FAT
		Total kcal =	1741 per bag of TPN

CLINICAL ALERT!

Begin TPN at a slow rate of 40 to 60 mL per hour and gradually increase by 25 mL per hour every 6 hours to the ordered rate, according to agency protocol. Maintain a steady rate of infusion (within 10% of the ordered dose) to reduce the chance of a sudden onset of hyperglycemia. TPN should never be abruptly stopped because this may precipitate sudden, severe hypoglycemia.

CLINICAL RELEVANCE

- Patients receiving TPN must be monitored for hyperglycemia and serum potassium level as well as for all electrolytes.
- The TPN and lipid administration set should be changed every 24 hours. When administering lipids only, change tubing every 12 hours.
- The fat emulsions filter should be a 1.2-micron size.
- The TPN and lipid solutions should be refrigerated at 39° F or 4° C until time of administration.
- TPN solutions should be filtered with a 0.22-micron filter.
- It is not recommended to administer other medications via the Y port line or piggyback before consulting with the pharmacist for compatibility. There can be many metabolic complications as the result of the type of additives in the TPN solution.

CLINICAL ALERT!

The admixture of fat emulsions with the dextrose and amino acids may produce bacterial growth. Discard the solution after 24 hours.

Answers on page 376

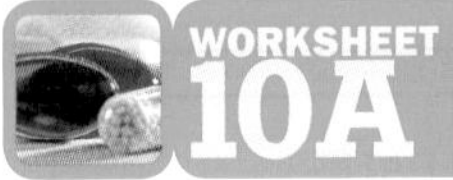

WORKSHEET 10A Central Parenteral Nutrition Calculations

Use Figure 10.10 to answer the following questions.

1. What are the total grams per bag of:
   a. Amino acids (AA)
   b. CHO
   c. Lipids

2. What are the percentages of concentration per bag of:
   a. AA
   b. Dextrose
   c. Lipids

3. How many kilocalories are there per bag of:
   a. CHO
   b. AA
   c. Lipids
   d. What is the total number of kilocalories per bag?

4. For how many mL per hour will you set the infusion device?

5. 1500 mL of D50W provides how many grams of dextrose?

A sample MAR for parenteral nutrition is shown in Figure 10.11.

TPN ORDER SHEET

HOME HEALTH		DATE
PATIENT	ADDRESS	

TPN FORMULA:

AMINO ACIDS: ☑ 5.5% ☐ 8.5% ☐ 10% ☐ WITH STANDARD ELECTROLYTES	400 mL
DEXTROSE: ☑ 10% ☐ 20% ☐ 40% ☐ 50% ☐ 70% (check one)	350 mL
LIPIDS: ☑ 10% ☐ 20% FOR ALL-IN-ONE FORMULA	200 mL

FINAL VOLUME qsad STERILE WATER FOR INJECTION 400 mL	1350 mL

Calcium Gluconate	0.465 mEq/mL	5 mEq
Magnesium Sulfate	4 mEq/mL	10 mEq
Potassium Acetate	2 mEq/mL	mEq
Potassium Chloride	2 mEq/mL	20 mEq
Potassium Phosphate	3 mM/mL	mM
Sodium Acetate	2 mEq/mL	mEq
Sodium Chloride	4 mEq/mL	30 mEq
Sodium Phosphate	3 mM/mL	mM
TRACE ELEMENTS CONCENTRATE	☐ 4 ☐ 5 ☐ 6	mL

Patient Additives:

☐ MVC 9 + 3 10 mL Daily

☐ HUMULIN-R 10 units DAILY

☐ FOLIC ACID ________ mg ______ times weekly

☐ VITAMIN K ________ mg ______ times weekly

☐ OTHER: MVI 12 10 mL/daily

☐ OTHER: ____________

Directions:

INFUSE: ☑ DAILY

☐ _____ TIMES WEEKLY

OTHER DIRECTIONS:

Rate: ☐ CYCLIC INFUSION: OVER _____ HOURS (TAPER UP AND DOWN) " ☐ CONTINUOUS INFUSION: AT _____ mL PER HOUR " ☑ STANDARD RATE: AT _____ mL PER HOUR FOR 12 HOURS

LAB ORDERS:

☐ STANDARD LAB ORDERS
SMAC-20, CO2, Mg+2 TWICE WEEKLY
CBC WITH AUTO DIFF WEEKLY
UNTIL STABLE, THEN:
SMAC-20, CO2, Mg+2 WEEKLY
CBC WITH AUTO DIFF MONTHLY

☐ OTHER: ____________

VALIDATION:

____
PROVIDER'S SIGNATURE

Print Name: ____________

Office Address: ____________

Phone: ____________

WHITE: Home Health CANARY: Provider

FIGURE 10.10 Sample provider's order form for TPN for Worksheet 10A.

Acct: Admitted: Att Phys: Diagnosis: Allergies:	MR#: Age: HT: WT:	M A R **MEDICATION ADMINISTRATION RECORD** Page: 3 From: 10/10/18 0730 Thru: 10/11/18 0730

Start Date/Time	Stop Date/Time	RN/ LPN	Medication	0731-1530	1531-2330	2331-0730
10/10/18 1800	10/11/18 1759		PICC Line Flush (1 Inject) FLush Q12H IV #022 Flush PICC Q 12 HRS with NS 10 ML when PICC line used for TPN		1800	0600
10/10/18 1800	10/11/18 1759		Amino Acid 8.5% 600 ML (600 ML) Dextrose 50% 600 ML (600 ML) Sodium Chloride CO 58 MEQ (14.5 ML) Potassium Acetate 12 MEQ (6 ML) Magnesium Sulfate 6 MEQ (1.5 ML)		1800	
			Calcium Gluconate 6 MEQ (12.84 ML) Infuvite Multivitamin 10 ML (10 ML) Trace Elements 1 ML (1 ML) Sodium Phosphate 26 MEQ (6.5 ML) Insulin Humulin Regu 21 units (0.21 ML)			
			50 ML/HR Q24H #047 IV Central			
			Store in Refrigerator			

The preprinted MAR from the pharmacy shows the contents of the TPN, the time it is to be started, and the times and amount of NS to be used to flush the central and PICC lines. The nurse will initial next to the preprinted time as well as initial and sign the bottom of the MAR. The MAR is for 24 hours only.

Order Date	RN INIT.	Date/Time To Be Given	One Time Orders and Pre-Operatives Medication-Dose-Route	Actual Time Given

Site Codes			Dose Omission Code
Arm	LA	RA	A = pt absent
Deltoid	LD	RD	H = hold
Ventrogluteal	LVG	RVG	M = med absent
Gluteal	LG	RG	N = NPO
Abdomen	LUQ	RUQ	O = other
Abdomen	LLQ	RLQ	R = refused
			U = unable to tolerate

INIT	Signature	INIT	Signature

60321 (8/98)A CHART

FIGURE 10.11 Sample medication administration record (MAR).

Answers on page 376

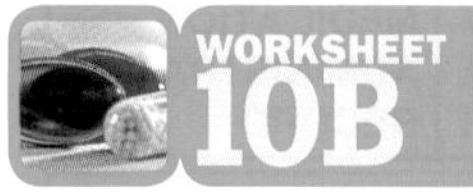

WORKSHEET 10B Peripheral Parenteral Nutrition Calculations

Use Figure 10.12 to answer the following questions.

1. What are the total grams per bag of:
   a. Amino acids (AA)
   b. Dextrose
   c. Lipids

2. What are the percentages of concentration per bag of:
   a. AA
   b. Dextrose
   c. Lipids

3. How many kilocalories are there per bag of:
   a. PRO
   b. CHO
   c. FAT
   d. What is the total number of kilocalories per bag?

4. For how many mL per hour will you set the infusion device?

5. How many kilocalories are in 750 g of dextrose?

HOME HEALTH		DATE
PATIENT	ADDRESS	

TPN FORMULA:

AMINO ACIDS: ☐ 5.5% ☑ 8.5% ☐ 10% ☐ WITH STANDARD ELECTROLYTES	500 mL
DEXTROSE: ☐ 10% ☐ 20% ☐ 40% ☑ 50% ☐ 70% (check one)	500 mL
LIPIDS: ☑ 10% ☐ 20% FOR ALL-IN-ONE FORMULA	250 mL

FINAL VOLUME qsad STERILE WATER FOR INJECTION	1500 mL

Calcium Gluconate	0.465 mEq/mL	5 mEq
Magnesium Sulfate	4 mEq/mL	15 mEq
Potassium Acetate	2 mEq/mL	8.3 mEq
Potassium Chloride	2 mEq/mL	mEq
Potassium Phosphate	3 mM/mL	35 mM
Sodium Acetate	2 mEq/mL	mEq
Sodium Chloride	4 mEq/mL	35 mEq
Sodium Phosphate	3 mM/mL	mM
TRACE ELEMENTS CONCENTRATE	☐ 4 ☐ 5 ☐ 6	mL

Patient Additives:

☐ MVC 9 + 3 10 ml Daily

☐ HUMULIN-R 10 units DAILY

☐ FOLIC ACID _______ mg
_____ times weekly

☐ VITAMIN K _______ mg
_____ times weekly

☑ OTHER: MVI 12 1.5mL/daily

☐ OTHER: _______

Directions:

INFUSE: ☑ DAILY
☐ _____ TIMES WEEKLY

OTHER DIRECTIONS:

Rate:

☐ CYCLIC INFUSION:	☐ CONTINUOUS INFUSION:	☑ STANDARD RATE:
OVER 12 HOURS	AT _____ mL PER HOUR	AT _____ mL PER HOUR
(TAPER UP AND DOWN)		FOR 12 HOURS

LAB ORDERS:

☑ STANDARD LAB ORDERS
SMAC-20, CO2, Mg+2 TWICE WEEKLY
CBC WITH AUTO DIFF WEEKLY
UNTIL STABLE, THEN:
SMAC-20, CO2, Mg+2 WEEKLY
CBC WITH AUTO DIFF MONTHLY

☐ OTHER: _______

VALIDATION:

____
PROVIDER'S SIGNATURE

Print Name: _______

Office Address: _______

Phone: _______

WHITE: Home Health CANARY: Provider

FIGURE 10.12 Sample provider's order for Worksheet 10B.

Answers on page 377

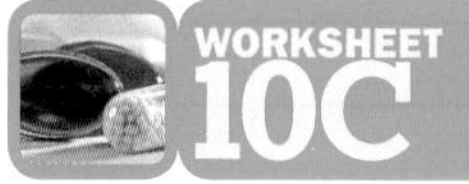

WORKSHEET 10C Central Parenteral Nutrition Calculations

Use Figure 10.13 to answer the following questions. Use the formulas on pages 364 and 365.

1. Total grams per bag:
  a. How many total grams of amino acids (AA) are there per bag?
  b. How many total grams of dextrose are there per bag?

2. Percentages of concentration per bag:
  a. What is the percentage of amino acids per bag?
  b. What is the percentage of dextrose per bag?

3. Kilocalories per bag:
  a. AA
  b. CHO
  c. Total number of kilocalories

4. How many hours will it take for the contents of the parenteral nutrition bag to be infused?

5. 8.5% AA in 1000 mL provides how many grams of AA?

Amino Acid 10%	**(900 ML)**
Dextrose 70%	**(430 ML)**
Sterile Water For Injection	**(70 ML)**
Sodium Chloride Conc 140 MEQ	**(35 ML)**
Potassium Phosphate 41 MEQ	**(9.318 ML)**
Potassium Chloride 43 MEQ	**(21.5 ML)**
Magnesium Sulfate 7 MEQ	**(1.75 ML)**
Calcium Gluconate 7 MEQ	**(14.98 ML)**
Insulin Humulin Regular 20 units	**(0.2 ML)**
Infuvite Multivitamin A 10 ML	**(10 ML)**
	Total: 1492.748

**** Continued ****

DO NOT START AFTER 24 HOURS

Rate: 55 mL/hr Freq: Q24H

Modified Central TPN
Hang Date/Time: 1800 11/19/18

Expir:
Init: DF
Refrigerate
Prep. By: /_________

DO NOT START AFTER 24 HOURS

FIGURE 10.13 Sample CPN label for Worksheet 10C.

Answers on page 377

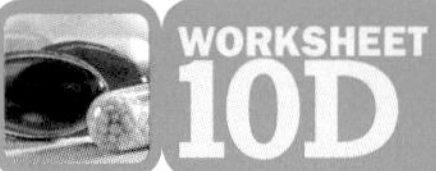

WORKSHEET 10D Peripheral Parenteral Nutrition Calculations

Use Figure 10.14 to answer the following questions. Use the formulas on pages 364 and 365.

1. Total grams per bag:
   a. Amino acids (AA)
   b. Dextrose

2. Percentages of concentration per bag:
   a. Amino acids
   b. Dextrose

3. Kilocalories per bag:
   a. AA
   b. CHO
   c. Total number of kilocalories
   d. What is the total number of kilocalories per bag?

4. How many hours will it take for the contents to be infused?

5. 20% of lipids in 500 mL provides how many kilocalories?

Amino Acid 8% (Hepatic)	**(600 ML)**
Dextrose 20%	**(600 ML)**
Sodium Chloride Conc 42 MEQ	**(10.5 ML)**
Potassium Phosphate 26 MEQ	**(5.909 ML)**
Potassium Acetate 10 MEQ	**(5 ML)**
Calcium Gluconate 6 MEQ	**(12.84 ML)**
Magnesium Sulfate 6 MEQ	**(1.5 ML)**
Infuvite Multivitamin A 10 ML	**(10 ML)**
Insulin Humulin Regular 24 units	**(0.24 ML)**
	Total: 1245.989

**** Continued ****

DO NOT START AFTER 24 HOURS

Rate: 50 mL/hr   Freq: Q24H
Peripheral
Hang Date/Time: 1800 11/19/18
Expir:
Init: MM
Prep. By: /________

DO NOT START AFTER 24 HOURS

FIGURE 10.14 Sample PCN label for Worksheet 10D.

Answers on page 378

WORKSHEET 10E Multiple-Choice Practice

1. Have: A three-in-one TPN solution with 20% lipids in 175 mL. The total volume (TV) is 1200 mL. How many grams of lipids are in the solution?
   a. 42 g per bag **b.** 48 g per bag **c.** 52 g per bag **d.** 36 g per bag

2. What is the percentage of concentration of grams per bag for lipids in question 1?
   a. 2.7% **b.** 3.5% **c.** 5.6% **d.** 7%

3. Have: Potassium acetate 12 mEq/L. The TV is 1385 mL. What is the percentage of potassium acetate in the bag?
   a. 2.2% **b.** 3.6% **c.** 1.2% **d.** 2.6%

4. The TV of the parenteral nutrition (PN) solution is 1275 mL. The infusion rate is 110 mL per hour. The infusion is started at 1800 hr. What time will it be completed?
   a. 0659 hr **b.** 0459 hr **c.** 0535 hr **d.** 0345 hr

5. Have: CPN solution with 8.5% AA in 375 mL. The TV is 1500 mL. How many grams of protein are in the solution?
   a. 50 g per bag **b.** 77.7 g per bag **c.** 62 g per bag **d.** 47.8 g per bag

6. What is the percentage of concentration of grams per bag of the AA in question 5?
   a. 4.6% **b.** 3% **c.** 8.2% **d.** 4.7%

7. Have: Calcium gluconate additive of 6 mEq/L. The TV of the TPN is 1350 mL. What is the percentage of calcium gluconate in the bag?
   a. 0.3% **b.** 1% **c.** 0.4% **d.** 0.6%

8. Have: Magnesium sulfate additive 10 mEq/L. The TV is 1258 mL. What is the percentage of magnesium sulfate in the bag?
   a. 1% **b.** 10.2% **c.** 1.8% **d.** 11%

9. Have: CPN solution with 40% dextrose in 400 mL. The TV is 1450 mL. How many grams of dextrose are in the bag?
   a. 232 g per bag **b.** 130 g per bag **c.** 160 g per bag **d.** 260 g per bag

10. What is the percentage of concentration per bag for dextrose in question 9?
    a. 1.6% **b.** 16% **c.** 2.3% **d.** 23%

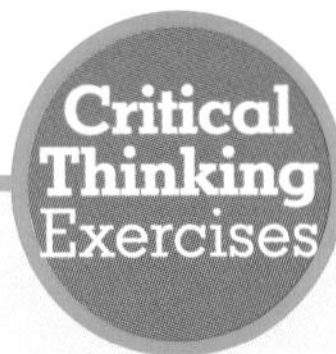

Critical Thinking Exercises provide math and medication-related patient safety issues for student discussion. Answers are not provied.

Analyze the following scenarios.

1. Your patient, Mary Braun, is receiving peripheral parenteral nutrition (PPN). On assessment, she complains that the IV site burns. When the site is checked, the solution is infusing well at the correct rate. The label on the solution is 8.5% amino acids and 70% dextrose.

   Error(s):

   Causes of error(s):

   Nursing interventions:

   Preventive measures:

   Discussion

   What will be your first action?

   Why are the percentages of amino acids and dextrose important to know?

   What is the percentage difference for PPN and CPN infusion?

   How can this situation be reconciled to reduce potential risks?

2. Mrs. S. had been hospitalized for 5 days for ulcerative colitis that was not responding to the treatment. During this time she was receiving a TPN solution with 8.5% amino acids and 40% dextrose with multivitamins 1.5 mL daily. She was then scheduled for a total colectomy. After the surgery, Mrs. S. was returned to the surgical unit. The postoperative orders were PCA 1.5 mg morphine every 6 minutes, Ambien 10 mg prn for sleep, and continue daily TPN with Aminosyn II 15%, dextrose 40%, multivitamins 10 mL, and 10 units of Humulin R added to the bag. After 3 days, Mrs. S. complained of nausea and her skin appeared flushed.

   What would be your first reaction to her signs and symptoms?

   What medication is she receiving that might cause an adverse reaction?

   What are the side effects of Aminosyn?

   If this is an adverse reaction, do you think the benefit of the medication outweighs the reaction?

   How can you make Mrs. S. more comfortable to alleviate the signs and symptoms?

3. A 1500-mL TPN infusion of 5% amino acids, 40% dextrose, and 10% lipids is ordered to be infused in 12 hours. The infusion was started at 1430 hr. At 630 hr, the nurse checked the infusion and found that it still had 300 mL in the bag. She checked the infusion pump, which was set at 100 mL per hour.

Ordered:

Error:

Discussion:

What would be your first action?

Why do you think the infusion time of 12 hours is important?

How was the patient's safety jeopardized?

At what rate should the TPN be infusing?

You are the person who found the error. Will you make out the incident report?

How would an error like this be reconciled in the future?

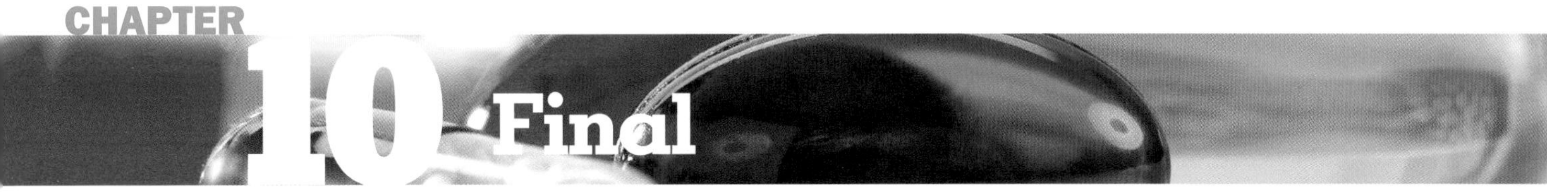

Calculate and solve the following problems using a calculator, moving decimals, reducing ratios, and labeling your answers. Prove your work.*

1. Why is a 50% dextrose solution infused via a central line?

2. What is the major difference between a PPN line and a CPN line?

3. A three-in-one TPN solution has lipids 20% in 110 mL. The total volume is 1145 mL.
   a. How many grams of lipids will the patient receive?
   b. How many kilocalories of fat will the patient receive?

4. The TPN order reads: Dextrose 40% in 400 mL. The TV is 1325 mL.
   a. How many grams of dextrose will the patient receive?
   b. How many kilocalories of carbohydrate will the patient receive?

5. A TPN order reads: Amino acids 8.5% in 550 mL. The TV of the TPN infusion is 1430 mL.
   a. How many grams of AA will the patient receive through the central line?
   b. How many kilocalories of protein will the patient receive?

6. A TPN order reads dextrose 10% in 475 mL.
   a. How many grams of dextrose will be infused?
      The total volume is 1550 mL in the peripheral line.
   b. How many kilocalories of dextrose will the patient receive?

7. A TPN solution has 48 g of protein, 255 g of carbohydrate, and 38.6 g of fat. How many total kilocalories will the patient receive?

8. A PPN order reads: Amino acids 5% in 350 mL. The TV is 1280 mL.
   a. How many grams of AA will the patient receive?
   b. How many kilocalories of protein will the patient receive?

9. The TPN of 1420 mL is to start at 1800 hr. The rate is 108 mL per hour. What time will the infusion be completed?

10. A TPN of 1320 mL is infusing at 120 mL per hour. How many hours will it take to infuse?

Refer to the Advanced Calculations section of Drug Calculations Companion, version 5 on Evolve for additional practice problems.

*It may be acceptable to withdraw small amounts of large-volume IV solutions equal to the number of milliliters of drug to be added so as to simplify calculations and flow rates. Follow your hospital's policy.

Answer Key

10 Parenteral Nutrition

WORKSHEET 10A (page 365)

1. Total grams per bag:
   % × mL = g/L | **g/L × TV/L = g/bag**
   a. AA 0.055 × 400 = 22 g/L | 22 × 1.350 = 29.7 g/bag
   b. Dextrose 0.10 × 350 = 35 g/L | 35 × 1.350 = 47.25 g/bag
   c. Lipids 0.10 × 200 = 20 g/L | 20 × 1.350 = 27 g/bag

2. Percentage of concentration:
   g/bag ÷ TV = % of concentration
   a. AA 29.7 g ÷ 1350 = 2.2%
   b. Dextrose 47.25 ÷ 1350 = 3.5%
   c. Lipids 27 ÷ 1350 = 2%

3. kcal per bag:
   a. CHO 47.25 × 4 = 189 | PRO = 4 kcal/g
   b. PRO 29.7 × 4 = 118.8 | CHO = 4 kcal/g
   c. FAT 27 × 9 = 243 | FAT = 9 kcal/g
   d. Total kcal 550.8

4. mL/hr to set infusion device
   $\frac{TV}{TT}$ = mL/hr | $\frac{1350}{12}$ = 112.5 = 113 mL/hr

   Percentage is based on 100
5. 0.50 × 1500 = 750 g CHO

WORKSHEET 10B (page 368)

1. Total grams per bag:
   % × mL = g/L | **g/L × TV/L = g/bag**
   a. 0.085 × 500 = 42.5 g/L AA | 42.5 × 1.5 = 63.75 g/bag
   b. 0.50 × 500 = 250 g/L DEX | 250 × 1.5 = 375 g/bag
   c. 0.10 × 250 = 25 g/L LIP | 25 × 1.5 = 37.5 g/bag

2. Percentage of concentration
   g/bag ÷ TV = % of concentration
   a. 63.75 ÷ 1500 = 4.25% AA
   b. 375 ÷ 1500 = 25% DEX
   c. 37.5 ÷ 1500 = 2.5% LIP

3. **kcal per bag**
   a. 63.75 × 4 = 255 kcal PRO | CHO = 4 kcal/g
   b. 375 × 4 = 1500 kcal CHO | PRO = 4 kcal/g
   c. 37.5 × 9 = 337.5 kcal FAT | FAT = 9 kcal/g
   d. Total kcal = 2092.5

4. mL/hr to set infusion device

$\frac{\textbf{TV}}{\textbf{TT}} = \textbf{mL/hr}$ $\frac{1500}{12} = 125$ mL/hr

5. 750 g × 4 = 3000 kcal CHO

WORKSHEET **10C** (page 370)

1. Total grams per bag

Formula: % × mL = g/L **Formula: g/L × TV/L = g/bag**

Shortcut method: % × mL = g/L × TV/L = g/bag

AA 0.10 × 900 = 90 × 1.492 = 134.28 g/bag

Dex 0.70 × 430 = 301 × 1.492 = 449 g/bag

Percentage of concentrate per bag

2. Formula: $\frac{\textbf{g/bag}}{\textbf{TV}} = \textbf{\%/bag}$

AA $\frac{134.28}{1492.74} = 0.0899 = 9\%$

Dex $\frac{449}{1492.74} = 0.30 = 30\%$

3. Total kcal per bag
   a. Protein 134.28 g × 4 = 537 kcal
   b. Carbohydrate 449 g × 4 = 1796 kcal
   c. Total kcal = 2333

4. KNOW WANT TO KNOW

55 mL : 1 hr = 1492 mL : x hr

$55x = 1 \times 1492 = 1492$

$x = 27.127 = 27$ hr

27 hr 8 min

PROOF

55 mL × 27.127 = 1491.9 = 1492

1 × 1492 = 1492

5. 1000 × 0.085 = 85 g of AA

WORKSHEET **10D** (page 371)

1. Total grams per bag

Formulas: % × mL = g/L

g/L × TV/L = g/bag

Shortcut method: % × mL = g/L × TV/L = g/bag

AA 0.08 × 600 = 48 × 1.246 = 59.8 = 60 g/bag

Dex 0.20 × 600 = 120 × 1.246 = 149.5 = 150 g/bag

Percentage of concentrate per bag

2. Formula: $\frac{\textbf{g/bag}}{\textbf{TV}} = \textbf{\%/bag}$

AA $\frac{60}{1246} = 0.048 = 4.8\%$/bag

Dex $\frac{150}{1246} = 0.120 = 12\%$/bag

3. **Formula: 1 g of protein = 4 kcal; 1 g of dextrose = 4 kcal; 1 g of fat = 9 kcal**
   - **a.** AA 60 × 4 = 240 kcal
   - **b.** CHO 150 × 4 = 600 kcal
   - **c.** Total kcal = 840
   - **d.** 840 total kcal in bag

4. KNOW WANT TO KNOW

   50 mL : 1 hr = 1246 mL : x hr

   50x = 1 × 1246 = 1246

   x = 24.92 Convert .92 into minutes: 0.92 × 60 = 55 min

   x = 24 hr 55 min

   PROOF

   1 × 1246 = 1246

   50 × 24.92 = 1246

   FRACTION CROSS PRODUCT

   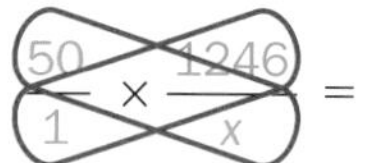

   $\frac{50}{1} \times \frac{1246}{x} =$

   50 x = 1246

   x = 24.96

   x = 24 hr 55 min

5. 500 mL × 0.20 = 100 g × 9 = 900 kcal

WORKSHEET **10E** (page 372)

1. **a.** 0.20 × 175 = 35 × 1.200 = 42 g lipids/bag

2. **b.** $\frac{42}{1200}$ = 0.035 = 3.5% conc. of lipids

3. **c.** 12 × 1.385 = 16.62 ÷ 1385 = 0.012 = 1.2% potassium

4. **c.** KNOW WANT TO KNOW

   110 mL : 1 hr = 1275 mL : x hr

   110x = 1275

   x = 11.59 hr = 11 hr 35 min

   OR

   FRACTION CROSS PRODUCT

   $\frac{110 \text{ mL}}{1 \text{ hr}} = \frac{1275 \text{ mL}}{x \text{ hr}}$

   110x = 1275

   x = 11.59 = 11 hr 35 min

   PROOF

   1 × 1275 = 1275

   110 × 11.59 = 1275

   IV started at 1800 hours plus 11 hr 35 min = 0535 hr

5. **d.** 0.085 × 375 = 31.8 × 1.500 = 47.8 g/bag of AA

6. **b.** $\frac{47.8}{1500}$ = 0.03 = 3% conc. of AA

7. **d.** 6 × 1.350 = 8.1 ÷ 1350 = 0.006 = 0.6% calcium gluconate

8. **a.** 10 × 1.258 = 12.5 ÷ 1258 = 0.01 = 1% magnesium sulfate

9. **a.** 0.40 × 400 = 160 × 1.450 = 232 g/bag of dextrose

10. **b.** $\frac{232}{1450}$ = 0.16 = 16% conc. of dextrose

CHAPTER 10 FINAL: PARENTERAL NUTRITION (page 375)

1. 50% dextrose has a high osmolarity that would be harmful to smaller veins.

2. The size and location of the veins. Central lines can tolerate higher percentages of dextrose and amino acids.

3. a. 25 g/bag of lipids
b. 225 kcal of fat

4. a. 212 g/bag of dextrose
b. 848 kcal of dextrose

5. a. 66.85 g/bag of AA
b. 267.4 kcal of PRO

6. a. 73.62 g/bag of dextrose
b. 294.5 kcal of CHO

7. 1559 total kcal

8. a. 22.4 g/bag of AA
b. 89.6 kcal of PRO

9. At 0709 hr the infusion will be completed

10. 11 hr to infuse

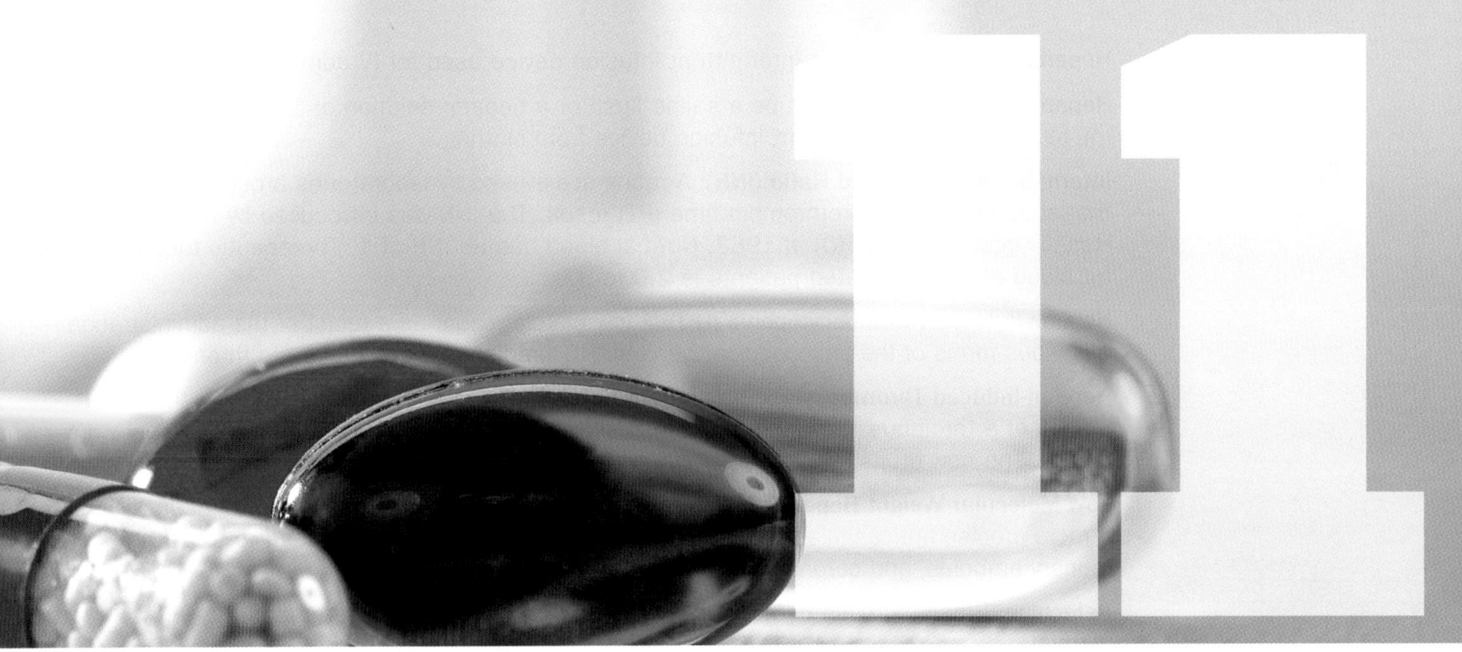

Anticoagulants

Objectives

- Compare the actions of oral, subcutaneous, and intravenous anticoagulants.
- Accurately measure a dose of an ordered anticoagulant medication in a tuberculin syringe.
- Accurately measure subcutaneous heparin doses using various concentrations.
- Titrate intravenous heparin for bolus dose, units per kg, units per hr, and mL per hr.
- Calculate the length of time to infuse the prescribed dose of anticoagulant.
- Analyze medication errors using critical thinking.

Introduction

Anticoagulant medications are administered subcutaneously, intravenously, or orally. They are all high-alert medications capable of doing great harm if a dose is measured incorrectly and administered. Anticoagulant drugs are designed to inhibit the coagulation cascade to decrease the chance for the formation of thrombi. Their purpose is to extend the clotting time of blood to prevent venous or arterial thrombosis, which could result in an embolus causing pulmonary or cerebral damage.

Vocabulary

Activated Partial Thromboplastin Time (aPTT): A shortened form of the prothrombin time (PT) test used to monitor heparin therapy. Normal control time is 30 to 40 seconds. This is not a standardized test like the INR, therefore results may vary depending on the agents used.

Anticoagulant: A drug that prevents or delays blood forming a clot.

Anti-Xa Assay: A test to measure heparin and low molecular weight heparin (LMWH) levels and to monitor anticoagulant therapy effectiveness. Dosages are titrated to maintain anticoagulant effectiveness.

Deep Vein Thrombosis (DVT): When a clot forms within one or more of the deep veins, such as those of the lower extremities (most common). Often a complication of immobilization, orthopedic surgery, or any type of surgery.

Embolus: A blood clot that travels from its original location, usually in the leg, to another part of the body, such as the lungs or brain.

Heparin: Heparin sodium or heparin calcium (unfractionated) is a parenteral drug that has a faster effect than oral warfarin or other oral medications. It is administered subcutaneously or intravenously. Heparin is usually administered in a care providing agency because the partial thromboplastin time must be monitored every 4 to 6 hours. Heparin inhibits coagulation by forming antithrombin, thereby preventing the conversion of prothrombin to thrombin. It is used as an anticoagulant in the prevention and treatment of thrombosis and embolism.

Heparin Lock (Heplock): An intermittent infusion device used for IV administration of drugs.

Heparin (Heplock) Flush: Can be a saline flush or a heparin solution of 10 to 100 units per mL to prevent the intermittent infusion device from clotting.

International Normalized Ratio (INR): A rating scale used by laboratories around the world that standardizes the prothrombin time (PT) result. The INR was introduced by the World Health Organization (WHO) in 1983. Normal blood has an INR of 1. Therapeutic target range for blood of anticoagulated patients is 2.0 to 3.0.

Heparin-Induced Thrombocytopenia (HIT): A low platelet count as a result of the administration of various forms of the anticoagulant heparin. HIT predisposes the patient to thrombosis.

Heparin-Induced Thrombocytopenia and Thrombosis (HITT): A low platelet count with the formation of a thrombus. Several drugs are available that will not reduce the platelet count any further. The new drugs are lepirudin and argatroban.

Low Molecular Weight Heparin: The most bioavailable fractionized product of heparin. It has a more precise anticoagulant effect than unfractionated heparin. It is used to treat DVT, pulmonary embolus, and coronary episodes.

Petechiae: Small, purplish hemorrhagic spots on the skin that appear in patients with platelet deficiencies.

Platelet Count: The number of platelets, or thrombocytes, in blood is normally 150,000 to 400,000 per mcL. A count of less than 200,000 platelets contributes to a risk for bleeding. Platelets release factors that initiate the first stages of clotting.

Protamine Sulfate: An antidote to reverse the effects of heparin and heparinoids.

Prothrombin Time (PT or Pro Time): Had been used for monitoring warfarin but is not as reliable as the standardized INR to monitor anticoagulated blood values. No longer used.

Pulmonary Embolus (PE): A blood clot that has traveled from its original source (possible DVT) and obstructs a pulmonary artery in the lungs. This is an extreme emergency.

Thrombocytopenia: An abnormal decrease in the number of platelets. Watch for signs of hemorrhage.

Thrombolytic Agent: An intravenous drug that lyses or dissolves clots to reverse a cerebral vascular accident (CVA) or a pulmonary embolus. Streptokinase is such a drug.

Vitamin K: An antidote to reverse the effects of warfarin (Coumadin).

Injectable Anticoagulants

Heparin sodium injection, USP, is a fast-acting drug used to interrupt the clotting process. It affects the ability of the blood to coagulate, thereby preventing clots from forming. It is used to treat deep vein thrombosis (DVT) and pulmonary embolism (PE); during cardiac surgery; during hemodialysis, myocardial infarction (MI), and disseminated intravascular coagulation (DIC); and prophylactically for immobilized patients. It may be given in therapeutic doses or in small, diluted doses to maintain the patency of IV or intraarterial (IA) lines.

Because it is inactive orally, heparin sodium is administered intravenously or subcutaneously. If administered intramuscularly, the drug produces a high level of pain and may cause hematomas. The orders for heparin are highly individualized and are based on the weight of the patient and coagulation values. Heparin comes in various strengths, including 1000, 5000, 10,000, 20,000, and 50,000 units per mL. Heparin also comes in 10 and 100 units per mL for IV patency flushes. The vial must be checked carefully before administration. Heparin is fast acting; therefore errors can be fatal.

Low molecular weight heparins (LMWH) are fractionalized heparin. They have replaced unfractionated heparin (UFH) to prevent and treat venous thrombosis, unstable angina, and pulmonary embolus. They are safer than UFH and just as effective. Once-daily subcutaneous dosing and a lower incidence of heparin-induced thrombocytopenia (HIT) and osteopenia make LMWH the choice drug. Natural or unfractionated heparin is less predictable than LMWH.

Differences between injectable (UFH) and LMWH (fractionated) include the following:

- The unfractionated weight of a heparin molecule is about 15 kDa.
- The fractionated weight of an LMWH molecule is about 4.5 kDa.

- Less frequent subcutaneous dosing is required for LMWH than UFH for postoperative prophylaxis of venous thromboembolism.
- With LMWH there is no need to monitor aPTT coagulation, which is necessary with UFH.
- Possibly a lower risk for bleeding.
- Lower risk of osteoporosis in long-term use.
- Less chance of heparin-induced thrombocytopenia.
- The anticoagulant effects of heparin are reversible with protamine sulfate.
- Protamine sulfate is less effective on LMWH.
- LMWH can inactivate factor Xa, activating (AT) antithrombin.
- UFH is unable to inactivate factor Xa, which can produce thrombocytopenia and osteoporosis.

The LMWH subcutaneous injectable drugs are Lovenox (enoxaparin), Arixtra (fondaparinux), Fragmin (dalteparin), and Innohep (tinzaparin). Figure 11.1 shows anticoagulant injection sites. Figure 11.2 demonstrates how subcutaneous heparin injections are documented.

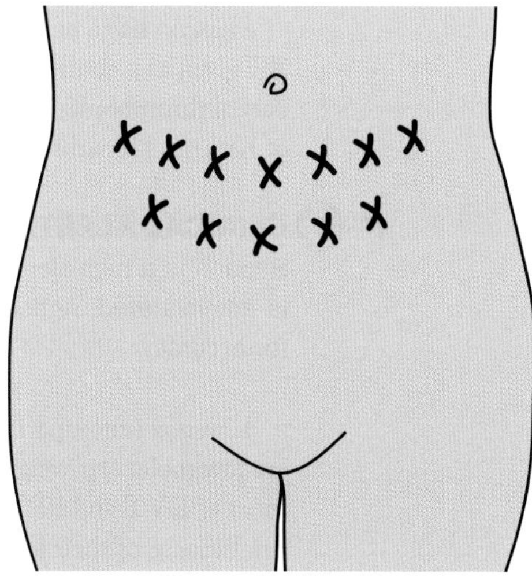

FIGURE 11.1 Subcutaneous injection sites. The abdominal sites are better for absorption of injectable anticoagulant.

MAR — MEDICATION ADMINISTRATION RECORD

ADM. DX :
DIET :
HT :
WT :
ALLERGIES:

Start Date/Time	Stop Date/Time	RN/ LPN	Medication	0731-1530	1531-2330	2331-0730
12/13/18		NB NB	Heparin sodium 5,000 units subcut Heparin sodium 5,000 units subcut	0800 RLQ 1400 LLQ		
		KR	Heparin sodium 5,000 units subcut	2000 RLQ		

Order Date	RN INIT.	Date/Time To Be Given	One Time Orders and Pre-Operatives Medication-Dose-Route	Actual Time Given

Site Codes		
Arm	LA	RA
Deltoid	LD	RD
Ventrogluteal	LVG	RVG
Gluteal	LG	RG
Abdomen	LUQ	RUQ
Abdomen	LLQ	RLQ

Dose Omission Code
A = pt absent
H = hold
M = med absent
N = NPO
O = other
R = refused
U = unable to tolerate

INIT	Signature	INIT	Signature
NB	Nancy Berg RN		
KR	Kay Rae RN		

FIGURE 11.2 Sample MAR. (Modified from Scottsdale Healthcare, Scottsdale, Ariz.)

Check laboratory values for clotting times before administering heparin. Heparin therapy must not be interrupted and is incompatible with other medications.

Heparin has a half-life of 1 to 6 hours. To maintain a therapeutic level in the blood, heparin is usually given as a continuous IV drip during care at an agency. The heparin level is titrated on the basis of partial thromboplastin time (PTT) levels, which are taken every 6 hours to correlate with the half-life of heparin. Heparin can be counteracted with protamine sulfate, the antidote.

CLINICAL ALERT!

Heparin is a high-alert medication that carries a risk of causing serious injury if the wrong dosage is administered. Anticoagulant dosages require two licensed nurses to verify the ordered dosage for accuracy.

Lovenox (enoxaparin) and Fragmin (dalteparin), Arixtra (fondaparinux), and Innohep (tinzaparin) are low molecular weight (LMWH) anticoagulants. They are prescribed for the prevention and treatment of DVT and PE and also after knee and hip surgery. LMWHs have a longer half-life than heparin. Because of their low level of activity in the blood, there is a reduced need for PTT tests. These four drugs have more predictable peaks and durations of action. The preferred sites for LMWH anticoagulants are the anterolateral abdominal wall.

CLINICAL ALERT!

Lovenox, Fragmin, Arixtra, and Innohep should never be given intramuscularly because they may cause large hematomas.

Example Ordered: Lovenox 30 mg subcutaneous q12h after hip replacement. The pharmacy has sent 40 mg per 0.4 mL in a prefilled syringe. How many milliliters will be administered? How many milliliters will be discarded?

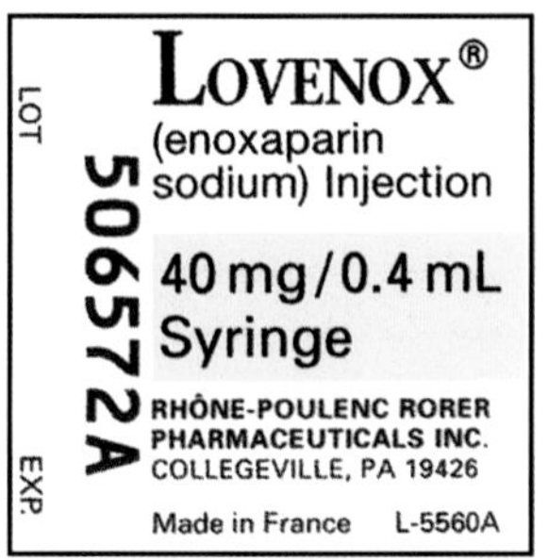

HAVE — WANT TO HAVE

$40 \text{ mg} : 0.4 \text{ mL} = 30 \text{ mg} : x \text{ mL}$

$40x = 0.4 \times 30 = 12$

$40x = 12$

$x = 0.3 \text{ mL}$

FRACTION CROSS PRODUCT

$\frac{40}{0.4} = \frac{30}{x \text{ mL}}$

$40x = 30 \times 0.4 = 12$

$x = 0.3 \text{ mL}$

PROOF	$40 \times 0.3 = 12$
	$0.4 \times 30 = 12$

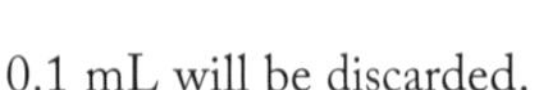
0.1 mL will be discarded.

Arixtra (fondaparinux sodium) is a nonheparin (fractionated) anticoagulant made by chemical synthesis and not from animal origin (Figure 11.3). It is a specific inhibitor of the activated factor X (Xa).

Arixtra is used for prophylaxis of venous thromboembolism (VTE), such as deep vein thrombosis (DVT), which may lead to pulmonary embolism (PE) in patients undergoing hip fracture surgery, knee replacement or hip replacement surgery, and for those at risk for thromboembolitic complications from abdominal surgery. Assess the patient's/family's religious practices to identify if medication of animal origin would be rejected. Fondaparinux sodium (Arixtra) could be considered by the provider if a conflict is identified.

Warfarin can be administered in conjunction with Arixtra for the treatment of acute DVT when initiated while the patient is in a care agency.

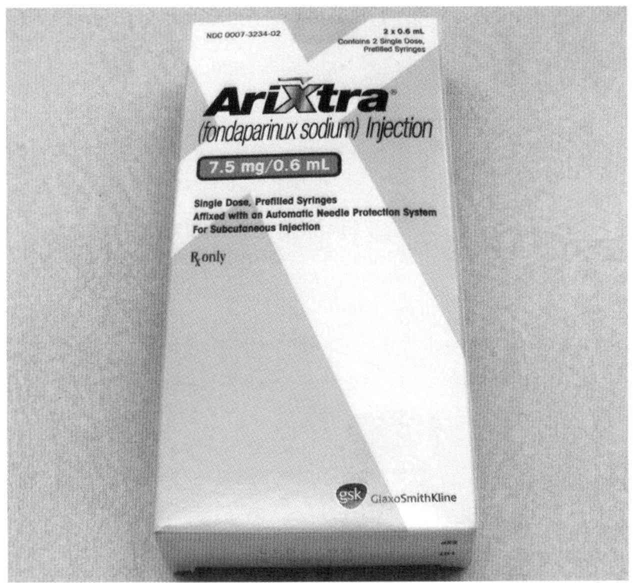

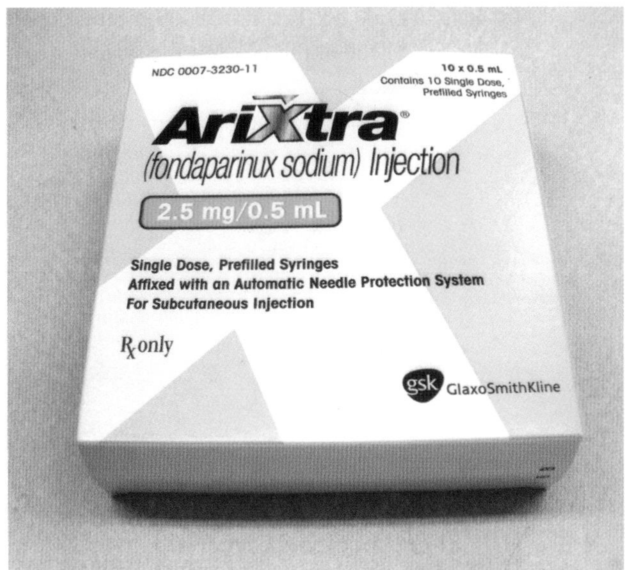

FIGURE 11.3 Arixtra single-dose syringes.

CLINICAL ALERT!

Arixtra is NOT intended for intramuscular use. It CANNOT be used interchangeably with heparin or other low molecular weight (LMW) heparinoids such as Lovenox (enoxaparin) and Fragmin (dalteparin).

There is a risk of hemorrhage for patients with impaired renal function and for those who are at increased risk of hemorrhage from thrombocytopenia. If the platelet count falls below 100,000/mm^3, discontinue Arixtra. This is known as heparin-induced thrombocytopenia (HIT) (see Vocabulary).

Subcutaneous Heparin Injections

Example Ordered: Heparin 3500 units subcutaneous q6h. Available: Vial containing 5000 units per mL. How many milliliters will the patient receive? Shade in the dose on the tuberculin syringe.

KNOW	WANT TO KNOW	FRACTION CROSS PRODUCT
5000 units : 1 mL = 3500 units : x mL		$\frac{5000}{1} = \frac{3500}{x \text{ mL}}$
$5000x = 3500$		$50x = 35$
$x = 0.7$ mL		$x = 0.7$ mL

PROOF $5000 \times 0.7 = 3500$
$1 \times 3500 = 3500$

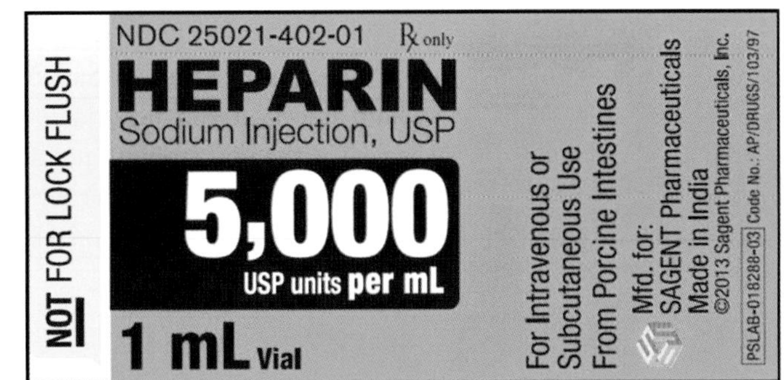

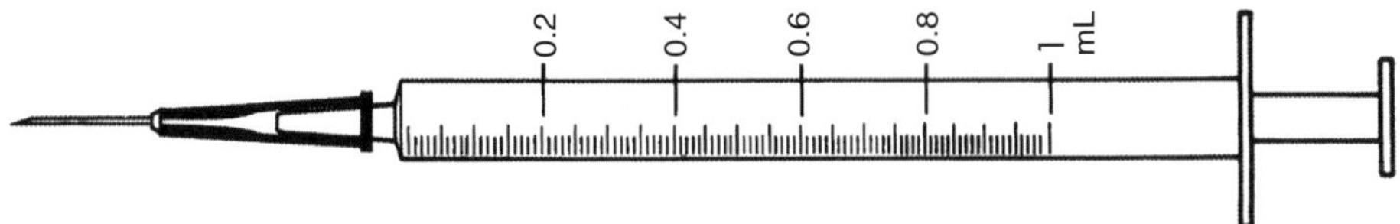

Example Ordered: Fragmin 8000 international units subcutaneous q6h. How many milliliters will you give? Shade in the dose on the syringe.

KNOW	WANT TO KNOW
10,000 international units : 1 mL =	8000 international units : x mL

FRACTION CROSS PRODUCT

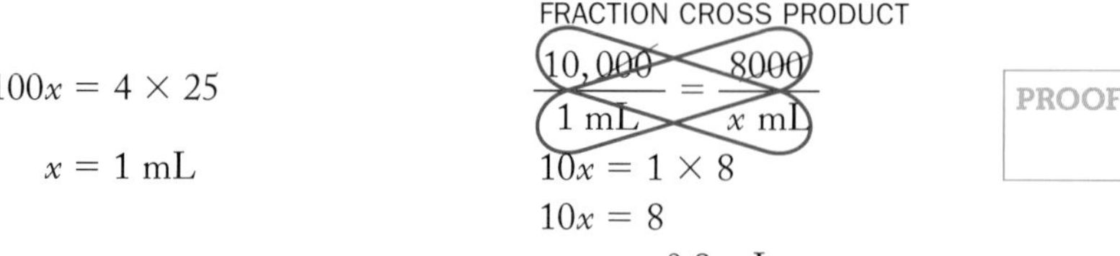

$$100x = 4 \times 25$$
$$x = 1 \text{ mL}$$

$$\frac{10{,}000}{1 \text{ mL}} = \frac{8000}{x \text{ mL}}$$
$$10x = 1 \times 8$$
$$10x = 8$$
$$x = 0.8 \text{ mL}$$

PROOF $1 \times 8000 = 8000$
$0.8 \times 10{,}000 = 8000$

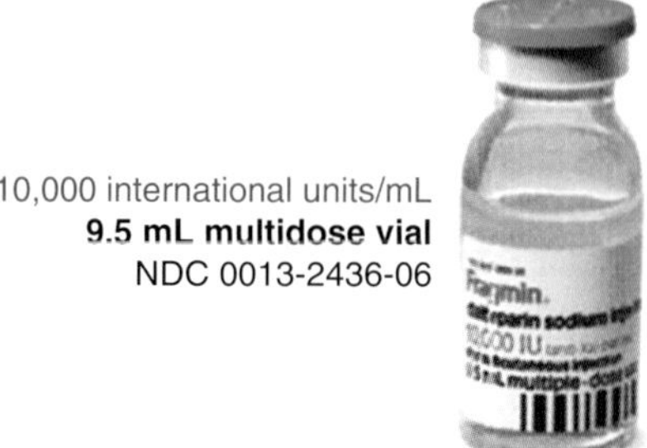

10,000 international units/mL
9.5 mL multidose vial
NDC 0013-2436-06

The product, as depicted in this label, is no longer available. This image was authorized for use by Pfizer Inc. for educational purposes only.

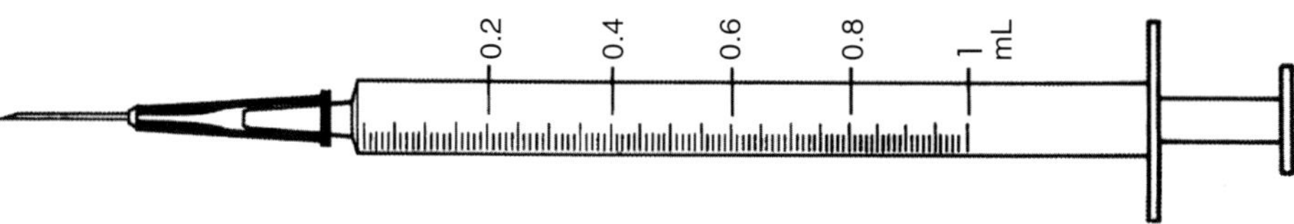

CLINICAL ALERT!

Do not substitute insulin syringes for tuberculin syringes. Insulin syringes are calibrated in 100 units per mL and tuberculin syringes are calibrated in tenths per mL.

CLINICAL RELEVANCE

Do not massage the injection site after injecting any anticoagulant because this increases the incidence of bleeding and hematoma development.

The U.S. Pharmacopeia (USP) and the Institute for Safe Medication Practices (ISMP) require that manufacturers of heparin sodium injection and heparin lock flush solutions clearly state the total strength per volume per vial as well as the unit strength per milliliter for the heparin sodium injection. Care agencies may have both types of labels available as they transition to all new labels. Compare the old label and the new label (see Worksheet 11A, question 1).

Answers on page 406

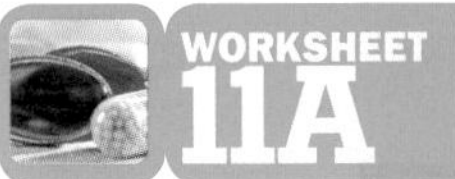

WORKSHEET 11A Subcutaneous Injections

Multidose vials are available in 10, 100, 1000, 5000, 10,000, 20,000, and 50,000 units per mL. Read the labels carefully. Answer the following questions and show your proofs (carry out to nearest hundredth). Shade in doses on syringes.

1. Ordered: Heparin 6000 units subcutaneous. Available: Heparin 10,000 units/mL. How many milliliters will the patient receive?

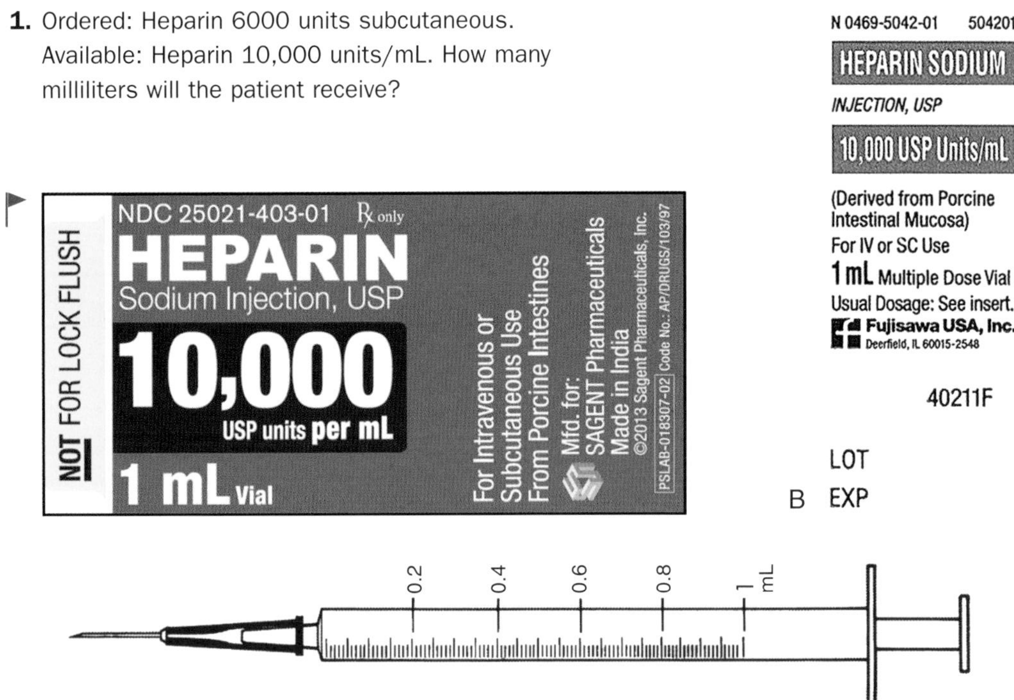

2. Ordered: Lovenox 35 mg subcut daily following hip replacement surgery. How many milliliters will the patient receive?

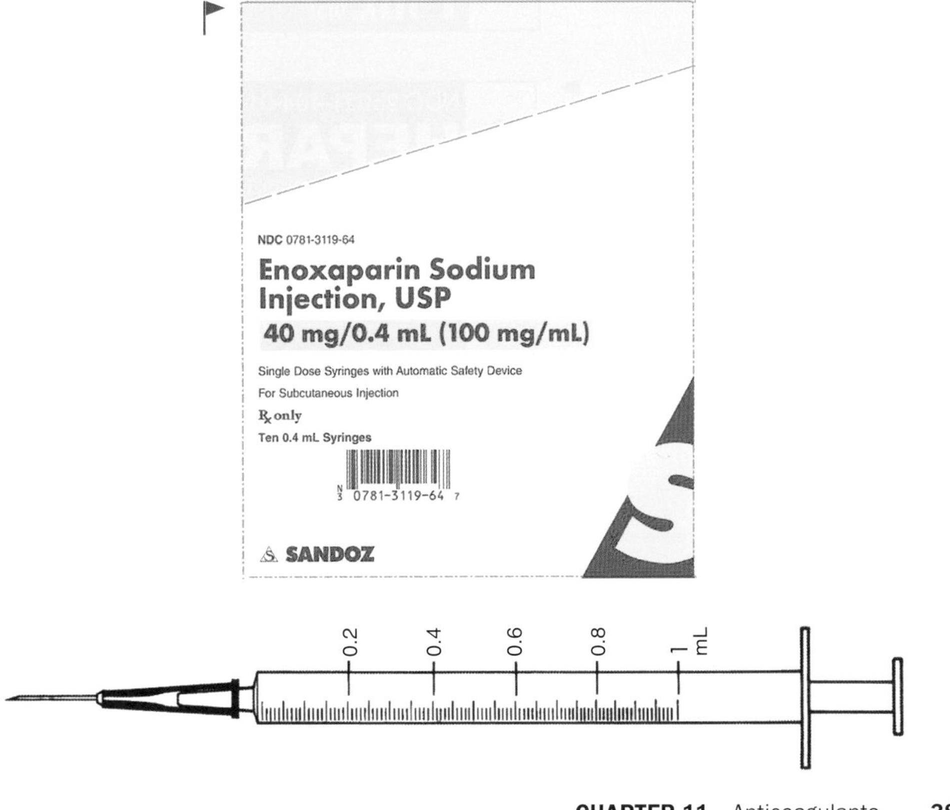

3. Ordered: Heparin 15,000 units subcutaneous q8h. Available: Heparin 20,000 units/mL. How many milliliters will the patient receive?

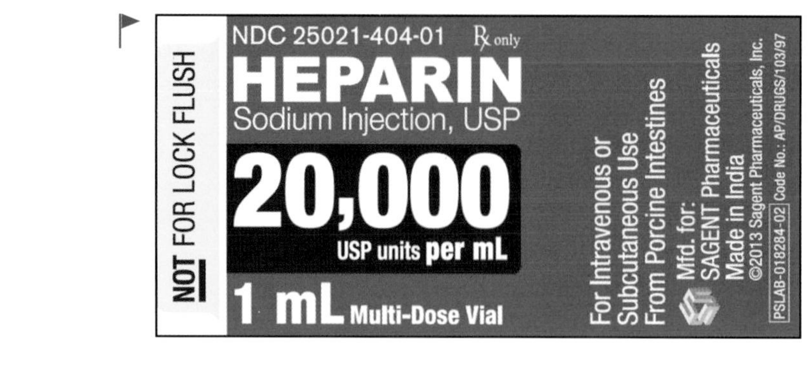

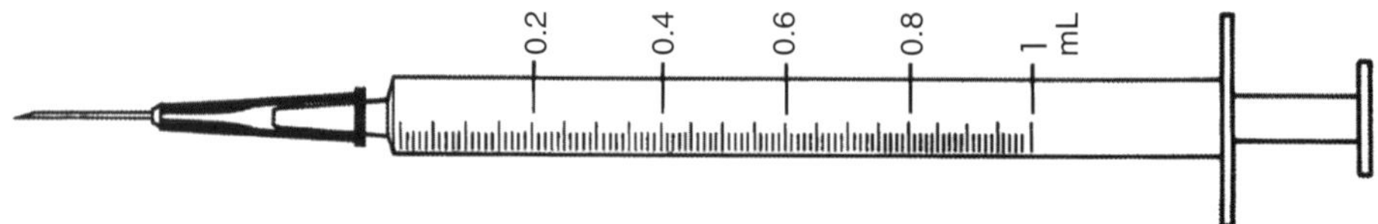

4. Ordered: Heparin 17,000 units subcutaneous stat dose. Available: Heparin 10,000 units/mL and 20,000 units/mL. Which strength will you choose? How many milliliters will the patient receive? Shade the amount on the syringe.

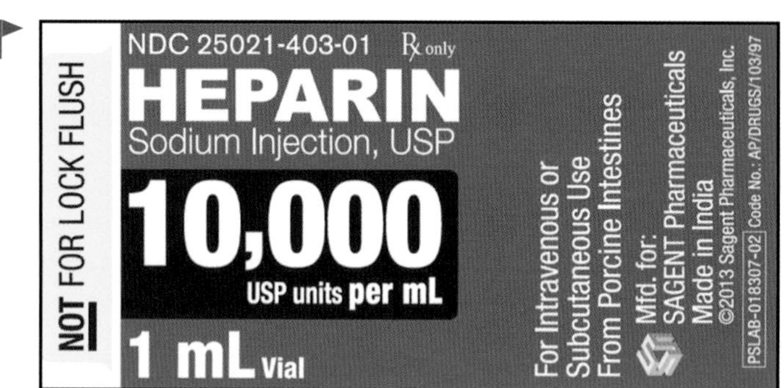

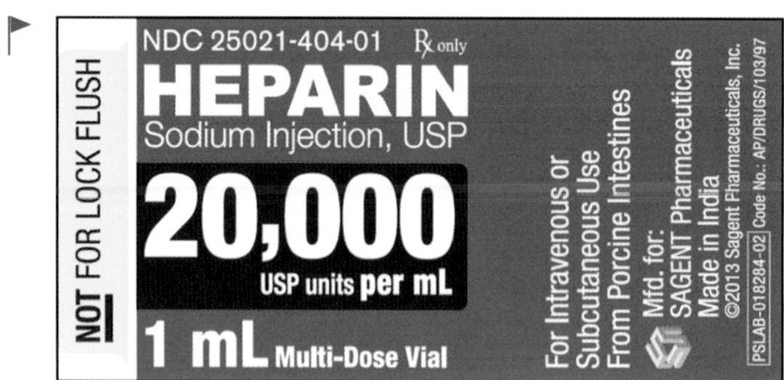

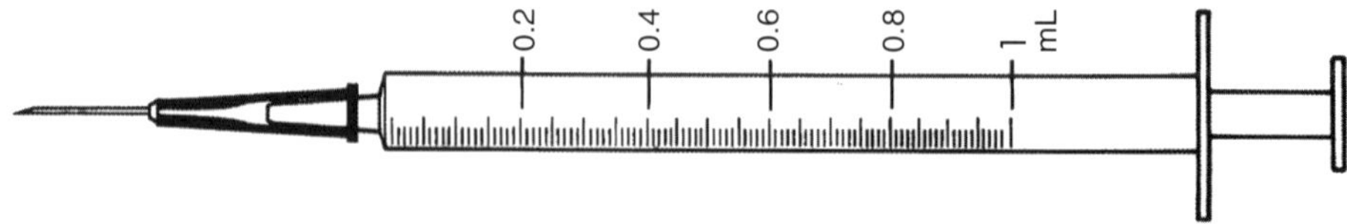

CLINICAL ALERT!

The subcutaneous dosage of heparin should not exceed 1 mL.

5. Ordered: Heparin 750 units subcutaneous q4h. Available: Heparin 1000 units/mL. How many milliliters will the patient receive? Shade the amount on the syringe.

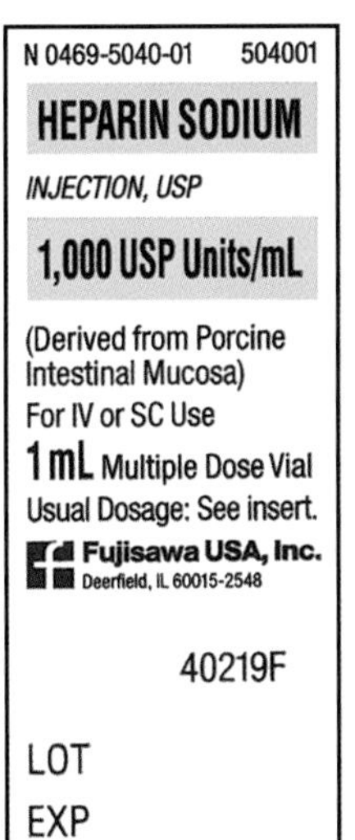
N 0469-5040-01 504001
HEPARIN SODIUM
INJECTION, USP
1,000 USP Units/mL
(Derived from Porcine Intestinal Mucosa)
For IV or SC Use
1 mL Multiple Dose Vial
Usual Dosage: See insert.
Fujisawa USA, Inc.
Deerfield, IL 60015-2548
40219F
LOT
EXP

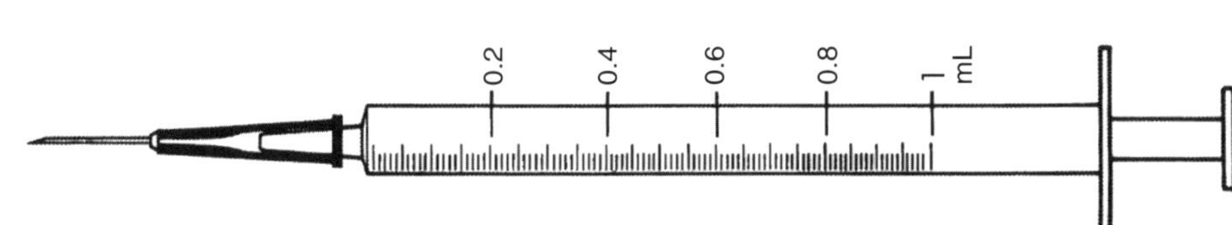

6. Ordered: Heparin 800 units subcutaneous q8hr. Available: Heparin 1000 units/mL in a multidose vial. How many milliliters will the patient receive? Shade the amount on the syringe.

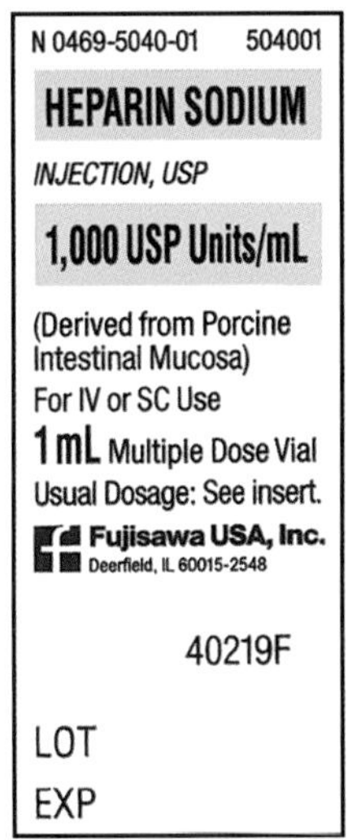
N 0469-5040-01 504001
HEPARIN SODIUM
INJECTION, USP
1,000 USP Units/mL
(Derived from Porcine Intestinal Mucosa)
For IV or SC Use
1 mL Multiple Dose Vial
Usual Dosage: See insert.
Fujisawa USA, Inc.
Deerfield, IL 60015-2548
40219F
LOT
EXP

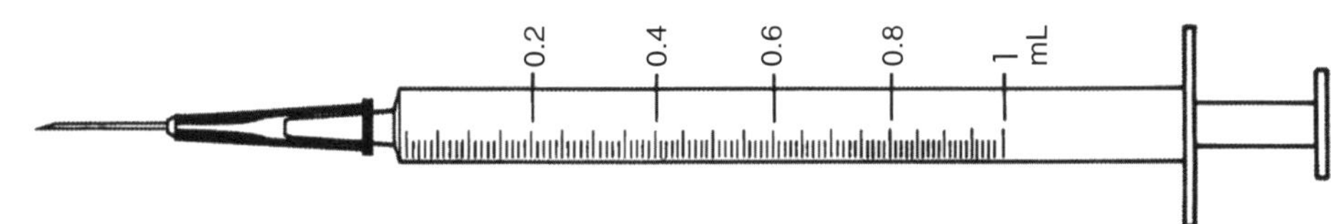

CLINICAL ALERT!

Check your patient's chart for allergies. Heparin is made from pork and beef. Remember to check with your patient/family about religious practices that may prohibit the administration of animal-based medications.

7. Ordered: Heparin 3000 units subcutaneous q8h. Available: Heparin 5000 units/mL in a multidose vial. How many milliliters will the patient receive? Shade the amount on the syringe.

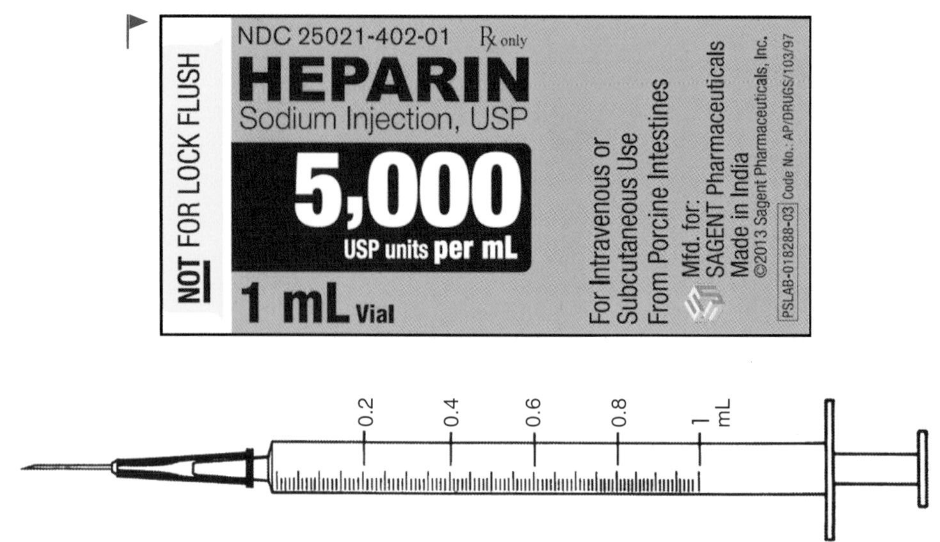

IV Flushes

8. Ordered: Heparin flush 5 units after each medication administration to prevent clot formation in the heparin lock. Available: Heparin 10 units/mL. How many units of medication are in the vial? How many milliliters will the patient receive? Shade the amount on the syringe.

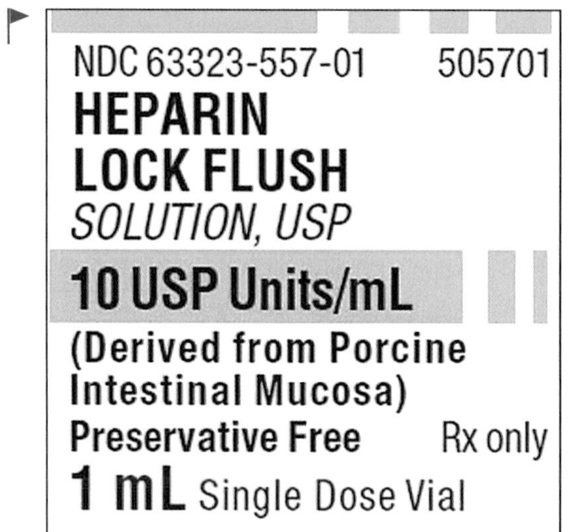

Follow agency protocol for saline and heparin flushes after medication administration.

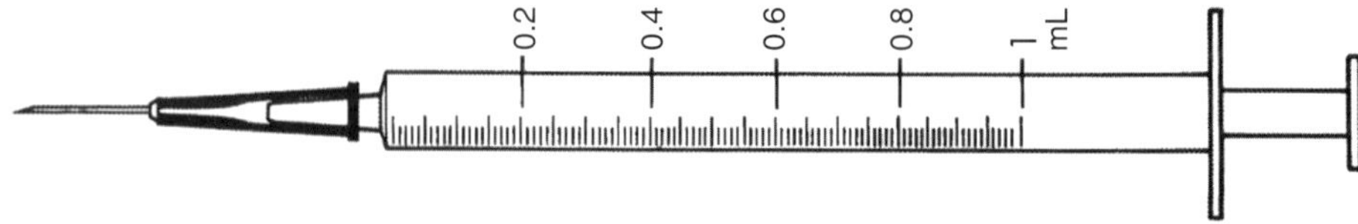

CLINICAL RELEVANCE

Heparin resistance has been documented in elderly patients; therefore larger than expected doses may be ordered. Verify with provider and monitor elderly patients closely for complications.

CLINICAL ALERT!

Symptoms of overdose are nosebleed, bleeding gums, tarry stools, petechiae, and easy bruising. An electric razor should be used for shaving. Make sure protamine sulfate is available.

9. Ordered: Heparin flush 50 units q12h for IV site patency. Available: Heparin 100 units/mL. How many milliliters will the patient receive? Shade the amount on the syringe.

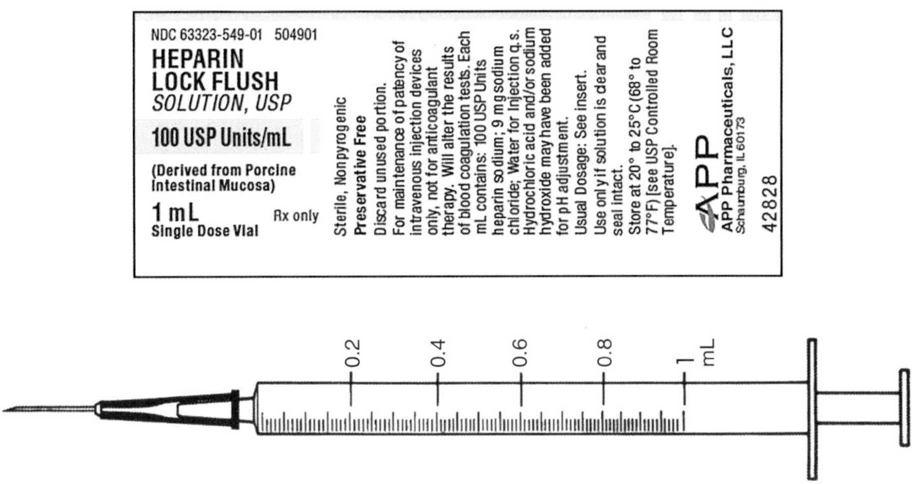

IV Flushes

Peripheral lines are gently flushed with 2 to 3 mL of normal saline.

Heparin locks provide patients with mobility while they are receiving IV medications. Heparin flushes are used to prevent clot formation in the central line. Central lines are used for access to large veins. Hyperosmolarity solutions can be used without causing vein damage. Heparin flushes for central lines come in prefilled 12-mL syringes with 5 mL of 10 units per mL of heparin. Heparin flushes are also available in prefilled 12-mL syringes with 10 mL of 100 units per mL of heparin. Multiple-dose vials of various strengths are also available.

CLINICAL ALERT!

Heparin IV flushes are available in many different strengths and multiple-dose vials. READ LABELS CAREFULLY. Agency protocol will specify the strength and the amount to administer.

Polypharmacy

Many people who take prescription drugs also take over-the-counter (OTC) medication. Researchers from the University of Chicago found that about 91% of older adults use at least one medication, and nearly 30% have at least five prescriptions. The study also indicated that many of these older people are taking anticoagulants or antiplatelet agents, which puts them at high risk for adverse drug reactions. It is imperative that all OTC and prescription drugs be charted and the provider notified.

IV Heparin

When intermittent or continuous IV therapy is used, blood should be drawn for a PTT and a hematocrit level to determine the course of therapy. Therapeutic anticoagulant dosage is regulated according to the results of the PTT and the patient's weight.

Pharmacies are standardizing IV heparin preparations in concentrations of 25,000 units/500 mL and 25,000 units/250 mL. Dispensing charts indicating mL/hr and units/hr are available for each concentration. This should reduce overdosing and underdosing but the nurse must still verify all medication orders, perform proper calculations, and validate proper working of infusion devices. Protamine sulfate is the antagonist for heparin. It is the nurse's responsibility to have protamine sulfate available.

The usual dosage for protamine sulfate is 1 mg for every 100 IU of active heparin, not to exceed 50 mg, given slowly over a 10-minute interval. This is used to reverse large doses of heparin administered IV during surgery, especially heart surgery. Monitor aPTT 5 to 15 minutes after the dose is administered, then again in 2 to 8 hours.

CLINICAL RELEVANCE

Patients receiving IV heparin may experience a complex of symptoms (systemic reaction) when the infusion is started. The symptoms include fever, chills, high blood pressure, fast heart rate, shortness of breath, and chest pain. This happens in about 25% of people who have HIT. Others may develop a skin rash consisting of red spots.

Answers on page 408

WORKSHEET 11B | IV Heparin Calculations: mL per hr

Answer the following questions and show your proofs (carry out to the nearest hundredth). The heparin will be administered with an infusion device.

Example Ordered: Heparin 1400 units per hr IV. Available: 500 mL of NS with 25,000 units of heparin sodium.

a. How many mL per hr will deliver 1400 units per hr?

b. How many hours will it take to infuse?

KNOW — WANT TO KNOW

500 mL : 25,000 units = x mL : 1400 units

$250x = 500 \times 1400 = 7000$

$250x = 7000$ units

$x = 28$/mL per hr. Set infusion pump to deliver 28 mL per hr.

FRACTION CROSS PRODUCT

$$\frac{500}{25000 \text{ units}} \times \frac{x \text{ mL}}{1400 \text{ units}}$$

$250x = 5 \times 1400 = 7000$

$x = 28$ mL

PROOF $500 \times 1400 = 7000$
$250 \times 28 = 7000$

KNOW — WANT TO KNOW

28 mL : 1 hr = 500 mL : x hr

$28x = 1 \times 500 = 500$

$28x = 500$

$x = 17.85$ hr

$60 \times 0.85 = 51$. The IV will take 17 hr 51 minutes to infuse.

FRACTION CROSS PRODUCT

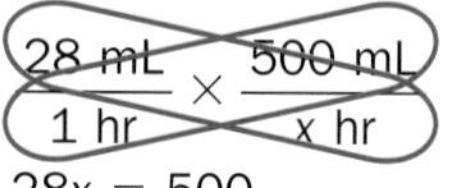

$$\frac{28 \text{ mL}}{1 \text{ hr}} \times \frac{500 \text{ mL}}{x \text{ hr}}$$

$28x = 500$

$x = 17.85$

PROOF $500 \times 1 = 500$
$28 \times 17.85 = 499.8 = 500$

1. Ordered: Heparin 2500 units per hr IV. Available: 50,000 units per 1000 mL 0.9% NS.

a. How many mL per hr will deliver 2500 units per hr?

b. How many hours will it take to infuse?

2. Ordered: Heparin 10,000 units in 15 hr. Pharmacy has sent 1000 mL NS with 10,000 units of heparin.

a. How many units per hr will the patient receive?

b. How many mL per hr will be infused?

c. 300 mL have been infused at 0700. When will the infusion finish? How many hours remain for the infusion?

3. Ordered: Heparin 1500 units per hr IV. Pharmacy has sent 1 L 0.9% saline with 20,000 units of heparin.
   a. How many mL per hr will deliver 1500 units?
   b. How many hours will it take to infuse this bag?

4. Ordered: Heparin sodium 20,000 units IV in 12 hr. Pharmacy has sent 1000 mL of 0.9% normal saline with 20,000 units heparin sodium.
   a. At how many mL per hr should the IV infuse?
   b. How many units per hr will infuse?
   c. The shift report states that 250 mL have been infused. How many hours remain for the infusion?

5. Ordered: Heparin 1200 units per hr. Available: 500 mL NS with 10,000 units of heparin.
   a. How many mL per hr will infuse 1200 units per hr?
   b. How many hours will it take to infuse this bag?

6. Ordered: Heparin sodium 1000 units/hr IV. Available: 1 L of 0.9% saline with 20,000 units of heparin.
   a. How many mL per hr will deliver 1000 units?
   b. How many hours will it take to infuse the bag?

7. Ordered: Heparin 1000 units per hr. Your patient is on fluid restrictions. The pharmacy has sent 20,000 units per 250 mL of NS.
   a. How many mL per hr will deliver 1000 units per hr?
   b. How many hours will it take to infuse?

8. Ordered: Heparin 1300 units per hr IV. Available: 500 mL with 25,000 units of heparin sodium.
   a. How many mL per hr will deliver 1300 units per hr?
   b. How long will it take to infuse?

9. Ordered: Heparin 1800 units per hr IV. Your patient is on fluid restrictions; therefore the pharmacy has sent a concentrated solution of 25,000 units per 250 mL of NS.
   a. How many mL per hr will deliver 1800 units per hr?
   b. How many hours will it take to infuse?

10. Ordered: Heparin 1500 units per hr IV. Available: 25,000 units per 500 mL.
   a. How many mL per hr will deliver 1500 units per hr?
   b. How many hours will it take to infuse?

Answers on page 410

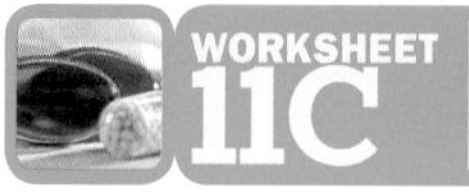

WORKSHEET 11C IV Heparin Calculations Titrated to Kilograms

All intravenous anticoagulants are based on the PTT results. Loading (bolus) doses are individualized and are titrated to weight in kilograms. Agency protocol is usually standardized for each institution. It is important that the nurses know what the protocol standards are and where they are located. Protocols and literature may vary, but the loading doses are usually between 70 and 100 units per kg. Infusion rates for heparin sodium also vary but are usually between 15 and 25 units per kg per hr.

Example Ordered: IV heparin loading dose to infuse at 15 units per kg per hr. The patient weighs 190 lb.
Available: 20,000 units of heparin sodium in 1000 mL of D5W.
At what rate will you set the IV infusion pump?

Change 190 lb to kg. 190 divided by 2.2 = 86.36 = 86 kg.
Multiply units per hr by the patient's weight in kg. 15 × 86 = 1290 units per hr.

Ratio and Proportion Method

KNOW | WANT TO KNOW | FRACTION CROSS PRODUCT

15 units : 1 kg = x units : 86 kg

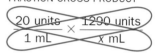

$$\frac{15 \text{ units}}{1 \text{ kg}} \times \frac{x \text{ units}}{86 \text{ kg}}$$

$x = 15 \times 86 = 1290$
$x = 1290$ units per hr

$x = 15 \times 86 = 1290$
$x = 1290$ units per hr

PROOF $15 \times 86 = 1290$
$1 \times 1290 = 1290$

KNOW | WANT TO KNOW | FRACTION CROSS PRODUCT

20,000 units : 1000 mL = 1290 units : x mL

$$\frac{20 \text{ units}}{1 \text{ mL}} \times \frac{1290 \text{ units}}{x \text{ mL}}$$

$20x = 1 \times 1290 = 1290$
$20x = 1290$
$x = 64.5$ mL per hr = 65 mL per hr. Set infusion pump to deliver 65 mL per hr.

$20x = 1290$
$x = 64.5 = 65$

PROOF $1 \times 1290 = 1290$
$20 \times 64.5 = 1290$

Directions: Follow the above example to calculate the loading dose, units per hr, and mL per hr.

1. Ordered: Heparin sodium 90 units per kg as a loading dose. Infuse at 25 units per kg per hr. Available: 1000 mL 0.45% NS with 25,000 units of heparin. The patient weighs 210 lb.
   a. How many units is the loading dose?
   b. How many units per hr will the patient receive?
   c. At what rate will you set the mL per hr?

2. Ordered: 80 units per kg of heparin as a loading dose. Set infusion rate to deliver 1500 units per hr. Available: 1000 mL NS with 30,000 units of heparin. The patient weighs 160 lb.
   a. Calculate the loading dose.
   b. Calculate the mL per hr.

CLINICAL ALERT!
Always have protamine sulfate available as an antidote for heparin.

3. Ordered: Heparin sodium 70 units per kg bolus loading dose. Infusion rate to run at 20 units per kg per hr. Available: 1000 mL D5W with 25,000 units of heparin. The patient weighs 176 lb.
   a. Calculate the loading dose.
   b. Calculate the units per hr based on weight.
   c. Calculate the mL per hr.

4. Ordered: Loading dose of 75 units per kg; then infuse at 20 units per kg per hr. Available: 1000 mL 0.9% NS with 50,000 units of heparin. The patient weighs 300 lb.
   a. Calculate the loading dose.
   b. How many units per hr will the patient receive?
   c. At what rate will you set the infusion device?

5. Ordered: A bolus dose of heparin at 70 units per kg. Run the infusion at 18 units per kg per hr. Available: 1000 mL D5W with 30,000 units of heparin. The patient weighs 194 lb.
   a. How many units will you give as the bolus dose?
   b. How many units per hr will infuse?
   c. At what rate will you set the infusion device?

6. Ordered: Loading dose of 65 units per kg. Set the infusion to run at 15 units per kg per hr. Available: 500 mL 0.45% NS with 30,000 units of heparin. The patient weighs 145 lb.
   a. How many units is the loading dose?
   b. How many units per hr will infuse?
   c. At what rate will you set the infusion device?

7. Ordered: Bolus dose of heparin at 80 units per kg. Titrate infusion to run at 1000 units per hr. Available: 1000 mL D5W with 25,000 units of heparin. The patient weighs 120 kg.
   a. Calculate the number of units for the bolus dose.
   b. Calculate mL per hr to infuse 1000 units per hr.

8. Ordered: Loading dose of heparin 75 units per kg. Infuse at 17 units per kg per hr. Available: 1000 mL D5W with 20,000 units of heparin. The patient weighs 185 lb.
   a. How many units is the loading dose?
   b. How many units per hr will the patient receive?
   c. At what rate will you set the infusion device?

9. Ordered: A loading dose of heparin at 95 units per kg. Pharmacy has sent 1000 mL 0.9% NS with 20,000 units of heparin. Run the infusion at 20 units per kg per hr. The patient weighs 136 kg.
   a. How many units is the loading dose?
   b. How many units per hr will infuse?
   c. At what rate will you set the infusion device?

10. Ordered: Heparin 1000 units/kg bolus dose. Infuse at 18 units per kg per hr. Available: 1000 mL 0.45% NS with 35,000 units of heparin. The patient weighs 108 kg.
    a. How many units is the loading dose?
    b. How many units per hr will infuse?
    c. At what rate will you set the infusion device?

Answers on page 412

WORKSHEET 11D

Dosing Guidelines

The sequence of IV administration usually follows a process of bolus or loading dose, the titrated dose, and a rebolus rate adjusted to the aPTT result.

Directions:

Use the Dosing Guidelines for (DVT-PE) Treatment Chart (Table 11.1) to calculate the units per hour for the IV rate for a patient who weighs 70 kg. The standard infusion bag holds 25,000 units per 250 mL (100 units per mL).

Table 11.1 Dosing Guidelines for (DVT-PE) Treatment Chart

(Based on Raschke[1] nomogram)
Obtain baseline aPTT, prothrombin time (PT), CBC, platelet count.
Check for contraindications to heparin therapy.

Patient name: **Location:**
Height: 70 inches **Weight:** 70 kg **Dosing weight:** 70 kg

Standard infusion bag concentration: 25,000 units per 250 mL (100 units per mL).
Also, all infusion rates below are rounded to the nearest **100** units.

Initial bolus dose (80 units per kg): 5600 units
Initial infusion rate (18 units per kg per hr): 1300 units per hr (13 mL per hr)

aPTT (seconds)*	Dose Change (units per kg per hr)	Additional Action	Next aPTT
<35 (1.2 × mean normal)	Increase by 4 units per kg per hr (300 units) or 3 mL per hr	Rebolus with 80 units per kg (5600 units)	6 hours
35 to 45 (1.2 to 1.5 × mean normal)	Increase by 2 units per kg per hr (100 units) or 1 mL per hr	Rebolus with 40 units per kg (2800 units)	6 hours
46 to 70 (1.5 to 2.3 × mean normal)	No change		6 hours†
71 to 90 (2.3 to 3.0 × mean normal)	Decrease by 2 units per kg per hr (100 units) or 1 mL per hr		6 hours
>90 (>3 × mean normal)	Decrease by 3 units per kg per hr (200 units) or 2 mL per hr	Stop infusion 1 hour	6 hours

*The therapeutic range in seconds should correspond to a plasma heparin level of 0.2 to 0.4 IU per mL by protamine sulfate or 0.3 to 0.6 IU per mL by amidolytic assay.
†Repeat aPTT every 6 hours during the first 24 hours; thereafter, monitor aPTT once every morning, unless it is outside the therapeutic range.

1. Calculate the initial bolus dose of 80 units per kg for the patient who weighs 70 kg.

2. Calculate the units per hour.

3. Calculate the infusion rate.

The 6-hour aPTT is 30. Rebolus with 80 units per kg (5600 units) and increase the rate by 4 units per kg.

4. a. Calculate the increased units per hour.
b. What is the new units-per-hour rate?

5. Calculate the new infusion rate.

The 6-hour aPTT is 40. Increase the IV rate by 2 units per kg per hour. Rebolus with 40 units per kg.

6. Calculate the bolus dose.

7. **a.** Calculate the increased units per hour.
   b. What is the new units-per-hour rate?

8. Calculate the new infusion rate.

The 6-hour aPTT is 55 = no change
The 6-hour aPTT is 85 = decrease the rate by 2 units per kg per hour.

9. **a.** Calculate the decreased units per hour.
   b. What is the new units-per-hour rate?

10. Calculate the new infusion rate.

The 6-hour aPTT is 95 = decrease the rate by 3 units per kg per hour.

11. **a.** Calculate the decreased units per hour.
    b. What is the new units-per-hour rate?

12. Calculate the new infusion rate.

13. What will be your next action?

Oral Anticoagulants

Warfarin (Coumadin) (Figure 11.4) is used as prophylaxis after an episode of thrombolytic complications and for atrial fibrillation to prevent blood coagulation. The drug inhibits the activity of vitamin K, which is required for the activation of clotting factors. Patients receiving heparin therapy are converted to an oral anticoagulant in the care agency while still receiving heparin injections. The level of warfarin in the blood is monitored by the laboratory value of the international normalized ratio (INR). The INR is a standardized measurement of the prothrombin time (PTT). The INR should be maintained at 2 to 3 for best results, depending on the illness being treated. Dosing for all anticoagulants is individualized. The antidote for warfarin is vitamin K (Figure 11.5), plasma, or whole blood.

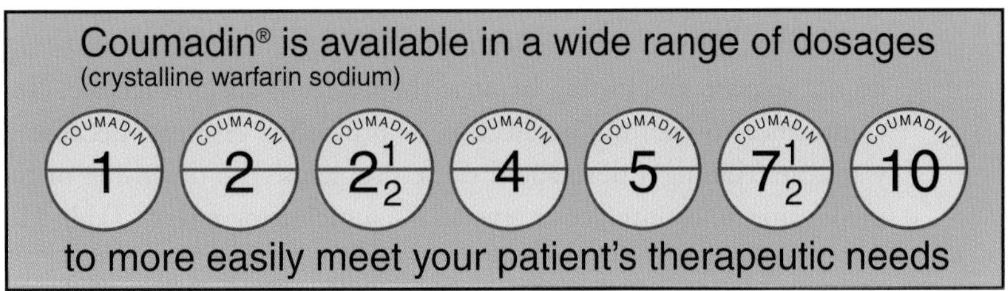

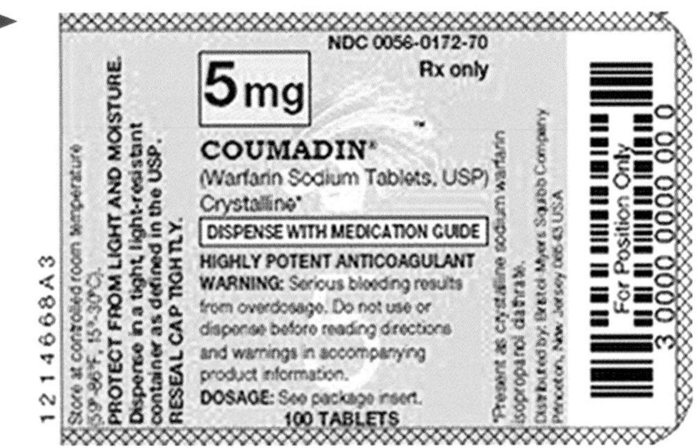

FIGURE 11.4 Coumadin tablets come in a variety of dosages. (From *Mosby's Drug Consult 2007,* St Louis, 2007, Mosby.)

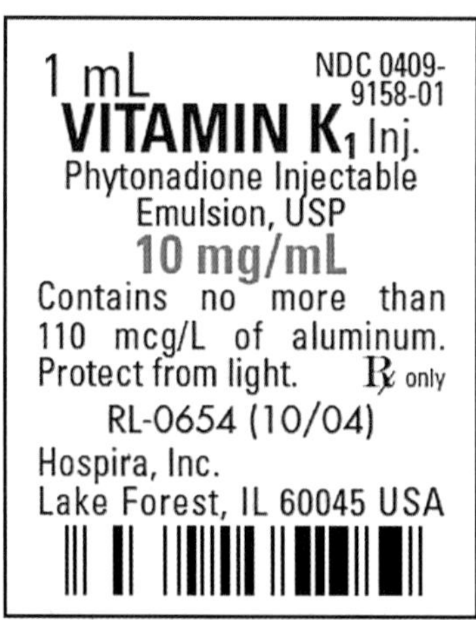

FIGURE 11.5 Vitamin K may be given as an antidote for warfarin.

CLINICAL RELEVANCE

When discharging a patient who will be going home on Coumadin (warfarin), it is extremely important that the patient is knowledgeable about medications that can potentiate the anticoagulation effect of Coumadin. A list of these medications is available from the pharmacist. Also, there are medications that can inhibit the effect of the Coumadin and over-the-counter medications that can increase the effects of the anticoagulant. Foods high in vitamin K should be avoided once the INR level has been stabilized. Compliance to daily dosage and diet restrictions is essential.

Because of the potential harmful effects of anticoagulants, these medications deserve special protocols for use and compliance with the blood-testing regimen. The importance must be stressed that all PT/INR tests be taken at the scheduled times. Signs and symptoms of bleeding or clotting must be reported immediately.

Oral anticoagulant warfarin (Coumadin) has been used to treat atrial fibrillation (AF) for many years. People with defibrillation have had to rely on warfarin to control their blood clotting cascade. The major drawback with warfarin use is the weekly or monthly blood testing to monitor the INR. A strict diet is necessary, and some medications may interfere with the anticoagulant property of warfarin. The effects of warfarin can be counteracted with vitamin K.

The new class of oral medications called *target-specific oral anticoagulants* (TSOACs) act rapidly and do not require monitoring because their actions are predictable. No special diet is required; however, compliance to take the medication as ordered is essential because they have a shorter half-life than warfarin. Missing a dose could cause problems. The downside of the newer drugs is that there is no medication to counteract or reverse the anticlotting effect (Table 11.2).

CLINICAL RELEVANCE

It is important for the nurse to be familiar with the agency's preferred clotting factor protocols to treat bleeding associated with TSOACs.

Table 11.2 Warfarin Oral Anticoagulant vs. New Oral Anticoagulants (TSOACs)

Drug Name (Brand Name)	Pros	Cons
Warfarin (Coumadin)	Predictable benefits and risks Take once daily Can be reversed rapidly with vitamin K	Weekly or monthly blood test to monitor prothrombin time (PT) and INR
Dabigatran (Pradaxa)	No blood monitoring required Lower risk of stroke or brain bleeding than warfarin	Take twice daily, making missed doses more likely More likely than warfarin to cause stomach upset
Rivaroxaban (Xarelto)	Take once daily Lower rates of brain bleeding than warfarin	Slightly higher risk of gastrointestinal bleeding than with apixaban or warfarin
Apixaban (Eliquis)	Lower risk of brain bleeding than with warfarin Major bleeding rate lower than with warfarin Lower rate of upset stomach than with dabigatran	Take twice daily Missed doses can become a problem

Patients taking Coumadin are at increased risk for medication interactions. The patient must always report to the health care provider all medications, including over-the-counter medications being taken.

Clopidogrel (Plavix) is an antiplatelet agent that blocks the formation of blood clots by preventing the clumping of platelets. Plavix is used for the prevention of heart attacks, unstable angina, recent stroke, or peripheral vascular disease. As with warfarin, there are many drug interactions associated with the efficacy of this drug. Atorvastatin (Lipitor) may potentiate the action of Plavix. A proton pump inhibitor (PPI) may subject the patient to another heart attack. The only PPI found to be safe for patients taking Plavix is pantoprazole (Protonix).

Missed doses: Warfarin and Plavix are usually taken once a day. If a dose is missed at the patient's usual dosing time, he or she should take it as soon as possible afterward. If it is missed closer to the 24-hour period, then the patient should resume his or her regular dose the next day. DO NOT DOUBLE THE DOSE.

Acetylsalicylic acid (aspirin) is also an antiplatelet agent that prevents the formation of blood clots. Sometimes a low dose of aspirin is prescribed for concurrent use along with warfarin, as these two drugs work in different ways. Warfarin prevents clotting of blood, and aspirin prevents clumping of platelets that can form blood clots.

CLINICAL ALERT!

There are many over-the-counter and prescribed medications that can adversely affect the efficacy of warfarin (Coumadin) and clopidogrel (Plavix). A list of medications and foods that interact with Coumadin and Plavix must be discussed with the patient and family or caregiver (if appropriate) before discharge. It is essential that the patient and family/caregiver (if appropriate) understand the necessity of compliance.

Answers on page 414

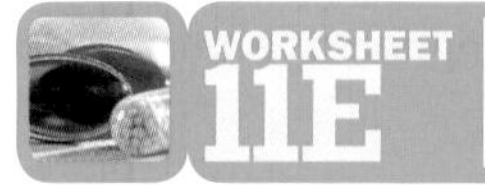

WORKSHEET 11E Multiple-Choice Practice

1. Ordered: Administer a bolus of heparin sodium IV. The hospital protocol is 80 units per kg. The patient weighs 160 lb. How many units will you give?
a. 5840 units **b.** 6620 units **c.** 4320 units **d.** 2420 units

2. Ordered: IV heparin to infuse at 18 units per kg per hr. Available: 1000 mL D5W with 20,000 units heparin. The patient weighs 175 lb. How many units per hr will the patient receive?
a. 1220 units per hr **b.** 880 units per hr **c.** 1280 units per hr **d.** 1440 units per hr

At what rate will you set the infusion device?
a. 110 mL per hr **b.** 85 mL per hr **c.** 68 mL per hr **d.** 72 mL per hr

3. Ordered: Fragmin subcutaneous q12h titrated to kg. Titrate Fragmin to 120 international units per kg subcutaneous. The patient weighs 132 lb. How many kilograms does the patient weigh?
a. 50 kg **b.** 120 kg **c.** 60 kg **d.** 45 kg

How many international units of Fragmin will you prepare?
a. 7000 international units **b.** 5000 international units
c. 83,000 international units **d.** 7200 international units

4. Refer to question 3. How many milliliters of Fragmin will you give? Available: 10,000 IU per mL multidose vial.
a. 0.7 mL **b.** 0.5 mL **c.** 1 mL **d.** 1.2 mL

5. Ordered: Fragmin subcutaneous. Titrate to 120 international units per kg q12h for 3-5 days. The patient weighs 185 lb. How many international units of Fragmin will you administer for each dose?
a. 5800 international units **b.** 1800 international units
c. 10,080 international units **d.** 6400 international units

6. Refer to question 5. Available: 25,000 IU per mL multidose vial of Fragmin. How many milliliters of Fragmin will you give?
a. 2.2 mL **b.** 0.4 mL **c.** 4.4 mL **d.** 0.2 mL

7. Ordered: Heparin drip at 40 units per kg. Available: 25,000 units of heparin in 1000 mL of D5W. The patient weighs 75 kg. At what rate will you set the infusion device?
a. 100 mL per hr **b.** 120 mL per hr **c.** 75 mL per hr **d.** 82 mL per hr

8. Ordered: Heparin IV drip at 500 units/hr. Available: 500 mL 0.9% NS with 10,000 units of heparin. At what hourly rate will you set the infusion?
a. 50 mL per hr **b.** 75 mL per hr **c.** 100 mL per hr **d.** 25 mL per hr

9. Ordered: Fragmin subcutaneous titrated to 120 international units per kg q12h for 3-8 days. Begin treatment at 0800 hr. The patient weighs 220 lb. How many kg does the patient weigh?

a. 100 kg **b.** 120 kg **c.** 110 kg **d.** 60 kg

How many international units of Fragmin will the patient receive per dose?

a. 10,000 international units **b.** 15,000 international units
c. 8000 international units **d.** 12,000 international units

10. Refer to question 9. Available: Fragmin 10,000 international units per mL and Fragmin 25,000 international units per mL multidose vials. Which multidose vial will you use? How many mL will you give?

a. 1 mL **b.** 0.75 mL **c.** 0.48 mL **d.** 0.66 mL

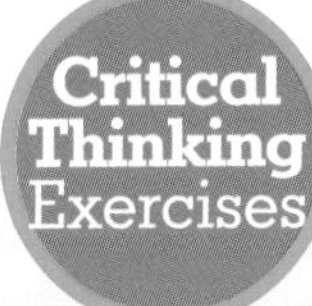

Critical Thinking Exercises provide math and medication-related patient safety issues for student discussion. Answers are not provided.

Analyze the following scenarios.

1. Mrs. Smith, a 76-year-old woman, was recuperating after abdominal surgery. The provider wrote the following order: *2000 units heparin subcut stat.* The nurse administered a 1-mL dose taken from a multidose vial labeled 20,000 units/mL. Later that day, the provider reduced the heparin order. He wrote: *Reduce heparin to 1000 units q8h.* While the nurse is preparing the 1000-unit dose from the multidose vial of 20,000 units/mL, she realizes the error when the first dose of heparin was administered.

Order:

Given:

Error(s):

Potential injuries:

Preventive measures:

Discussion

What factors contributed to the error?
How many units of heparin did Mrs. Smith receive for the first dose?
How was the patient's safety jeopardized?
What medication should always be on hand when a patient is receiving heparin?
What safety measures should have been implemented?
How can this type of error be reconciled?

2. Mr. G., an 80-year-old man, was admitted with a diagnosis of pulmonary embolism. He was given a bolus dose of 80 units of heparin and then was started on an IV drip of 25,000 units of heparin in 500 mL of D5W for 3 days. He has an order to start Coumadin 10 mg daily 72 hours before being discharged. Mr. G.'s discharge orders are for Coumadin (warfarin) 10 mg daily and blood tests for INR status once a week for the first 2 weeks. What precautions will Mr. G. need to be aware of while taking Coumadin?

Discussion:

What types of food might interfere with the desired effects of Coumadin?

What safety precautions should Mr. G. be aware of concerning possible bleeding?

What are some of the OTC medications that could enhance the effect of Coumadin?

What is the need for INR blood tests every week for the first 2 or 3 weeks?

How do you think that noncompliance with diet, medications, lifestyle, and blood testing could interfere with the patient's safety?

3. A 68-year-old woman who had a hip replacement just returned to the general surgery floor. The woman is a type 1 diabetic. The provider wrote a new order that read: *Start IV drip with 500 units of insulin in 1 liter of NS. Infuse over 24 hr. Heparin 250 units subcut q6h.* The nurse charted on the MAR: 500 units of heparin subcut. 250 units of insulin R added to the liter of NS. The nurse on the next shift noticed that the wrong medication and the wrong amount of heparin and insulin were charted for the IV and the subcut injection.

Order:

Given:

Discussion:

What factors contributed to the error?

What measures could be implemented for patient safety?

Why is it important to have another licensed nurse check the order?

What agency protocols should be addressed to remediate these types of errors?

Do you think that the first nurse was aware of the error?

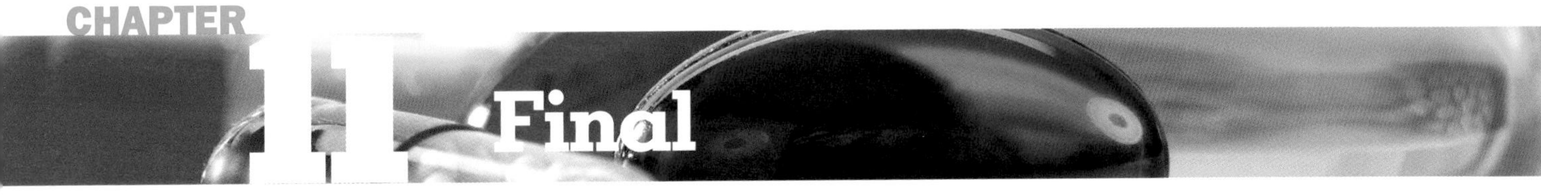

CHAPTER 11 Final

1. Ordered: Heparin 3000 units subcutaneous for prophylaxis of cerebral thrombosis. Available: 5000 units/mL. How many milliliters will the patient receive?

2. Ordered: Heparin 2500 units q4h subcutaneous to prevent thrombi from recurring. Available: 10,000 units/mL vial. How many milliliters will the patient receive?

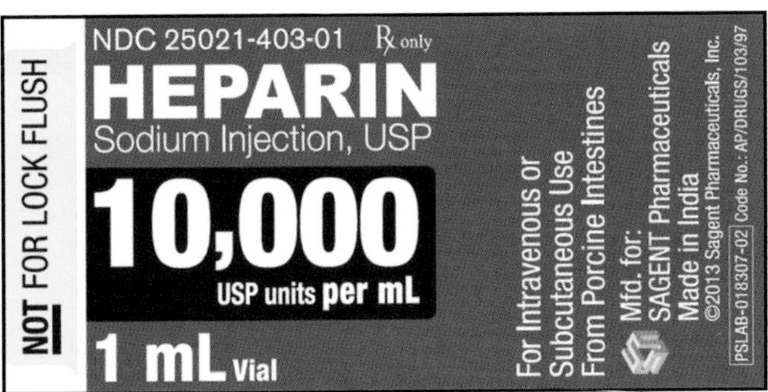

3. Ordered: Heparin 2000 units q4h subcutaneous for venous stasis. Available: 5000 units/mL and 10,000 units/mL. Which vial will you choose? If a tuberculin syringe is used, how many milliliters will the patient receive?

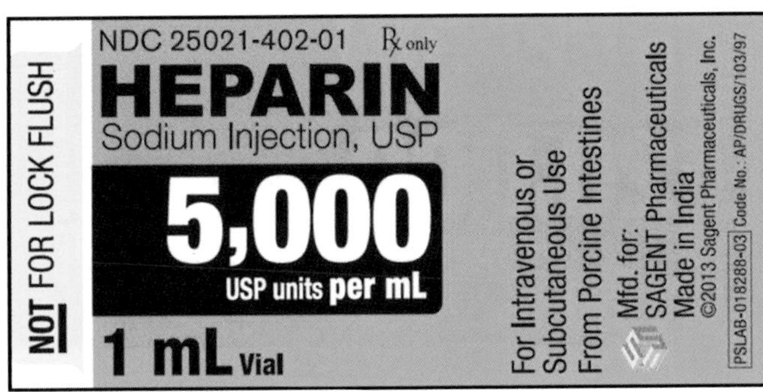

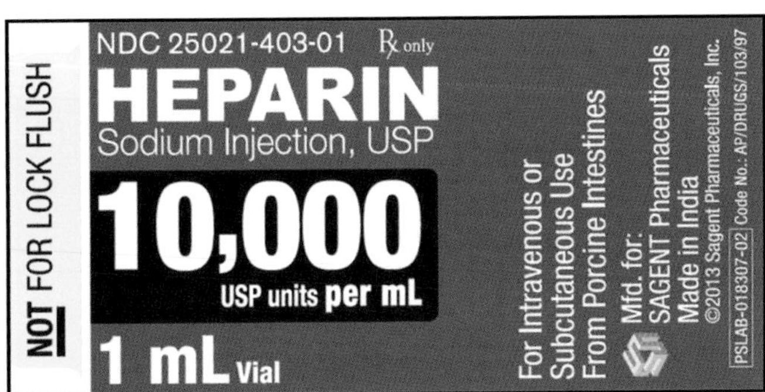

4. Ordered: Heparin 7000 units subcutaneous q8h before initiating a heparin infusion for a venous thromboembolism. Available: 5000, 10,000, and 20,000 units per mL. Which one will you choose? How many milliliters will the patient receive?

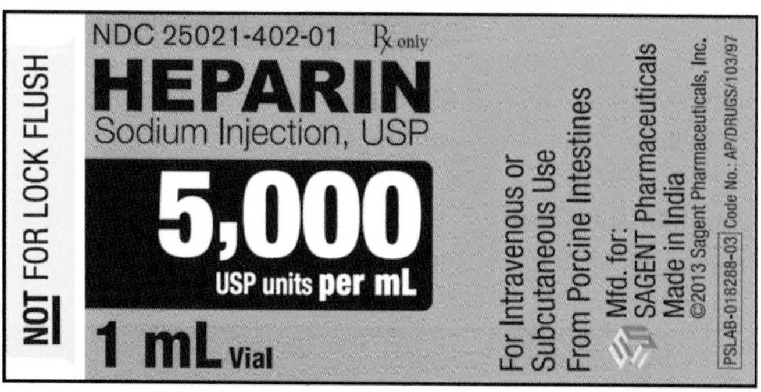

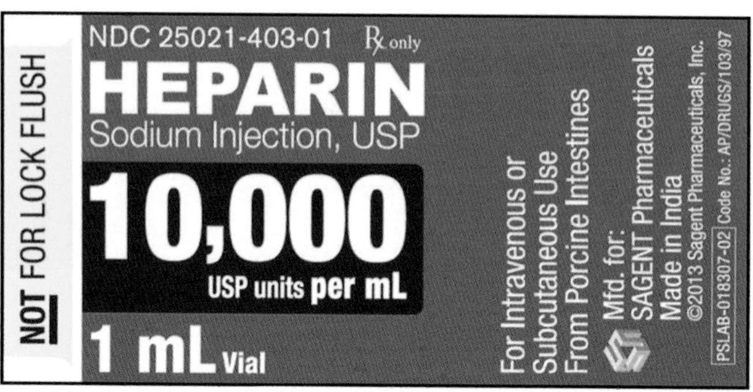

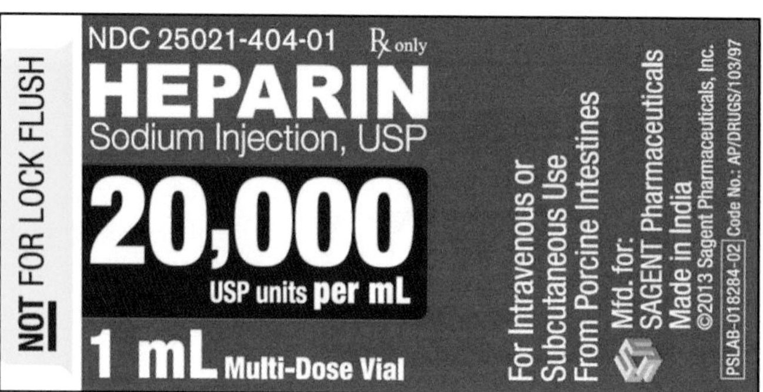

5. Ordered: Heparin 650 units subcutaneous every 4 hours as a prophylaxis for immobility. Available: Heparin 1000 units per mL. How many milliliters will the patient receive?

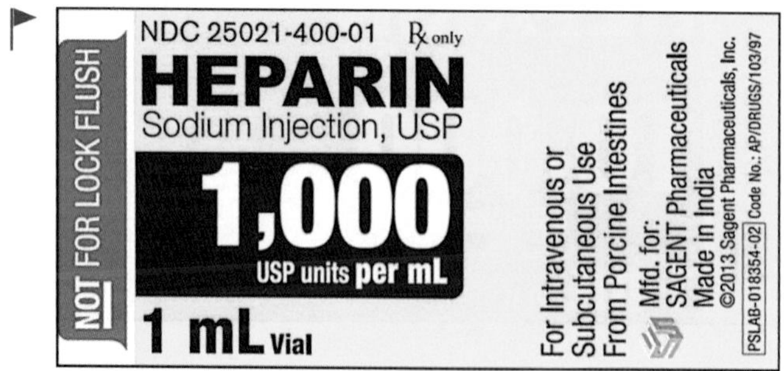

6. Ordered: 700 units per hr IV to infuse. Available: 20,000 units per 500 mL. How many mL per hr will provide 700 units per hr? For how many hours will the IV infuse?

7. Ordered: 1500 units per hr IV for hyperlipidemia. Available: 25,000 units per 500 mL. How many mL per hr will provide 1500 units per hr? For how many hours will the IV infuse?

8. Ordered: Heparin 35,000 units IV in 24 hr for atrial fibrillation. Available: 1000 mL 0.9% NS with 35,000 units of heparin sodium. How many mL per hr will the patient receive? How many units per hr will the patient receive?

9. Ordered: Heparin 2000 units per hr IV for pulmonary emboli. Available: Heparin 20,000 units in 1000 mL 0.9% NS. How many mL per hr will be delivered via the infusion device? For how long will the IV infuse?

10. Ordered: Heparin 25,000 units IV in 24 hr for peripheral arterial embolization. Available: 1000 mL with 25,000 units of heparin sodium. How many mL per hr will give 25,000 units in 24 hr? How many units per hr will infuse?

Refer to the Advanced Calculations section of Drug Calculations Companion, version 5 on Evolve for additional practice problems.

Answer Key

11 Anticoagulants

WORKSHEET **11A** (page 387)

1. KNOW — WANT TO KNOW

10,000 units : 1 mL = 6000 units : x mL

$10x = 6$

$x = 0.6$ mL

FRACTION CROSS PRODUCT

$$\frac{10{,}000}{1 \text{ ml}} = \frac{6000}{x \text{ mL}}$$

$10x = 6$

$x = 0.6$ mL

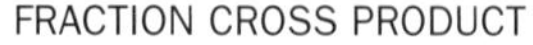

PROOF

$1 \times 6000 = 6000$

$10{,}000 \times 0.6 = 6000$

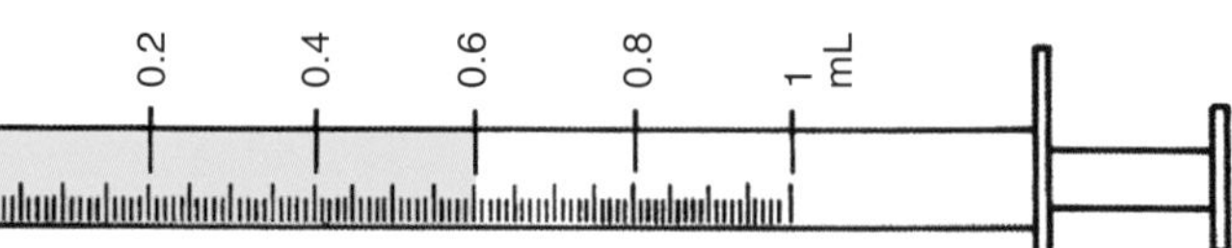

2. KNOW — WANT TO KNOW

40 mg : 0.4 mL = 35 mg : x mL

$40x = 0.4 \times 35 = 14$

$x = 0.35$

FRACTION CROSS PRODUCT

$$\frac{40 \text{ mg}}{0.4} = \frac{35 \text{ mg}}{x \text{ mL}}$$

$40x = 0.4 \times 35 = 14$

$x = 0.35$

PROOF

$40 \times 0.35 = 14$

$0.4 \times 35 = 14$

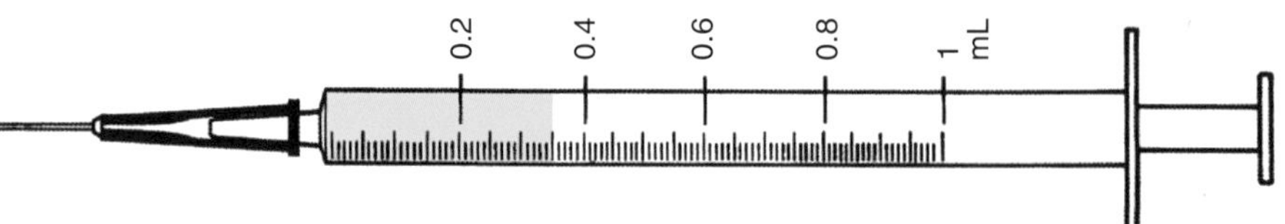

3. KNOW — WANT TO KNOW

20,000 units : 1 mL = 15,000 units : x mL

$20x = 15$

$x = 0.75$ mL

FRACTION CROSS PRODUCT

$$\frac{20{,}000}{1} = \frac{15000}{x \text{ mL}}$$

$20x = 15$

$x = 0.75$ mL

PROOF

$1 \times 15{,}000 = 15{,}000$

$20{,}000 \times 0.75 = 15{,}000$

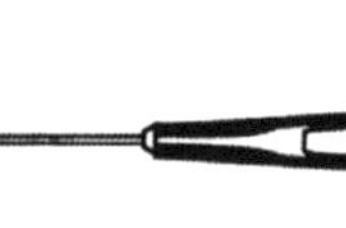

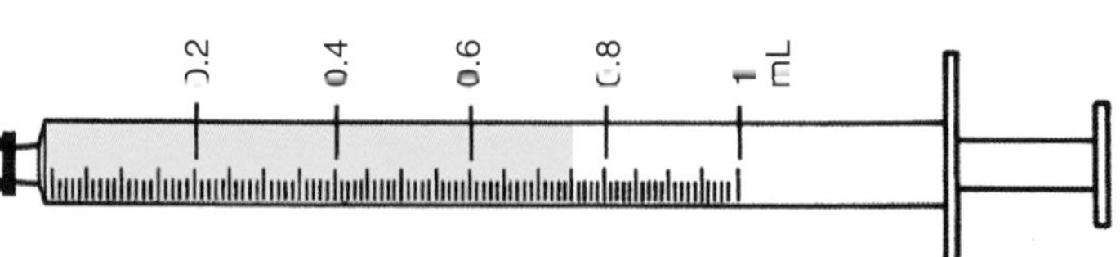

4. KNOW — WANT TO KNOW

20,000 units : 1 mL = 17,000 units : x mL } use 20,000 units per mL to keep injection less than 1 mL

FRACTION CROSS PRODUCT

$$\frac{20{,}000}{1} = \frac{17{,}000}{x \text{ mL}}$$

$20x = 17$

$x = 0.85$ mL

PROOF

$1 \times 17 = 17$

$20 \times 0.85 = 17$

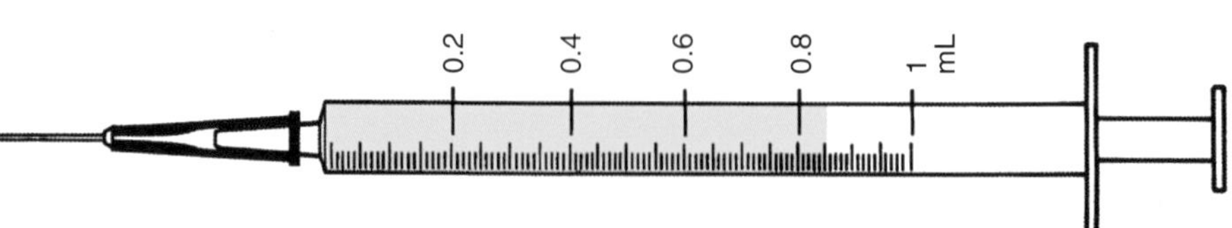

5. KNOW WANT TO KNOW

1000 units : 1 mL = 750 units : x mL

$100x = 75$

$x = 0.75$ mL

PROOF

$1000 \times 0.75 = 750$

$1 \times 750 = 750$

6. KNOW WANT TO KNOW

1000 units : 1 mL = 800 units : x mL

$10x = 8$

$x = 0.8$ mL

PROOF

$10 \times 0.8 = 8$

$1 \times 8 = 8$

7. KNOW WANT TO KNOW

5000 units : 1 mL = 3000 units : x mL

$5x = 3$

$x = 0.6$ mL

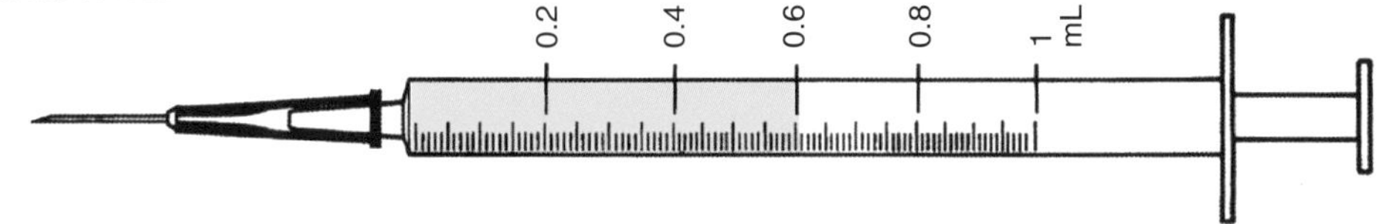

PROOF

$1 \times 3 = 3$

$5 \times 0.6 = 3$

8. The vial contains 10 units of heparin.

KNOW WANT TO KNOW

10 units : 1 mL = 5 units : x mL

$10x = 5$

$x = 0.5$ mL

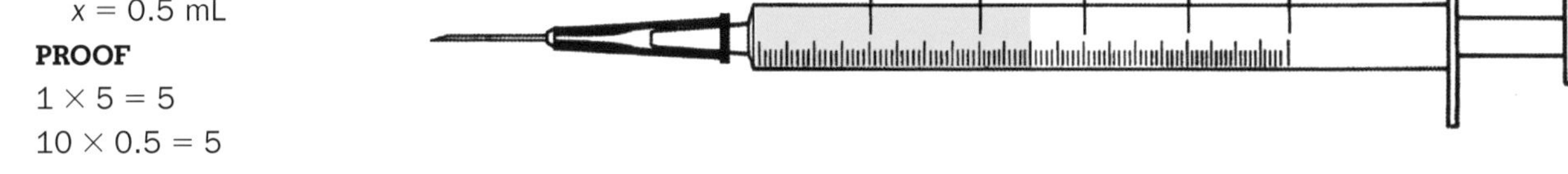

PROOF

$1 \times 5 = 5$

$10 \times 0.5 = 5$

9. KNOW WANT TO KNOW

100 units : 1 mL = 50 units : x mL

$10x = 5$

$x = 0.5$ mL

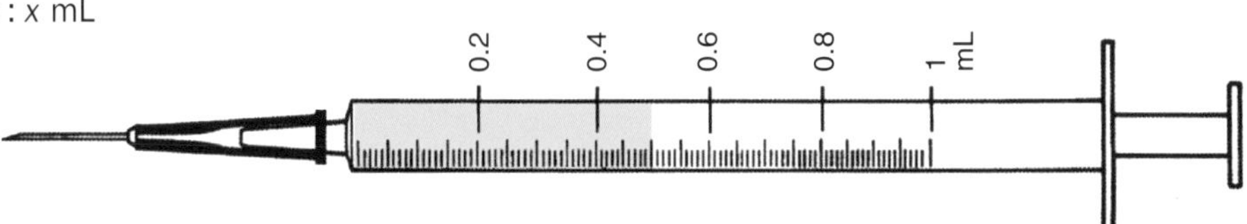

PROOF

$1 \times 5 = 5$

$10 \times 0.5 = 5$

WORKSHEET **11B** (page 392) SETTING UP THE FRACTION CROSS PRODUCT WILL ASSIST YOU IN SOLVING THESE PROBLEMS SUCCESSFULLY

1. a. KNOW WANT TO KNOW

50,000 units : 1000 mL = 2500 units : x mL

$500x = 25 \times 1000 = 25{,}000$

$5x = 250$

$x = 50$ mL per hr

PROOF

$500 \times 50 = 25{,}000$

$1000 \times 25 = 25{,}000$

b. KNOW WANT TO KNOW

50 mL : 1 hr = 1000 mL : x hr

$50x = 1000$

$x = 20$ hr

PROOF

$50 \times 20 = 1000$

$1 \times 1000 = 1000$

2. a. KNOW WANT TO KNOW

10,000 units : 15 hr = x units : 1 hr

$15x = 10{,}000$

$x = 666.6$ units per hr = 667 units per hr

PROOF

$15 \times 666.6 = 9999$

$10{,}000 \times 1 = 10{,}000$

b. $\frac{1000}{15} = 66.6$ or 67 mL per hr

c. KNOW WANT TO KNOW

67 mL : 1 hr = 700 mL : x hr

$67x = 700$

$x = 10.45$ hr or 10 hr 27 min remaining

The IV will be infused at 1727 hours.

PROOF

$1 \times 700 = 700$

$67 \times 10.45 = 700$

3. a. KNOW WANT TO KNOW

20,000 units : 1000 mL = 1500 units : x mL

$200x = 15{,}000$

$x = 75$ mL per hr = 1500 units heparin

PROOF

$200 \times 75 = 15{,}000$

$1000 \times 15 = 15{,}000$

b. KNOW WANT TO KNOW

75 mL : 1 hr = 1000 mL : x hr

$75x = 1000$

$x = 13.33$ hr or 13 hr, 20 min

PROOF

$1 \times 1000 = 1000$

$75 \times 13.33 = 999.75$

4. a. $\frac{1000}{12} = 83.3$ or 83 mL per hr

b. KNOW WANT TO KNOW

20,000 units : 12 hr = x units : 1 hr

$12x = 20{,}000$

$x = 1666.6$ units per hr = 1667 units per hr

PROOF

$20{,}000 \times 1 = 20{,}000$

$12 \times 1666 = 19{,}992$

c. KNOW WANT TO KNOW

83 mL : 1 hr = 750 mL : x hr

$83x = 750$

$x = 9$ hr remaining

PROOF

$1 \times 750 = 750$

$83 \times 9 = 747$

5. a. KNOW WANT TO KNOW

10,000 units : 500 mL = 1200 units : x mL

$100x = 6000$

$x = 60$ mL per hr

PROOF

$500 \times 12 = 6000$

$100 \times 60 = 6000$

b. KNOW WANT TO KNOW

60 mL : 1 hr = 500 mL : x hr

$60x = 500$

$x = 8.33$ hr or 8 hr 20 min

PROOF

$60 \times 8.33 = 499.8$

$1 \times 500 = 500$

6. a. KNOW WANT TO KNOW

20,000 units : 1000 mL = 1000 units : x mL

$20x = 1000$

$x = 50$ mL per hr = 1000 units heparin

PROOF

$20 \times 50 = 1000$

$1000 \times 1 = 1000$

b. KNOW WANT TO KNOW

50 mL : 1 hr = 1000 mL : x hr

$50x = 1000$

$x = 20$ hr

PROOF

$1 \times 1000 = 1000$

$50 \times 20 = 1000$

7. a. KNOW WANT TO KNOW

20,000 units : 250 mL = 1000 units : x mL

$20x = 250$

$x = 12.5$ mL per hr or 13 mL per hr

PROOF

$20 \times 12.5 = 250$

$250 \times 1 = 250$

b. KNOW WANT TO KNOW

13 mL : 1 hr = 250 mL : x hr

$13x = 250$

$x = 19.23$ hr or 19 hr 14 min

PROOF

$1 \times 250 = 250$

$13 \times 19.23 = 249.9$

8. a. KNOW WANT TO KNOW

25,000 units : 500 mL = 1300 units : x mL

$250x = 6500$

$x = 26$ mL per hr

PROOF

$26 \times 250 = 6500$

$500 \times 13 = 6500$

b. KNOW WANT TO KNOW

26 mL : 1 hr = 500 mL : x hr

$26x = 500$

$x = 19.23$ hr or 19 hr 14 min

PROOF

$1 \times 500 = 500$

$26 \times 19.23 = 499.98$

9. a. KNOW WANT TO KNOW

25,000 units : 250 mL = 1800 units : x mL

$250x = 250 \times 18 = 4500$

$250x = 4500$

$x = 18$ mL per hr

PROOF

$250 \times 18 = 4500$

$250 \times 18 = 4500$

b. KNOW WANT TO KNOW

18 mL : 1 hr = 250 mL : x hr

$18x = 250$

$x = 13.88$ hr or 13 hr 53 min

PROOF

$1 \times 250 = 250$

$18 \times 13.8 = 248.4$

10. a. KNOW WANT TO KNOW

25,000 units : 500 mL = 1500 units : x mL

$250x = 500 \times 15 = 7500$

$25x = 750$

$x = 30$ mL per hr

PROOF

$250 \times 30 = 7500$

$500 \times 15 = 7500$

b. KNOW WANT TO KNOW

30 mL : 1 hr = 500 mL : x hr

$30x = 500$

$3x = 50$

$x = 16.66 = 16$ hr 40 min

PROOF

$1 \times 500 = 500$

$30 \times 16.66 = 499.8$

WORKSHEET **11C** (page 394) SETTING UP THE FRACTION CROSS PRODUCT WILL ASSIST YOU IN SOLVING THESE PROBLEMS SUCCESSFULLY

1. lb to kg = 210 lb divided by 2.2 = 95.5 = 96 kg

a. KNOW WANT TO KNOW

90 units : 1 kg = x units : 96 kg

$x = 90 \times 96 = 8640$

x = 8640 units loading dose

PROOF

$1 \times 8640 = 8640$

$90 \times 96 = 8640$

b. KNOW WANT TO KNOW

25 units : 1 kg/hr = x units : 96 kg/hr

$x = 25 \times 96 = 2400$

x = 2400 units per hr

PROOF

$25 \times 96 = 2400$

$1 \times 2400 = 2400$

c. KNOW WANT TO KNOW

1000 mL : 25,000 units = x mL : 2400 units

$25x = 1 \times 2400 = 2400$

$25x = 2400 = 96$

x = 96 mL per hr

PROOF

$96 \times 25 = 2400$

$1 \times 2400 = 2400$

2. lb to kg = 160 lb divided by 2.2 kg = 72.7 = 73 kg

a. KNOW WANT TO KNOW

80 units : 1 kg = x units : 73 kg

$x = 80 \times 73 = 5840$

x = 5840 units loading dose

PROOF

$1 \times 5840 = 5840$

$73 \times 80 = 5840$

b. KNOW WANT TO KNOW

1000 mL : 30,000 units = x mL : 1500 units

$30x = 1 \times 1500 = 1500$

$30x = 1500$

$3x = 150$

x = 50 mL per hr

PROOF

$50 \times 300 = 15,000$

$15 \times 1000 = 15,000$

3. lb to kg = 176 ÷ 2.2 = 80 kg

a. KNOW WANT TO KNOW

70 units : 1 kg = x units : 80 kg

$x = 70 \times 80 = 5600$ units loading dose

PROOF

$1 \times 5600 = 5600$

$70 \times 80 = 5600$

b. KNOW WANT TO KNOW

20 units : 1 kg per hr = x units : 80 kg per hr

$x = 20 \times 80 = 1600$

x = 1600 units per hr

PROOF

$1 \times 1600 = 1600$

$20 \times 80 = 1600$

c. KNOW WANT TO KNOW

1000 mL : 25,000 units = x mL : 1600 units

$250x = 1000 \times 16 = 16,000$

x = 64 mL/hr

PROOF

$64 \times 250 = 16,000$

$16 \times 1000 = 16,000$

4. lb to kg = 300 lb divided by 2.2 = 136.3 = 136 kg

a. KNOW WANT TO KNOW

75 units : 1 kg = x units : 136 kg

$x = 75 \times 136 = 10,200$

x = 10,200 units bolus dose

PROOF

$1 \times 110,200 = 10,200$

$75 \times 136 = 10,200$

b. KNOW WANT TO KNOW

20 units : 1 kg = x units : 136 kg

$x = 20 \times 136 = 2720$

x = 2720 units per hr

PROOF

$1 \times 2720 = 2720$

$20 \times 136 = 2720$

c. KNOW WANT TO KNOW

1000 mL : 50,000 units = x mL : 2720 units

$50x = 1 \times 2720 = 2720$

$50x = 2720$

$x = 54.4 = 54$ mL per hr

PROOF

$1 \times 2720 = 2720$

$54.4 \times 50 = 2720$

5. lb to kg = 194 divided by 2.2 = 88 kg

a. KNOW WANT TO KNOW

70 units : 1 kg = x units : 88 kg

$x = 70 \times 88 = 6160$

$x = 6160$ units bolus dose

PROOF

$1 \times 6160 = 6160$

$70 \times 88 = 6160$

b. KNOW WANT TO KNOW

18 units : 1 kg = x units : 88 kg

$x = 18 \times 88 = 1584$

$x = 1584$ units per hr

PROOF

$1 \times 1584 = 1584$

$18 \times 88 = 1584$

c. KNOW WANT TO KNOW

1000 mL : 30,000 units = x mL : 1584 units

$30x = 1584 \times 1 = 1584$

$30x = 1584$

$x = 52.8 = 53$ mL per hr

PROOF

$30 \times 52.8 = 1584$

$1 \times 1584 = 1584$

6. lb to kg = 145 divided by 2.2 = 65.9 = 66 kg

a. KNOW WANT TO KNOW

65 units : 1 kg = x units : 66 kg

$x = 65 \times 66 = 4290$

$x = 4290$ units loading dose

PROOF

$1 \times 4290 = 4290$

$65 \times 66 = 4290$

b. KNOW WANT TO KNOW

15 units : 1 kg per hr = x units : 66 kg per hr

$x = 15 \times 66 = 990$ units

$x = 990$ units per hr

PROOF

$1 \times 990 = 990$

$15 \times 66 = 990$

c. KNOW WANT TO KNOW

500 mL : 30,000 units = x mL : 990 units

$300x = 5 \times 990 = 4950$

$30x = 495$

$x = 16.5 = 17$ mL per hr

PROOF

$990 \times 500 = 495{,}000$

$30{,}000 \times 16.5 = 495{,}000$

7. a. KNOW WANT TO KNOW

80 units : 1 kg = x units : 120 kg

$x = 80 \times 120 = 9600$

$x = 9600$ units bolus dose

PROOF

$1 \times 9600 = 9600$

$80 \times 120 = 9600$

b. KNOW WANT TO KNOW

1000 mL : 25,000 units = x mL : 1000 units

$25x = 1000$

$x = 40$ mL per hr

PROOF

$25 \times 40 = 1000$

$1 \times 1000 = 1000$

8. lb to kg = 185 divided by 2.2 = 84.09 = 84 kg

a. KNOW WANT TO KNOW

75 units : 1 kg = x units : 84 kg

$x = 75 \times 84 = 6300$

$x = 6300$ units loading dose

PROOF

$1 \times 6300 = 6300$

$75 \times 84 = 6300$

b. KNOW WANT TO KNOW

17 units : 1 kg per hr = x units : 84 kg per hr

$x = 17 \times 84 = 1428$

$x = 1428$ units per hr

PROOF

$1 \times 1428 = 1428$

$17 \times 84 = 1428$

c. KNOW WANT TO KNOW

1000 mL : 20,000 units = x mL : 1428 units

$20x = 1 \times 1428 = 1428$

$20x = 1428$

$x = 71.4 = 71$ mL per hr

PROOF

$1 \times 1428 = 1428$

$20 \times 71.4 = 1428$

9. a. KNOW WANT TO KNOW

95 units : 1 kg = x units : 136 kg

$x = 95 \times 136 = 12{,}920$

x = 12,920 units loading dose

PROOF

$1 \times 12{,}920 = 12{,}920$

$95 \times 136 = 12{,}920$

b. KNOW WANT TO KNOW

20 units : 1 kg per hr = x units : 136 kg per hr

$x = 20 \times 136 = 2720$

x = 2720 units per hr

PROOF

$1 \times 2720 = 2720$

$20 \times 136 = 2720$

c. KNOW WANT TO KNOW

1000 mL : 20,000 units = x mL : 2720 units

$20x = 1 \times 2720 = 2720$

$20x = 2720$

x = 136 mL per hr

PROOF

$2000 \times 136 = 272{,}000$

$1000 \times 272 = 272{,}000$

10. a. KNOW WANT TO KNOW

1000 units : 1 kg = x units : 108 kg

$x = 1000 \times 108 = 108{,}000$

x = 108,000 units loading dose

PROOF

$1 \times 108{,}000 = 108{,}000$

$1000 \times 108 = 108{,}000$

b. KNOW WANT TO KNOW

18 units : 1 kg = x units : 108 kg

$x = 18 \times 108 = 1944$

x = 1944 units per hr

PROOF

$1 \times 1944 = 1944$

$18 \times 108 = 1944$

c. KNOW WANT TO KNOW

1000 mL : 35,000 units = x mL : 1944 units

$35x = 1944$

$x = 55.54 = 56$ mL per hr

PROOF

$35 \times 55.54 = 1943.9$

$1944 \times 1 = 1944$

WORKSHEET **11D** (page 396) SETTING UP THE FRACTION CROSS PRODUCT WILL ASSIST YOU IN SOLVING THESE PROBLEMS SUCCESSFULLY

1. Give initial bolus dose = 80 units/kg

KNOW WANT TO KNOW

80 units : 1 kg = x units : 70 kg

$x = 70 \times 80 = 5600$

x = 5600 units initial bolus dose

PROOF

$80 \times 70 = 5600$

$1 \times 5600 = 5600$

2. Initial infusion rate: 18 units per kg per hr

KNOW WANT TO KNOW

18 units : 1 kg per hr = x units : 70 kg

$x = 70 \times 18 = 1260$

x = 1260 units per hr. Round off units to nearest whole number = 1300 units per hr

PROOF

$18 \times 70 = 1260$

$1 \times 1260 = 1260$

3. KNOW WANT TO KNOW

250 mL : 25,000 units = x mL : 1300 units

$250x = 250 \times 13 = 3250$

x – 13 mL per hr

PROOF

$250 \times 1300 = 325{,}000$

$13 \times 25000 = 325{,}000$

After 6 hours the aPTT is 30. Rebolus with 80 units/kg (5600 units). Increase the rate by 4 units per kg per hr.

4. a. KNOW WANT TO KNOW

4 units : 1 kg = x units : 70 kg

$x = 4 \times 70 = 280$ units round to 300 units

PROOF

$4 \times 70 = 280$

$1 \times 280 = 280$

b. 1300 units/hr increased by 300 units = 1600 units/hr

5. Reset infusion rate to:

KNOW WANT TO KNOW

250 mL : 25,000 units = x mL : 1600 units

$25{,}000x = 250 \times 1600 = 4{,}000$

$250x = 4000$

$25x = 400$

x = 16 mL per hr is the new rate for the infusion

PROOF

$250 \times 1600 = 400{,}000$

$16 \times 25{,}000 = 400{,}000$

After 6 hours the aPTT is 40. Increase IV rate by 2 units per kg per hr. Rebolus with 40 units per kg.

6. KNOW WANT TO KNOW

40 units : 1 kg = *x* units : 70 kg
x = 40 × 70 = 2800
x = 2800 units bolus dose

PROOF
40 × 70 = 2800
1 × 2800 = 2800

7. KNOW WANT TO KNOW

a. 2 units : 1 kg = *x* units : 70 kg
x = 2 × 70 = 140
x = 140 units per hr rounded to 100 units

b. 1600 units per hr increased by 100 units = 1700 units per hr

Reset infusion rate to:

PROOF
2 × 70 = 140
1 × 140 = 140

8. KNOW WANT TO KNOW

250 mL : 25,000 units = *x* mL : 1700 units
250*x* = 250 × 17 = 4250
x = 17 mL per hr is the new rate for the infusion
6-hour aPTT is 55 = no change in the rate.
6-hour aPTT is 85. Decrease rate by 2 units per kg per hr.

PROOF
250 × 1700 = 425,000
17 × 25,000 = 425,000

9. KNOW WANT TO KNOW

a. 2 units : 1 kg = *x* units : 70 kg
x = 2 × 70 = 140
x = 140 rounded to 100 units per hr decrease

b. 1700 units/hr decreased by 100 units/hr = 1600 units per hr new rate
Reset infusion rate to:

PROOF
2 × 70 = 140
1 × 140 = 140

10. KNOW WANT TO KNOW

250 mL : 25,000 units = *x* mL : 1600 units
250 = 250 × 1600 = 4,000
25*x* = 400
x = 16 mL per hr new rate to set the IV pump
6-hr aPTT is 95. Decrease rate by 3 units per kg per hr.

PROOF
250 × 1600 = 400,000
16 × 25,000 = 400,000

11. KNOW WANT TO KNOW

a. 3 units : 1 kg = *x* units : 70 kg
x = 3 × 70 =210
x = 210 units = 200 units/hr decrease

b 1600 units per hr decreased by 200 units per hr = 1400 units per hr new rate
Reset infusion rate to:

PROOF
3 × 70 = 210
1 × 210 =210

12. KNOW WANT TO KNOW

250 mL : 25,000 units = *x* mL : 1400 units
250*x* = 250 × 14 = 3500
250*x* = 3500
x = 14 mL per hr new IV rate.

PROOF
250 × 1400 = 350,000
25,000 × 14 = 350,000

13. Stop infusion for 1 hour before resuming IV rate. Next aPTT in 6 hours.

WORKSHEET **11E** (page 400) SETTING UP THE FRACTION CROSS PRODUCT WILL ASSIST YOU IN SOLVING THESE PROBLEMS SUCCESSFULLY

1. a. KNOW WANT TO KNOW

80 units : 1 kg = x units : 73 kg

$x = 80 \times 73 = 5840$

x = 5840 units of heparin

PROOF

$1 \times 5840 = 5840$

$80 \times 73 = 5840$

2. d. KNOW WANT TO KNOW

18 units : 1 kg = x units : 80 kg

$x = 18 \times 80 = 1440$

x = 1440 units/hr

PROOF

$1 \times 1440 = 1440$

$18 \times 80 = 1440$

d. KNOW WANT TO KNOW

1000 mL : 20,000 units = x mL : 1440 units

$20,000x = 1000 \times 1440 = 1,440$

x = 72 mL per hr

PROOF

$1000 \times 1440 = 1,440,000$

$72 \times 20,000 = 1,440,000$

3. c. KNOW WANT TO KNOW

1 kg : 2.2 lb = x kg : 132 lb

$2.2x = 132$

x = 60 kg

PROOF

$1 \times 132 = 132$

$2.2 \times 60 = 132$

d. KNOW WANT TO KNOW

120 international units : 1 kg = x international units : 60 kg

$x = 60 \times 120$

x = 7200 international units q12h

PROOF

$1 \times 7200 = 7200$

$60 \times 120 = 7200$

4. a. KNOW WANT TO KNOW

10,000 international units : 1 mL = 7200 international units : x mL

$10,000x = 7200$

$x = 0.72 = 0.7$ mL

PROOF

$7200 \times 1 = 7200$

$10,000 \times 0.72 = 7200$

5. c. KNOW WANT TO KNOW

120 international units : 1 kg = x international units : 84 kg

$x = 120 \times 84 = 10,080$

x = 10,080 international units of Fragmin

PROOF

$120 \times 84 = 10,080$

$1 \times 10,080 = 10,080$

6. b. KNOW WANT TO KNOW

25,000 international units : 1 mL = 10,080 : x mL

$25,000x = 10,080$

x = 0.4 mL

PROOF

$1 \times 10,080 = 10,080$ (units can be rounded up or down)

$0.4 \times 25,000 = 10,000$

7. b. KNOW WANT TO KNOW

1000 mL : 25,000 units = x mL : 3000 units

$25,000x = 3,000,000$

$25x = 3000 = 120$ mL per hr

PROOF

$25 \times 120 = 3000$

$1000 \times 3 = 3000$

8. d. KNOW WANT TO KNOW

10,000 units : 500 mL = 500 units : x mL

$10,000x = 250,000$

x = 25 mL per hr

PROOF

$25 \times 10,000 = 250,000$

$500 \times 500 = 250,000$

9. a. 220 divided by 2.2 = 100 kg

d. KNOW WANT TO KNOW

120 international units : 1 kg = x international units : 100 kg

$x = 120 \times 100 = 12{,}000$

x = 12,000 international units Fragmin

PROOF

$1 \times 12{,}000 = 12{,}000$

$100 \times 120 = 12{,}000$

10. c. KNOW WANT TO KNOW

25,000 international units : 1 mL = 12,000 international units : x mL

$25{,}000x = 12{,}000$

$x = 0.48$ mL

PROOF

$1 \times 12{,}000 = 12{,}000$

$25{,}000 \times 0.48 = 12{,}000$

CHAPTER 11 FINAL: ANTICOAGULANTS (page 403)

1. 0.6 mL

2. 0.25 mL

3. 0.2 mL using the 10,000 units per mL strength or 0.4 mL using the 5000 units per mL strength Give 0.2 mL the smallest amount. Use the 10,000 units per mL vial

4. 0.35 mL using the 20,000 units per mL strength or 0.7 mL using the 10,000 units per mL strength or 1.4 mL using the 5,000 units per mL strength Give 0.35 mL, the smallest amount.

5. 0.65 mL

6. 17.5 mL/hr or 18 mL/hr
27 hr, 46 min

7. 30 mL per hr
16 hr, 40 min

8. 42 mL per hr
1458 units per hr

9. 100 mL per hr via infusion device
10 hr to infuse

10. 42 mL per hr
1042 units per hr

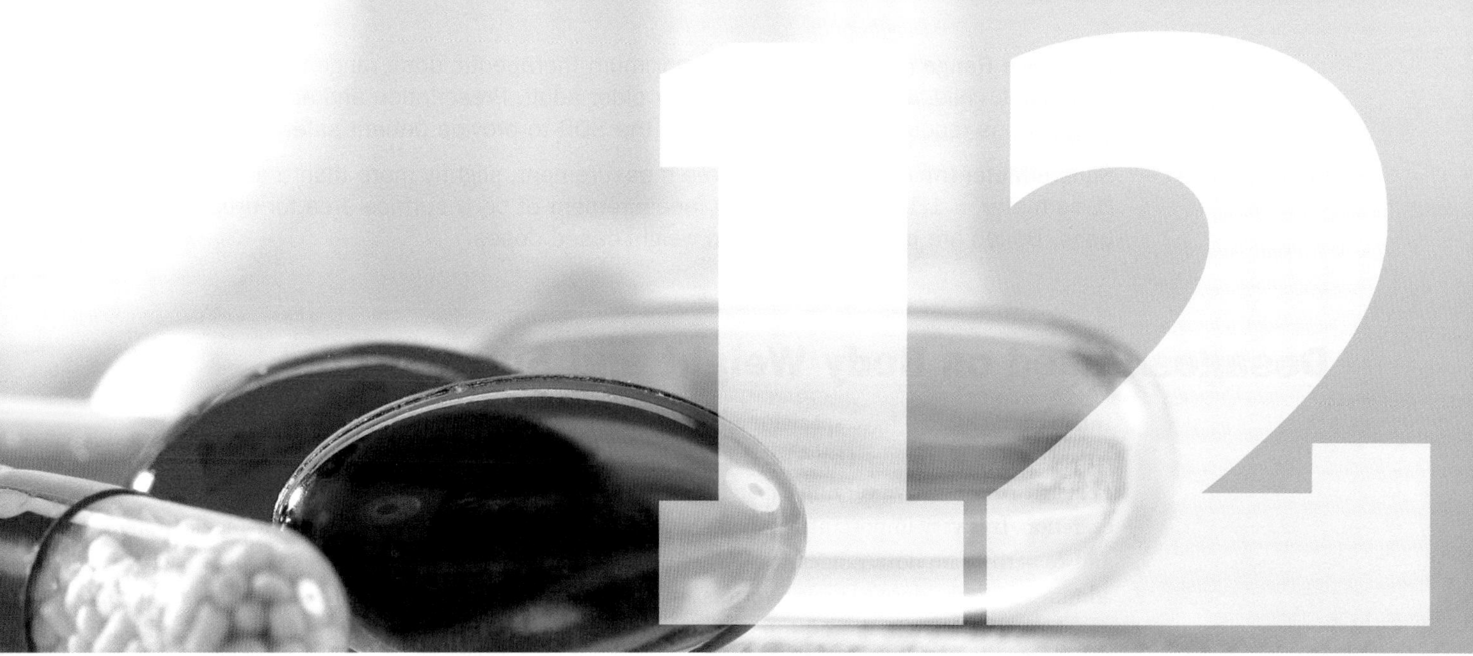

Pediatric Dosages

Objectives

- Evaluate drug doses for safe dose range (SDR).
- Accurately calculate doses in mcg per kg and mg per kg and square meters of body surface area (BSA).
- Calculate 24-hour drug doses and divided doses for specific weights for oral and parenteral medications.
- Identify medication-related safety precautions with calculating and administering medications for pediatric patients.
- Analyze medication errors using critical thinking.

Introduction

The trend for increased safety in medication administration for pediatric patients is to provide pediatric customized doses and supplies. The usual medication doses and supplied amounts for adults have resulted in adverse drug events (ADE) for pediatric patients. Pediatric patients often receive very small (fractional) medication doses compared to an adult. Nurse competency for safe medication administration is essential to protect this at-risk population that cannot protect itself. Communication about the medications with the family caretaker(s) is also essential. Mentoring with an experienced, intuitive pediatric nurse is ideal during the clinical experience phase.

Vocabulary

Anaphylactic Shock: An extreme life-threatening inflammatory allergic reaction that can occur in any age group. Immediate medication is needed en route to an emergency facility. A few of the common offenders are medications such as penicillin, sulfa drugs, aspirin; foods such as tree nuts, shellfish, and eggs; and insect bites and bee stings. The patient's history—including prior mild allergic reactions—must be documented on the MAR and rechecked before each medication is administered.

Body Surface Area (BSA): Square meters (m^2) of external skin area used to calculate drug dosages for specific drugs and patient conditions.

Milligrams or Micrograms per kilogram (mg per kg; mcg per kg): Metric measurement of drug dose per body weight in kilograms (kg). Common units of measurement for medications for pediatric and adult patients, particularly for parenteral medications.

Nomogram: A chart used to prescribe medication based on the patient's weight and height.

Safe Dose Range (SDR): Minimum-to-maximum therapeutic dose range for a target population: adult, child, infant, neonate, and/or older adult. Prescription and administration of medications requires prior knowledge of the SDR to provide patient safety.

Square Meter (m^2): Metric unit of area measurement, slightly more than a square yard (1 sq meter = 1.19 sq yd), used in measurement of body surface area for drug calculations. Doses are much smaller than weight-based doses.

Dosages Based on Body Weight and Surface Area

Infants and children have special medication needs because of their smaller size and weight as well as larger body surface area (BSA) per kilogram of body weight, which is larger than that of an adult. Pediatric patients have varying capabilities of drug absorption, digestion, distribution, metabolism, and excretion. It is very important for the nurse to check current references for pediatric medication orders and to verify safe dose ranges (SDRs) with current, reliable drug references or a pharmacist before administering the dose to prevent errors and injury. Minute doses that require scrupulous mathematics may be ordered. Pediatric and intensive care nurses use written pediatric drug guidelines and calculators to determine weights and verify SDRs.

Two methods currently used for calculating safe pediatric and adult doses are based on (1) *body weight* in milligrams per kilogram (mg per kg) or micrograms per kilogram (mcg per kg) and (2) *body surface area* in square meters (m^2) using a scale called a *nomogram.*

mg per kg Method (Weight-Based Dosing)

The most *frequently* used calculation method for customized dosing is *mg per kg.* References usually state the safe amount of drug in mg per kg for a 24-hour period to be given in one or more divided doses. You may also see *mcg per kg* cited for therapeutic doses when very small amounts of medication are to be given.

Because kilograms are required for weight-based medications, the nurse does not usually have to convert pounds and ounces to kilograms. In the event that only a pound/ounce weight is available, the nurse needs to know how to convert pounds and ounces to kilograms.

Steps to Solving mg per kg Problems

Step 1

a. **Estimate** the weight in kilograms by dividing the pounds in half*; then *calculate* the weight in kilograms using 2.2 lb = 1 kg equivalency (divide pounds by 2.2). Use a calculator. Check your estimate with the answer.

b. If a weight is in *pounds* and *ounces,* convert the ounces to the nearest tenth of a pound and *add* this to the total pounds. Then convert the total pounds into kilograms to the nearest tenth (two-step calculation). (Refer to page 419 for kilogram-to-pound conversions and page 16 for rounding instructions.)

Step 2 **Calculate** the safe dose range (SDR) using a calculator and current safe dose recommendations found in current, reliable drug literature for this child's weight in mg per kg or mcg per kg.

Step 3 **Compare** and **evaluate** the 24-hr ordered dose with the recommended SDR. Be sure the comparisons are for the *same* dosing frequency!

Step 4 If safe, **calculate** the actual dose to be administered using written ratio and proportion. If the ordered dose is *less* than or *more* than the SDR, hold the medication and clarify the order promptly.

Shortcut Steps

1. Weight in kg to nearest tenth of a kilogram
2. SDR per 24 hours and per dose
3. Compare with order
4. Calculate whether or not dose is safe to give

*Estimation helps prevent major math errors; it must be followed by calculation and verification.

RULE **All pediatric medication administration begins with an accurate kilogram weight (Step 1) and a calculation of the SDR (Step 2).**

Example **Ordered:** erythromycin oral suspension 150 mg po q6h for an infant allergic to penicillin who has an infection. Patient weight: 15 lb, 6 oz today. The literature states that the SDR is 30 to 100 mg per kg per day in four divided doses for severe infections.

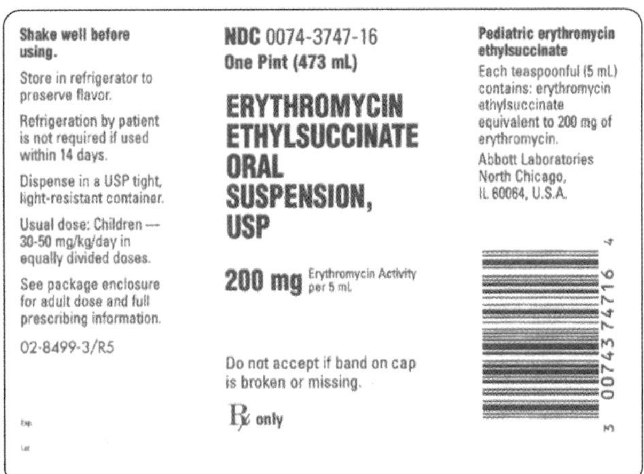

Step 1 **Estimate** the infant's weight.

a. *Pounds to kilograms:* 15 lb ÷ 2 = 7.5 kg

Calculate the actual weight.

b. Two-step conversion because ounces are involved.

Ounces to pounds: 6 oz ÷ 16 = 0.37 lb. Add part of pound to total pounds. The infant thus weighs 15.4 lb.

Pounds to kilograms: 15.4 lb ÷ 2.2 = 7 kg (close to estimate)

Step 2 The **SDR** recommended for children more than 1 month of age is 30 to 100 mg per kg per day po in four divided doses.

Low-range calculation: 30 mg × 7 kg = 210 mg (low SDR) per day ÷ 4 = 52.5 mg per dose

High-range calculation: 100 mg × 7 kg = 700 mg (high SDR) per day ÷ 4 = 175 mg per dose

Step 3 **Compare** and **evaluate:** The **SDR** recommended for this child's weight is 210 to 700 mg total q24h in four divided doses.

Ordered: 150 mg q6h or 150 mg × 4 or 600 mg total in 24 hr.

Step 4 **Decision:** Give medication. Administering 600 mg for the day is within the SDR of 210 to 700 mg in four divided doses. Administer with an oral syringe.

Calculate the individual dose (write out and prove).

KNOW | WANT TO KNOW | FRACTION CROSS PRODUCT

200 mg : 5 mL = 150 mg : x mL

$$\frac{200}{5} = \frac{150}{x}$$

$$\frac{\cancel{200}}{\cancel{200}}x = \frac{750}{200} \quad (5 \times 150)$$

$$x = 3.75 \text{ mL}$$

PROOF
200 × 3.75 = 750
5 × 150 = 750

ANSWER
Give 3.75 mL*

Hint Review and analyze the logic of these four steps.

CLINICAL ALERT!

Avoid two potential errors when converting pounds and ounces to kilograms. First, ounces must be converted to part of a pound *before* converting total pounds to kilograms; for example, 6 oz does not convert to 0.6 lb. Second, 15.4 lb does not equal 15.4 kg.

Do not forget the second step—convert the total pounds to kilograms.

*Use a 1-mL syringe to add 0.75 mL if the exact dose or calibrated dropper is not supplied by the pharmacy.

Answers on page 444

WORKSHEET 12A Calculator Practice

RULE Calculators are used in pediatric and adult care units for long division and multiplication problems. Dividing ounces by 16 will give the pound equivalent in the first step of two-step problems. Dividing or multiplying by 2.2 will give pound and kilogram equivalents. Note: Knowing your own weight in kilograms is a helpful reminder of the difference between pound and kilogram weight.

1. Estimate the weight conversions, then use a calculator to convert from pounds to kilograms or kilograms to pounds. Round to the *nearest tenth.* Double-check all work.

a. 14 lb (1 or 2 steps?)
Estimate:
Actual:

b. 12 lb, 2 oz (1 or 2 steps?)
Estimate:
Actual:

c. 10 lb
Estimate:
Actual:

d. 14 kg
Estimate:
Actual:

e. 10 kg
Estimate:
Actual:

2. Calculate the 24-hr total dose in milligrams.

a. 150 mg q8h
b. 200 mg q6h
c. 400 mcg q4h
d. 50 mg tid
e. 750 mcg q12h

3. Calculate the unit dose.

a. 1 g in 4 equally divided doses
b. 750 mg divided in 3 equal doses
c. 2 g in 4 to 6 equally divided doses
d. 16 g a day in 2 to 4 divided doses
e. 500 mg in 4 divided doses

4. Calculate the SDR in milligrams for the following weights. Note that the answers will only be in milligrams or micrograms because *x*, the unknown, is a *dosage* measurement not a weight measurement. You want to know how many milligrams a day and milligrams per dose are safe for this patient. (2.2 lb = 1 kg)

SDR per kg; Weight	SDR for This Weight
a. 10 mg per kg; weight is 5 kg	________ Safe total mg per day
b. 5 to 8 mg per kg; weight is 7.3 kg	________ SDR for the day in mg
c. 6 to 8 mg per kg; weight is 8 lb	________ SDR for the day in mg
d. 3 to 6 mg per kg; weight is 5 lb, 8 oz	________ SDR for the day in mg
e. 200 to 400 mcg per kg; weight is 4 lb, 6 oz	________ SDR for the day in mg

5. **Ordered:** Drug X, 50 mg tid. **SDR:** 2 to 3 mg per kg given in three divided doses. Patient weight: 18 kg.

a. SDR for 24 hr
b. SDR per dose
c. Total ordered dose for day and per dose
d. Evaluation and decision: Safe or unsafe to give? Why?

Answers on page 445

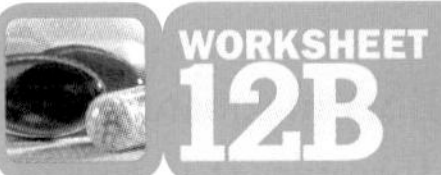

WORKSHEET 12B Safe Dose Range (SDR) Practice

For each problem, use a calculator to calculate the SDR, and compare it with the order. If the total dose for 24 hours is excessive, the unit dose is automatically excessive. Evaluate the order and make a decision.

1. Give medication (within SDR for unit dose and 24-hr dose).
2. Hold and clarify promptly (overdose or underdose).

1. Weight: 9.1 kg
SDR in literature: 2 to 4 mg per kg per day
Ordered: 50 mg daily
a. SDR for this child:
b. Dose ordered:
c. Evaluation and decision:

2. Weight: 15 kg
SDR in literature: 100 to 200 mcg per kg per day in divided doses
Ordered: 0.5 mg tid
a. SDR for this child:
b. Dose ordered:
c. Evaluation and decision:

3. Weight: 11.5 kg
SDR in literature: 10 to 30 mg per kg per day in divided doses*
Ordered: 100 mg tid
a. SDR for this child:
b. Dose ordered:
c. Evaluation and decision:

4. Weight: 38.6 kg
SDR: 10 to 15 mg per kg per day in 4 to 6 divided doses
Ordered: 100 mg q6h
a. SDR for this child:
b. Dose ordered:
c. Evaluation and decision:

5. Weight: 2.3 kg
SDR: 10 to 20 mcg per kg per day
Ordered: 0.03 mg four times daily
a. SDR for this child:
b. Dose ordered:
c. Evaluation and decision:

---

*In divided doses, the total dose must be divided into two or more doses.

BSA Method (mg per m^2)

The term "body surface area" refers to the total external body area. The estimated BSA in square meters (m^2) is derived from height and weight measurements by using a mathematical formula. It is considered the most reliable way to calculate therapeutic dosages.

This method may be used to calculate safe dosages of antineoplastic drugs, of new drugs, and of drugs for special populations such as infants, children, frail elderly patients, and patients with cancer.

Example Child weighs 33 lb (15 kg) and has a BSA of 0.55 m^2.

Ordered: 20 mg per kg	vs	**Ordered:** 20 mg per m^2	vs	**Ordered:** 20 mg per lb
20 mg : 1 kg = x mg : 15 kg		20 mg : 1 m^2 = x mg : 0.55		20 mg : 1 lb = x mg : 33 lb
$x = 20 \times 15 = 300$ mg		$x = 20 \times 0.55 = 11$ mg		$x = 20 \times 33 = 660$ mg

As seen, the doses calculated range from 11 mg to 660 mg and, depending on the unit of measurement, reflect extremely large differences. This illustrates the need to check not only the numbers but also the units of measurement.

The West nomogram in Figure 12.1 allows the user to plot the *estimated* square meters of BSA by using height and weight measurements.

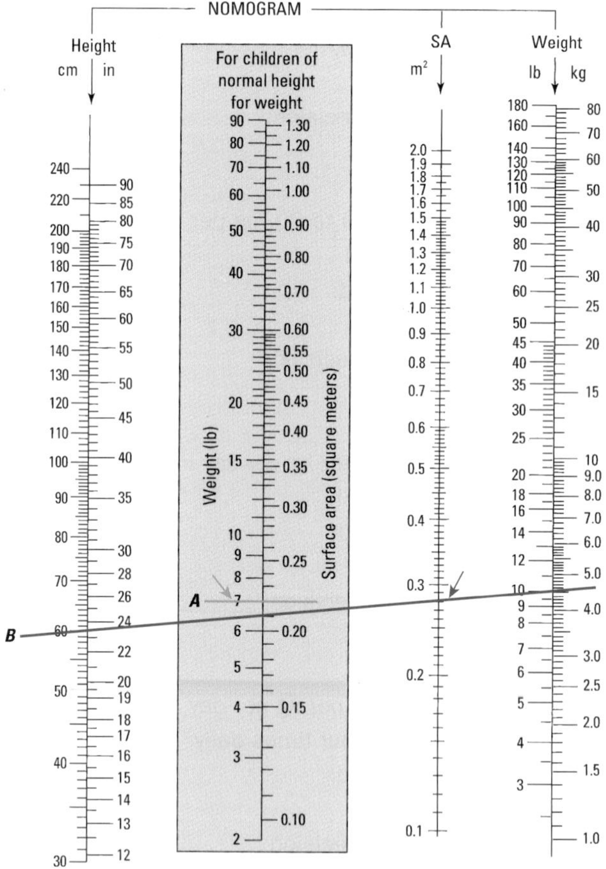

FIGURE 12.1 West nomogram for estimation of body surface area (BSA). *A,* The estimated BSA in square meters for children of normal height for weight is determined by reading the m^2 at the alignment point with the child's weight in pounds in the highlighted column. The blue line denoted by the arrow reveals that an infant weighing 10 lb has an approximate BSA of 0.27 m^2. *B,* The BSA in square meters for children who are *under*weight or *over*weight (refer to pediatric standard growth charts and development grids for normal height and weight ranges for pediatric groups) is determined by connecting the child's plotted weight in the left column and plotted height in the right column with a straight line and reading the intersection point on the SA (surface area) column, as indicated by the arrow on the red line. This illustrates an estimated BSA of 0.28 m^2 for an infant of 60 cm height weighing 4.5 kg. Reading the SA column requires that height and weight be plotted in the same system of measurement—metric or pounds/inches. (From Kliegman RM, Stanton BF, St. Geme JW, et al: *Nelson textbook of pediatrics,* ed. 19, Philadelphia, 2011, Saunders.)

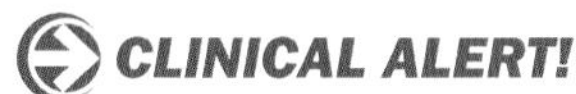

CLINICAL ALERT!

Nurses are not expected to calculate BSA. The pharmacy provides the BSA calculations. Nurses *do* have a critical responsibility to distinguish the difference in a medication order based on mg per **kg** of weight and an order based on mg per **m²** of BSA (e.g., 20 mg per kg vs 20 mg per m^2).

Calculating BSA (m^2) Using a Mathematical Formula

There are two formulas for calculating BSA (m^2), and both use height and weight dimensions. A. Formula using only metric system. B. Formula using only pounds and inches

$$\sqrt{\frac{\text{Weight (kg)} \times \text{Height (cm)}}{3600}} = \text{m}^2 \text{ BSA} \qquad \sqrt{\frac{\text{Weight (lb)} \times \text{Height (in)}}{3131}} = \text{m}^2 \text{ BSA}$$

Note the differences in the divisors. The formulas must be used exactly as shown.

Example Using a calculator and the metric formula, determine the BSA in square meters for a child with a weight of 20 kg and a height of 95 cm.

Step 1 Multiply the kilograms by centimeters first and *divide* the result by 3600 ($20 \times 95 = 900/3600 = 0.527$)

Step 2 Obtain the *square root* of 0.527 by pushing the square root button. *Round* your answer to the *nearest* hundredth.

$$\frac{20 \times 95}{3600} = 0.527 \qquad \sqrt{0.527} = 0.725 = 0.73 \text{ m}^2$$

Compare this answer with the West nomogram (see Figure 12.1). Create a straight line between 20 kg and 95 cm and read the result in the surface area (SA) column on the nomogram. Take care to plot the height and weight on the metric graph—the outside columns. When reading the results (m^2) columns, be sure to note the value of each calibrated line on the scale at the intersection point. The formula method is more accurate.

A square meter is slightly larger than a square yard. Visualize a square meter or a square yard of skin. As seen on the nomogram, a child of 90 lb has only about 1 square meter of BSA (1 m^2). Use one of the formulas to calculate your own BSA.

Answers on page 445

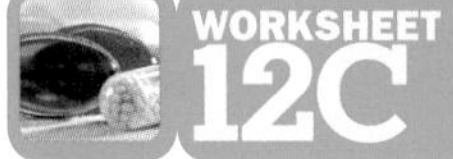

WORKSHEET 12C | Comparing BSA-Based (mg per m^2) Dosages With mg per lb and mg per kg Orders

Use the West nomogram (see Figure 12.1), highlighted section for children of normal height and weight, to obtain the BSA (m^2) based on weight.

Calculate the dose to be given based on the mg per m^2 and dose ordered. Compare the doses to be given. All the weights are the same.

	Wt in lb	BSA in m^2	Dose Ordered	Dose to be Given
1.	4 lb	0.15	10 mg per m^2	10×0.15 = 1.5 mg
2.	6 lb	_____	15 mg per m^2	____________
3.	10 lb	_____	5 mg per m^2	____________

Calculate the dose to be given in mg per kg measurements. Divide lb by 2.2 to obtain kilogram weight.

	Wt in kg (to nearest tenth)	Dose Ordered	Dose to be Given
4.	4 lb = 1.8 kg	10 mg per kg	10×1.8 = 18 mg
5.	6 lb = _____ kg	2 mg per kg	____________
6.	20 lb = _____ kg	5 mg per kg	____________

Calculate the dose for the same-weight children in mg per lb measurements.

	Wt in lb	Dose Ordered	Dose to be Given
7.	4 lb	10 mg per lb	$4 \times 10 = 40$ mg
8.	6 lb	15 mg per lb	______________
9.	20 lb	5 mg per lb	______________

10. Using the appropriate BSA formula on page 423, obtain the BSA in m^2 for a child who weighs 70 lb and is normal height for weight.

CLINICAL ALERT!

Consider the patient safety implications when mg per m^2, mg per lb, and mg per kg are erroneously interchanged. This mistake has resulted in serious errors. The nurse must understand the differences among these three terms and focus to ensure that the correct values are being used when calculating the dose.

Answers on page 445

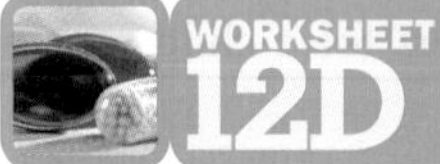

WORKSHEET 12D Additional Pediatric Safe Dose Range (SDR) Practice

Calculate SDRs and doses. Evaluate the order. If dose is within the SDR, calculate and prove the answer.

1. SDR: 1 to 2 g per day in 4 divided doses
Ordered: 500 mg q6h
a. SDR for this child:
b. Dose to be administered:
c. Evaluation and decision:

2. Weight: 44 lb, normal weight for height
SDR: 5 to 8 mg per m^2* daily
Ordered: 4 mg daily
a. SDR for this child:
b. Dose ordered:
c. Evaluation and decision:

3. Weight: 8.6 kg
SDR: 0.1 to 0.3 mg per kg per day in 2 divided doses
Ordered: 2500 mcg bid
a. SDR for this child:
b. Dose ordered:
c. Evaluation and decision:

4. Weight: 4.1 kg
SDR 1 to 5 mcg per kg per day
Ordered: 0.01 mg daily
a. SDR for this child:
b. Dose ordered:
c. Evaluation and decision:

5. Weight: 6.4 kg
SDR: 0.02 to 0.05 mg per kg per day
Ordered: 150 mcg bid
a. SDR for this child:
b. Dose ordered:
c. Evaluation and decision:

---

*For BSA conversion, refer to West nomogram (see Figure 12.1).

CLINICAL ALERT!

Estimating the approximate dose of a medication before doing the actual calculation is a valuable safety check for calculation errors. Estimation can alert you to major math errors. Verify your estimate with calculations.

The trend is to supply the appropriate calibrated equipment with pediatric medications to reduce potential dosing errors caused by using household equipment (Figure 12.2).

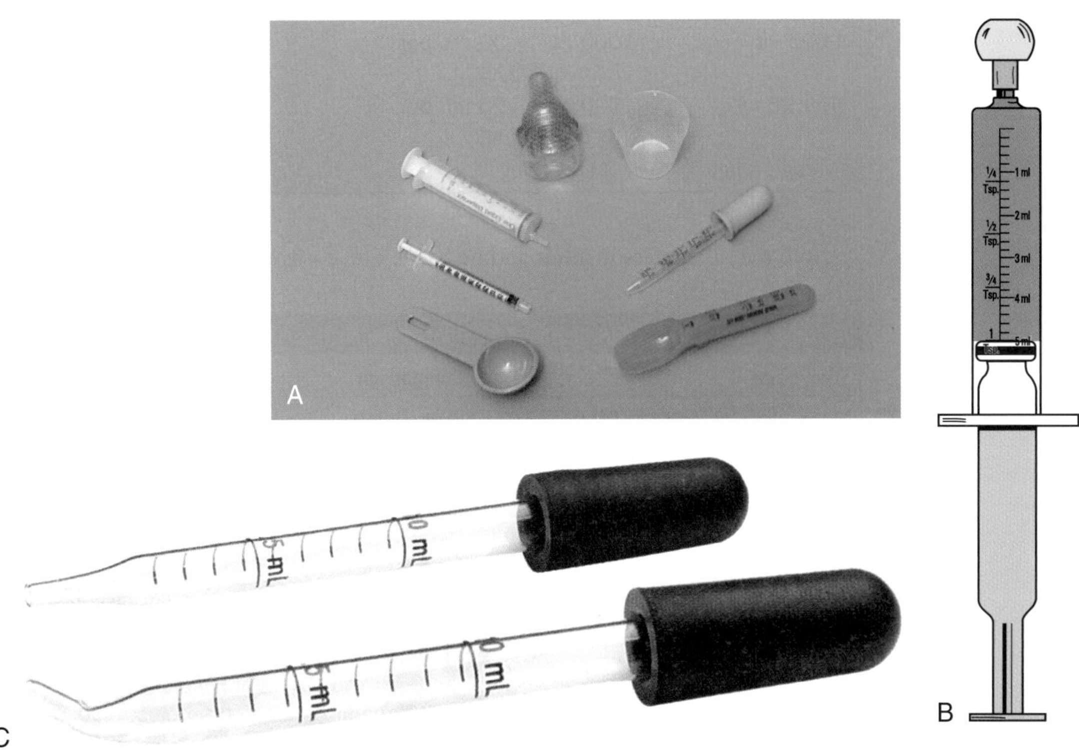

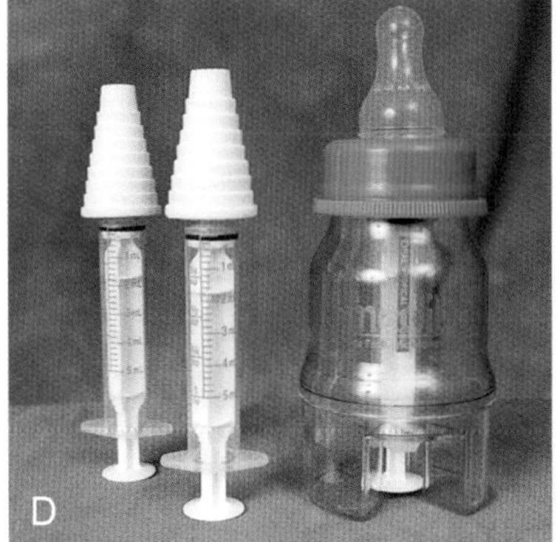

FIGURE 12.2 **A,** Acceptable devices for measuring and administering oral medication to children (clockwise): measuring spoon, plastic syringes, calibrated nipple, plastic medicine cup, calibrated dropper, hollow-handled medicine spoon. **B,** Prefilled oral syringe. **C,** Calibrated droppers. **D,** Medibottle. (**A,** From Wong DL et al: *Wong's nursing care of infants and children,* ed 7, St. Louis, 2005, Mosby. **C,** From Macklin D, Chernecky C, Infortuna H: *Math for clinical practice,* ed 2, St. Louis, 2011, Mosby.)

Fluid Requirements

CLINICAL ALERT!

Volume needs for infants and children are very different from those of adults. Overhydration and dehydration can present grave risks to pediatric patients. The nurse must be aware of the fluid orders, including fluid restriction orders, in relation to the current intake and output when administering liquid medications. This is a critical responsibility. Infants have a higher fluid volume as a percentage of body weight than do older children and adults. They lose more water through the skin and a higher percentage of fluids from the lungs and excrete more urine, which is less concentrated.

Contrast the differences between the normal requirements of a healthy adult and a child (Table 12.1).

Table 12.1 Fluid Requirements of Healthy Children and Adults

Weight	Normal Fluid Volume Need	Sample Weight (kg)	Average Fluid Intake Requirement Daily (mL)	Hourly (mL)
Neonate	90 mL per kg per 24 hr	3	270	11
Up to 10 kg	120 mL per kg per 24 hr after age 7 days	8	960	40
11-20 kg	1000 mL + 50 mL per kg over 10 kg	15	1250	52
Over 20 kg	1500 mL + 20 mL per kg over 20 kg	25	1600	67
Average adult	2-3 L per day	68	2000-3000	125

Note the differences in adult and pediatric safe dosages in Table 12.2.

Table 12.2 Drug Dosage Comparison by Age-Group

Drug Name	Dosage Comparison
Potassium chloride (KCl)*	SDR, **Adult,** individualized: IV 20-60 mEq q24h 200 mEq per 24 hr for hypokalemia is usually not exceeded. 40 mEq dilution per liter preferred. SDR, **Child,** individualized: IV 1-4 mEq per kg of body weight per 24 hr. *or* 10 mEq per hr, whichever is **less,** not to exceed 40 mEq per 24 hr. Must be at least 40 mEq dilution per liter. Monitor serum potassium levels. Contact prescriber if patient is fluid restricted. Monitor ECG for symptoms of hypokalemia and hyperkalemia. Pediatric: KCL must be infused on electronic infusion pump. Obtain written order for *each* infusion.
Morphine sulfate	
Pain relief	**Adult,** IV: 2.5-15 mg q4h
Postoperative analgesia	**Child,** IV: 0.01 -0.04 mg per kg per hr **Neonate,** IV: 015-0.02 mg per kg per hr†
Severe chronic cancer pain	**Child,** IV: 0.025-2.6 mg per kg per hr
Amoxicillin	**Adult,** PO: 250-500 mg q8h **Child,** PO: 25-50 mg per kg per day (max 60-80 per kg per day divided q8h)
Digoxin IV injection	Initial loading (digitalizing) dose **Premature:** 15-25 mcg per kg **2-5 yr:** 25-35 mcg pr kg **Over 10 yr:** 8-12 mcg per kg

*All formulations of KCl must always be diluted and well mixed before administration and before placing it on an IV apparatus.

†A neonate refers to an infant in the first 4 weeks of life. Consult drug references for child age-related dosage guidelines; they vary.

Slashes (/) will be seen in printed drug references. Write out "per" for slashes to avoid misinterpretation and medication errors.

Answers on page 446

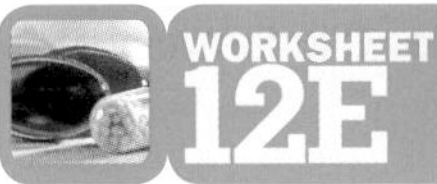

WORKSHEET 12E Pediatric Oral Medications

These medications can be given to infants and children with a dropper or in an oral medication syringe. Small amounts may be given to an infant in a nipple.

For each problem, use a calculator to determine the child's weight in kilograms or pounds if required, calculate the SDR, and compare it with the order. Evaluate the order and make a decision:

1. Give medication (within SDR for unit dose and 24-hr dose).

2. Hold and clarify promptly (overdose or underdose).

CLINICAL ALERT!

If a nipple is used to deliver medication, rinse the nipple with water first so that the medicine will flow rather than stick to the nipple. Family may be very helpful with oral medication administration by holding the child or by giving the oral medication or something pleasant-tasting following the medication.

For decisions 1 and 2 only, calculate the medication amount to be administered using *written ratio and proportion.* Prove your work. Do *not* calculate overdose or underdose orders. Hold them and clarify promptly.

1. **Ordered:** acetaminophen children's oral suspension 160 mg po for a 4-year-old child who weighs 14 kg today.
   a. Estimated weight in lb:
   b. Actual weight in lb:
   c. SDR for this child:
   d. Dose ordered:
   e. Evaluation and decision:
   f. Amount to be given in mL if applicable:

Drug Facts (continued)

- use only enclosed dosing cup designed for use with this product. Do not use any other dosing device.
- if needed, repeat dose every 4 hours while symptoms last
- do not give more than 5 times in 24 hours
- do not give for more than 5 days unless directed by a doctor
- **this product does not contain directions or complete warnings for adult use**

Weight (lb)	Age (yr)	Dose (tsp or mL)
under 24	under 2 years	ask a doctor
24-35	2-3 years	1 tsp or 5 mL
36-47	4-5 years	1 1/2 tsp or 7.5 mL
48-59	6-8 years	2 tsp or 10 mL
60-71	9-10 years	2 1/2 tsp or 12.5 mL
72-95	11 years	3 tsp or 15 mL

Attention: use only enclosed dosing cup specifically designed for use with this product. Do not use any other dosing device.

Other information
- **each teaspoon contains:** sodium 3 mg
- store at 20°-25°C (68°-77°F)
- do not use if printed neckband is broken or missing

Inactive ingredients anhydrous citric acid, butylparaben, carboxymethylcellulose sodium, carrageenan, D&C red no. 33, FD&C blue no. 1, flavor, glycerin, high fructose corn syrup, hydroxyethyl cellulose, microcrystalline cellulose, propylene glycol, purified water, sodium benzoate, sorbitol solution

***Questions?* Call 1-800-910-6874**

*This product is not manufactured or distributed by the Tylenol Company, owner of the registered trademark Tylenol®.

094 01 0137 ID209441
Distributed by Target Corporation
Minneapolis, MN 55403
© 2009 Target Brands, Inc.
All Rights Reserved Shop Target.com

NDC 11673-130-26

children's acetaminophen
oral suspension

80 mg per ½ teaspoon
(160 mg per 5 mL)
fever reducer/pain reliever

Compare to active ingredient in Children's Tylenol® Oral Suspension*

see new warnings information

alcohol free
ibuprofen free
aspirin free

up&up™

grape flavor

AGE **2-11** YEARS

4 FL OZ (118 mL)

2. **Ordered:** Clindamycin HCl pediatric solution 300 mg q8h po. The child weighs 30 kg today. The SDR is 10 to 30 mg per kg per day in 3 to 4 divided doses. **Available:** Clindamycin palmitate pediatric oral solution 75 mg per 5 mL.
   a. SDR for this child:
   b. Dose ordered:
   c. Evaluation and decision:
   d. Amount to be given in mL if applicable:

CLINICAL ALERT!

Avoid mixing medicines in essential foods such as formula or milk. A changed taste may result in long-term refusal of that food. Gelatin, applesauce, or sherbet in small amounts may be used to mix the medications if the diet allows. The medicine may be followed immediately with formula, juice, or an ice pop as the diet permits. Keep in mind that if not all of the mixture is ingested, all of the medication will not be administered.

3. **Ordered:** Tegretol (carbamazepine) oral suspension 0.25 g po tid for a child with seizures. The SDR for maintenance in a child over 12 years of age is 400 to 800 mg per day in 3 to 4 divided doses. **Available:** carbamazepine 100 mg per 5 mL.
   a. SDR for this child:
   b. Dose ordered in mg:
   c. Evaluation and decision:
   d. Amount to be given if applicable:

4. **Ordered:** leucovorin calcium 5 mg q6h po. The child weighs 24 lb and has normal weight and height. The SDR according to the literature is 10 mg per m^2 q6h for 72 hr. For BSA calculation, refer to the West nomogram (see Figure 12.1). The BSA is determined by pounds, not kilograms. **Available:** leucovorin calcium tablets 5mg.
   a. SDR for this child:
   b. Dose ordered:
   c. Evaluation and decision:
   d. Amount to be given if applicable:

5. **Ordered:** Augmentin 200 mg q8h po for a child with an infection who weighs 12.3 kg. The SDR is 20 to 40 mg per kg per day in 3 divided doses. **Available:** Augmentin oral suspension 125 mg per 5 mL.
   a. SDR for this child:
   b. Dose ordered:
   c. Evaluation and decision:
   d. Amount to be given in mL if applicable:

CLINICAL ALERT!

Monitor for allergic-type reactions: rash, diarrhea, or increased respiratory difficulty.

Multiple subcutaneous and intramuscular injections are not preferred for pediatric patients because of limited sites and potential emotional and physical trauma. Nevertheless, some vaccines, analgesics, and single-dose medicines or daily hormones are given using this route. The technique must be practiced in a clinical laboratory setting under supervision.

- The vastus lateralis can be used from birth to adulthood but is a *preferred injection* site for IM injections for babies younger than 7 months (Figure 12.3).
- The ventrogluteal muscle is an *alternate site* for IM injections for children over 7 months and for adults (Figure 12.4).
- The deltoid site may be used for small-volume, nonirritating IM medications, 0.5 to 1 mL, in older children and adults with *well-developed* deltoid muscles (Figure 12.5).
- Needle lengths and gauges and fluid amounts are much smaller for pediatric patients.

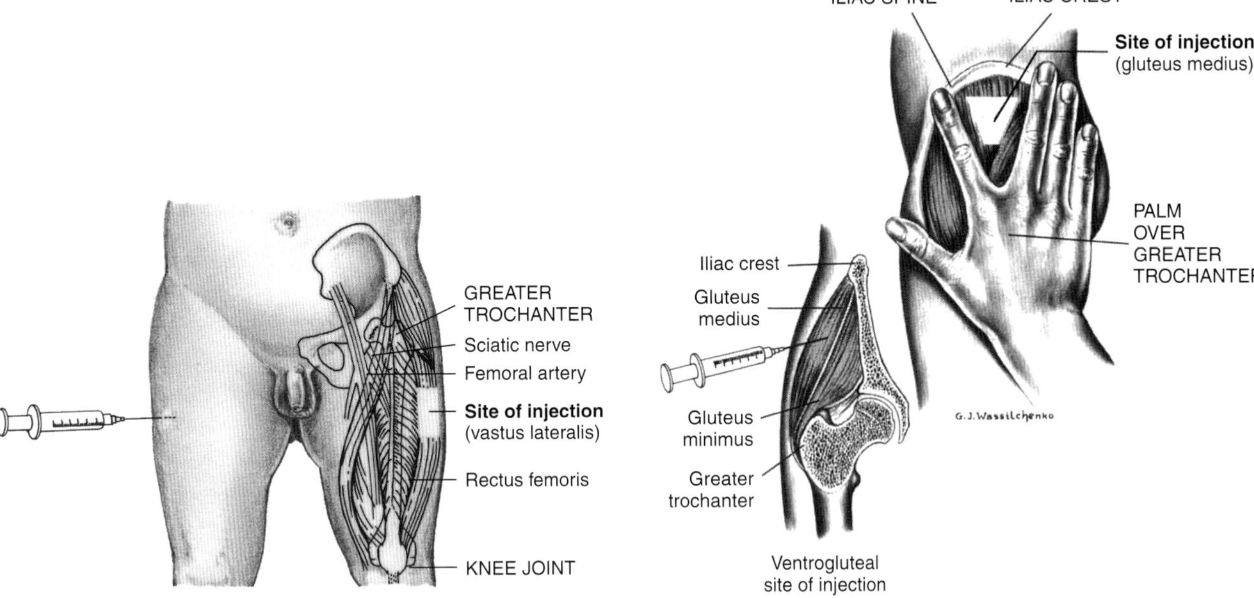

FIGURE 12.3 Vastus lateralis intramuscular injection site. (From Wilson D, Hockenberry MJ: *Wong's clinical manual of pediatric nursing,* ed. 9, St. Louis, 2011, Mosby.)

FIGURE 12.4 Ventrogluteal intramuscular injection site. (From Wilson D, Hockenberry MJ: *Wong's clinical manual of pediatric nursing,* ed. 9, St. Louis, 2011, Mosby.)

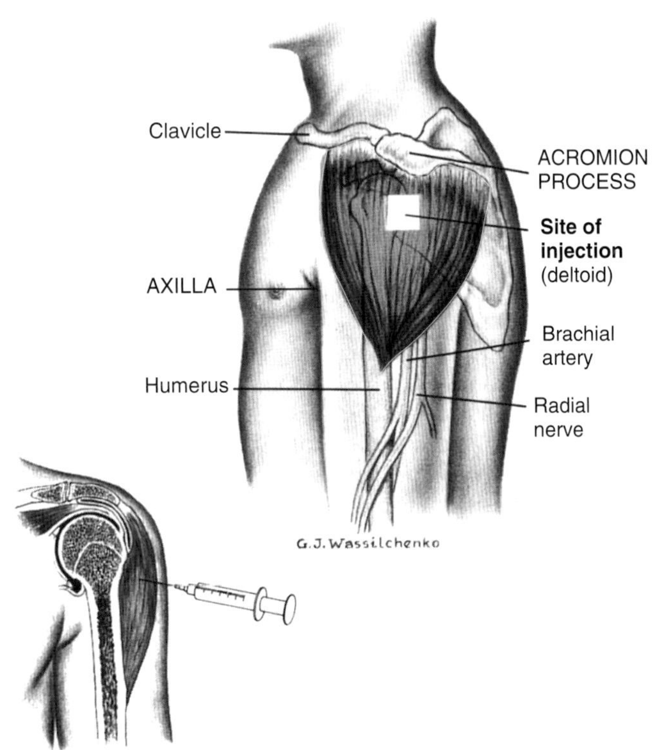

FIGURE 12.5 Deltoid intramuscular injection site. (From Wilson D, Hockenberry MJ: *Wong's clinical manual of pediatric nursing,* ed. 9, St. Louis, 2011, Mosby.)

CLINICAL ALERT!

The dorsogluteal site is not a recommended injection site because of the dangers both in children and adults of damaging the sciatic nerve and striking blood vessels.

Subcutaneous injections are given in the anterolateral thigh (upper outer thigh portion) of infants up to age 1 and adults. The mid-lateral thigh can be used for children and adults with a sufficient fatty layer. The size of needle and angle of injection is adjusted for the depth of the fatty layer that can be pinched up. Parents are asked to comfort the child after the staff perform a painful procedure.

Answers on page 447

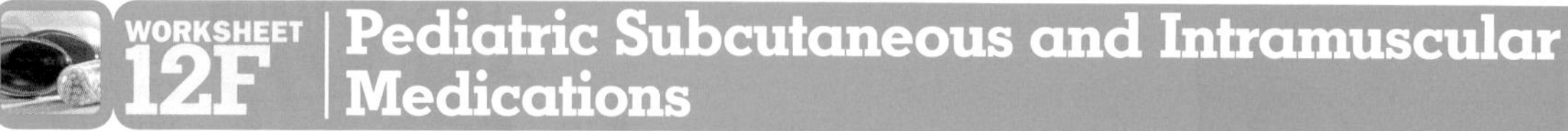

WORKSHEET 12F | Pediatric Subcutaneous and Intramuscular Medications

Subcut and IM injections are rarely ordered on a regular basis for pediatric patients. Calculate the SDR, and compare it with the order. Evaluate the order and make a decision:

1. Give medication (within SDR for unit dose and 24-hr dose).

2. Hold and clarify promptly (overdose or underdose).

For decisions 1 and 2 only, calculate the medication amount to be administered *using written ratio and proportion.* Double-check and prove your work. Do *not* calculate overdose orders.

1. **Ordered:** morphine sulfate 4 mg subcut stat to treat a child with pain (Figure 12.6) who weighs 25.2 kg. The SDR is 0.1 to 0.2 mg per kg per dose.

a. SDR for this child:

b. Dose ordered:

c. Evaluation and decision:

d. Volume to be administered if applicable:

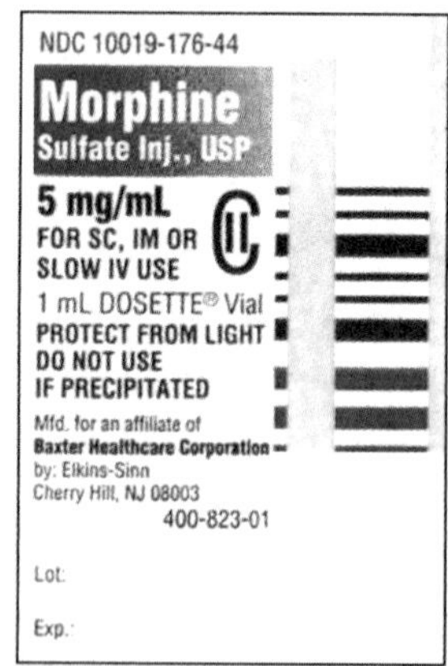

NDC 10019-176-44
Morphine
Sulfate Inj., USP
5 mg/mL
FOR SC, IM OR
SLOW IV USE
1 mL DOSETTE® Vial
PROTECT FROM LIGHT
DO NOT USE
IF PRECIPITATED
Mfd. for an affiliate of
Baxter Healthcare Corporation
by: Elkins-Sinn
Cherry Hill, NJ 08003
400-823-01
Lot:
Exp.:

Asking children and adults to point with one finger where it hurts the most is helpful for localizing specific areas.

CLINICAL ALERT!

Do not confuse morphine with hydromorphone. Do not use the popular abbreviation MS for morphine sulfate or magnesium sulfate even if only one of the two is used in a specific clinical area. One can be misread for the other. Clarify any MS order with the prescriber.

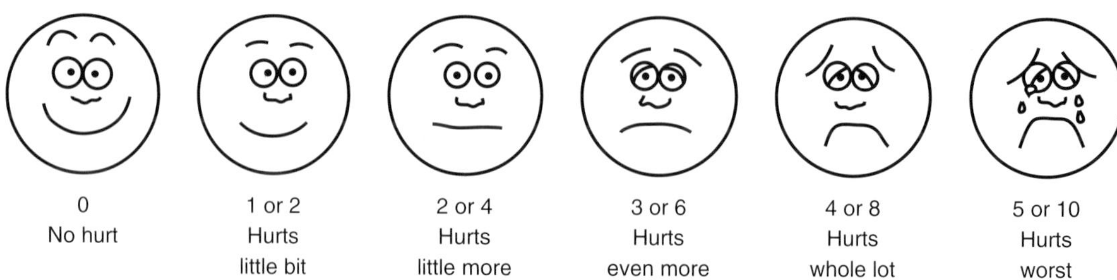

FIGURE 12.6 Wong-Baker FACES pain rating scale for children over 3 years of age and adults. (From Hockenberry MJ, Wilson D, Winkelstein ML: *Wong's essentials of pediatric nursing,* ed. 9, St Louis, 2013, Mosby.)

2. **Ordered:** atropine sulfate 0.2 mg subcutaneous preoperatively for a child who weighs 8.6 kg. The SDR for a child weighing 7 to 9 kg is 0.2 mg, 30 to 60 min before surgery.

- **a.** SDR for this child:
- **b.** Dose ordered:
- **c.** Evaluation and decision:
- **d.** Volume to be administered if applicable:

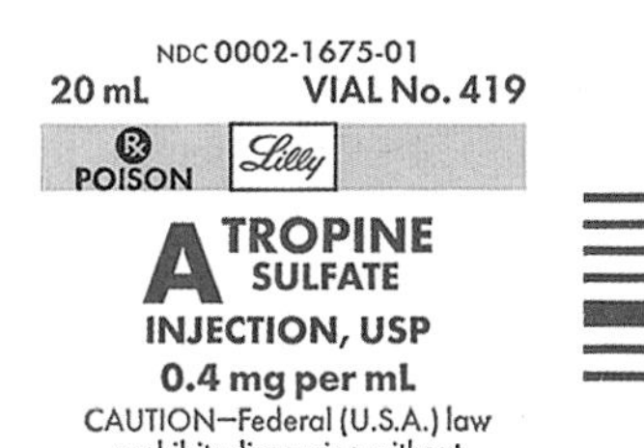

3. **Ordered:** ampicillin sodium 500 mg IM q12h for a 3.2-kg infant with septicemia. SDR is 100 to 200 mg per kg per day in 2 divided doses.

- **a.** SDR for this child:
- **b.** Dose ordered:
- **c.** Evaluation and decision:
- **d.** Volume to be administered if applicable:

4. **Ordered:** glycopyrrolate 0.16 mg IM 60 minutes before anesthesia induction. Patient's weight: 40 kg. SDR: 0.004 mg per kg IM.

- **a.** SDR for this child:
- **b.** Dose ordered:
- **c.** Evaluation and decision:
- **d.** Volume to be administered if applicable:

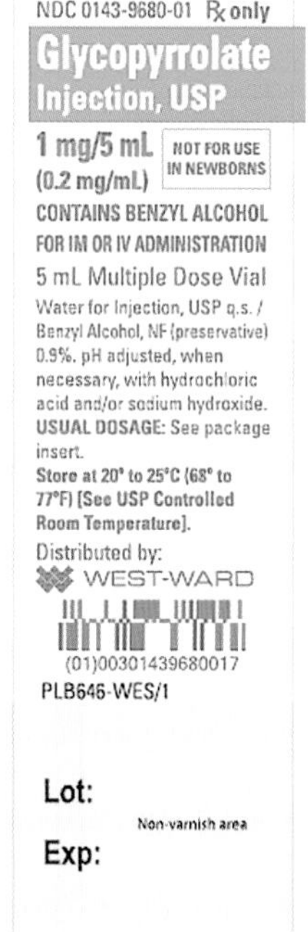

5. **Ordered:** EpiPen (adrenalin)* 2 pack subcut single-use autoinjector with trainer 0.3 mg for a child who is being discharged after an anaphylactic reaction. Patient's weight: 30 kg. SDR is 0.3 mg, 1:1000 for a patient weighing ≥30 kg. **Available:** EpiPen single-use autoinjectors 0.3 mg, 1:1000 and EpiPen 0.15 mg, 1:2000.

- **a.** What are the metric terms for the concentrations: 1:1000? 2:2000? (Hint: they are the same as for basic IV solutions taught in Chapter 7)
- **b.** How is an autoinjector different from other syringes?
- **c.** How many mg per mL are in a 1:1000 concentration?
- **d.** How many mg per mL are in a 1:2000 concentration?
- **e.** Is the dose ordered safe?

*Do not confuse EpiPen with Epifrin.

The pen must be kept near the child at all times and plans made with responsible people when the child is away from home. Nurses and family need to be very well informed on all aspects of this type of allergic reaction and how to use the pen, including practice with the trainer. Encourage the family to read all the literature and to have follow-up visits with the provider or referred allergist. Recommended reference for the nurse and family: https://www.epipen.com.

CLINICAL RELEVANCE

Only the **middle** of the autoinjector is held. It does not have a plunger. The ends are not to be touched.

The **orange end** contains the needle and is immediately pressed against the *middle of the upper outer* (anterolateral) *thigh*—NO OTHER LOCATION—*through clothing if necessary* for both children and adults. On contact with the skin, the autoinjector releases the hidden fine needle to the subcutaneous layer. The **blue end** is touched to deactivate the autoinjector after use.

CLINICAL RELEVANCE

Discharge planning needs to start when the EpiPen is ordered.

Children's IV Medications: Reconstitution, Dilution, and Flow Rate Information

Agency pharmacies and pediatric drug references provide directions for dilution and rates of administration of IV medications for children. The volumes are smaller than those for adults. After determining that the ordered dose is within the SDR, the nurse may have to dilute the medication in a prescribed ratio, withdraw the ordered amount, then further dilute it using a compatible IV solution, and administer it directly or by an infusion pump in a volume-control device. Devices used to administer IV medications to children are shown in Figure 12.7. Volume-control devices help prevent fluid and/or drug overdoses.

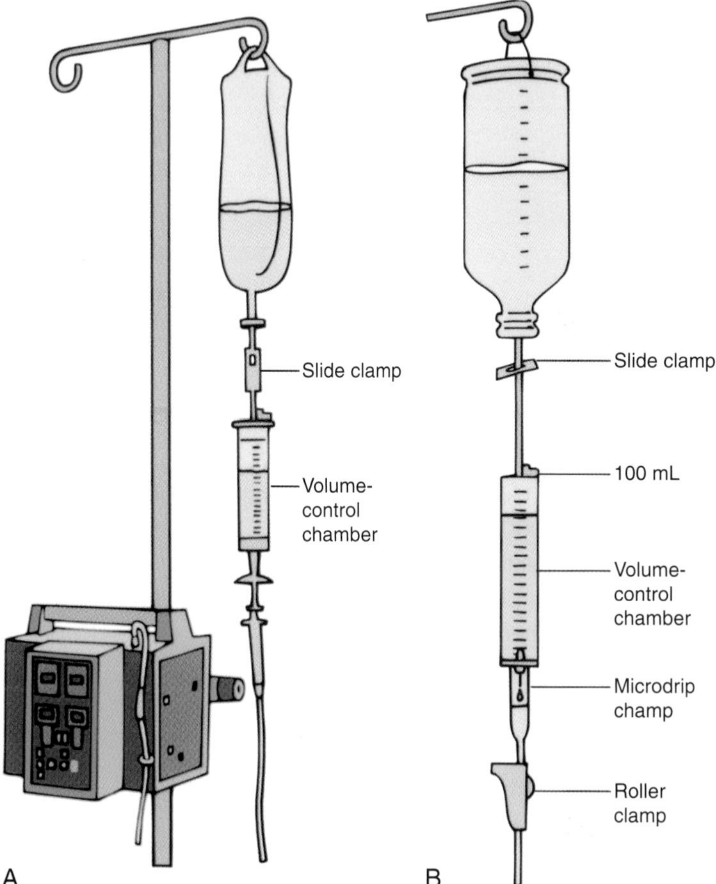

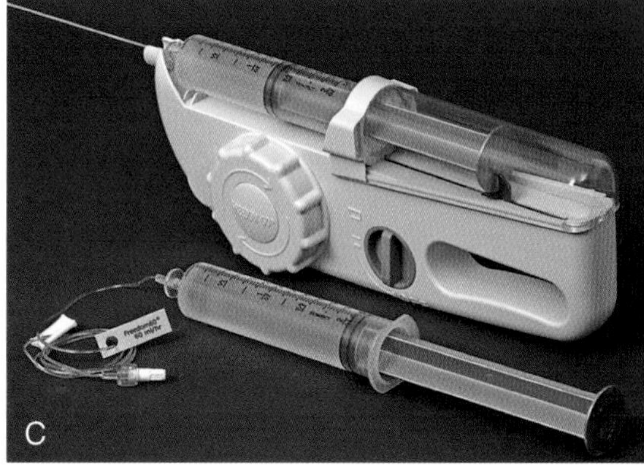

FIGURE 12.7 A, Electronic infusion pump with volume-control device. **B,** Gravity infusion with microdrip tubing (60 gtt per mL delivered through a needle) and volume-control device. Electronic infusion devices with volume-control devices are preferred for the administration of IV fluids to infants and children. If one of these is not available, microdrip (60-drop factor) tubing should be used with a volume-control device to prevent fluid or drug overload. Small volumes to be delivered IV within a short period may be administered directly through a syringe or a syringe pump. **C,** Freedom 60-syringe infusion pump. This portable reusable manual infusion uses standard 60-mL syringes and can be filled from 1 to 60 mL. It offers flow rates with rate-controlled tubing from 0.5 to 1200 mL per hr. It does not permit free flow. (**C,** From A B Repro-Med Systems, Inc., Chester, N.Y.)

Example **Ordered:** Antibiotic 1 g q6h IV. Supplied: A powdered form of antibiotic that requires reconstitution. Pediatric directions from pharmacy: *Dilute to 100 mg per mL, withdraw ordered amount, then further dilute to 30 mL, and administer over 20 min.* The label reads 2 grams (2 g).

Step 1 Dilute to 100 mg per mL. The label reads 2 g. (Change to milligrams for dilution: 2 g = 2000 mg.)

KNOW WANT TO KNOW

100 mg : 1 mL = 2000 mg : x mL

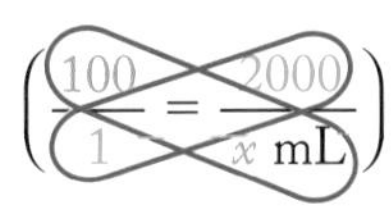

$$\frac{\text{Drug}}{\text{Volume}} = \frac{\text{Drug}}{\text{Volume}}$$

$$\frac{\cancel{100}}{\cancel{100}}x = \frac{2000}{100}$$

$$x = 20 \text{ mL}$$

PROOF
100 × 20 = 2000
1 × 2000 = 2000

Reconstitute antibiotic with 20 mL compatible solution.*

Step 2 Withdraw ordered amount (1 g).

KNOW WANT TO KNOW

2 g : 20 mL = 1 g : x mL

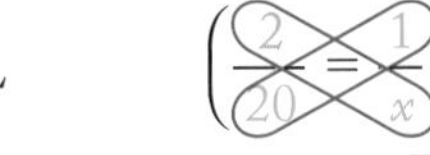

$$2x = 20$$

$$x = 10 \text{ mL} = 1 \text{ g}$$

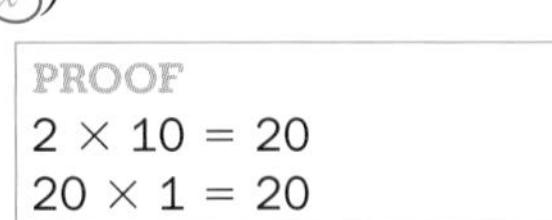

PROOF
2 × 10 = 20
20 × 1 = 20

ANSWER
10 mL

Step 3 Place the medication in a volume-control device, adding a compatible IV solution to 30 mL. Set the flow rate. Consult a procedure book for use of volume-control devices. Flow rate:

KNOW WANT TO KNOW

30 mL : 20 min = x mL : 60 min

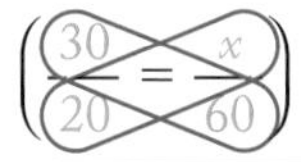

$$\frac{\cancel{20}}{\cancel{20}}x = \frac{1800}{20}$$

$$x = 90 \text{ mL per hour}$$

PROOF
30 × 60 = 1800
20 × 90 = 1800

ANSWER
Set rate at 90 mL per hr for 20 min

RULE

To *estimate* hourly IV flow rates for amounts to be delivered in less than 60 minutes by a pump: for 10 minutes, multiply the volume by 6 because there are six 10-minute periods in an hour; for 15 minutes, multiply the volume by 4; for 20 minutes, multiply the volume by 3; and for 30 minutes, multiply the volume by 2. This will work only for 10-, 15-, 20-, and 30-minute orders.

To *calculate* the setting for mL per hr on a pump for medications to be delivered in less than 1 hour, set up a ratio and proportion of milliliters to minutes. The final dilution may be made with an existing IV solution if it is compatible with the medication.

Example To give 10 mL in 15 min with a pump, *estimate* (10 × 4 = 40 mL per hr).
Calculate:

KNOW WANT TO KNOW

10 mL : 15 min = x mL : 60 min

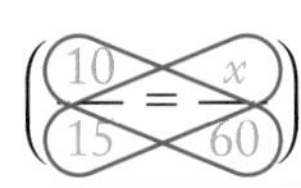

$$\frac{\cancel{15}}{\cancel{15}}x = \frac{600}{15}$$

$$x = 40 \text{ mL}$$

PROOF
10 × 60 = 600
15 × 40 = 600

ANSWER
40 mL per hr

*For information and practice reconstituting medications, refer to Chapter 6.

Example **Ordered:** Antibiotic 250 mg q4h IV.

The label reads: *Mix (dilute) with 4.2 mL sterile water for injection to yield 5 mL of 100 mg per mL.*

Amount of ordered antibiotic to be withdrawn after mixing:

KNOW WANT TO KNOW

100 mg : 1 mL = 250 mg : x mL $\left(\frac{100}{1} = \frac{250}{x}\right)$

$$\frac{\cancel{100}}{\cancel{100}}x = \frac{250}{100}$$

$$x = 2.5 \text{ mL}$$

PROOF
100 × 2.5 = 250
1 × 250 = 250

ANSWER
2.5 mL

Directions for pediatric administration: *Further dilute to 25 mL and administer over 30 minutes.* Total volume to be administered: 25 mL.

Example Flow rate in volume-control device, estimate (2 × 25 = 50 mL per hr):

KNOW WANT TO KNOW

25 mL : 30 min = x mL : 60 min $\left(\frac{\overset{5}{\cancel{25}}}{\underset{6}{\cancel{30}}} = \frac{x}{60}\right)$

$$30x = 25 \times 60 \text{ or } 1500$$

$$x = 50 \text{ mL}$$

PROOF
26 × 60 = 1500
30 × 50 = 1500

ANSWER
50 mL per hr

Answers on page 448

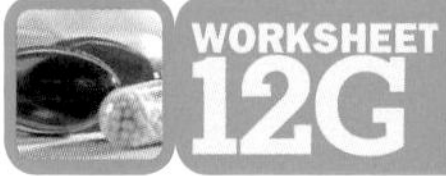

WORKSHEET 12G Pediatric IV Medications

For each problem, use a calculator to determine the child's weight in kg if required, calculate the SDR, and compare it with the order. Round oz, lb, and kg to the nearest tenth. Evaluate the order and make a decision:

1. Give medication (within SDR for unit dose and 24-hr dose).
2. Hold and clarify promptly (overdose or underdose).

Calculate the medication amount to be administered based on the label provided. Use written ratio and proportion and prove your answer even if you use a calculator to verify it. Calculate the IV pump flow rate in mL per hr if medication is to be administered for more than 5 min. Round ounces and kilograms to the nearest tenth. Enter calculator data twice for verification.

1. **Ordered:** phenobarbital sodium 50 mg IV preoperative sedation.
   Patient's weight: 28.2 kg. The SDR for sedation is 1 to 3 mg per kg, 1 to 1½ hr before procedure.
   a. SDR for this child:
   b. Dose ordered:
   c. Evaluation and decision:
   d. Dose in mL to the nearest hundredth to be withdrawn before dilution:

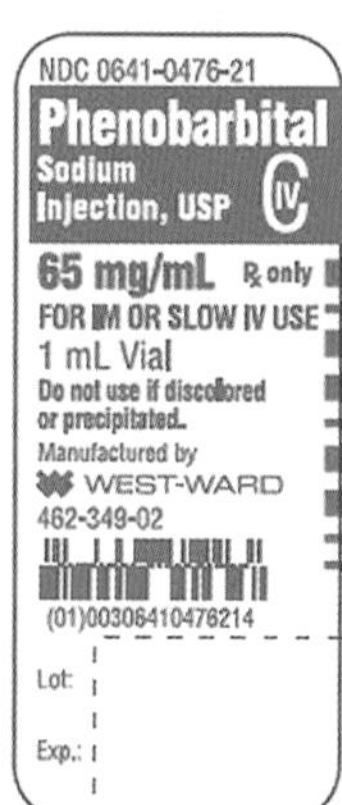

2. **Ordered:** Initial dose of furosemide 25 mg IV stat for a child with urinary retention. The SDR is 1 mg per kg to titrate gradually in 1 mg per kg increments to desired response, not to exceed 6 mg per kg. The child weighs 25 kg today.

a. SDR for this child:

b. Dose ordered:

c. Evaluation and decision:

d. Volume to be administered if applicable:

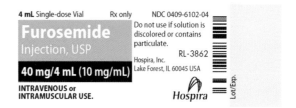

3. **Ordered:** Garamycin 15 mg IV q8h for a child with an infection. Patient weight: 6 kg today. The SDR is 2 to 2.5 mg per kg q8h. Directions from the pharmacy say to dilute *to* 50 mL with 0.9% NaCl and administer over 60 minutes. **Available:** Garamycin pediatric injectable 20 mg per 2 mL.

a. SDR for this child:

b. Dose ordered:

c. Evaluation and decision:

d. Amount withdrawn from vial:

e. How should the 50 mL volume be infused and what should the nurse monitor?

CLINICAL ALERT!

Many of the generic antibiotics, particularly the cephalosporins, have very similar names, such as ceftizoxime, ceftriaxone, and cephradine. However, the uses and the SDRs are very different!

4. **Ordered:** digoxin 0.5 mg IV stat for a child with congestive heart failure. SDR: 0.015 to 0.35 mg per kg. Patient's weight: 11.1 kg. **Directions:** Administer IV over 5 minutes. Dilute each mL of drug in 4 mL SW to permit small amounts of drug to be infused over 5 minutes. Use a calculator to determine SDR.

a. SDR for this child:

b. Dose ordered:

c. Evaluation and decision:

d. How many mL of digoxin will you prepare before dilution?

e. What flow rate per minute will you administer after dilution?

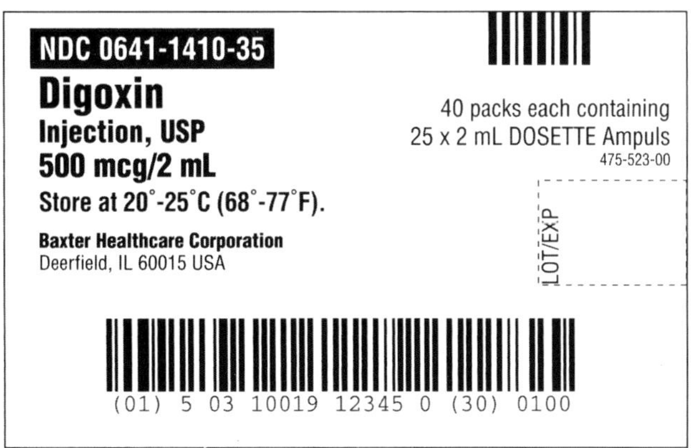

5. **Ordered:** Geopen (carbenicillin disodium) 2 g IV q6h for a child with an infection. The SDR is 50 to 500 mg per kg q24h in divided doses every 4 to 6 hr. Dilute to 200 mg per mL with compatible solution and administer at rate of 1 per 10 min. Patient weight: 11.8 kg.

a. SDR for this child:

b. Dose ordered:

c. Evaluation and decision:

d. Amount withdrawn after reconstitution:

e. Flow rate in mL per hr if applicable:

CLINICAL ALERT!

Pediatric IV flow rates carry a high potential for errors. Consult current, reliable pediatric IV drug references and the pharmacy for pediatric IV dilutions and rates of administration. Note that liquids added to solids result in a higher total volume than just the amount of liquid added. Instructions to dilute ***with*** *x mL* result in more volume than instructions to dilute ***to*** *x mL*. Dilute *to* limits a total volume for the mixture. Dilute ***with*** is just stating the amount of liquid to be added to the solid. When in any doubt about IV dilutions and flow rates, consult the pharmacy and document the verification. The prescriber may have to be contacted, too.

Answers on page 449

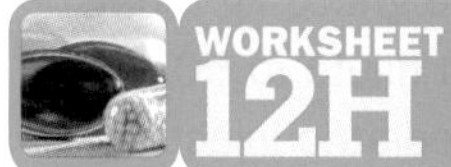

WORKSHEET 12H Multiple-Choice Practice

For the following problems, estimate kilograms, then calculate kilograms to the *nearest* tenth when a pound-to-kilogram conversion is needed, and estimate the answers before solving each step.

1. A child weighs 50 lb. What is a rough estimate of the equivalent kg?

a. 200 **b.** 50 **c.** 100 **d.** 25

2. Ordered: methotrexate sodium 30 mg per m^2 po daily maintenance for a child with leukemia. The child's BSA is 1.20 m^2.* How much medication will you administer?

a. 1.20 mg **b.** 30 mg **c.** 36 mg **d.** 30.12 mg

3. Ordered: 1.5 tsp of acetaminophen suspension liquid po stat for a child with fever. How many milliliters will you administer?

a. 5 mL **b.** 7.5 mL **c.** 8 mL **d.** 10 mL

4. Which foods are best to administer with medications for infants and children?

a. Their favorite fruit juices
b. Formula or milk
c. High-protein shakes
d. Applesauce, sherbet, gelatin

5. Which of many instructions is accurate to give a parent of a child who is being discharged with a prescription for an EpiPen?

a. Always keep the EpiPen in the refrigerator or a cooler.
b. Have an unexpired EpiPen in a convenient location near the child at all times.
c. If the EpiPen is not used before its expiration date, it will not be necessary to spend the money on another one.
d. Use the EpiPen as a backup when you cannot transport the child to an emergency department.

6. Which IM route is not recommended for infants and children and patients with undeveloped gluteal muscles?

a. Vastus lateralis
b. Ventrogluteal
c. Dorsogluteal
d. Deltoid

*Note: Trailing zeros appear in BSA m^2 measurements. Delete them for math calculations.

7. **Ordered:** Phenytoin oral suspension 15 mg bid po for a 6-kg child with seizures. The SDR is 5 mg per kg in 2 to 3 divided doses. Label reads: Dilantin pediatric suspension 30 mg per 5 mL. Your decision:
   a. Hold and clarify the order with the physician. It is an overdose.
   b. The order is safe. Give 2.5 mL.
   c. Clarify the order with an experienced supervisor.
   d. The order is safe. Give 15 mL.

8. Which muscle is recommended for IM injections for infants less than 7 months of age or for underweight infants?
   a. Vastus lateralis
   b. Ventrogluteal
   c. Dorsogluteal
   d. Deltoid

9. Which medication order would result in the largest dose?
   a 20 mg
   b. 20 mg per kg
   c. 20 mg per m^2
   d. 20 mg per lb

10. In addition to distracting a young pediatric patient, how is it best to involve a parent when administering an injection?
   a. Have the parent assist with restraining the child to avoid movement during the injection.
   b. Ask the parent to comfort the child after the procedure.
   c. Have the parent(s) leave the room during the procedure.
   d. Ask the parent to visit children who do not have visitors until the child has calmed down.

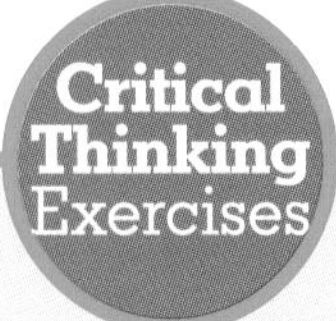

Critical Thinking Exercises provide math and medication-related patient safety issues for student discussion. Answers are not provided.

Analyze the following scenarios.

1. Baby Louise is in your unit with a diagnosis of congestive heart failure secondary to a congenital heart defect. She weighs 8.4 kg at age 18 months. Her orders include lanoxin 0.05 mg po bid. The orders include temporary fluid restriction to 500 mL per 24-hr period. On hand is furosemide oral solution 10 mg per mL. Given this a.m. by the reporting nurse: 2 mL. During report, the nurse tells you that for the past 24 hours the intake exceeded 500 mL by 120 mL because the baby wouldn't take the medicine without a lot of juice.

   Is there a problem with mathematics?

   What error in concepts of arithmetic rounding might have led to an error?

   Which knowledge bases are insufficient?

   Medication error(s) and possible causes:

   Fluid intake error:

   Potential injuries:

   Nursing actions:

   Recommendations for the nurse and for patient safety if you were on a hospital committee studying this incident:

2. John, a 3-year-old boy weighing 20 kg, has an order for IV anticoagulation. Heparin *25 units per kg per hr* continuous infusion is ordered until the next laboratory checks. Pharmacy supplies a premixed drug concentration (12,500 International Units in 250 mL D5W). Pharmacy instruction is to infuse at 10 mL per hr. Nurse A has calculated that the child needs 500 units per hr, that 50 units per mL (12,500 per 250) are in the solution, and that the flow rate should be 50 mL per hr.

How many units per hr are needed based on John's kg weight? How many units of heparin per mL are there in the solution?

How many mL per hour should be infused? Who is correct, the pharmacist or the nurse?

Potential ADE/sentinel events:

What would you do if you were Nurse A?

Recommendations for the agency Safety Committee if you were on the committee:

Do you believe that nurses should also double-check the SDR for all drug orders?

3. A 10-kg child admitted with hyperglycemia, patient of Nurse A, has an order for Regular insulin 0.05 units per kg per hr. The agency requires a second independent nurse check for all high-risk drugs. Nurse A and Nurse B agree that the order is safe. Nurse B, the independent check nurse, leaves. Nurse A programs 0.5 units Regular insulin per kg per hr on the IV Smart Pump. An overdose alarm alert sounds. There is also an option on the pump to override the visual and auditory alert and administer the IV. Nurse A needs to decide whether to override or recheck.

How much of an error was programmed?

Why do you think this happened?

Potential ADE from this event?

Under what circumstances do you believe an agency should or should not permit an override of a pump alert?

What sort of procedure should a hospital have for an override?

Do you have any recommendations for Nurse B, the independent check nurse?

Web reference: www.ihi.org

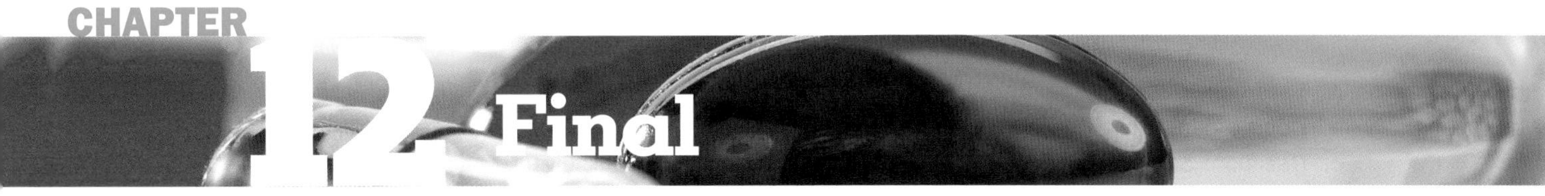

Use a calculator to find the SDR for each child. Compare it with the order. Make a decision: Safe to give or hold and contact prescriber. If safe, calculate the dose.

1. **Ordered:** Cephalexin capsules* 2 g per day in 4 divided doses po q6h × 7 days for John, a 14-year-old with a respiratory infection. The SDR for adults and teenagers is 1000 to 4000 mg per day in divided doses.
   a. Dose ordered:
   b. SDR:
   c. Decision: Safe to give or hold and contact prescriber?
   d. If safe, how many capsules will you give?

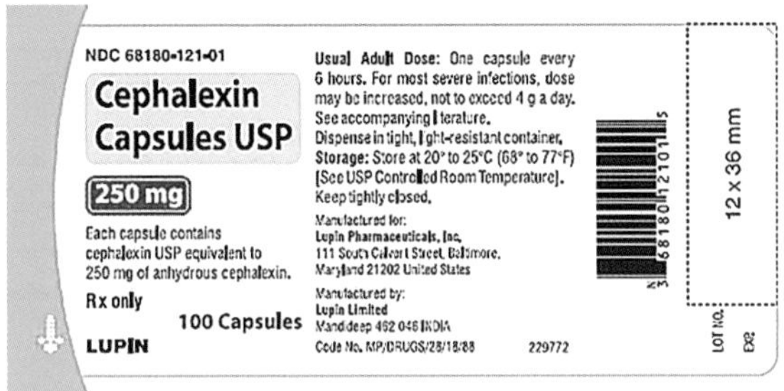

2. **Ordered:** levothyroxine† sodium tablets 0.15 mg po daily to John's 16-year-old sister, who has hypothyroidism. The SDR for patients more than 12 years old, 2 to 3 mcg per kg. Patient's weight: 60 kg.
   a. SDR:
   b. Dose ordered:
   d. Decision: Safe to give or hold and contact prescriber? If unsafe, state reason.
   e. How many tablets will you give?

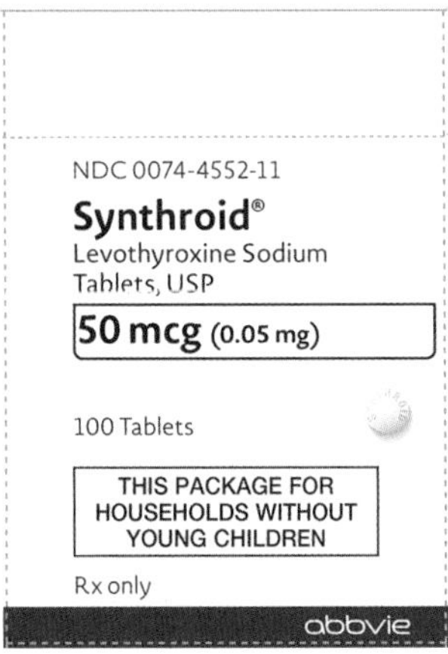

*Read the antibiotic labels that begin with *C* very carefully. Many of the generic versions look alike and sound alike (e.g., cefazolin, cefaclor, cefepime, cefotaxime, cefotetan) but have different purposes and dosing. For more information, visit www.ismp.org/tools/confuseddrugnames.pdf.

†Do not confuse levothyroxine with levofloxacin, an antibiotic.

3. **Ordered:** Benadryl Allergy Liquid (diphenhydramine HCl) 25 mg po tid and at bedtime × 3 days for John's pruritus. Johnny is 8 years old. Read the label and make your decision.
   a. Safe daily dose maximum for this child:
   b. Dose ordered for 24 hr:
   c. Decision: Safe to give or hold and contact prescriber? If unsafe, state reason.
   d. Dose to be administered:

NDC 0501-2050-04

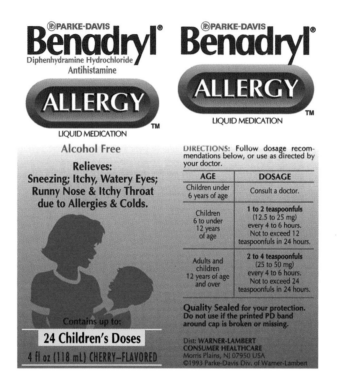

CLINICAL ALERT!

Approximately 15% of people, or 1 in 6 persons, with an allergy to penicillin will have an allergy to the cephalosporins.

4. Ordered amoxicillin clavulanate potassium* oral suspension 700 mg po q8h for Marissa, a 13-year-old with otitis media. Patient's weight: 35 kg. The SDR for children less than 40 kg is 20 to 40 mg per kg per day in divided doses q8h.
   a. SDR for this child:
   b. Dose ordered:
   c. Decision: Safe to give or hold and contact prescriber?
   d. If safe, how many mL will you give? If unsafe, state reason.

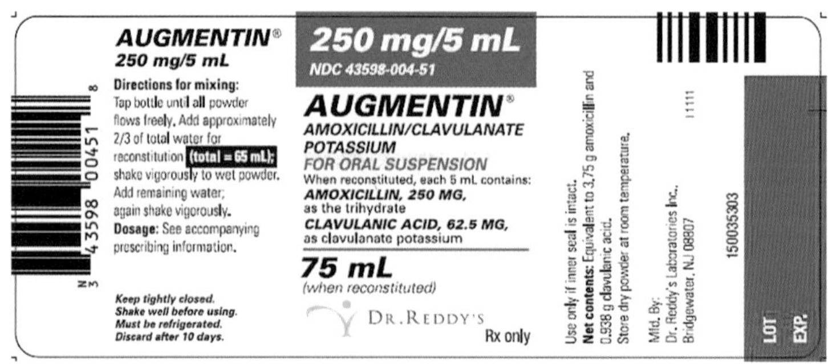

*Do not confuse amoxicillin with the compound drug amoxicillin clavulanate potassium or amoxipine. They are different drugs for different uses.

5. Karen, age 3, is admitted to the hospital with a compound fracture of the femur incurred during an automobile accident. **Ordered:** atropine sulfate 0.3 mg preop IM. The SDR for children weighing 12 to 16 kg is 0.3 mg 30 to 60 min before surgery. Karen weighs 35 lb.
   a. SDR for this child:
   b. Dose ordered:
   c. Decision: Safe to give or hold and contact prescriber?
   d. Dose to be administered:

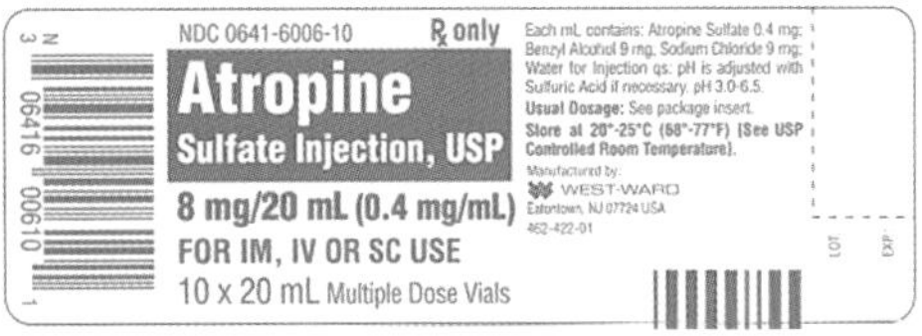

6. **Ordered:** valproic acid* oral solution 0.1 g po bid for a child with a seizure disorder. The SDR for initial administration is 10 to 15 mg per kg per day in 2 or 3 divided doses. Patient's weight: 20 kg. *Directions:* immediately before use, dilute the medication with distilled water, acidified tap water, or juice.
   a. SDR for this child:
   b. Decision: Safe to give or hold and contact prescriber?
   c. If safe, how many mL will you give?

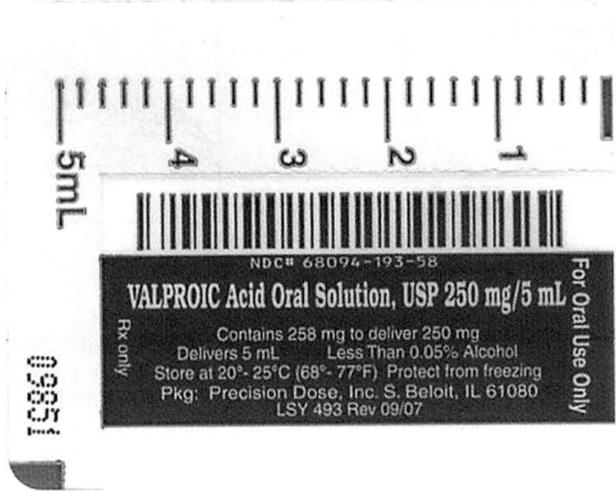

CLINICAL ALERT!

Check compatibility with the other medications ordered for the patient. Double-check the eMAR for orders for more than one antiseizure medication and clarify before administration. Usually a patient is on only one antiseizure medication. Note: Many antiseizure medications are incompatible with several other drugs.

7. **Ordered:** Nystatin 200,000 units 4 times a day for a 3-month-old infant with oral candidiasis (thrush). The SDR is 100,000 units to each side of the mouth 4 times a day. Directions: this suspension must be well mixed before administration. For children and adults, have the patient swish the solution around the inside of the mouth and retain in the mouth for several minutes if possible. For infants, paint the solution in recesses of the mouth, inside cheeks, and on the tongue.
   a. If the order is safe, how many milliliters will you place on each side of the mouth?
   b. Which device in Figure 12.2 would you use to administer this medication if a "brush" was not available to coat the inside of the mouth?

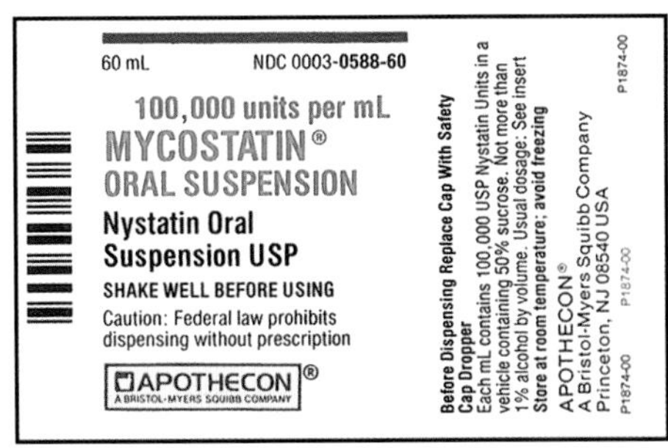

*The brand name equivalent of valproic acid is Depakote. Do not confuse Depakote with Depakene.

8. **Ordered:** epinephrine 0.01 mg per kg 1:1000* subcut stat (not to exceed 0.5 mg) for a child brought to an outpatient clinic with an anaphylactic reaction, bronchospasm/airway obstruction caused by an insect bite. May repeat in 20 minutes, not to exceed 0.5 mg for bronchospasm/airway obstruction. Patient weight: 20 kg. The patient has a history of eczema and asthma.
   a. 1:1000 solution = _____ mg per mL; 1:10,000 solution = _____ mg per mL
   b. What is the numerical difference between the solutions?
   c. How many milliliters will you administer subcut?
   d. What would be the difference in dose if the nurse prepared a 0.1 mg per kg instead of 0.01 mg because of misreading the order or a decimal calculation error?

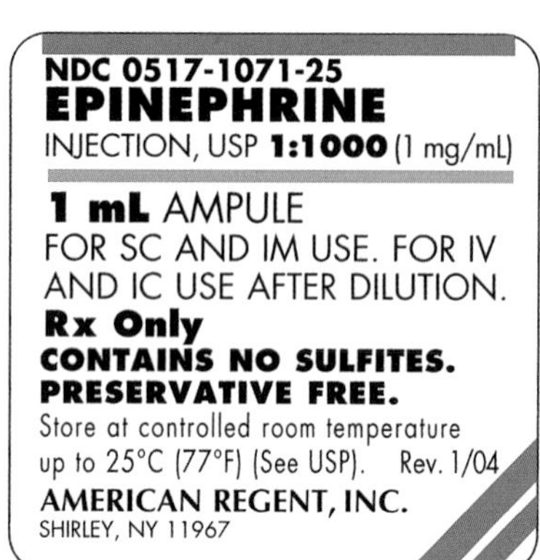

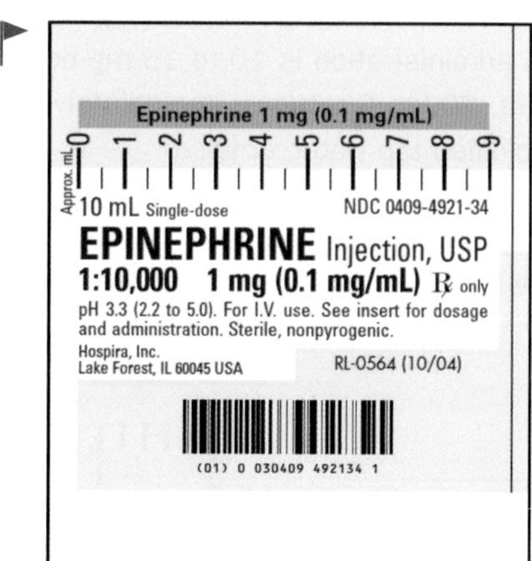

CLINICAL ALERT!

Clarify any questions about the order with the provider or the supply with the pharmacist.

CLINICAL RELEVANCE

Epinephrine orders vary depending on the use, the route of administration, and the age of the patient. Because there is less familiarity with these types of solutions, the nurse needs to take time to study the usual orders and labels of acute lifesaving medications so that when an emergency arises, the label and contents will be familiar.

CLINICAL ALERT!

Review agency policies for verbal orders. These occur with emergency situations. Repeating the order with the medication label in hand while facing the person who ordered the medication is very important.

9. **Ordered:** leucovorin calcium 0.01 g q6h po for a child with toxic effects resulting from an antineoplastic agent. The child weighs 70 lb and has normal height for weight. The SDR for children is up to 10 mg per m^2 q6h for 72 hr. Use the West nomogram* to determine the BSA for this child's weight.
   a. BSA in m^2:
   b. SDR for this child:
   c. Dose ordered:
   d. Evaluation and decision:
   e. Amount to be given if applicable:

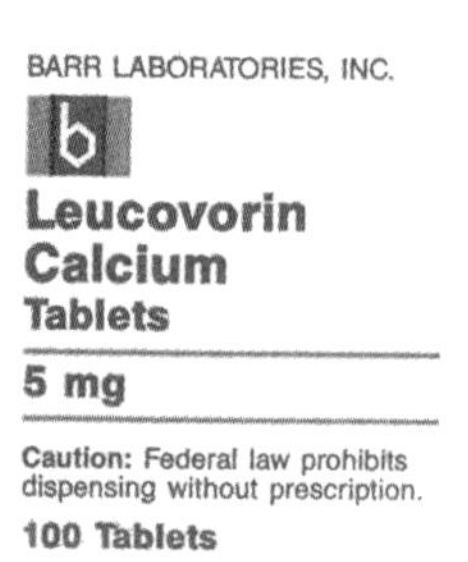

*Refer to Figure 12.1 for the West nomogram.

10. Ordered for a child with hemophilia: a recommended dose of NovoSeven 90 mcg per kg, IV bolus, q3h until hemostasis is achieved or until the treatment has been judged to be inadequate. The child's weight is 22 kg. Directions: Administer over 2 to 5 minutes slow bolus. This bolus will be administered over 3 minutes with the syringe provided. These are single-dose vials that must be discarded 3 hours after reconstitution. Use a calculator for long division and multiplication.

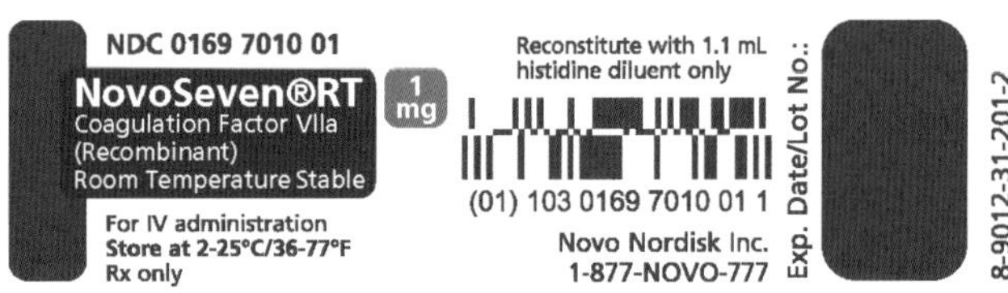

a. Dose in mcg ordered for this child:
b. Equivalent dose in mg:
c. Total mL to be administered:
d. How many vials of medication will the nurse need?
e. Total calibrations to be occupied by the volume (refer to syringe):
f. mL per minute:
g. Draw a line on the syringe to indicate the total dose.

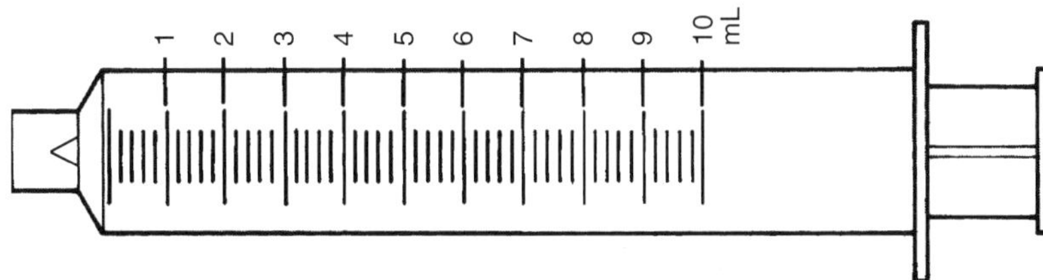

h. How many mL will remain after a. 1 minute; b. 2 minutes; c. 3 minutes?

CLINICAL ALERT!

Beware of medication orders for "T" and "t" and "tsp"—for example, 1 T daily or 1 tsp daily. Teaspoon and tablespoon abbreviations can easily be confused. Also, dosage strength may vary per teaspoon among infant, child, and adult preparations and may also vary among manufacturers. Call the provider and clarify the specific strength desired in milligrams, milliequivalents, or units.

Refer to the Pediatric Calculations section of Drug Calculations Companion, version 5 on Evolve, for additional practice problems.

Answer Key

12 Pediatric Dosages

WORKSHEET **12A** (page 420)

1. a. Estimate: 7 kg
Actual: 6.4 kg
b. Estimate: 6 kg
Actual: 12.1 lb (2 steps)
5.5 kg
c. Estimate: 5 kg
Actual: 4.5 kg
d. Estimate: 28 lb
Actual: 30.8 lb
e. Estimate: 20 lb
Actual: 22 lb

2. a. 150 mg × 3 = 450 mg
b. 200 mg × 4 = 800 mg
c. 400 mcg × 6 = 2400 mcg or 2.4 mg
d. 50 mg × 3 = 150 mg
e. 750 mcg × 2 = 1500 mcg or 1.5 mg

3. a. 1 g or 1000 mg ÷ 4 = 250 mg
b. 750 mg ÷ 3 = 250 mg
c. 2 g or 2000 mg ÷ 4 = 500 mg
2 g or 2000 mg ÷ 6 = 333.3 mg
d. 16 g a day ÷ 2 = 8 g
16 g a day ÷ 4 = 4 g
e. 500 mg ÷ 4 = 125 mg

4. a. 10 × 5 = 50 mg
b. 5 × 7.3 = 36.5 mg (low dose)
8 × 7.3 = 58.4 mg (high dose)
SDR is 36.5 to 58.4 mg.
c. 8 lb = approximately 4 kg estimated
Step 1: 8 lb = 3.6 kg actual
Step 2: *Low dose:* 6 × 3.6 = 21.6 mg
High dose: 8 × 3.6 = 28.8 mg
SDR is 21.6 to 28.8 mg.
d. 5 lb, 8 oz = approximately 2.5 kg
Step 1: *oz to lb:* 8 oz/16 = 0.5 lb
Step 2: *lb to kg:* 5.5 lb ÷ 2.2 = 2.5 kg
Step 3: *Low dose:* 3 × 2.5 = 7.5 mg
High dose: 6 × 2.5 = 15 mg
SDR is 7.5 to 15 mg.
e. 4 lb, 6 oz = approximately 2 kg
Step 1: *oz to lb:* 6 oz/16 = 0.37 rounded to 0.4 lb
Step 2: *lb to kg:* 4.4 lb ÷ 2.2 = 2 kg
Step 3: *Low dose:* 200 mcg × 2 = 400 mcg or 0.4 mg
High dose: 400 mcg × 2 = 800 mcg or 0.8 mg
SDR is 400 to 800 mcg or 0.4 to 0.8 mg.

5. a. 36 to 54 mg ($2 \times 18 = 36$)
($3 \times 18 = 54$)
 b. 12 to 18 mg ($36 \div 3$)
($54 \div 3$)
 c. 150 mg per day; 50 mg per dose
(50×3) ($150 \div 3$)
 d. Unsafe to give. Overdose ordered. Hold and clarify promptly with the physician.

WORKSHEET 12B (page 421)

1. a. SDR for this child: 18.2 to 36.4 mg per day
$2 \times 9.1 = 18.2$ mg
$4 \times 9.1 = 36.4$ mg
 b. Dose ordered: 50 mg daily
 c. Evaluation and decision: Hold and clarify promptly (overdose)

2. a. SDR for this child: 1500 to 3000 mcg per day or 1.5 to 3 mg per day
15×100 mcg $= 1500$ mcg or 1.5 mg
15×200 mcg $= 3000$ mcg or 3 mg
 b. Dose ordered: 0.5 mg tid or 1.5 mg per day
 c. Evaluation and decision: Safe to give

3. a. SDR for this child: 115 to 345 mg per day
$10 \times 11.5 = 115$ mg
$30 \times 11.5 = 345$ mg
 b. Dose ordered: 100 mg tid or 300 mg per day
 c. Evaluation and decision: Safe to give

4. a. SDR for this child: 386 mg to 579 mg per day in divided doses
 b. Dose ordered: 100 mg q6h or
$100 \times 4 = 400$ mg per day
 c. Evaluation and decision: Safe to give

5. a. SDR for this child: 23 to 46 mcg per day
$10 \times 2.3 = 23$ mcg
$20 \times 2.3 = 46$ mcg
 b. Dose ordered: 0.03 mg $\times$ 4 = 0.12 mg per day or 120 mcg per day
 c. Evaluation and decision: Hold and clarify promptly (overdose)

WORKSHEET 12C (page 423)

1. 0.15 m^2
$10 \times 0.15 = 1.5$ mg

2. 0.20 m^2*
$15 \times 0.2 = 3$ mg

3. 0.27 m^2
$5 \times 0.27 = 1.35$ mg

4. $10 \times 1.8 = 18$ mg

5. 2.72 kg
$2 \times 2.7 = 5.4$ mg

6. $5 \times 9.1 = 45.5$ mg

7. $4 \times 10 = 40$ mg

8. $15 \times 6 = 90$ mg

9. $20 \times 5 = 100$ mg

10. 1.10 m^2

WORKSHEET 12D (page 424)

1. a. SDR: 1000 to 2000 mg in 4 divided doses
 b. Dose ordered: 500 mg $\times$ 4 or 2000 mg
 c. Evaluation and decision: Safe to give
Total dose is divided by 4.

2. a. SDR for this child: 4.0 to 6.4 mg 4 times daily
$5 \times 0.8\ m^2 = 4.0$ mg (low safe dose)
$8 \times 0.8\ m^2 = 6.4$ mg (high safe dose)
 b. Dose ordered: 4 mg daily
 c. Evaluation and decision: Safe to give

*Note: Trailing zeros are seen in BSA square meters. Delete them for math calculations.

3. a. SDR for this child: 0.9 to 2.6 mg in 2 divided doses or 860 to 2600 mcg in 2 divided doses
   $0.1 \times 8.6 = 0.86$ mg rounded to 0.9 mg (low safe dose)
   $0.3 \times 8.6 = 2.58$ rounded to 2.6 mg (high safe dose)
   b. Dose ordered: 2500 mcg bid or 2.5 mg $\times$ 2 = 5 mg per day
   c. Evaluation and decision: Hold and clarify promptly (overdose)

4. a. SDR for this child: 4.1 to 20.5 mcg per day
   $1 \times 4.1 = 4.1$ mcg
   $5 \times 4.1 = 20.5$ mcg
   b. Dose ordered: 0.01 mg or 10 mcg daily
   c. Evaluation and decision: Safe to give

5. a. SDR for this child: 0.13 to 0.32 mg per day
   $0.02 \times 6.4 = 0.128$ mg (low safe dose)
   $0.05 \times 6.4 = 0.32$ mg (high safe dose)
   b. Dose ordered: 150 mcg $\times$ 2 = 300 mcg per day or 0.3 mg per day
   c. Evaluation and decision: Safe to give

WORKSHEET **12E** (page 427)

1. a. Estimated wt in lb: 14×2 or 28 lb
   b. Actual wt in lb: 30.8 lb
   c. SDR for this child: For 24 to 35 lb, 1 tsp
   d. Dose ordered: 160 mg
   e. Evaluation and decision: Safe to give
   f. Give: 1 tsp or 5 mL (80 mg per ½ tsp)

2. a. SDR for this child: 300 to 900 mg per day in 3 to 4 doses
   $10 \times 30 = 300$ mg (low safe daily dose)
   $30 \times 30 = 900$ mg (maximum safe daily dose)
   b. Dose ordered: $300 \times 3 = 900$ mg per day.
   c. Evaluation and decision: Safe to give
   d. Give

   HAVE / WANT TO HAVE
   75 mg : 5 mL = 300 mg : x mL
   $$\frac{\cancel{75}}{\cancel{75}}x = \frac{1500}{75}$$
   $x = 20$ mL

   PROOF
   $75 \times 20 = 1500$
   $1 \times 1500 = 1500$

3. a. SDR for this child: 400 to 800 mg per day in 3 to 4 doses
   b. Dose ordered in mg:
   0.25 g = 250 mg $\times$ 3 = 750 mg per day

   HAVE / WANT TO HAVE
   1 g : 1000 mg = 0.25 g : x mg
   $x = 1000 \times 0.25$ or 250 mg

   PROOF
   $1 \times 250 = 250$
   $1000 \times 0.25 = 250$
   c. Evaluation and decision: Safe to give
   d. Give 12.5 mL

   HAVE / WANT TO HAVE
   100 mg : 5 mL = 250 mg : x mL
   $$\frac{\cancel{100}}{\cancel{100}}x = \frac{125\cancel{0}}{10\cancel{0}}\ (5 \times 250)$$
   $x = 12.5$ mL

   PROOF
   $100 \times 12.5 = 1250$
   $5 \times 250 = 1250$

4. a. SDR for this child:
   $10 \times 0.5 \times 4 = 20$ mg per day
   b. Dose ordered: 5 mg four times a day.
   c. Evaluation and decision: Safe to give
   d. Give 1 tab

5. a. SDR for this child: 246 mg to 492 mg per day
   b. Dose ordered: 200 mg per dose × 3 = 600 mg per day
   c. Overdose. Hold and clarify promptly with prescriber.
   d. N/A

WORKSHEET 12F (page 430)

1. a. SDR for this child: 2.52 to 5.04 mg q4h-6h
   $0.1 \times 25.2 = 2.52$ mg
   $0.2 \times 25.2 = 5.04$ mg
   b. Dose ordered: 4 mg subcut
   c. Evaluation and decision: Safe to give
   d. Give 0.8 mL
   HAVE WANT TO HAVE
   5 mg : 1 mL = 4 mg : x mL
   $$\frac{\cancel{5}x}{\cancel{5}} = \frac{4}{5}$$
   $x = 0.8$ mL
   PROOF
   $5 \times 0.8 = 4$
   $1 \times 4 = 4$

2. a. SDR for a child between 7 and 9 kg: 0.2 mg
   b. Dose ordered: 0.2 mg
   c. Evaluation and decision: Safe to give
   d. Give 0.5 mL
   HAVE WANT TO HAVE
   0.4 mg : 1 mL = 0.2 mg : x mL
   $$\frac{\cancel{0.4}}{\cancel{0.4}}x = \frac{0.2}{0.4}$$
   $x = 0.5$ mL
   PROOF
   $0.4 \times 0.5 = 0.2$
   $1 \times 0.2 = 0.2$

3. a. SDR for this child: 320 to 640 mg per day (based on 3.2 kg wt)
   b. Dose ordered: 1000 mg per day
   c. Evaluation and decision: Overdose. Hold and clarify promptly. Also ask whether IV route is preferred.
   d. Not applicable.

4. a. SDR: 0.004×40 kg = 0.16 mg
   b. Dose ordered: 0.16 mg
   c. Evaluation and decision: Safe to give
   d. HAVE WANT TO HAVE
   0.2 mg : 1 mL = 0.16 mg : x mL
   $$\frac{\cancel{0.2}}{\cancel{0.2}}x = \frac{0.16}{0.2}$$
   $x = 0.8$ mL
   PROOF
   $0.2 \times 0.8 = 0.16$
   $1 \times 0.16 = 0.16$

5. a. 1 gram: 1000 mL; 2 grams per 2000 mL
   b. There is no plunger. It injects a hidden needle upon contact.
   c. 1 mg per mL (1000 mg = 1 g; 1000 mg : 1000 mL = 1 : 1
   d. 0.5 mg per mL
   e. Safe to give

WORKSHEET **12G** (page 434)

1. a. SDR for this child: 28.2 to 84.6 mg q24h

b. Dose ordered: 50 mg IV

c. Evaluation and decision: Safe to give

d. Dose withdrawn from vial: 0.77 mL

65 mg : 1 mL = 50 mg : x mL

$65x = 50$

$x = 0.769$ rounded to 0.77 mL

PROOF

$65 \times 0.769 = 49.9$

$1 \times 50 = 50$

2. a. SDR for this child: 25 to 150 mg (1 to 6 mg per kg)

$1 \times 25 = 25$

$6 \times 25 = 150$

b. Dose ordered: 25 mg IV stat

c. Evaluation and decision: Safe to give (The initial dose for this drug must not exceed the lowest dose in the SDR.)

d. Give 2.5 mL

HAVE WANT TO HAVE

40 mg : 4 mL = 25 mg : x mL

$\frac{40}{40}x = \frac{100}{40} (4 \times 25)$

$x = 2.5$ mL

PROOF

$40 \times 2.5 = 100$

$4 \times 25 = 100$

3. a. SDR for this child: 12 to 15 mg q8h

$2 \text{ mg} \times 6 \text{ kg} = 12 \text{ mg}$

$2.5 \text{ mg} \times 6 \text{ kg} = 15 \text{ mg}$

b. Dose ordered: 15 mg q8h

c. Evaluation and decision: Safe to give

d. Amount withdrawn from vial: Give 1.5 mL

HAVE WANT TO HAVE

20 mg : 2 mL = 15 mg : x mL $\left(\frac{10}{1} = \frac{15}{x}\right)$

$\frac{20}{20}x = \frac{30}{20}$

$x = 1.5$ mL

e. The 50 mL can be administered with a syringe pump or a volume-control device. Monitor urinary output hourly and during visits to bedside.*

4. a. SDR IV for this child: 0.17 mg to 3.9 mg per day

$0.015 \times 11.1 = 0.166$ rounded to 0.17 mg per day

$0.35 \times 11.1 = 3.88$ rounded to 3.9 mg per day

b. Dose ordered: 0.5 mg IV

c. Evaluation and decision: Safe to give. 0.5 mg is within the SDR

d. 2 mL (0.5 mg = 500 mcg) Label states 0.5 mg per 2 mL

e. Infuse at 1.6 mL per minute for 5 minutes

HAVE WANT TO HAVE

8 mL : 5 minutes = x mL : 1 minute

$5x = 8$ $\left(\frac{8 \text{ mL}}{5 \text{ minutes}} = \frac{x \text{ mL}}{1 \text{ minute}}\right)$

$x = 1.6$ mL

PROOF

$5 \times 1.6 = 8$

$8 \times 1 = 8$

5. a. SDR for this child: 590 to 5900 mg divided into 4 doses = 1475 mg maximum unit dose

$50 \times 11.8 = 590$

$500 \times 11.8 = 5900$

b. Dose ordered: 2 g or 2000 mg q6h

c. Evaluation and decision: Hold and clarify promptly (overdose)

d. Not applicable

e. Not applicable

---

*Dilute *"to"* is interpreted as, "Add diluent to the prepared medicine to make 50 mL total volume."
Dilution *"with"* a substance adds to the volume. Dilution "to" an amount does not add to the volume.

WORKSHEET 12H (page 436)

1. d 25 kg (lb ÷ 2 = rough estimate of kg)

2. c

$30 \text{ mg} : 1 \text{ m}^2 = x \text{ mg} : 1.20 \text{ m}^2$
$x = 30 \times 1.20$ or 36 mg

PROOF
$30 \times 1.2 = 36$
$1 \times 36 = 36$

3. b

5 mL = 1 tsp
5 mL : 1 tsp = x mL : 1.5 tsp
x = 7.5 mL
Measure 7.5 mL

PROOF
$5 \times 1.5 = 7.5$
$1 \times 7.5 = 7.5$

4. d If the taste is unpleasant or unfamiliar, the child may refuse the essential food.

5. b Administer the EpiPen first, then call 911; consult provider for any questions about use, how long to retain, and read the accompanying information and practice with the trainer.

6. c The sciatic nerve and blood vessels are close together in undeveloped gluteal muscles. Occasionally they may also be located in a different quadrant than the upper outer.

7. b

SDR
5 mg : 1 kg = x mg : 6 kg
$x = 5 \times 6$ or 30 mg

PROOF
$5 \times 6 = 30$
$1 \times 30 = 30$

Compare the SDR with the order. 30 mg ÷ 2 = 15 mg bid. The order is 15 mg bid.
The order is safe.

Step 3: Calculate the unit dose.
30 mg : 5 mL = 15 mg : x mL
$30x = 75 \times 2.5$ mL

PROOF
$30 \times 2.5 = 75$
$5 \times 15 = 75$

Give 2.5 mL using a syringe to measure, if necessary.

8. a Vastus lateralis is the largest developed muscle at that age.

9. d 20 mg per pound. Refer to the examples on page 420.

10. b The child associates the parent with the inflicted pain.

CHAPTER 12 FINAL: PEDIATRIC DOSAGES (page 439)

1. a. Ordered: 2 g per day = 2000 mg in 4 divided doses of 500 mg each
b. SDR: 1000 to 4000 mg per day in divided doses
c. Safe to give
d. 2 capsules four times a day

2. a. SDR: 120 to 180 mcg daily
b. Ordered: 0.15 mg daily
c. Safe to give, 0.15 mg = 150 mcg
d. 3 tablets

3. a. SDR for this child: 150 mg maximum (6×25 mg) in 24 hr in 4 to 6 divided doses
b. Dose ordered: 25 mg × 4 or 100 mg per day
c. Evaluation and decision: Safe to give
d. Dose to be administered: 2 tsp or 25 mg per dose

4. **a.** SDR: 233.3 to 466.67 mg per dose every 8 hr
   b. Ordered: 700 mg q8h
   c. Decision: Overdose; contact prescriber promptly
   d. Not applicable

5. **a.** SDR for this child: 0.3 mg (for 12- to 26-kg child)
   b. Dose ordered: 0.3 mg
   c. Decision: Safe to give (35 lb = 15.9 kg)
   d. Give 0.75 mL in anterolateral thigh.

6. **a.** SDR: 200 to 300 mg ÷ 2 = 100 mg to 175 mg per dose
   b. Decision: Safe to give
   c. 2 mL = 100 mg per dose at 50 mg per mL

7. **a.** 100,000 units (1 mL) each side of mouth
   b. the dropper; flow could be controlled and directed to desired areas more easily than the other devices, permitting a couple of applications over a few minutes

8. **a.** 1 : 1000 = 1 mg per mL (1 g per 1000 mL) = (1000 mg per 1000 mL), commonly ordered IM or subcut for allergic reactions; 1 : 10,000 = 0.1 mg per mL (1 g per 10,000 mL) = (1000 mg per 10,000 mL), more commonly order IV (more dilute)*
   b. Ten times difference
   c. 0.2 mL = 0.2 mg dose ordered (0.01 mg × 20 kg)
   d. Child would receive 10 times the ordered dose

9. **a.** BSA in m^2: 1.10 m^2
   b. SDR for this child: Up to 44 mg per day
   $1.10 \times 10 \times 4 = 44$
   c. Dose ordered: 40 mg per day
   d. Evaluation and decision: Safe to give.
   e. Give 2 tab.

10. **a.** 1980 mcg (90 mcg × 22 kg)
    b. 1.98 mg rounded to 2 mg

    KNOW WANT TO KNOW

    $$\frac{\cancel{1000}}{\cancel{1000}} x = \frac{198\cancel{0}}{100\cancel{0}}$$

    $x = 1.98$ mg rounded to 2 mg

    c. 2.2 mL
    1 mg : 1.1 mL = 2 mg : x mL
    $x = 2.2$ mL
    d. 2 vials
    e. 11 calibrations
    f. 0.7 mL per minute
    2.2 mL : 3 minutes = x mL : 1 minute
    $2.2x = 3$
    $x = 0.73$ mL per minute or approximately 0.7 mL per minute

    g.

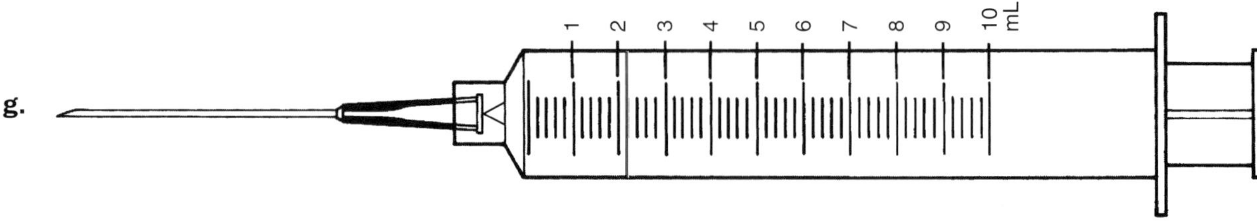

    h. a. 1.5 mL; b. 0.8 ml; c. 0

*Only use commercially prepared correct dilutions.

Multiple-Choice Final

Estimate reasonable answers when possible. Round kg to the nearest tenth. Round liquid oral and injection doses to the nearest tenth of a mL. Round IV flow rates to the nearest whole mL. Answers can be found on page 460.

1. **Ordered:** cimetidine 0.4 g tablet po twice daily for a patient with a gastric ulcer.
   Available: cimetidine 200 mg tablets. **Give how many tablet(s) each dose:**
   a. 0.5 tablet
   b. 1 tablet
   c. 2 tablets
   d. 4 tablets

2. **Ordered:** Klonopin (clonazepam) 1 mg tablet po stat for a patient who has seizures.
   Available: Klonopin (clonazepam) 0.5 mg tablets. **Give:**
   a. 0.5 tablet
   b. 1 tablet
   c. 2 tablets
   d. 4 tablets

3. **Ordered:** lanoxin 250 mcg tablet po daily in the a.m. for a patient with heart failure.
   Available: lanoxin 0.125 mg tablets, scored. **Give:**
   a. 2 tablets
   b. 1 tablet
   c. 0.5 tablet
   d. 0.25 tablet

4. What is the purpose of the Tall-Man Lettering promoted by the FDA, TJC, ISMP, and Clinical Pharmacology Organizations?*
   a. All prescription drug names are to be written legibly in tall letters so that pharmacy can input the correct orders on the EMAR.
   b. Drugs that have similar names need adjacent sections of letters that are written in uppercase to reduce confusion and errors.
   c. PRN drug orders must be written in capital letters to distinguish them from scheduled drugs.
   d. Patients who are over 6 feet tall must have their identification distinguished by Tall Man letters.

5. **Ordered:** naloxone HCl 0.6 mg IM stat to reverse effects of a narcotic overdose.
   Available: naloxone 400 mcg per mL. How many mL will you administer?
   a. 0.8 mL
   b. 1.1 mL
   c. 1.3 mL
   d. 1.5 mL

---

*Refer to http://ismp.org/tools/tallmanletters.pdf.

6. **Ordered:** Cipro (ciprofloxacin) 1.5 g tablets po bid for a patient with an infection. **Available:** Cipro (ciprofloxacin HCl) 500 mg tablets. **Give:**
   a. 0.5 tablet
   b. 1 tablet
   c. 2 tablets
   d. 3 tablets

7. **Ordered:** morphine sulfate 6 mg IM q4h prn for a patient with severe pain. **Give:**

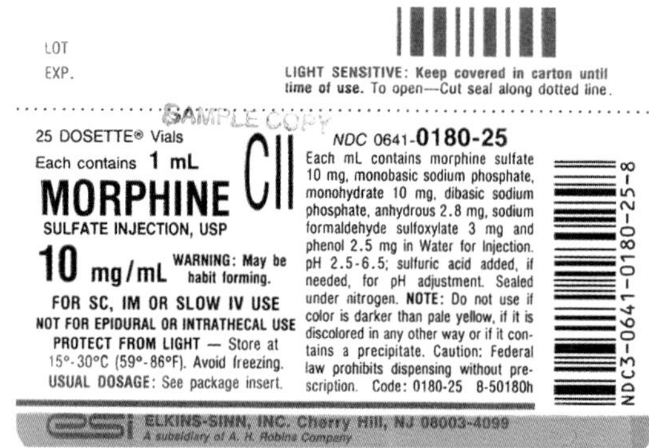

   a. 0.6 mL
   b. 0.8 mL
   c. 1 mL
   d. 1.2 mL

8. **Ordered:** glycopyrrolate 0.3 mg IM at 8 a.m. preoperatively to reduce excessive pharyngeal secretions and protect the heart from vagal stimulation. **Available:** glycopyrrolate injection 200 mcg per mL. Will you give more or less than the available unit dose? **Give:**
   a. 0.5 mL
   b. 0.7 mL
   c. 1.5 mL
   d. 2 mL

9. The nurse is trying to interpret a provider order that is illegible. What is the best action to take?
   a. Ask a staff nurse who works regularly on the floor.
   b. Check to see if something similar has been given before to the patient.
   c. Call the pharmacy.
   d. Call the provider.

10. **Ordered:** promethazine 25 mg IM stat for a patient with nausea. **Available:** promethazine HCl injection 75 mg per mL. **Give:**
   a. 0.3 mL
   b. 0.5 mL
   c. 1.25 mL
   d. 3 mL

11. Ordered: Ativan (lorazepam) 3 mg IM stat for an agitated patient. **Give** (to the nearest tenth of a milliliter):

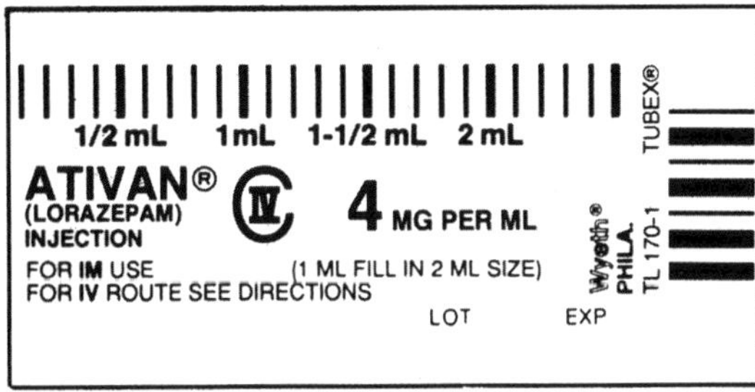

a. 0.8 mL
b. 1.2 mL
c. 1.3 mL
d. 1.4 mL

12. Ordered: oxacillin sodium 250 mg IM q6h for a patient with an upper respiratory infection. After reconstituting with sterile water for injection, what is the strength of the medication?

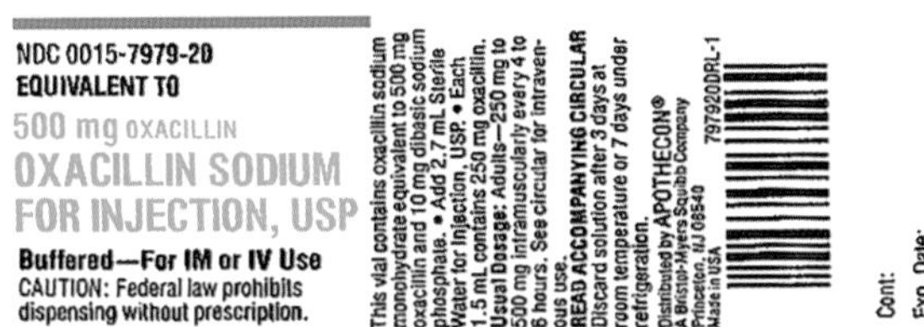

a. 250 mg per mL
b. 500 mg per mL
c. 2.7 mg per mL
d. 250 mg per 1.5 mL

How many milliliters will you administer?
a. 1.0 mL
b. 1.5 mL
c. 2.0 mL
d. 2.5 mL

13. Ordered: ampicillin 0.5 g IM q6h for a patient with an infected leg ulcer. After reconstituting with the accompanying diluent, how many milliliters will you administer?

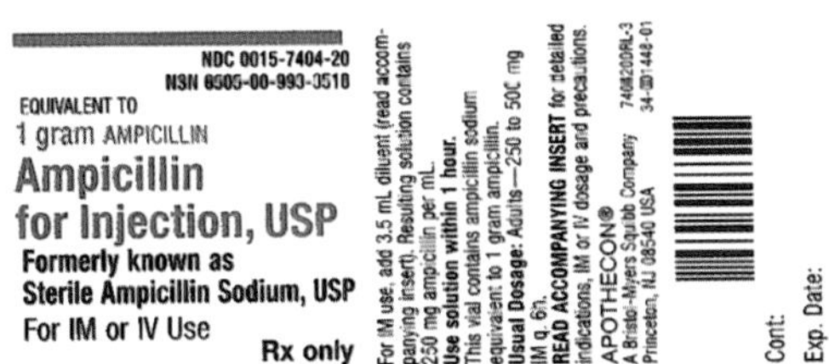

a. 1.6 mL
b. 2.0 mL
c. 1.5 mL
d. 3.5 mL

What is the shelf life of the medication?
a. 24 hours
b. 1 week, refrigerated
c. 1 hour
d. 48 hours

14. Ordered: penicillin G potassium 300,000 units IM q6h for a patient with tonsillitis. Available: Pfizerpen 1 million units for reconstitution for injection. If you add 4.0 mL of diluent, how many milliliters of medication will you give?

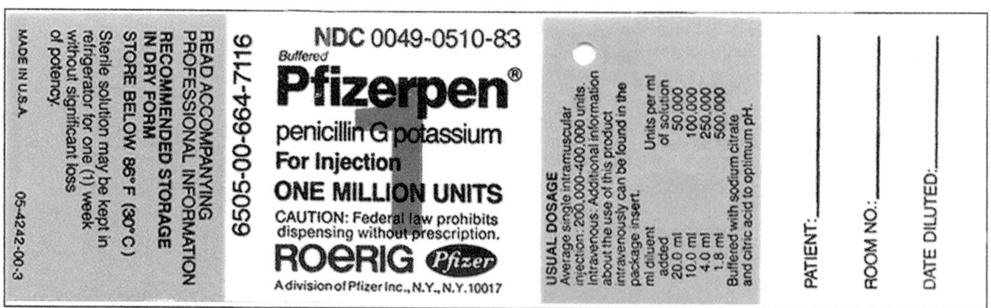

a. 2.0 mL
b. 2.4 mL
c. 1.2 mL
d. 0.5 mL

15. The IV is infusing at 30 gtt per minute. The drop factor is 20 gtt per mL. The IV label reads 500 mL 5% dextrose and 0.45% sodium chloride. The IV had been infusing for 1½ hours when you came on duty. How much longer does the IV have to infuse?

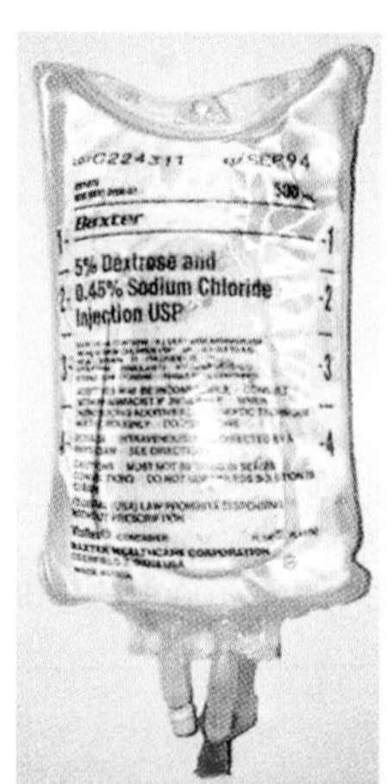

LOT EXP

2B1073
NDC 0338-0085-03 – 1

5% Dextrose and 0.45% Sodium Chloride Injection USP – 2

500 mL – 3

EACH 100 mL CONTAINS 5 g DEXTROSE HYDROUS USP 450 mg SODIUM CHLORIDE USP pH 4.0 (3.2 TO 6.5) mEq/L SODIUM 77 CHLORIDE 77 HYPERTONIC OSMOLARITY 406 mOsmol/L (CALC) STERILE NONPYROGENIC SINGLE DOSE CONTAINER ADDITIVES MAY BE INCOMPATIBLE CONSULT WITH PHARMACIST IF AVAILABLE WHEN INTRODUCING ADDITIVES USE ASEPTIC TECHNIQUE MIX THOROUGHLY DO NOT STORE DOSAGE – 4 INTRAVENOUSLY AS DIRECTED BY A PHYSICIAN SEE DIRECTIONS CAUTIONS SQUEEZE AND INSPECT INNER BAG WHICH MAINTAINS PRODUCT STERILITY DISCARD IF LEAKS ARE FOUND MUST NOT BE USED IN SERIES CONNECTIONS DO NOT USE UNLESS SOLUTION IS CLEAR FEDERAL (USA) LAW PROHIBITS DISPENSING WITHOUT PRESCRIPTION STORE UNIT IN MOISTURE BARRIER OVERWRAP AT ROOM TEMPERATURE (25°C/77°F) UNTIL READY TO USE AVOID EXCESSIVE HEAT SEE INSERT

Baxter
BAXTER HEALTHCARE CORPORATION
DEERFIELD IL 60015 USA
MADE IN USA

VIAFLEX® CONTAINER
PL 146® PLASTIC
FOR PRODUCT INFORMATION CALL 1-800-933-0303

a. 4 hours
b. 50 minutes
c. 3 hours
d. 3½ hours

16. Ordered: Monocid 600 mg IM. **Available:** cefonicid 1 g for reconstitution. How many milliliters will you administer?

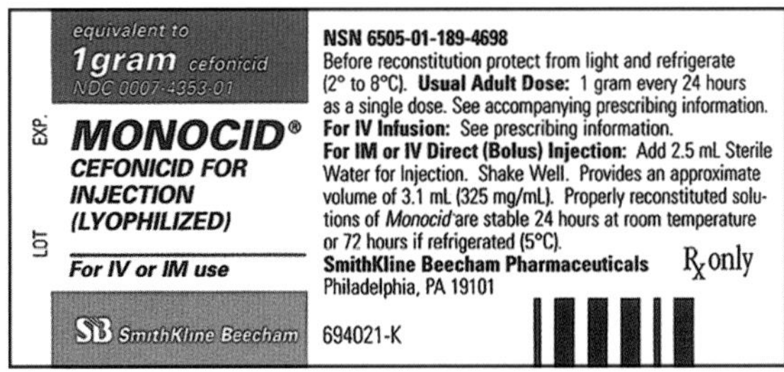

a. 1.8 mL
b. 0.7 mL
c. 1.3 mL
d. 1.5 mL

17. Ordered: 1000 mL D5W IV to infuse at 125 mL per hr on admission. The drop factor is 20. How many gtt per min will you set the IV to infuse?

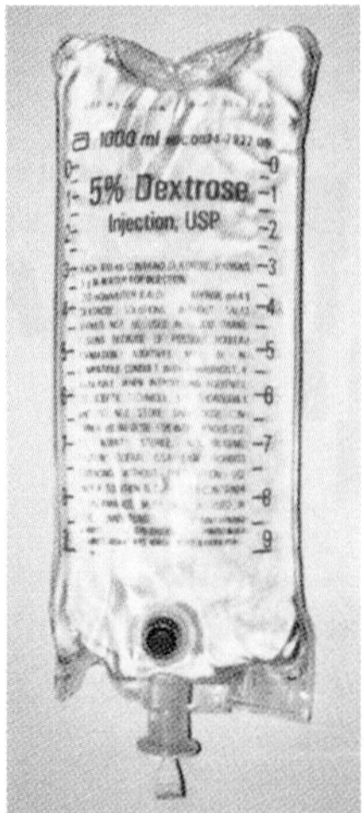

a. 12 gtt per min
b. 22 gtt per min
c. 20 gtt per min
d. 42 gtt per min

18. Ordered: ampicillin 1 g IV bid. **Available:** ampicillin 1 g for IV use. **Directions:** Add 4.5 mL of sodium chloride diluent to yield 5 mL. Dilute with normal saline to 50 mL and infuse in 30 minutes. On hand you have a microdrip infusion set. At how many drops per min will you set the IV?

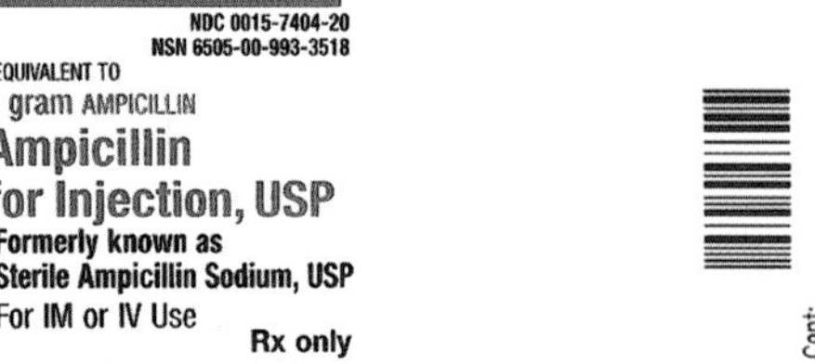

a. 100 drops per minute
b. 150 drops per minute
c. 200 drops per minute
d. 250 drops per minute

19. The pharmacy standard insulin drip is 100 units of Humulin Regular in 250 mL of normal saline. 1 unit = 2.5 mL. The patient's blood sugar level is 218 mg per dL. Use the following chart to determine the correct insulin rate for the IV. How many units per hr should the patient receive?

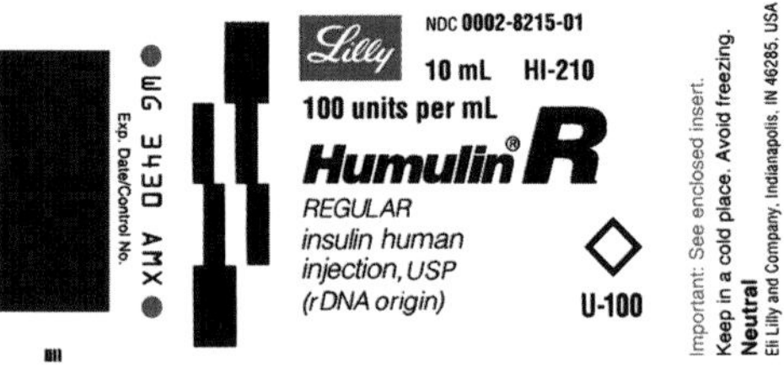

Blood Sugar (BS) per dL	Standard Rate in units per hr
101-140	1.0
141-180	1.5
181-220	2.0
221-260	2.5
261-300	3.0

a. 1.5 units per hr
b. 2.5 units per hr
c. 2.0 units per hr
d. 3.0 units per hr

At what rate will you set the IV infusion device?
a. 3 mL per hr
b. 4 mL per hr
c. 5 mL per hr
d. 6 mL per hr

20. Ordered: Novolin R insulin 15 units per hr IV for a patient having surgery. **Available:** 250 mL of sodium chloride 0.9% with 100 units of Humulin R insulin. At how many mL per hr will you need to set the electronic infusion device?

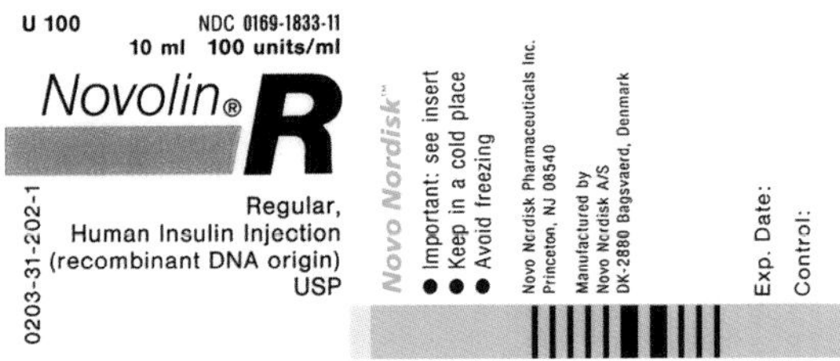

a. 56 mL per hr
b. 38 mL per hr
c. 33 mL per hr
d. 58 mL per hr

How many hours will it take to infuse the 250 mL?
a. 5 hr 30 min
b. 6 hr 36 min
c. 9 hr 40 min
d. 8 hr

21. Ordered: heparin sodium 10,000 units IV in 15 hr for a patient after hip surgery. **Available:** pharmacy has sent 1000 mL of normal saline solution with 10,000 units of heparin sodium. At how many mL per hr will you set the IV infusion device?
a. 67 mL per hr
b. 125 mL per hr
c. 83 mL per hr
d. 100 mL per hr

If the IV described above was started at 2000 hr on 10/21, when should it be finished?
a. 10/22 at 0900 hr
b. 10/23 at 0200 hr
c. 10/23 at 1000 hr
d. 10/22 at 1100 hr

22. Ordered: Fragmin 15,000 units subcutaneous for a patient with a deep venous thrombosis (DVT). **Available:** Fragmin in 9.5-mL multidose vial. The label reads: 1 mL = 10,000 units. How many milliliters will you give?

10,000 international units/mL
9.5 mL multidose vial
NDC 0013-2436-06

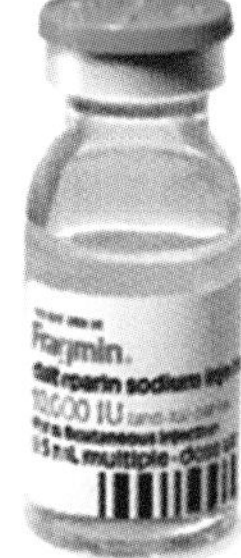

(Used with permission from Pfizer, Inc.)

a. 1.8 mL
b. 2 mL
c. 1.5 mL
d. 1.2 mL

23. A blood sugar level (BS) of 120 mg per dL is desired. **Ordered:** give 1 unit Regular insulin for every 8 mg above 120 mg per dL; give 1 unit of Regular insulin for each 8 g of CHO consumed. The BS is 200 mg per dL. The amount of CHO consumed is 112 g. How many total units of insulin will the patient receive?

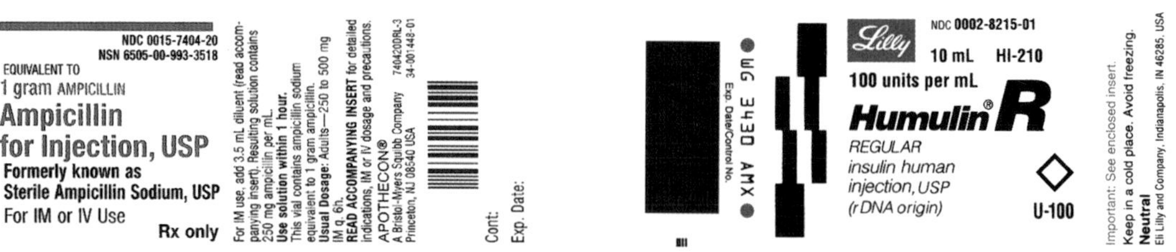

a. 10 units
b. 13 units
c. 24 units
d. 28 units

24. **Ordered:** IV heparin to infuse at 20 units per kg per hr. **Available:** 1000 mL D5W with 25,000 units of heparin sodium. Patient's weight: 176 lbs. How many units per hour will the patient receive on the electronic infusion device?
a. 160 units
b. 1600 units
c. 1620 units
d. 1640 units

At how many mL per hr will you set the infusion device?
a. 58 mL per hr
b. 48 mL per hr
c. 66 mL per hr
d. 64 mL per hr

25. **Ordered:** 90 units per kg of heparin for a loading dose. After the loading dose has been administered, set the maintenance continuous infusion to run at 1200 units per hr. **Available:** 500 mL NS with 25,000 units of heparin. Patient's weight: 176 lb (80 kg). How many units will you give as the loading dose?
a. 5700 units
b. 6900 units
c. 7000 units
d. 7200 units

At how many mL per hr will you set the continuous infusion?
a. 84 mL per hr
b. 60 mL per hr
c. 64 mL per hr
d. 24 mL per hr

26. The patient has a TPN solution for nutritional therapy with 8.5% amino acids in 375 mL. The total volume (TV) is 1500 mL. How many grams of protein will the patient receive? Use the following formula for calculating the amino acids.
Step 1: % × mL = g per L
Step 2: g per L × TV per L = g per bag
a. 8.5 g per bag
b. 47.8 g per bag
c. 478 g per bag
d. 31.8 g per bag

27. **Ordered:** A maintenance dose of methotrexate 30 mg per m^2 po for a child with lymphocytic leukemia. Patient's weight: 30 lb, which is equivalent to a BSA of 0.6 m^2. **Give:**

a. 12 mg
b. 15 mg
c. 18 mg
d. 20 mg

28. **Ordered:** Dobutrex HCl to be infused at 4 mcg per kg per minute for a patient with cardiac decompensation. Patient's weight: 50 kg. **Available:** Dobutrex solution (dobutamine HCl solution) 500 mg in 250 mL (2 mg per mL). Given the total drug in mg to total solution ratio, how many mL per hr should be infused?

a. 12 mL per hr
b. 10 mL per hr
c. 8 mL per hr
d. 6 mL per hr

29. **Ordered:** morphine sulfate 5 mg IV push for a patient in severe pain. **Directions:** Dilute to 5 mL with NS or sterile water for injection and administer over 5 minutes. Identify the correct total dose and mL per minute to inject.

a. Administer 5 mL at 1 mL per minute
b. Administer 5 mL at 0.4 mL per minute
c. Administer 6 mL at 0.4 mL per minute
d. Administer 8 mL at 0.03 mL per minute

SEAL
NDC 10019-179-63

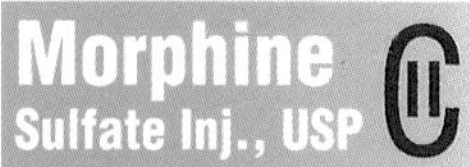

15 mg/mL ℞ only
FOR SC, IM OR
SLOW IV USE
NOT FOR EPIDURAL OR
INTRATHECAL USE
20 mL
Multiple Dose Vial

Baxter ESILEDERLE™
Mfd. for an affiliate of
Baxter Healthcare Corporation
Deerfield, IL 60015 USA
by: Elkins-Sinn
Cherry Hill, NJ 08003

30. **Ordered:** A diuretic, furosemide 15 mg IV stat for a child with edema. Dosing is based on weight in kilograms; patient's weight: 14 kg. SDR: 1 to 2 mg per kg per dose IV every 6 to 12 hours. Your decision:

a. Give 15 mg. The order is within the safe dose range.
b. Hold. Contact the physician promptly and clarify. The order is an underdose.
c. Hold. Contact the physician promptly and clarify. The order is an overdose.
d. Hold. The order is unclear.

Answer Key

Multiple-Choice Final

1. c
2. c
3. a
4. b
5. d
6. d
7. a
8. More; c
9. d
10. a
11. a
12. d; b
13. b; c
14. c
15. a
16. a
17. d
18. a
19. c; c
20. b; b
21. a; d
22. c
23. c
24. b; d
25. d; d
26. b
27. c
28. d
29. a
30. a

Comprehensive Final

Estimate answers and then solve the following problems. Prove your answers. Answers can be found on page 472.

1. **Ordered:** Nitrostat 600 mcg SL tablets every 5 minutes × 3, prn angina (chest pain). Call provider if relief not obtained with 3 tablets.
   a. What is the dose in milligrams?
   b. What route is ordered?

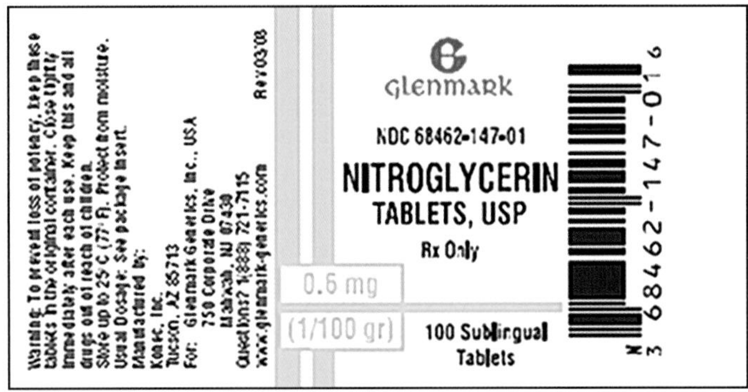

Glenmark
NDC 68462-147-01
NITROGLYCERIN
TABLETS, USP
Rx Only
0.6 mg
(1/100 gr)
100 Sublingual Tablets

2. **Ordered:** Septra DS 80/400 tab PO daily for a urinary tract infection.
   a. How many tablets will you give?
   b. How is DS different from abbreviations such as E-R, X-L, S-R, D-R, and so forth?

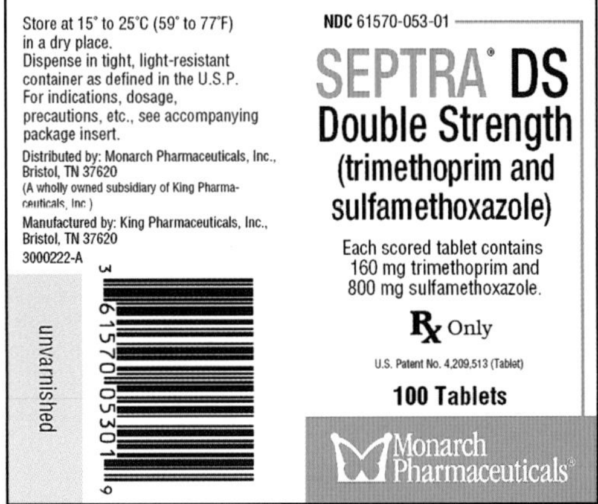

Store at 15° to 25°C (59° to 77°F) in a dry place.
Dispense in tight, light-resistant container as defined in the U.S.P.
For indications, dosage, precautions, etc., see accompanying package insert.
Distributed by: Monarch Pharmaceuticals, Inc., Bristol, TN 37620
(A wholly owned subsidiary of King Pharmaceuticals, Inc.)
Manufactured by: King Pharmaceuticals, Inc., Bristol, TN 37620
3000222-A
unvarnished
NDC 61570-053-01
SEPTRA® DS
Double Strength
(trimethoprim and sulfamethoxazole)
Each scored tablet contains 160 mg trimethoprim and 800 mg sulfamethoxazole.
Rx Only
U.S. Patent No. 4,209,513 (Tablet)
100 Tablets
Monarch Pharmaceuticals

3. **Ordered:** carbamazepine chewable tablet 0.3 g daily for a patient with seizures. **Available:** carbamazepine 100 mg chewable tablets. How many tablets will you give?

4. **Ordered:** diltiazem HCl 0.12 g at bedtime daily for a patient with high blood pressure. How many tablets will you give?

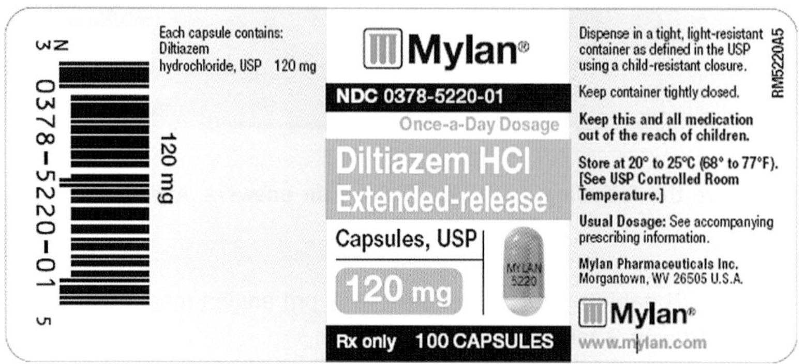

5. **Ordered as a discharge prescription:** zidovudine syrup 0.2 g po bid for a patient who is HIV positive. **Available:** zidovudine syrup 50 mg per 5 mL.
   a. How many mL will you instruct the patient to take?
   b. What kind of equipment should the patient use to measure the medication?

6. **Ordered:** isoniazid 0.6 g po daily for 9 months as preventive therapy for an adult patient with a positive test result for latent tuberculosis infection (LTBI); patient has positive test results for presence of TB bacteria without any active signs and symptoms. Patient weighs 264 lb. SDR for patients with LTBI ages 11 to adult is 5 mg per kg daily for 9 months. **Available:** isoniazid tablets 300 mg.
   a. Is the ordered dosage safe?
   b. How many tablets will you give?

7. **Ordered:** fluoxetine hydrochloride (Prozac) oral solution 30 mg po for a patient with anxiety. **Available:** Prozac oral solution 20 mg per 5 mL. How many mL will you administer? Shade in the medicine cup with the nearest measurable dose. Mark the syringe provided with the additional amount needed to the nearest measurable dose.

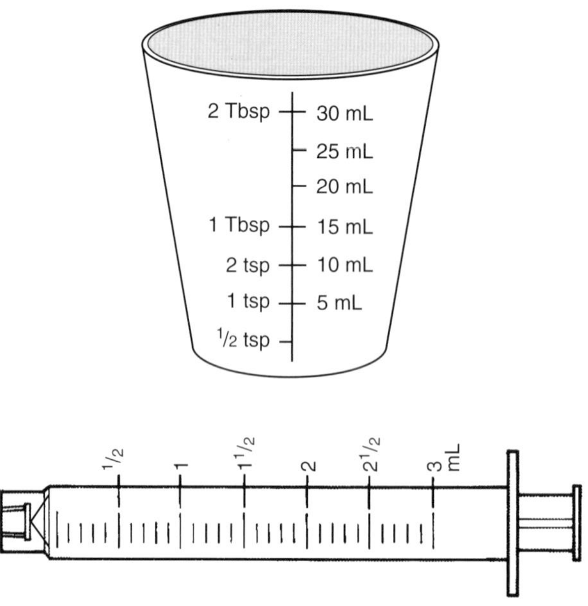

8. **Ordered:** butorphanol tartrate 0.8 mg IM stat for a patient with a severe migraine headache. **Available:** butorphanol tartrate 2 mg per mL.

   a. Would you give *more* or *less* than 1 mL?

   b. How many mL (to the nearest measurable amount) will be needed? Indicate the amount on the syringe.

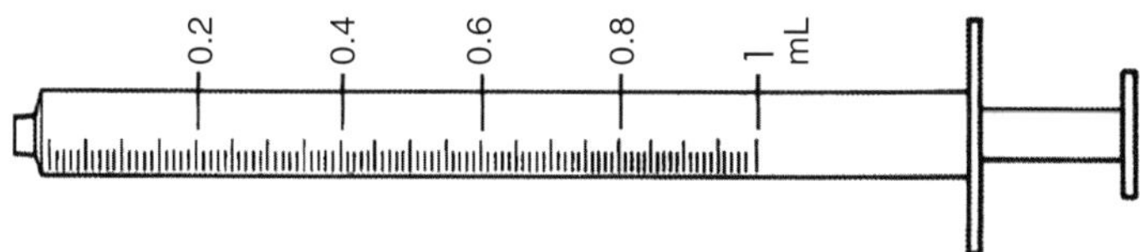

9. **Ordered:** morphine sulfate, an opioid narcotic, 10 mg IM q4h prn pain; last administered by Nurse A, according to the MAR, at 0800 hr.
Given: Morphine 10 mg IM at 0845 hr by Nurse B, a busy staff nurse who covered Nurse A's patient during Nurse A's break.
Error:
Nurse actions:
How could this error have occurred? What are some ways it might have been prevented?

10. **Ordered:** haloperidol decanoate LA 60 mg IM every 28 days for an adult patient with schizophrenia. SDR for monthly dosing not to exceed 100 mg. **Available:** haloperidol decanoate LA inj 75 mg per mL. How many mL will you give? Mark on syringe.

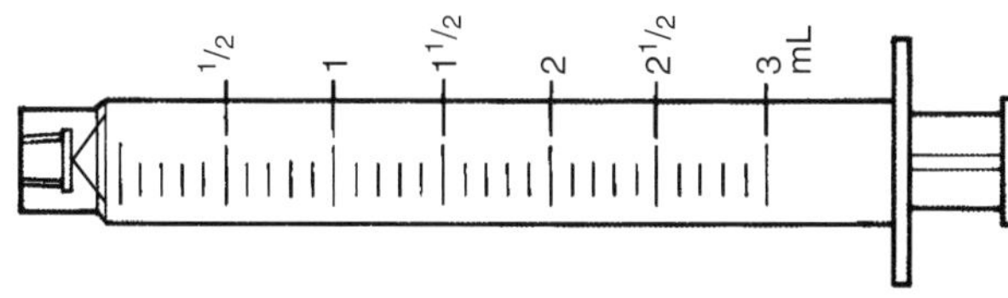

11. **Ordered:** atropine sulfate 0.6 mg IV for a patient with bradycardia, an apical pulse 40 beats per minute. **Available:** atropine sulfate inj 0.4 mg per mL. How many mL (to the nearest tenth of a mL) will you administer? Mark on syringe.

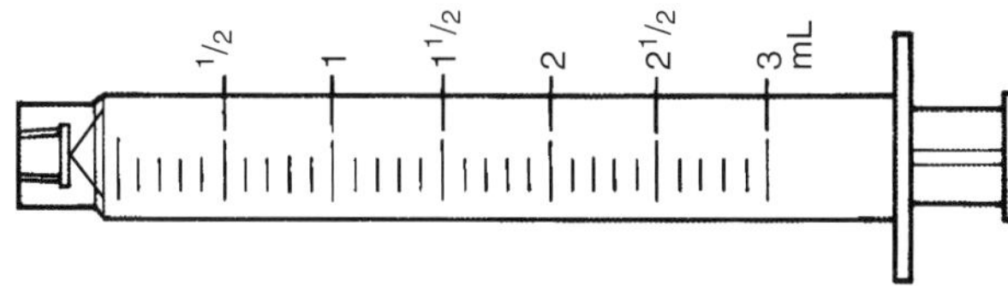

12. Ordered: ceftriaxone 300 mg IM q4h for a patient with pelvic inflammatory disease. **Available:** ceftriaxone 500 mg for reconstitution. How many milliliters will you give? Shade in the amount on the syringe.

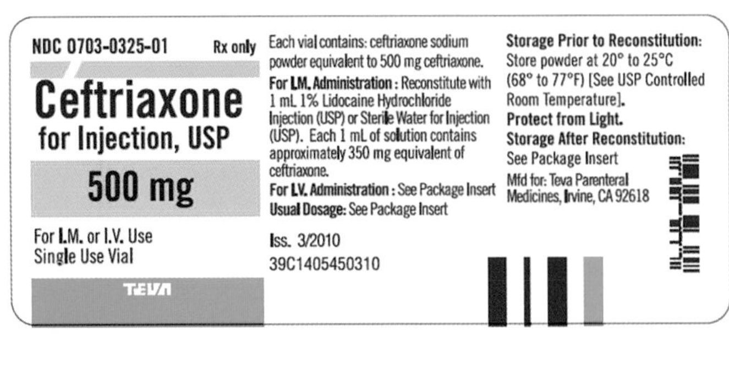

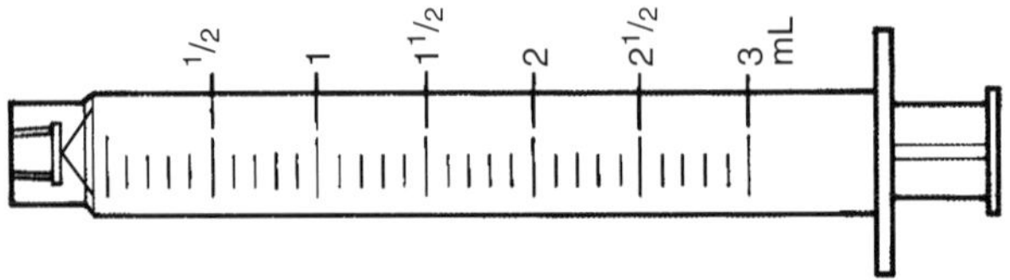

13. Ordered: Cefadyl 500 mg IM q8h for a patient with cellulitis. **Available:** Cefadyl 1 g for reconstitution.

a. How much diluent will you add?

b. How many milliliters will you give per dose? Shade in the syringe.

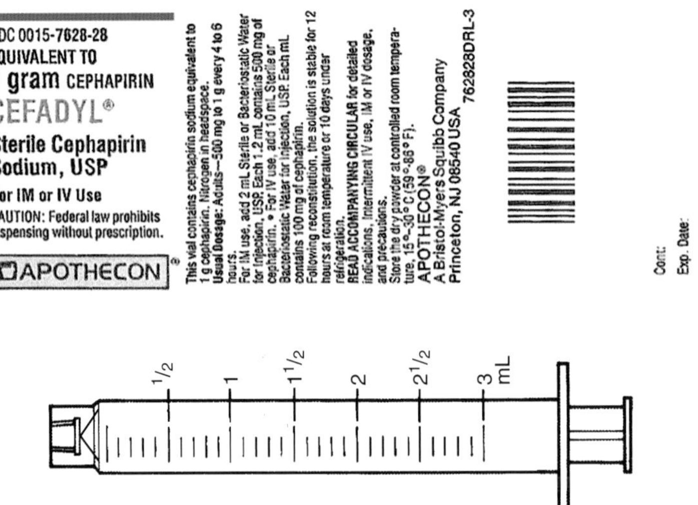

14. Ordered: MethylPREDNISolone 20 mg IM daily for 7 days for a patient with lumbar pain.
Available: MethylPREDNISolone sodium 40 mg for reconstitution.

a. How many milliliters of bacteriostatic water will you use to reconstitute?

b. How many milliliters will you give? Fill in amount on syringe.

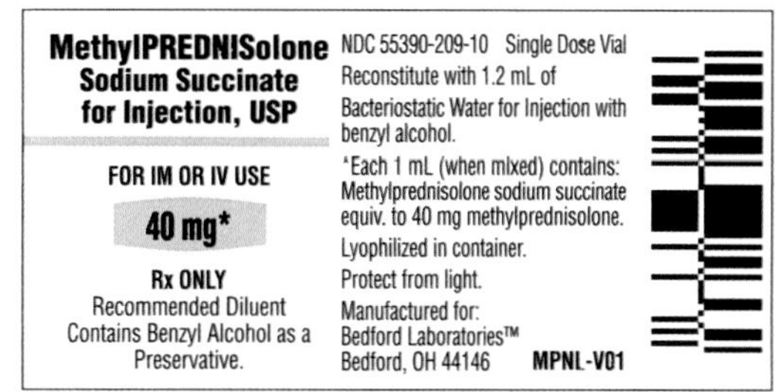

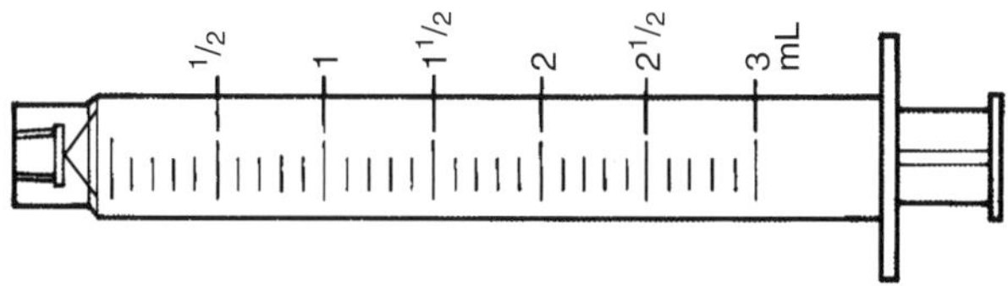

15. Ordered: 2000 mL D5/Ringer's lactate solution to be infused in 24 hr for hydration. The drop factor is 10.

a. How many gtt per min will be infused via gravity infusion?

b. How many mL per hr will be infused by an electronic device?

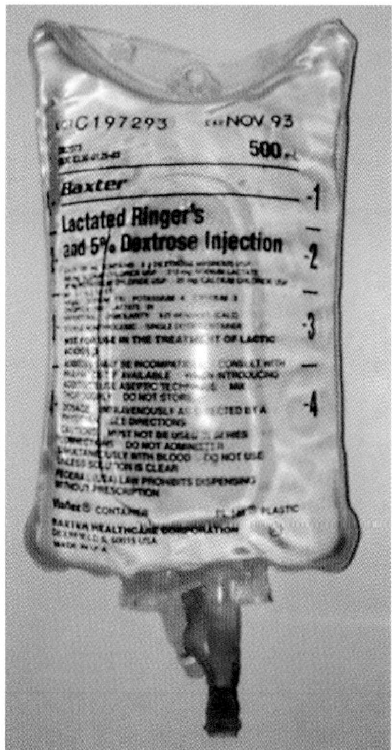

16. Ordered: Gentamicin 60 mg in 50 mL, IVPB for pneumonitis. Infuse in 40 minutes.

a. At how many mL per hr will you set the electronic infusion device?

b. How many gtt per min will be infused by a microdrip set?

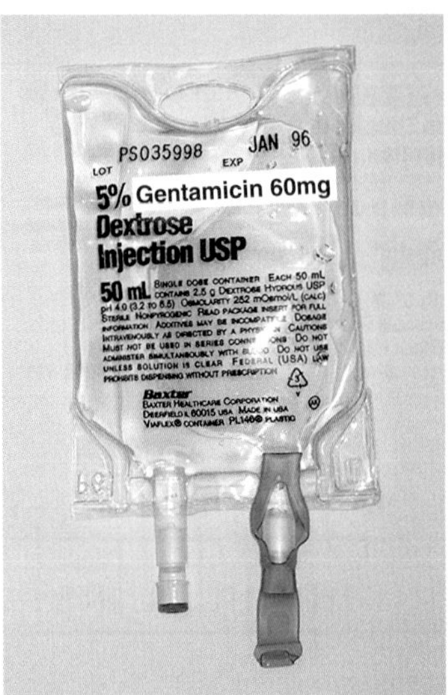

17. Ordered: 1000 mL D5NS followed by 1000 mL D5W, then 500 mL NS to infuse in 24 hr for hydration. The drop factor is 15.

a. At how many mL per hr will you set the electronic infusion device to deliver 2500 mL in 24 hr?

b. At how many gtt per min will you regulate the IV?

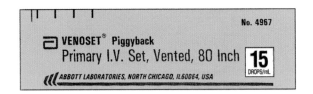

18. The patient's blood sugar (BS) at 0600 hr is 176 mg per dL. According to the titration schedule, Lantus will be increased to how many units per day? Shade in the amount on the insulin syringe.

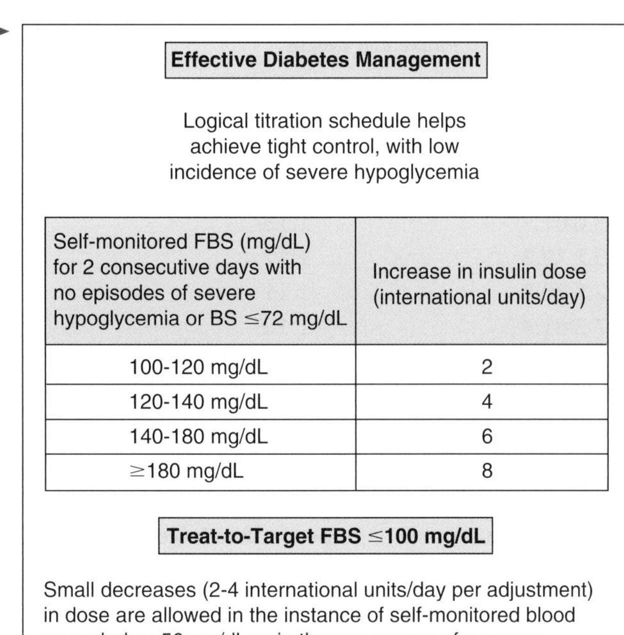

Effective Diabetes Management

Logical titration schedule helps achieve tight control, with low incidence of severe hypoglycemia

Self-monitored FBS (mg/dL) for 2 consecutive days with no episodes of severe hypoglycemia or BS ≤72 mg/dL	Increase in insulin dose (international units/day)
100-120 mg/dL	2
120-140 mg/dL	4
140-180 mg/dL	6
≥180 mg/dL	8

Treat-to-Target FBS ≤100 mg/dL

Small decreases (2-4 international units/day per adjustment) in dose are allowed in the instance of self-monitored blood sugar below 56 mg/dL or in the occurrence of a severe hypoglycemic episode.

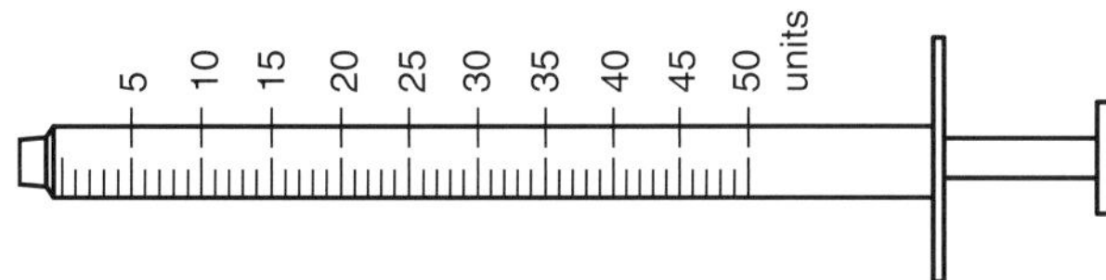

19. Ordered: Humulin R insulin 50 units in 500 mL of 0.9% NS IV to infuse at 2 units per hr. At what rate will you set the IV infusion device?

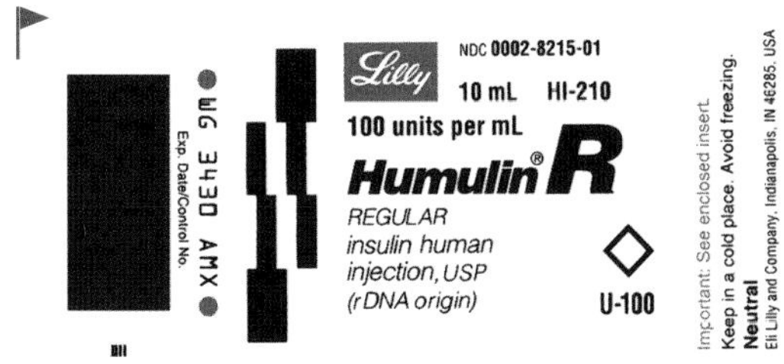

20. Ordered: The patient consumed 25 g CHO for breakfast, 95 g CHO for lunch, and 35 g CHO for dinner. Patient weight: 83 kg. How many total units of R has the patient received based on the units-to-CHO ratio chart?

Insulin Units Required Based on CHO Intake and Weight

Weight in Pounds	Weight in kg	Unit: grams of CHO
100-109	45.5-49.5	1:16
110-129	50-58.6	1:15
130-139	59-63.2	1:14
140-149	63.6-67.7	1:13
150-159	68.2-72.3	1:12
160-169	72.7-76.8	1:11
170-179	77.3-81.4	1:10
180-189	81.8-85.9	1:9
190-198	86.4-90	1:8
200-239	90.9-108.6	1:7
240+	109.1+	1:6

21. Ordered: Regular Humulin insulin to infuse at 3 units per hr. **Available:** 250 mL NS with 40 units of Humulin R insulin.

a. At how many mL per hr will you set the electronic infusion device?

b. The IV was started at 0830. At what hour will the IV be complete?

22. Ordered: Heparin injection 4000 units subcutaneous q12h before surgery. **Available:** A multi-dose vial of Heparin sodium injection. How many milliliters will you give? Shade in the amount on the syringe.

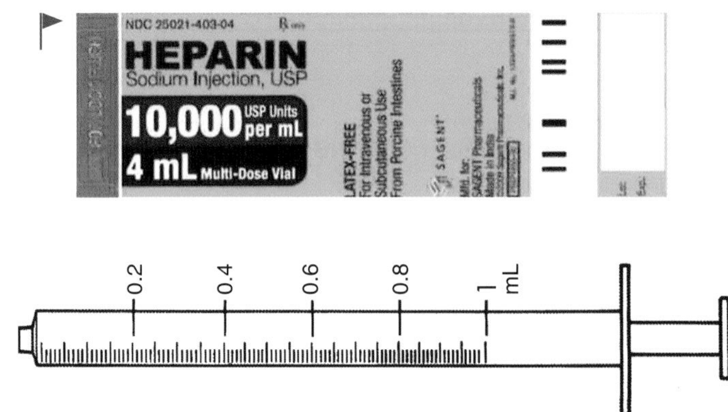

23. Ordered: heparin sodium 1000 units per hr IV. The pharmacy sent 1000 mL of 0.9% sodium chloride with 20,000 units of heparin sodium for a patient with a DVT.

a. At what rate will you set the infusion device?

b. What is the antidote for heparin?

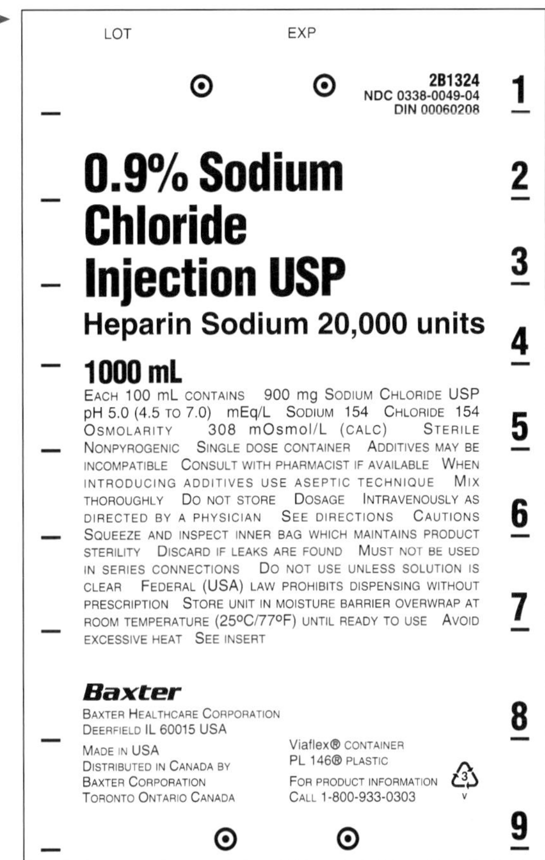
LOT
EXP
2B1324
NDC 0338-0049-04
DIN 00060208
0.9% Sodium Chloride Injection USP
Heparin Sodium 20,000 units
1000 mL
EACH 100 mL CONTAINS 900 mg SODIUM CHLORIDE USP pH 5.0 (4.5 TO 7.0) mEq/L SODIUM 154 CHLORIDE 154 OSMOLARITY 308 mOsmol/L (CALC) STERILE NONPYROGENIC SINGLE DOSE CONTAINER ADDITIVES MAY BE INCOMPATIBLE CONSULT WITH PHARMACIST IF AVAILABLE WHEN INTRODUCING ADDITIVES USE ASEPTIC TECHNIQUE MIX THOROUGHLY DO NOT STORE DOSAGE INTRAVENOUSLY AS DIRECTED BY A PHYSICIAN SEE DIRECTIONS CAUTIONS SQUEEZE AND INSPECT INNER BAG WHICH MAINTAINS PRODUCT STERILITY DISCARD IF LEAKS ARE FOUND MUST NOT BE USED IN SERIES CONNECTIONS DO NOT USE UNLESS SOLUTION IS CLEAR FEDERAL (USA) LAW PROHIBITS DISPENSING WITHOUT PRESCRIPTION STORE UNIT IN MOISTURE BARRIER OVERWRAP AT ROOM TEMPERATURE (25°C/77°F) UNTIL READY TO USE AVOID EXCESSIVE HEAT SEE INSERT
Baxter
BAXTER HEALTHCARE CORPORATION
DEERFIELD IL 60015 USA
MADE IN USA
DISTRIBUTED IN CANADA BY
BAXTER CORPORATION
TORONTO ONTARIO CANADA
Viaflex® CONTAINER
PL 146® PLASTIC
FOR PRODUCT INFORMATION
CALL 1-800-933-0303
1
2
3
4
5
6
7
8
9

24. Ordered: Loading dose of IV heparin at 82 units per kg. Set continuous maintenance infusion to follow at 18 units per kg per hr. **Available:** 500 mL D5W with 20,000 units of heparin. The patient weighs 160 lb. 160 divided by 2.2 = 72.7 rounded to 73kg. Round kg to nearest whole number.

a. How many units of heparin will you give for the bolus loading dose?

b. How many units per hr will infuse?

c. How many hours will it take to infuse?

d. At what rate will you set the infusion device to deliver 18 units per kg per hr?

25. Calculate the grams of amino acids, dextrose, and lipids per bag the patient on nutritional therapy will receive. Use the following formulas on the TPN label below. The total volume is 1158 mL.

Step 1: % × mL = g per L

Step 2: g per L × TV per L = g per bag

TPN Label

a. Ordered: amino acids 5.5% in 300 mL for a patient needing hyperalimentation.

b. Ordered: dextrose 10% in 250 mL for a patient needing hyperalimentation.

c. Ordered: lipids 15% in 125 mL for a patient needing hyperalimentation.

26. Using the answers from Problem 25, how many total kilocalories will the patient receive?

27. The pharmacy has supplied potassium chloride (KCl) 15 mEq in an IV of 500 mL D5W.

a. How many mEq per mL are there on the available label for concentrated KCl?

b. How many mg per mL are there on the available label?

c. How many mL of the concentrated KCl would the pharmacy have added to prepare the IV solution?

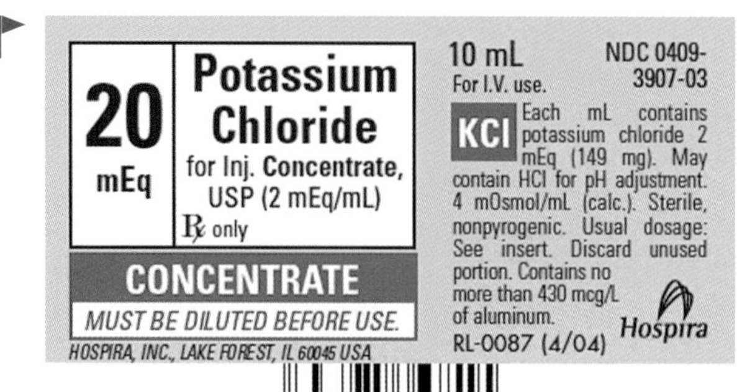

28. Ordered: Thorazine 2 mg IV injection for an agitated patient. **Directions:** Dilute each 25 mg (1 mL) with 24 mL of sterile NS for injection. Each mL will contain 1 mg. Give at slow rate of 1 mg per min.

NSN 6505-01-156-1981
Dilute before I.V. use. Store below 86°F
Do not freeze. Protect from light.
Each mL contains, in aqueous solution, chlorpromazine hydrochloride, 25 mg; ascorbic acid, 2 mg; sodium bisulfite, 1 mg; sodium sulfite, 1 mg; sodium chloride, 1 mg. Contains benzyl alcohol, 2%, as preservative. See accompanying prescribing information. For deep I.M. injection.
Caution: Federal law prohibits dispensing without prescription.
Manufactured by **SmithKline Beecham Pharmaceuticals**, Philadelphia, PA 19101
Marketed by SCIOS NOVA INC.
LOT EXP.
693897-AE

25mg/mL
NDC 0007-5062-01
THORAZINE®
CHLORPROMAZINE HCl INJECTION
10 mL Multi-Dose Vial
SB SmithKline Beecham

a. Total milliliters to be injected (shade in amount on syringe)

b. Total time in *seconds* to be injected

c. mL per min to be injected for how many minutes

d. Seconds to be injected per calibration

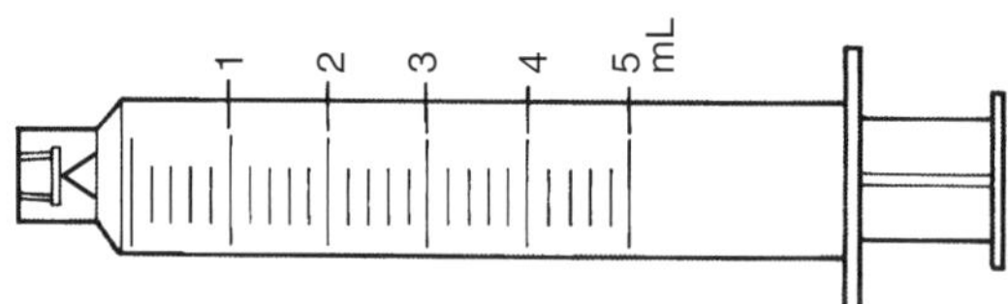

29. Ordered: Leucovorin calcium tablets 0.01 g po for a child who has delayed excretion of the anticancer drug methotrexate. The SDR is 10 mg/m^2. Patient weight: 70 lb with a BSA of 1.10 m^2. **Available:** Leucovorin calcium tablets 5 mg.

a. How many tablets (to the nearest whole number) will you give?

b. Which of the following orders would yield the lowest dose? mg per m^2, mg per lb, or mg per kg?

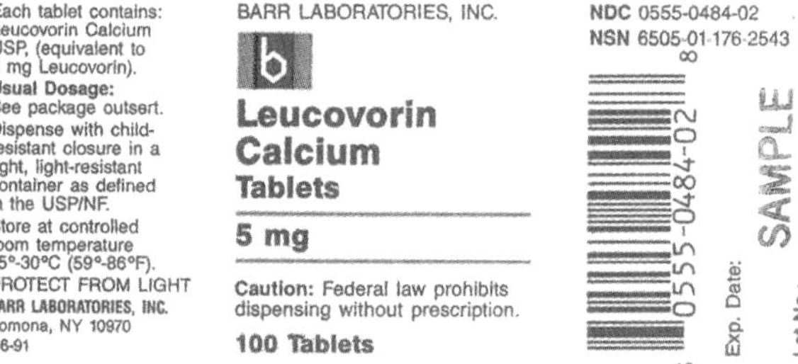

30. Ordered: DOPAmine IV infusion 5 mcg per kg per min for an adult with cardiac decompensation. The dopamine is infusing at 30 mL per hr on an infusion pump with an IV container of 200 mg per 250 mL D5W. Patient weight: 80 kg.

a. How many mcg per hr are ordered?

b. How many mg per hr are ordered?

c. How many mg per mL are in the solution (to the nearest tenth of a mg)?

d. Is the flow rate correct?

Answer Key

Comprehensive Final

1. a. 0.6 mg
   b. sublingual (SL) (under the tongue)

2. a. Give ½ tablet
   b. DS only refers to double strength/concentration compared to the regular strength. Note that DS medication is released *as soon as it is dissolved.* Extended-release medications are *released slowly (extended)* over a *longer* period of time and often are characterized by separate small, coated sprinkles. Extended-release formulation reduces the number of medications the patient has to take each day. Delayed-release medications are coated to avoid gastric irritation and are released *as soon as the coating dissolves.* Underdosing and overdosing ADE have been made because of confusion about these abbreviations.

3. 3 tablets

4. None. The order called for regular-strength tablets. Extended-release tablets were supplied. Reconfirm the order and contact pharmacy if there is a mismatch.

5. a. 20 mL.
   b. Instruct the patient to use a metric-calibrated medicine cup and to rinse it after use.

6. a. The ordered dose is safe.
   b. Give 2 tablets; emphasize adherence.

7. 7.5 mL

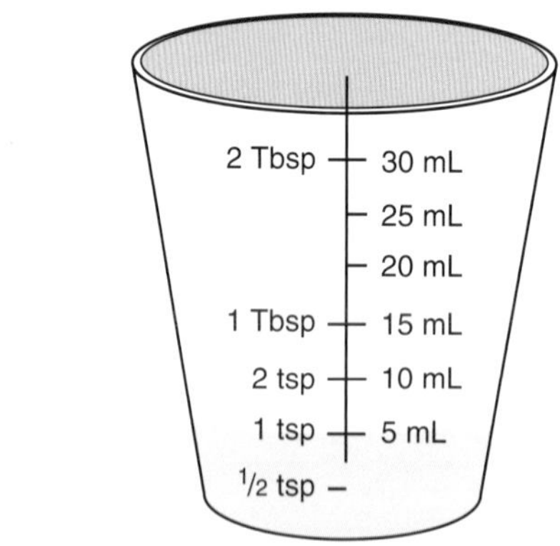

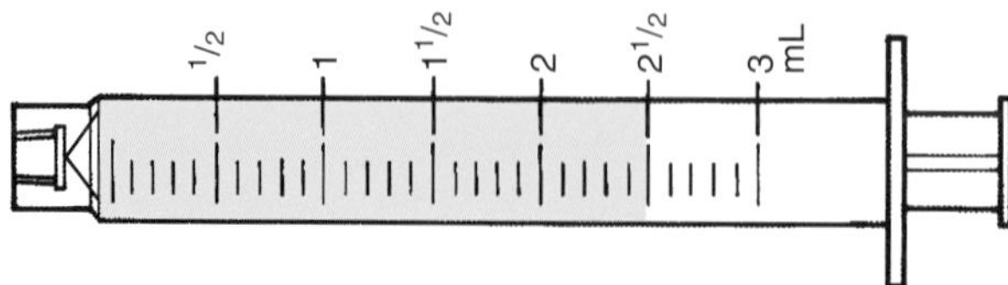

8. a. Less
b. Give 0.4 mL

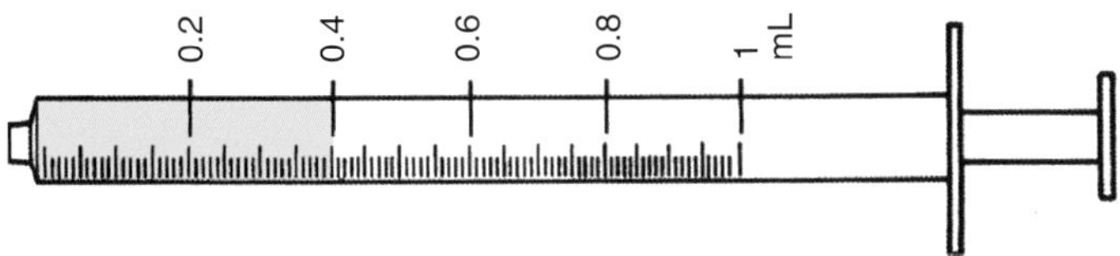

9. Error: 0845 Dose given 45 minutes after prior dose. Order stated q4h intervals prn.

Current Actions: Prescribe complete bed rest for patient, assess mental status and vital signs, notify supervising nurse or charge nurse and physician immediately, and obtain orders for medication to reverse.

Establish a patent IV line according to hospital policy in case emergency care may be needed.

Have crash cart close at hand. Document the error and to whom reported, patient evaluations, and all interventions, and continue to make the above assessments and evaluate. Fill out incident report. Continue to assess and evaluate patient every 5 to 15 minutes until patient is stabilized, then gradually extend assessment time.

Prevention: prn and stat medications must be charted as soon as possible after administration. Nurse A needed to report to Nurse B orally when her patients were due for their next prn medications. Nurse B needed to state she was too busy to care for additional patients beyond her own caseload. Nurse B needed to check record carefully to see when last medication for pain was given. Nurse B needed to ask patient when last medication for pain was received. (This is a recommended double-check but is not always reliable. The accuracy of response depends on the patient's mental status.) Refer to Hand-off Communication Report, Appendix A.

10. 0.8 mL

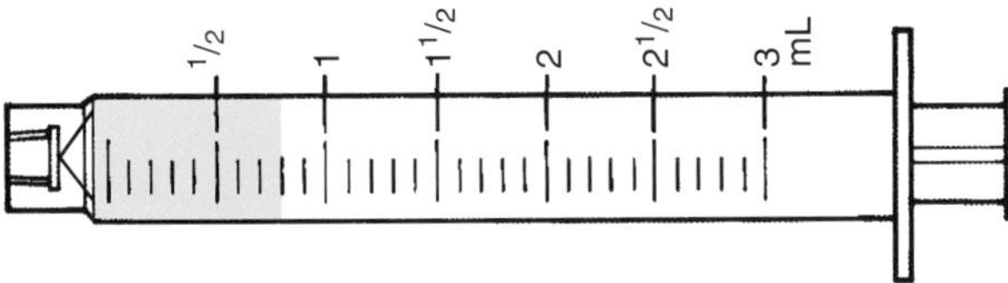

11. 1.5 mL

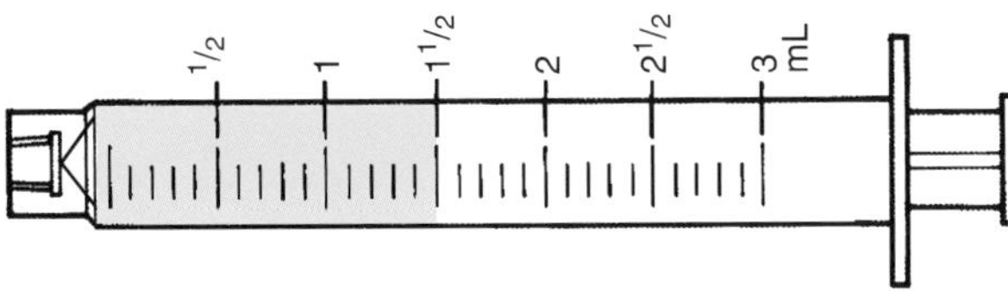

12. a. Give 0.9 mL

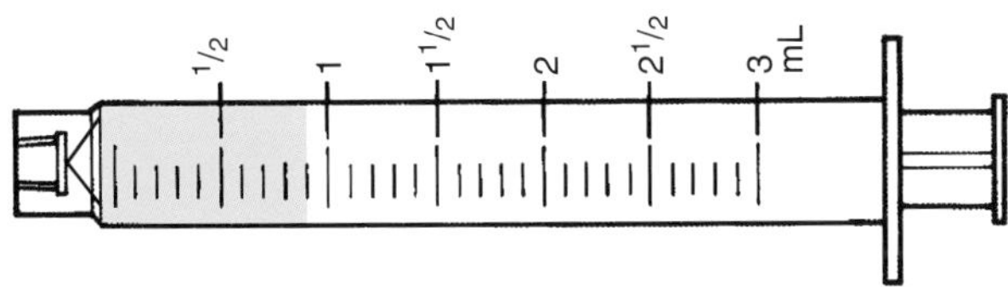

13. a. Add 2 mL of diluent
b. Give 1.2 mL per dose

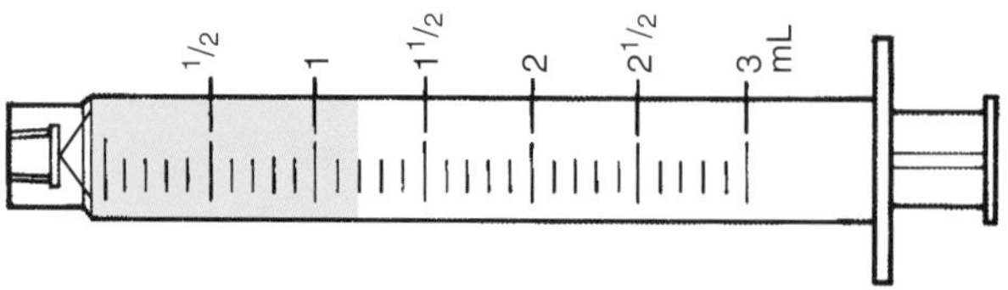

14. a. 1.2 mL bacteriostatic water for injection
b. Give 0.5 mL.

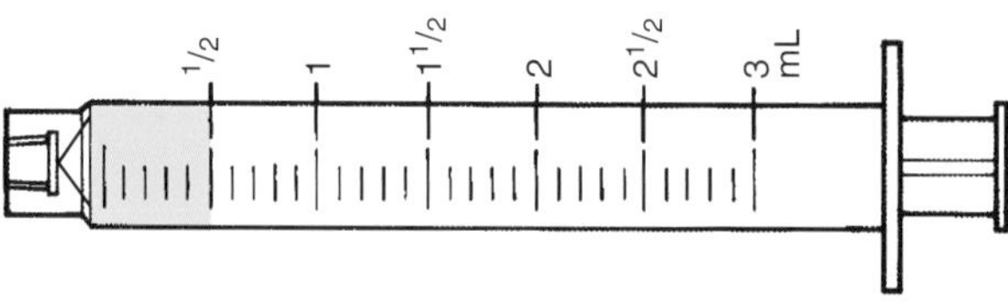

15. a. 14 drops per min
b. 83 mL per hr on infusion device

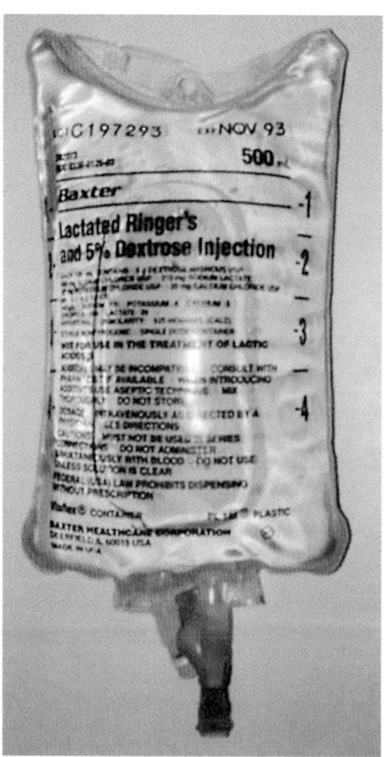

16. a. 75 mL per hr
b. 75 gtt per min

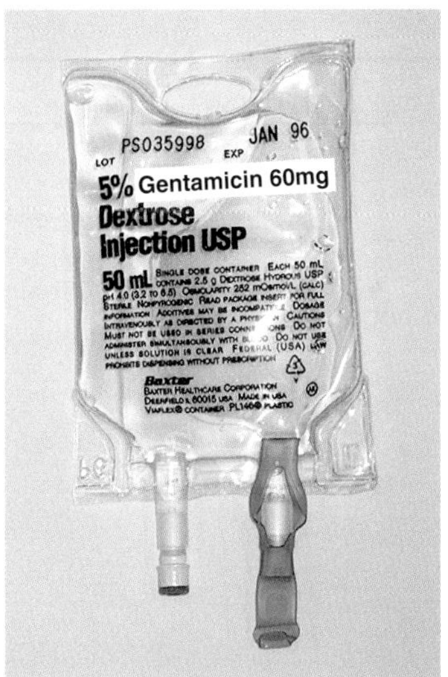

17. a. 104 mL per hr
b. 26 gtt per min

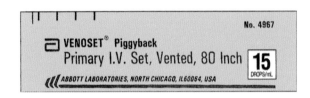

18. 6 units of Lantus

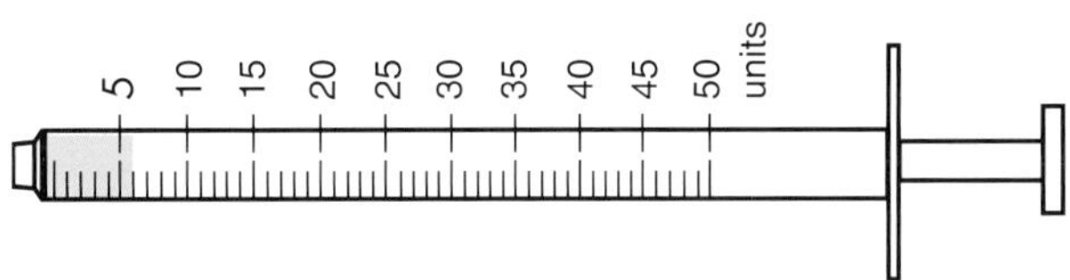

19. 20 mL per hr

20. 17 units of R insulin

21. a. Set infusion rate at 19 mL per hr
b. IV will be completed at 2139 hours

22. 0.4 mL Heparin

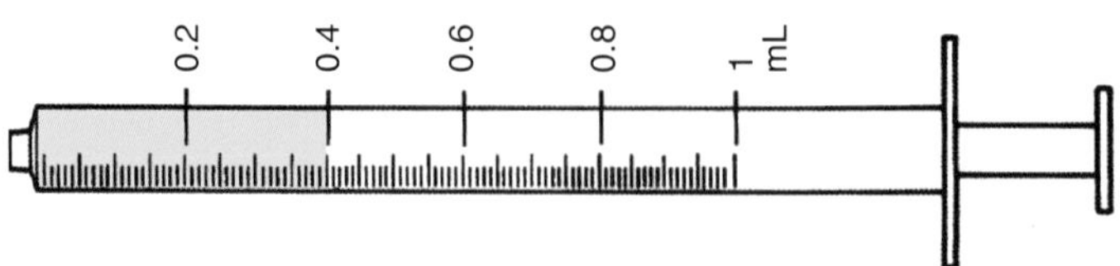

23. a. 50 mL per hr
b. Protamine sulfate is the antidote for heparin

24. a. Give 5986 units of heparin for the bolus dose.
b. 1314 units per hr will infuse
c. 15 hr 12 min
d. 33 mL per hr

25. a. 19 g per bag amino acids
b. 29 g per bag dextrose
c. 22 g per bag lipids

26. a. 76 protein kilocalories
b. 116 carbohydrate kilocalories
c. 198 fat kilocalories
d. Total kilocalories = 390

27. a. 2 mEq per mL
b. 149 mg per mL
c. 7.5 mL

28. a. 2 mL
b. 120 seconds
c. 1 mL per min for 2 min
d. 12 seconds per calibration based on 5 mL syringe on p 468.

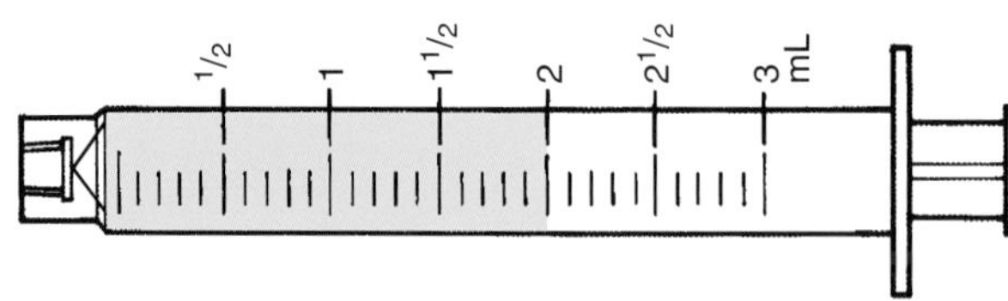

29. a. 10 mg; 2 tablets (based on approximate BSA of 1.10 m^2
b. mg per m^2 would yield the lowest dose

30. a. 24,000 mcg per hr (5 mcg × 80 kg × 60 min)
b. 24 mg per hr
c. 0.8 mg per mL (200 mg ÷ 250 mL)
d. Flow rate is correct

Note: Based on national agencies including TJC and ISMP recommendations to reduce medication errors with KCL administration, the pharmacy now supplies KCL premixed solutions. The nurse still needs to check the pharmacy label with the order to be sure the correct amount has been added.
Note: Many EID devices can deliver tenths of a mL per hr.

APPENDIX A

Institute for Safe Medication Practices (ISMP)

ISMP List of *High-Alert Medications in Acute Care Settings*

High-alert medications are drugs that bear a heightened risk of causing significant patient harm when they are used in error. Although mistakes may or may not be more common with these drugs, the consequences of an error are clearly more devastating to patients. We hope you will use this list to determine which medications require special safeguards to reduce the risk of errors. This may include strategies such as standardizing the ordering, storage, preparation, and administration of these products; improving access to information about these drugs; limiting access to high-alert medications; using auxiliary labels and automated alerts; and employing redundancies such as automated or independent double-checks when necessary. (Note: manual independent double-checks are not always the optimal error-reduction strategy and may not be practical for all of the medications on the list.)

Classes/Categories of Medications
adrenergic agonists, IV (e.g., **EPINEPH**rine, phenylephrine, norepinephrine)
adrenergic antagonists, IV (e.g., propranolol, metoprolol, labetalol)
anesthetic agents, general, inhaled and IV (e.g., propofol, ketamine)
antiarrhythmics, IV (e.g., lidocaine, amiodarone)
antithrombotic agents, including: ■ anticoagulants (e.g., warfarin, low molecular weight heparin, IV unfractionated heparin) ■ Factor Xa inhibitors (e.g., fondaparinux, apixaban, rivaroxaban) ■ direct thrombin inhibitors (e.g., argatroban, bivalirudin, dabigatran etexilate) ■ thrombolytics (e.g., alteplase, reteplase, tenecteplase) ■ glycoprotein IIb/IIIa inhibitors (e.g., eptifibatide)
cardioplegic solutions
chemotherapeutic agents, parenteral and oral
dextrose, hypertonic, 20% or greater
dialysis solutions, peritoneal and hemodialysis
epidural or intrathecal medications
hypoglycemics, oral
inotropic medications, IV (e.g., digoxin, milrinone)
insulin, subcutaneous and IV
liposomal forms of drugs (e.g., liposomal amphotericin B) and conventional counterparts (e.g., amphotericin B desoxycholate)
moderate sedation agents, IV (e.g., dexmedetomidine, midazolam)
moderate sedation agents, oral, for children (e.g., chloral hydrate)
narcotics/opioids ■ IV ■ transdermal ■ oral (including liquid concentrates, immediate and sustained-release formulations)
neuromuscular blocking agents (e.g., succinylcholine, rocuronium, vecuronium)
parenteral nutrition preparations
radiocontrast agents, IV
sterile water for injection, inhalation, and irrigation (excluding pour bottles) in containers of 100 mL or more
sodium chloride for injection, hypertonic, greater than 0.9% concentration

Specific Medications
EPINEPHrine, subcutaneous
epoprostenol (Flolan), IV
insulin U-500 (special emphasis)*
magnesium sulfate injection
methotrexate, oral, non-oncologic use
opium tincture
oxytocin, IV
nitroprusside sodium for injection
potassium chloride for injection concentrate
potassium phosphates injection
promethazine, IV
vasopressin, IV or intraosseous

*All forms of insulin, subcutaneous and IV, are considered a class of high-alert medications. Insulin U-500 has been singled out for special emphasis to bring attention to the need for distinct strategies to prevent the types of errors that occur with this concentrated form of insulin.

Background
Based on error reports submitted to the ISMP National Medication Errors Reporting Program, reports of harmful errors in the literature, studies that identify the drugs most often involved in harmful errors, and input from practitioners and safety experts, ISMP created and periodically updates a list of potential high-alert medications. During May and June 2014, practitioners responded to an ISMP survey designed to identify which medications were most frequently considered high-alert drugs by individuals and organizations. Further, to assure relevance and completeness, the clinical staff at ISMP, members of the ISMP advisory board, and safety experts throughout the US were asked to review the potential list. This list of drugs and drug categories reflects the collective thinking of all who provided input.

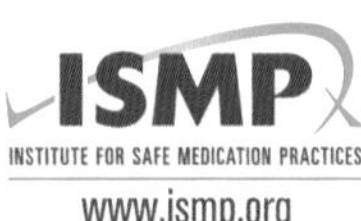

Institute for Safe Medication Practices

ISMP's List of *Error-Prone Abbreviations, Symbols,* and *Dose Designations*

The abbreviations, symbols, and dose designations found in this table have been reported to ISMP through the ISMP National Medication Errors Reporting Program (ISMP MERP) as being frequently misinterpreted and involved in harmful medication errors. They should **NEVER** be used when communicating medical information. This includes internal communications, telephone/verbal prescriptions, computer-generated labels, labels for drug storage bins, medication administration records, as well as pharmacy and prescriber computer order entry screens.

Abbreviations	Intended Meaning	Misinterpretation	Correction
µg	Microgram	Mistaken as "mg"	Use "mcg"
AD, AS, AU	Right ear, left ear, each ear	Mistaken as OD, OS, OU (right eye, left eye, each eye)	Use "right ear," "left ear," or "each ear"
OD, OS, OU	Right eye, left eye, each eye	Mistaken as AD, AS, AU (right ear, left ear, each ear)	Use "right eye," "left eye," or "each eye"
BT	Bedtime	Mistaken as "BID" (twice daily)	Use "bedtime"
cc	Cubic centimeters	Mistaken as "u" (units)	Use "mL"
D/C	Discharge or discontinue	Premature discontinuation of medications if D/C (intended to mean "discharge") has been misinterpreted as "discontinued" when followed by a list of discharge medications	Use "discharge" and "discontinue"
IJ	Injection	Mistaken as "IV" or "intrajugular"	Use "injection"
IN	Intranasal	Mistaken as "IM" or "IV"	Use "intranasal" or "NAS"
HS **hs**	Half-strength At bedtime, hours of sleep	Mistaken as bedtime Mistaken as half-strength	Use "half-strength" or "bedtime"
IU**	International unit	Mistaken as IV (intravenous) or 10 (ten)	Use "units"
o.d. or OD	Once daily	Mistaken as "right eye" (OD-oculus dexter), leading to oral liquid medications administered in the eye	Use "daily"
OJ	Orange juice	Mistaken as OD or OS (right or left eye); drugs meant to be diluted in orange juice may be given in the eye	Use "orange juice"
Per os	By mouth, orally	The "os" can be mistaken as "left eye" (OS-oculus sinister)	Use "PO," "by mouth," or "orally"
q.d. or QD**	Every day	Mistaken as q.i.d., especially if the period after the "q" or the tail of the "q" is misunderstood as an "i"	Use "daily"
qhs	Nightly at bedtime	Mistaken as "qhr" or every hour	Use "nightly"
qn	Nightly or at bedtime	Mistaken as "qh" (every hour)	Use "nightly" or "at bedtime"
q.o.d. or QOD**	Every other day	Mistaken as "q.d." (daily) or "q.i.d. (four times daily) if the "o" is poorly written	Use "every other day"
q1d	Daily	Mistaken as q.i.d. (four times daily)	Use "daily"
q6PM, etc.	Every evening at 6 PM	Mistaken as every 6 hours	Use "daily at 6 PM" or "6 PM daily"
SC, SQ, sub q	Subcutaneous	SC mistaken as SL (sublingual); SQ mistaken as "5 every;" the "q" in "sub q" has been mistaken as "every" (e.g., a heparin dose ordered "sub q 2 hours before surgery" misunderstood as every 2 hours before surgery)	Use "subcut" or "subcutaneously"
ss	Sliding scale (insulin) or ½ (apothecary)	Mistaken as "55"	Spell out "sliding scale;" use "one-half" or "½"
SSRI **SSI**	Sliding scale regular insulin Sliding scale insulin	Mistaken as selective-serotonin reuptake inhibitor Mistaken as Strong Solution of Iodine (Lugol's)	Spell out "sliding scale (insulin)"
i/d	One daily	Mistaken as "tid"	Use "1 daily"
TIW or tiw	3 times a week	Mistaken as "3 times a day" or "twice in a week"	Use "3 times weekly"
U or u**	Unit	Mistaken as the number 0 or 4, causing a 10-fold overdose or greater (e.g., 4U seen as "40" or 4u seen as "44"); mistaken as "cc" so dose given in volume instead of units (e.g., 4u seen as 4cc)	Use "unit"
UD	As directed ("ut dictum")	Mistaken as unit dose (e.g., diltiazem 125 mg IV infusion "UD" misinterpreted as meaning to give the entire infusion as a unit [bolus] dose)	Use "as directed"
Dose Designations and Other Information	**Intended Meaning**	**Misinterpretation**	**Correction**
Trailing zero after decimal point (e.g., 1.0 mg)**	1 mg	Mistaken as 10 mg if the decimal point is not seen	Do not use trailing zeros for doses expressed in whole numbers
"Naked" decimal point (e.g., .5 mg)**	0.5 mg	Mistaken as 5 mg if the decimal point is not seen	Use zero before a decimal point when the dose is less than a whole unit
Abbreviations such as mg. or mL. with a period following the abbreviation	mg mL	The period is unnecessary and could be mistaken as the number 1 if written poorly	Use mg, mL, etc. without a terminal period

ISMP's List of *Error-Prone Abbreviations, Symbols,* and *Dose Designations* (continued)

Dose Designations and Other Information	Intended Meaning	Misinterpretation	Correction
Drug name and dose run together (especially problematic for drug names that end in "l" such as Inderal40 mg; Tegretol300 mg)	Inderal 40 mg Tegretol 300 mg	Mistaken as Inderal 140 mg Mistaken as Tegretol 1300 mg	Place adequate space between the drug name, dose, and unit of measure
Numerical dose and unit of measure run together (e.g., 10mg, 100mL)	10 mg 100 mL	The "m" is sometimes mistaken as a zero or two zeros, risking a 10- to 100-fold overdose	Place adequate space between the dose and unit of measure
Large doses without properly placed commas (e.g., 100000 units; 1000000 units)	100,000 units 1,000,000 units	100000 has been mistaken as 10,000 or 1,000,000; 1000000 has been mistaken as 100,000	Use commas for dosing units at or above 1,000, or use words such as 100 "thousand" or 1 "million" to improve readability
Drug Name Abbreviations	**Intended Meaning**	**Misinterpretation**	**Correction**
To avoid confusion, do not abbreviate drug names when communicating medical information. Examples of drug name abbreviations involved in medication errors include:			
APAP	acetaminophen	Not recognized as acetaminophen	Use complete drug name
ARA A	vidarabine	Mistaken as cytarabine (ARA C)	Use complete drug name
AZT	zidovudine (Retrovir)	Mistaken as azathioprine or aztreonam	Use complete drug name
CPZ	Compazine (prochlorperazine)	Mistaken as chlorpromazine	Use complete drug name
DPT	Demerol-Phenergan-Thorazine	Mistaken as diphtheria-pertussis-tetanus (vaccine)	Use complete drug name
DTO	Diluted tincture of opium, or deodorized tincture of opium (Paregoric)	Mistaken as tincture of opium	Use complete drug name
HCl	hydrochloric acid or hydrochloride	Mistaken as potassium chloride (The "H" is misinterpreted as "K")	Use complete drug name unless expressed as a salt of a drug
HCT	hydrocortisone	Mistaken as hydrochlorothiazide	Use complete drug name
HCTZ	hydrochlorothiazide	Mistaken as hydrocortisone (seen as HCT250 mg)	Use complete drug name
MgSO4**	magnesium sulfate	Mistaken as morphine sulfate	Use complete drug name
MS, MSO4**	morphine sulfate	Mistaken as magnesium sulfate	Use complete drug name
MTX	methotrexate	Mistaken as mitoxantrone	Use complete drug name
NoAC	novel/new oral anticoagulant	No anticoagulant	Use complete drug name
PCA	procainamide	Mistaken as patient controlled analgesia	Use complete drug name
PTU	propylthiouracil	Mistaken as mercaptopurine	Use complete drug name
T3	Tylenol with codeine No. 3	Mistaken as liothyronine	Use complete drug name
TAC	triamcinolone	Mistaken as tetracaine, Adrenalin, cocaine	Use complete drug name
TNK	TNKase	Mistaken as "TPA"	Use complete drug name
TPA or tPA	tissue plasminogen activator, Activase (alteplase)	Mistaken as TNKase (tenecteplase), or less often as another tissue plasminogen activator, Retavase (retaplase)	Use complete drug names
ZnSO4	zinc sulfate	Mistaken as morphine sulfate	Use complete drug name
Stemmed Drug Names	**Intended Meaning**	**Misinterpretation**	**Correction**
"Nitro" drip	nitroglycerin infusion	Mistaken as sodium nitroprusside infusion	Use complete drug name
"Norflox"	norfloxacin	Mistaken as Norflex	Use complete drug name
"IV Vanc"	intravenous vancomycin	Mistaken as Invanz	Use complete drug name
Symbols	**Intended Meaning**	**Misinterpretation**	**Correction**
ʒ ♍	Dram Minim	Symbol for dram mistaken as "3" Symbol for minim mistaken as "mL"	Use the metric system
x3d	For three days	Mistaken as "3 doses"	Use "for three days"
> and <	More than and less than	Mistaken as opposite of intended; mistakenly use incorrect symbol; "< 10" mistaken as "40"	Use "more than" or "less than"
/ (slash mark)	Separates two doses or indicates "per"	Mistaken as the number 1 (e.g., "25 units/10 units" misread as "25 units and 110" units)	Use "per" rather than a slash mark to separate doses
@	At	Mistaken as "2"	Use "at"
&	And	Mistaken as "2"	Use "and"
+	Plus or and	Mistaken as "4"	Use "and"
°	Hour	Mistaken as a zero (e.g., q2° seen as q 20)	Use "hr," "h," or "hour"
Φ or ⦸	zero, null sign	Mistaken as numerals 4, 6, 8, and 9	Use 0 or zero, or describe intent using whole words

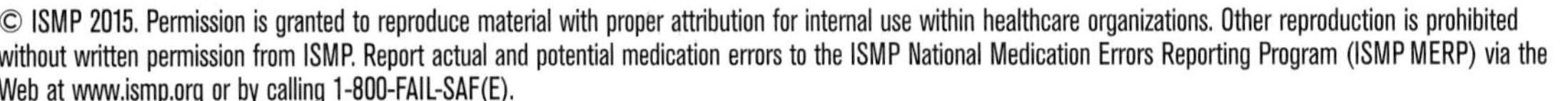

**These abbreviations are included on The Joint Commission's "minimum list" of dangerous abbreviations, acronyms, and symbols that must be included on an organization's "Do Not Use" list, effective January 1, 2004. Visit www.jointcommission.org for more information about this Joint Commission requirement.

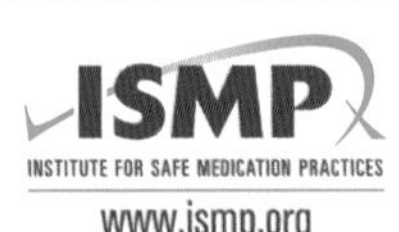

www.ismp.org

APPENDIX C

Sample Medication Administration Errors With Potential Clinical Outcomes

Medication errors may be made in each step of the process, including a prescription order error; pharmacy misinterpretation; pharmacy preparation, labeling, and dispensing; and finally, nurse interpretation, calculation, and administration. The nurse who administers the medication is the last protector of the patient. The nurse must review the order, patient allergies, and idiosyncrasies, followed by a check for drug interactions, before preparing and administering the medication. Each of the processes mentioned, including checking safe dose range, is necessary to protect the patient from an adverse drug event (ADE). Failure to do so not only may harm the patient but may result in disciplinary actions by the agency and/or the State Board of Nursing. There may be additional legal implications should an injury occur.

Sample Order	Error	Type of Error and Comments	Potential Outcomes
Morphine SO_4 10–20 mg q4h IM prn severe pain	Morphine SO_4 (10 mg per mL supplied in CarboJet) 20 mg given for initial dose	Lack of knowledge: initial dose should be lowest of the range Failure to monitor for side effects	Respiratory depression Coma Death
Blood administration	Administered with dextrose solution instead of normal saline Dextrose solution also administered through same line after transfusion	Lack of knowledge Failure to check the solutions for compatibility Failure to change line after transfusion	Hemolytic reaction (jaundice) and coagulation of blood in infusion line because of dextrose
Ordered: Furosemide, a diuretic, 0.05 mg per kg per hr, initial dose for a continuous IV for a 25-kg child	Programmed: Furosemide, 0.5 mg per kg per hr The nurse overrode the dose limit alarm on the smart pump, which resulted in a tenfold dosage error.	Lack of knowledge of initial safe dosage range and failure to focus Failure to double check the order and safe dosage range for this weight of child when the alarm sounded	Diuresis Dehydration Electrolyte imbalances Nephrocalcinosis Death
IV potassium chloride solution (KCl)	Administered undiluted or improperly diluted by nurse who obtained concentrated KCl 20 mEq per mL from pharmacy cabinet after hours per agency policy	Lack of knowledge related to potassium dilution and administration procedures when adding to IV solutions to ensure dilution is achieved	Burning pain Damage to the lining of the vein Arrhythmias Cardiac arrest

Continued

Sample Order	Error	Type of Error and Comments	Potential Outcomes
Gabapentin (Neurontin) for seizures	Two doses omitted because patient was nauseated Recorded on MAR Discovered by Pharmacy when medication cart returned and checked	Lack of knowledge of actions and dangers of omitted drugs Failure to report promptly to prescriber	Seizures Status epilepticus (continuous seizures) Prolonged hospitalization
Risperdal (risperidone) 4 mg bid po, an antipsychotic to treat a patient with schizophrenia Supplied: Requip (ropinirole) 2 mg tid po	Given: Requip (ropinirole) two 2-mg tablets A sound-alike/look-alike drug An antiparkinsonian drug also used for restless legs syndrome	Lack of knowledge regarding patient and drug: inappropriate medication Failure to check medication with prescriber order	Some side effects of Requip: Nausea Vomiting Low blood pressure Dizziness Relapse of psychotic behavior because of missed dose of Risperdal

Consequences depend on the history of errors; type of error; severity of error; whether corrective measures were sought and/or instituted promptly and by whom; patient outcome; and perceptions of those evaluating the incident, including the patient and family.

Action may be taken by the employing agency, the State Board of Nursing, and legal representatives of the patient. The actions can include a discussion; a letter of reprimand; required course(s) of study; probation with or without clinical supervision followed by reinstatement if probation period reflects competence; loss of employment; suspension of license; revocation of license; and lack of renewal of malpractice insurance. A civil and/or criminal lawsuit by the patient may be brought against the employee and the employer regardless of the previously mentioned actions.

Nurses should carry their own private malpractice insurance for personal representation, even if the employer "covers malpractice insurance." There may be occasional conflicts of interest when the nurse depends on the employer's insurance.

APPENDIX D
5-Minute Sample Verbal Communication From Nurses to Subsequent Caregivers

A hand-off report is the transfer and acceptance of critical patient information through effective communication between caregivers at shift change or for transfer between units or agencies, or when patients are discharged to home to ensure patient safety. Many errors, *including medication errors,* have been attributed to inadequate hand-off communication. The highlighted areas in the sample report presented here pertain to key medication-related information. Additional information would be given for discharge communication to home, including accompanying written materials about all medications and treatments and when to make appointments for checkups. Whereas only major medication issues are verbally reported for a shift change, complete medication resolution must be provided in writing for all physical patient transfers. Check agency procedures and forms for hand-off communication and medication resolution.

Nurse giving report to next caregiver at shift change on a medical-surgical unit

(Sex, Age, Mental/Emotional Status, Main Diagnoses, Dates of Admission and Transfers, Additional Diagnoses, Allergies)

Mr. G. is a 73-year-old, moderately hard-of-hearing, alert, oriented (to person, time, and place) cooperative, English-speaking male in no acute distress admitted to ICU with uncontrolled hypertension and acute bronchitis on the 3rd of October and transferred to our unit on the 6th. He also has chronic prostatitis, mild anemia, and an artificial hip replacement as of a year ago that requires use of a cane for stability. He has occasional asthmatic episodes controlled with an inhaler. He is allergic to penicillin and aspirin, reacting with hives and wheezing as well as diarrhea from penicillin, and is a fairly reliable historian. He lives with his daughter, so it is best to include her in all teaching, particularly because of the hearing loss.

(Vital Signs)

His vital signs are all stable today.

(Medications: Medication Changes, Medications Due, Related Orders)

He had a central line removed before transfer here. His main medications are: an intravenous antibiotic piggyback (IVPB) every 6 hr for 24 more hr for his bronchitis. His next one is due soon at 1700 hr. He is on digoxin every morning and two new blood pressure meds; one is a diuretic in the morning and the other is an ACE inhibitor in the evening. His blood pressure needs to be recorded each shift and after any complaint of weakness or extreme fatigue. Notify the healthcare provider if the systolic pressure exceeds 170. Make sure his inhaler is within reach and record his use.

(Labs)

His white blood count is still elevated at 13,000 but has been improving steadily. He is NPO after midnight for fasting blood work and also has a lung function test scheduled in the morning. His other labs are within normal limits. Hold the diuretic in the morning until the labs are completed.

(Treatments)

The discontinued central line site needs to be assessed once a day. He is receiving respiratory therapy every morning beween 0800 and 0900 and wants to bathe before the therapist arrives.

(Nutrition/Intake and Output)

He is now tolerating a regular diet well but needs encouragement to drink more fluids. Since he started on the diuretic, he self-limits fluids to try to reduce urination. The fluid intake and urinary output are to be recorded until discharge. Notify the healthcare provider if the intake or output drops below 1000 mL per day.

(Activity Level: Mobility)

He needs assistance and encouragement getting in and out of bed but does not need assistance walking as long as he has the cane. The doctor wants him to be out of bed most of the day if possible. Bedrails are up at bedtime and a urinal within reach at all times because of the diuretic and urinary frequency.

(Other Needs/Discharge Planning)

His discharge is tentatively planned for next Monday, so special emphasis needs to be given to teaching Mr. G about the new medication regimen and the need for fluids and activity. He lives with his daughter, who visits after work daily. Be sure to include her in all teaching and discharge planning because day shift does not see her often. A main issue is that he is unhappy about having to take "new pills," so we have already started reinforcing the importance of compliance with him and his daughter. Be sure to get feedback because he does not always mention that he did not hear everything.

Note: Although this seems like a lot of information, the nurse who cares for the patient for a full shift and who has established a sequential format for reporting information can communicate this information verbally on each assigned patient with ease. It helps to keep a checklist on hand with abbreviated cues (see the sample boldfaced subheadings) to ensure that the verbal hand-off report covers all the major areas. The receiving nurse refers to the written record for further details. There are many potential variations for reporting; for example, fasting could be included under Nutrition/Intake and Output instead of Labs.

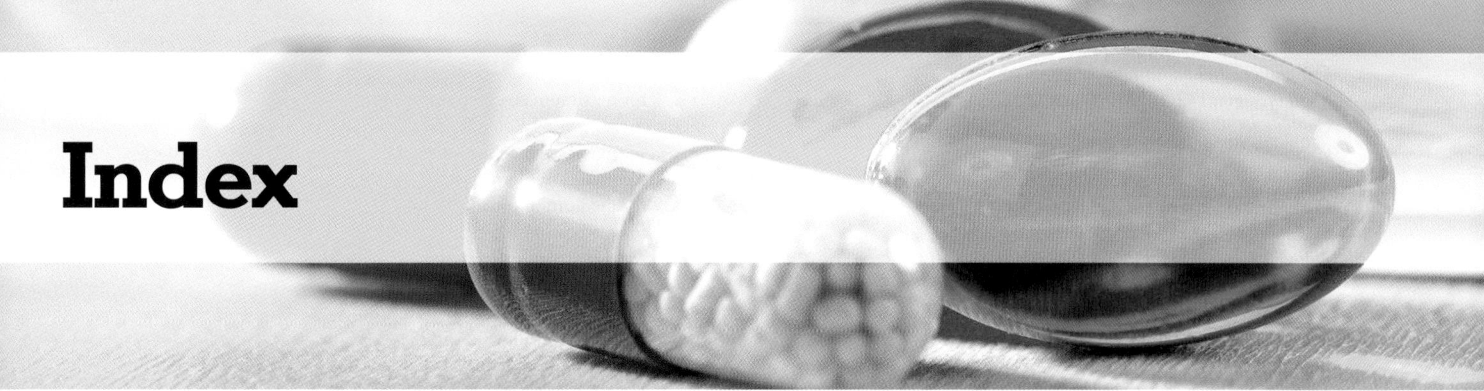

Index

A

Abbreviations
- for drug forms, 67
- error-prone, 60, 62*f*-63*f*, 479–480
- measurement, 69–70
- for medication administration, 60–64
- medication errors and, 314
- in metric system, 102
- for milliliters, 110
- for safe drug routes, 59
- for time and route, 69
- writing, 104

Acetaminophen, compared with aspirin products, 73
Acetylsalicylic acid (aspirin), 70, 399
Activated partial thromboplastin time (aPTT), 381
Addition
- of decimal, 19
- of fractions and mixed numbers, 10–11

ADD-Vantage system, 252, 253*f*
Adverse drug event (ADE), 57
- with medication administration routes, 68
- for pediatric patients, 417

Afrezza insulin, 310*t*
Alarms, in high-tech infusion devices, 287, 287*f*
Alerts. *see* Clinical Alerts
Allergic reaction, to antibiotics, 194
Ambulatory infusion device, 257, 257*f*
Ampules, 159, 159*f*
Amylin mimetics, 311*t*
Anaphylactic shock, 417
Antibiotics
- allergic reaction to, 194
- sound-alike and look-alike, 193

Anticoagulants, 381–405
- critical thinking exercises, 401–402
- injectable, 382–391
  - low molecular weight heparin, 382
  - subcutaneous heparin injections, 385–391
- IV flushes for, 391
- oral, 397–401
  - new class, 398
  - warfarin, 397
- polypharmacy and, 391
- vocabulary for, 381–382

Antiinfectives, Clinical Alert for, 201
Antiplatelet agents, 399
Anti-Xa assay, 381
Apidra, 310*t*
Apothecary system, 101
Aqueous suspensions, 65
Arixtra (fondaparinux), 384, 385*f*
Aspirin, 70, 399
Atrial fibrillation (AF), warfarin for, 397
Auto-injector, prefilled syringes, 150, 151*f*, 152
Automatic dose calculators, 361, 361*f*

B

Bar code, 83*f*
Basal rates, 342, 342*t*
Basic intravenous therapy calculations, 231–263
Baxter Mini-Bag Plus, 252, 252*f*
BD SafetyGlide™ needle, 242
Bedside monitor blood sugar (BMBS), 307
Bleb, formation of, 160*f*
Blood components, intravenous administration of, 255–257, 255*f*
Blood return, syringes and, 149
Blood sugar level, 307
- tracker, 336*f*

Blood transfusions, intravenous administration of, 255–257, 255*f*
Blood-borne illnesses, and needlestick injuries, 154
Body surface area (BSA), 417, 418
- for children, 422, 422*f*
- estimated, 422
- mathematical formula for, 423
- with mg per lb and mg per kg orders, 423–424

Bolus, defined, 231
Bolus dose, 307
Brand/trade name, 70, 71
Broviac catheter, 357*f*
Buccal administration, 68
Byetta, 314, 315*f*

C

CADD-Prizm, 254, 254*f*
Calculations
- dose
  - avoiding errors in, 126
  - errors in, 116
  - for injectable medications, 165–166
  - kilogram used for, 109
  - for liquid medications, 118, 118*f*, 121–123
  - for oral medications, 118
    - liquids, 119–123, 119*f*, 120*f*
    - solids, 113–116, 116
  - ratio and proportion methods, 104–107
- intravenous, 275–299
  - direct IV (bolus), 276–282, 277*f*, 278*f*
  - for hourly drug rate, 282–284
  - for hourly volume rate, 282–284
  - for medicated infusion, 282–284
  - medication errors in, 295–296
  - for medication orders, 284–287
  - for obstetrics, 293–294

Calculator practice, 420

Page references with *f* indicate figures; those with a *t*, tables.

Calibration, 147
  on syringes, 149, 149*f*
Caplets, 64
Capsules, 64, 65*f*
  delayed release (DR), 65, 65*f*
Carbohydrate intake
  insulin dosage based on, 336–341
  logbook based on, 336*f*
Carbohydrate ratio technique, 336
Caregivers, nurses and, verbal communication from, 483–484
Carpuject syringe holder, 151*f*
Centimeter scale, 111, 111*f*
Central line, 360, 360*f*
Central parenteral nutrition (CPN), 357, 370*f*
Cephalosporins, allergy to, 440
Chemical name, 70
Children
  diabetes in, 308
  dosages for, 417–443
    based on body weight and surface area, 418
    Clinical Alerts for, 423, 424, 425, 427, 428, 429
    contrasted with adult, 426, 426*t*
    for IV medications, 432–436, 432*f*
    for oral medications, 427
    vocabulary for, 417–418
    weight-based, 418–421
  fluid requirements for, 425, 426*t*
  subcutaneous and intramuscular medications for, 430–432, 430*f*
CHO. *see* Carbohydrate intake
Clinical Alerts
  for abbreviation confusion, 103, 110
  for administration, 87
  for allergy to penicillin, 440
  for antibiotic names, 435
  for antiinfectives, 201
  for antiseizure medications, 441
  for aspirin *vs.* acetaminophen products, 74
  for BSA calculations, 423
  checking ability to swallow, 120
  for checking orders, 123
  for clinical agency policy, 87
  for clinical facility, 88
  for compatibility, 250
  on compound drugs, 75
  for controlled substances, 130
  converting to kilograms, 419
  decimal errors on electronic IV device, 289
  for diluents, 191
  for dilution directions, 276, 299
  for documentation, 59
  for drops per minute, 243, 244*f*
  on DS (double-strength), 115
  for EID, 258
  for fatal errors, 87
  for fear of injections, 153
  for filter needles, 160
  for heparin, 384, 385, 386, 389, 391, 394
  for high-alert medications, 287, 288, 288*t*
  for incident reports, 84
  for incompatibility, 171
  for infusion alerts, 289
  for infusion device, 254
  for insulin administration, 317, 318
  for insulin syringes, 312
  insulin *vs.* tuberculin syringes, 386
  for interpretation, 86
  for intramuscular injections, 192, 204
  for IV insulin, 329, 329*f*
  for IV push, 277
  for IV solution, changing of, 292
  for MARs, 79
Clinical Alerts (*continued*)
  for maximum single injection, 196
  for measuring liquid medications, 189
  for medication administration, 59, 67, 68, 79
  for medication errors, 62
  for medication orders, 77, 443
  for medication reconciliation, 86
  for metric equivalents, 106
  for metric system, 106
  for microgram, and milligram, 286
  for mixing insulin, 324*f*, 325
  for morphine sulfate (MS) orders, 430
  for needlestick injuries, 154, 155
  for oral syringe use, 120
  for order dose, 87
  patient safety issue, 290
  for pediatric dosages, 423, 424, 425, 427, 428, 429
  for pediatric IV flow rates, 436
  for peripheral lines, 360
  for pharmacy data, 80
  for potassium chloride, 258
  preparing medications, 123
  problem solving, 113
  for recapping of needles, 154, 154*f*
  for reconstituted medications, 183
  for rounding decimals, 16
  for syringes, 148–149, 152
  for TPN, 357, 362, 365
  for unit-dose *vs.* multidose containers, 73
  for units of medication with milligrams, 199
  for using original labeled containers, 118
  for using unit measure, 124
  for value of decimals, 17
  for verbal orders, 442
  for warfarin, 399
Clock time, 78*f*, 79
Clopidogrel (Plavix), 399
Colons, using grammatical, 105, 112, 125
Common denominators, 8–9
Communication, verbal, from nurses to caregivers, 483–484
Compatibility, Clinical Alert for, 250
Compound drugs, Clinical Alerts for, 75
Computerized physician order entry (CPOE)
    systems, 64, 76
Container, sharps, 154, 154*f*
Continuous glucose monitoring (CGM) system device, 335
Continuous IV infusion, 231
Controlled drug schedules, 129–130, 130*f*
Controlled substances, Clinical Alert for, 130
CPN. *see* Central parenteral nutrition
Critical care IV practice, 291–292
Critical thinking exercises
  on anticoagulants, 401–402
  in basic intravenous therapy calculations, 262–263
  for high-alert medications, 296–297
  in injectable medications, 168–169
  for insulin administration, 344–345
  medication measurements, 132–133
  on parenteral nutrition, 373–374
  on pediatric dosages, 437–438
  for reconstitution of medications, 208–209
  on safety issues, 90–91
Crystals, reconstitution of medications from, 181–214
Cubic centimeter (cc), 110, 147
Cups, medicine, measuring with, 119, 119*f*

D

Decimal fractions
  definition of, 15
  reading, 15
Decimal point, 15

Decimals, 23–25
addition of, 19
avoiding errors with, 18
changing common fractions to, 23
changing to fractions, 22–23
changing to percentages, 22–23
Clinical Alert with, 16
comparison of, 15
converting to percentage, 24
division of, 20–22
with metric equivalents, 107–112, 107*f*
multiplication of, 20
percent numbers for, 24
rounding of, 16–17, 18
subtraction of, 19–20
value of, 15, 17
Deep vein thrombosis (DVT), 381
Dehydration, in pediatric patients, 425
Deltoid site, 161*f*
Denominators
definition of, 6
finding common, 8–9
Dextrose
in normal saline, 235*f*, 236*f*
in water, 234*f*
DF. *see* Drop factor (DF)
Diabetes mellitus, 308–309
complications of, 312
flow sheet, 332*f*
insulin for, 308
administration, 307–347
carbohydrate intake and, 336–341, 336*f*, 339*f*
critical thinking exercises and, 344–345
insulin measuring devices, 312
insulin-to-carbohydrate ratio, 342–344, 342*t*
intravenous, 329–332, 329*f*
labels for, 316–318
logbook for, 339*f*
mix, 317
mixing, 324–329, 324*f*
single-dose measures, 318–323
sliding-scale calculations for, 341
types of, 314–316, 316*f*
non-insulin injectables for, 311*t*
type 1, 308, 356
type 2, 308, 356
Diabetic ketoacidosis, 308
Dial-a-Flo tubing, 246, 247*f*
Dibasic sodium, 191
Diluents
Clinical Alert for, 191
definition of, 181
types of, 191
Dilution, 182, 436
Direct IV (bolus), 276–282, 277*f*, 278*f*
Displacement, definition of, 182
Division
of decimal, 20–22
of fractions and mixed numbers, 14
"Do Not Use" List (abbreviations), of TJC, 60, 61*t*, 64
Documentation
Clinical Alert for, 59
electronic, 59
and patient rights, 59
Dose calculations, 87
avoiding errors in, 126
errors in, 116
for injectable medications, 165–166
kilogram used for, 109
for liquid medications, 118, 118*f*, 121–123
Dose calculations (*continued*)
for oral medications, 118
liquids, 119–123, 119*f*, 120*f*
solids, 113–116, 116
and patient rights, 58
ratio and proportion, 104–107
Dose designations, error-prone, 60, 62*f*–63*f*, 479–480
Dosing guidelines, for (DVT-PE) treatment chart, 396, 396*t*
Drop factor (DF), 231
Droppers, medicine
calibrated, 118, 118*f*, 128
for pediatric dosages, 425
Drops per minute, by manufacturer, 242–243, 243*f*, 244*f*
Drug concentration (strength), 57
Drug forms, abbreviations for, 67
Drug names, types of, 70
DS medication, double checking, 75

E

EID. *see* Electronic infusion devices (EIDs)
Electronic infusion devices (EIDs), 232, 254, 254*f*, 361
Clinical Alert for, 258
rounding doses for, 244
Electronic infusion pump, for children, 432, 432*f*
Electronic medication administration records (EMARs), 79, 81*f*
Elixirs, 65
Embolus, 381
Emulsions, 65
Epidural administration, 68
Epipen, 151*f*, 431
Equivalent fractions, 8, 9
Errors, medication. *see* Medication errors
Estimates, compared with proofs, 46
Estimation, 101
Extracts, 65

F

Filter needles, 159, 159*f*
Flo Meter tape, IV delivery sets with, 244, 244*f*
Flow rates, 436
Fluid extracts, 65
Flush
with high-tech infusion devices, 287, 287*f*
ranges for, 360, 360*t*
SAS, 276
SASH, 276
solutions, 277
Food and Drug Administration (FDA), 57, 71
Fraction cross-product set up, using, 105, 112, 125
Fractions, 23–25
addition of, 10–11
change to percentage to make solutions, 25–26
changing to equivalent, 9
changing to higher terms, 10
changing to percentage, 24
common denominator for, 8–9
decimals
addition of, 19
avoiding errors with, 18
changing to, 22–23
comparison of, 15
definition of, 5–6
division of, 14
equivalent, 8
improper, 7
multiplication of, 13–14
ratio as, 41
reading, 15
reducing to lowest terms, 10

Fractions (*continued*)
  subtraction of, 12–13
  value of, 6
  whole number of, 6
Fragmin (dalteparin), 384
Free-flow, 232

G

Gastric administration, 68
Gel, delayed-release, 65
General mathematics, 5–31
  addition
    of decimal, 19
    of fractions and mixed numbers, 10–11
  changing common fractions to decimal, 23
  changing decimals to fractions, 22–23
  changing fractions to equivalent fractions, 8
  changing improper fractions to whole or mixed numbers, 7–8
  changing mixed numbers to improper fractions, 7–8
  common denominator for two or more fractions, 8–9
  comparison of decimal, 15
  division
    of decimal, 20–22
    of fractions and mixed numbers, 14
  fractions, 5–6
  multiplication
    of decimal, 20
    of fractions and mixed numbers, 13–14
  percentages, decimals, and fractions, 23–26
  reducing fractions to lowest terms, 10
  rounding of decimal, 16–17, 18
  subtraction
    of decimal, 19–20
    of fractions and mixed numbers, 12–13
  value of decimal, 15, 17
  value of fractions, 6
Generic drugs, 57, 71–76
  information about, 71
  labels for, 74–75
Generic name, 70
Glargine (Lantus), 310*t*
Glucagon, 308
Glucagon injection, emergency kits for, 308, 309*f*
Glucose gel, 308
Glucose tablet, 308
Glulisine (Apidra), 310*t*
Gram (g), 101
  abbreviation for, 102
  English system equivalent for, 102
  medications in, 108–110
Granules, extended-release, 64, 65*f*
Gravity infusions, 361
  for children, 432, 432*f*
  device for, 232
  drop factor calculations for, 244–249, 245*f*, 247*f*
  piggyback, 250–251, 251*f*
Gravity tubing, 246
Groshong catheter, 357*f*

H

Half-life, 275
Hand-off report, 483–484
Hard alert, 287, 287*f*
Heparin, 381
  antidote for, 384
  Clinical Alerts for, 384, 385, 386, 389, 391, 394
  as continuous IV drip, 384
  fractionalized *vs.* unfractionated, 382–383
  injection sites for, 383, 383*f*
Heparin (*continued*)
  intravenous, 391–397
    dosing guidelines for, 396–397, 396*t*
    mL per hr, 392–393
    titrated to kilograms, 394–395
  low molecular weight, 382
  MAR, 383, 383*f*
  multidose vials, 387
  subcutaneous injections of, 385–391
Heparin flushes, 249–250, 382, 391
Heparin lock, 249–250, 250*f*, 382
Heparin resistance, 390
Heparin sodium injection, USP, indications for, 382
Heparin-induced thrombocytopenia (HIT), 382
Hickman catheter, 357*f*
High-alert medications, 58, 381
  ISMP-identified, 129, 287, 288*t*, 477
Higher terms (fractions), 10
Home parenteral nutrition (HPN), 356
Hospira ADD-Vantage, 252, 252*f*, 253*f*
Hospira flush solutions, 277
Household measurements, metric measurements *vs.*, 117–118
Humalog insulin, 310*t*, 314
Human insulin, 314, 315*f*
Hyperglycemia, 308, 356
Hypertonic solution, 232, 237*t*
Hypodermic injection, 148
Hypoglycemia, 308, 356
  cause of, 308
  treatment of, 308
Hypothyroidism, testing for, 107
Hypotonic solution, 232, 237*t*

I

Improper fractions, 7
Incident reports, medication, 84, 85*f*
  Clinical Alerts for, 84
  example of, 85*f*
Incretin mimetics, 308, 311, 311*t*
  action of, 311
Infants
  drug doses for, 426*t*
  estimating weight of, 419
  fluid requirements for, 425–426, 426*t*
Information Management Standards, 64
Infusion devices, 260
  Clinical Alert for, 254
  high-tech, 287–295, 287*f*
  insulin, 335, 335*f*
  pressure-flow, 257, 257*f*
Infusion pumps
  for children, 432, 432*f*
  for parenteral nutrition, 358
Infusion syringe pump, Freedom, 281*f*
Inhalant administration, 68
Injectable medications, 147
  dose calculation for, 165–166
  intradermal, 160, 160*f*, 161*f*
  intramuscular, 153, 161, 161*f*
    for babies, 428, 429*f*
    for children, 428, 429*f*
  label interpretation for, 162–165
  parenteral, 160
  subcutaneous (subcut), 160, 160*f*
    for children, 430–432, 430*f*
    sites for, 161*f*
  unit-dose, 147
  vocabulary for, 147–148
Innohep (tinzaparin), 384
INR. *see* International normalized ratio

Institute for Safe Medication Practices (ISMP), 58, 386
high-alert medications, 129, 287, 288*t*, 477
List of Error-Prone Abbreviations, Symbols, and Dose Designations, 479–480
List of Error-Prone Abbreviations, Symbols, and Dose Designations of, 60, 62*f*-63*f*
Institute for Safe Medication Practices (ISMP), in PCA protocol, 256
Insulin, 308
administration, 307–347
injection sites for, 309, 309*f*
vocabulary in, 307–308
carbohydrate intake and, 336–341, 336*f*, 339*f*
critical thinking exercises and, 344–345
insulin measuring devices, 312
insulin-to-carbohydrate ratio, 342–344, 342*t*
intravenous, 329–332, 329*f*
labels for, 316–318
logbook for, 339*f*
mix, 317
mixing, 324–329, 324*f*
single-dose measures, 318–323
sliding-scale calculations for, 341
types of, 314–316, 316*f*
Insulin comparison chart, 310*t*
Insulin infusion chart, standard, 330, 330*t*
Insulin orders, 313–314
Insulin pens, 311–313, 315*f*
Insulin resistance, 308
Insulin shock, 308, 356
Insulin syringes, 311–313, 312*f*, 313*f*, 314*f*
Insulin therapy, complications of, 308
Insulin-to-carbohydrate ratio, estimating, 342–344, 342*t*
InterLink System Continu-Flo Solution Set, 245*f*
Intermittent IV lock, 250, 250*f*
Intermittent medication therapy, 249, 250*f*
International normalized ratio (INR), 382, 397
Intradermal (ID) administration, 68
Intradermal (ID) injections, 160, 160*f*, 161*f*
Intramuscular (IM) administration, 68
Intramuscular (IM) injections, 153, 161, 161*f*
for babies, 428, 429*f*
for children, 428, 429*f*
Intramuscular (IM) medications
for children, 430–432, 430*f*
Clinical Alert for, 192, 204
Intrathecal administration, 68
Intravenous (IV) administration, 68
blood transfusions in, 255–257
delivery sets, 242–244, 242*f*
drops per minute by manufacturer, 242–243, 243*f*, 244*f*
with Flo Meter tape, 244, 244*f*
direct IV in, 276–282, 277*f*, 278*f*
of insulin, 329–332, 329*f*
MAR for. *see* Medication administration records
Intravenous (IV) calculations, 231–263, 242, 247–249, 258–260, 259*f*, 275–299
critical thinking exercises, 262–263
direct IV (bolus), 276–282, 277*f*, 278*f*
drop factor calculations, for gravity infusions and rounding IV mL, 244–249, 245*f*, 247*f*
for hourly drug rate, 282–284
for hourly volume rate, 282–284
insulin, 330–332, 330*f*
for medicated infusion, 282–284
medication errors in, 295–296
for medication orders, 284–287
for obstetrics, 293–294
Intravenous (IV) flushes, 275, 391
Intravenous (IV) infusions, 249–260, 250*f*
blood and blood components in, 255–257, 255*f*
continuous, 231
electronic infusion devices in, 254, 254*f*
gravity piggyback infusions in, 250–251, 251*f*
nurse-activated piggyback systems in, 252–253, 252*f*, 253*f*
PCA protocol for, 256, 256*f*
piggyback infusions in, 257–258
piggyback premixed IVs in, 251–252, 251*f*
pressure-flow infusion device in, 257, 257*f*
Intravenous (IV) lines
flushing intermittent-access lock, 360, 360*t*
types of, 358–361, 359*f*, 360*f*, 360*t*, 361*f*
Intravenous (IV) liquid medications, rounding, drop factor calculations for, 244–249, 245*f*, 247*f*
Intravenous (IV) lock, intermittent, 250, 250*f*
Intravenous (IV) medications, for children, 432–436, 432*f*
Intravenous piggyback (IVPB) infusions, 232, 250, 260
Intravenous (IV) push medications, 276–282, 277*f*, 278*f*
piggyback, 277
timing of, 279–280
Intravenous (IV) solutions, 232
abbreviations for, 232–236, 233*f*, 234*f*, 235*f*, 236*f*
calculations, 238–241
osmolarity of, 237, 237*t*
percentage of solutes in, 236–237
Intravenous (IV) therapy, 232
medication administration record, 259*f*
vocabulary for, 231–232
ISMP. *see* Institute for Safe Medication Practices (ISMP)
Isotonic solution, 232, 237*t*
IVPB. *see* Intravenous piggyback (IVPB)

J

The Joint Commission (TJC), 58
"Do Not Use" list of, 60, 61*t*, 64
on medication reconciliation, 86
in PCA protocol, 256
Jordan Medical Count-a-Dose, 312

K

Kcal, 356
KCL. *see* Potassium chloride (KCL)
Ketoacidosis, 335
Kilograms, converting pounds to, 419

L

Labels
for CPN, 370*f*
for heparin sodium injection, 386
medication, 70–76
drug names on, 70
for generic drugs, 74–76
for injectable medications, 162–165
interpreting, 74–75
for reconstitution, 182–183, 183*f*, 190
types of print on, 72
oral antidiabetic drug, 333–334
PCN, 371*f*
TPN, 362, 362*f*, 363*f*
U-100 insulin, 316–318
intermediate- and rapid-acting mixtures, 318
intermediate-acting, 317
long-acting, 318
rapid-acting, 317
short-acting, 316, 316*f*
for warfarin (Coumadin), 397*f*
Lantus insulin, 316, 316*f*, 322*f*
Latex allergy, checking for, 159–160
Length, household *vs.* metric measurements for, 110
Levemir, 310*t*, 315*f*

Lidocaine, 191
Lifecare® Patient-controlled analgesia 3 Infusion System, 256*f*
Lipids
  delivery of, 358, 358*f*
  order for, 358*f*
Liposyn, 356, 358*f*
Liquid medications
  calculating dosage for, 121–123
  forms of, 65–67, 68*f*
  household and metric measurements for, 117
  measuring, 119–123, 119*f*, 120*f*, 183–190, 183*f*, 184*f*
    Clinical Alert for, 189
    practice in, 185–190
  from multidose bottle, 65
  rounding of, 118
    drop factor calculations for, 244–249
Liquids, measuring volume of, 109–110
Lispro (Humalog), 310*t*
Liter (L), 101, 109
  abbreviation for, 102
  English system equivalent for, 102
Lovenox (enoxaparin), 384
Low molecular weight heparin (LMWH)
  defined, 382
  indications for, 384
Lowest terms
  expressing ratios in, 42
  reducing fractions to, 10
Luer-Lok syringe tips, 155, 155*f*

M

Magni-Guide, for insulin syringe, 312
MARs. *see* Medication administration records
Mathematics, general, 5–31
  addition
    of decimal, 19
    of fractions and mixed numbers, 10–11
  changing common fractions to decimal, 23
  changing decimals to fractions, 22–23
  changing fractions to equivalent fractions, 8
  changing improper fractions to whole or mixed numbers, 7–8
  changing mixed numbers to improper fractions, 7–8
  common denominator for two or more fractions, 8–9
  comparison of decimal, 15
  division
    of decimal, 20–22
    of fractions and mixed numbers, 14
  fractions, 5–6
  multiplication
    of decimal, 20
    of fractions and mixed numbers, 13–14
  percentages, decimals, and fractions, 23–26
  reducing fractions to lowest terms, 10
  rounding of decimal, 16–17, 18
  subtraction
    of decimal, 19–20
    of fractions and mixed numbers, 12–13
  value of decimal, 15, 17
  value of fractions, 6
MEAC. *see* Minimal effective analgesic concentration (MEAC)
Measurement systems
  abbreviations for, 69–70
  household, 101
  metric, 102
    additional practice for, 126–129
    base units of, 101, 102
    calculation setup for, 104–107
    clinical relevance of, 107
    definition of, 102
    dose calculation, 112–116
    equivalent chart, 102
Measurement systems (*continued*)
    household measurements *vs.*, 117–118
    moving decimals for, 107–112, 107*f*
    notation review for, 106
    prefixes and values in, 103–104, 103*t*
    using ratio and proportion to find, 104–106
    for volume, 110
    for weight, 110
  units and milliequivalents, 124–130
Measuring cup, 183, 183*f*
Measuring teaspoon, 66*f*
MedFlo postoperative pain management system, 257*f*
Medibottle, for pediatric dosages, 425*f*
Medical terminology, 57
Medication administration
  abbreviations for, 60–64, 68–69
  Clinical Alert for, 59, 66, 67, 68, 84
  enteric-coated, 64
  medication errors and, 60, 481–482
  prioritizing, 84–86, 85*f*
  right to refuse, 59–60
  routes of, 68–69
  safe, 57–93
    patient rights, 58–60
Medication administration records (MARs), 79–83, 194*f*
  Clinical Alerts for, 79
  for heparin, 383, 383*f*
  interpreting, 82–83
  for IV therapy, 259*f*
  pharmacy-generated, 80
  for PRN orders, 81*f*
  sample, 80*f*
Medication carts, 83
Medication delivery, 83–84
Medication errors, 60
  abbreviating and, 314
  Clinical Alert for, 62
  IV, 295–296
  potential clinical outcomes of, 481–482
Medication forms, 64–67
  abbreviations for, 67
  liquid medications, 65–67, 68*f*
  solid oral medications, 64–65, 65*f*
Medication labels, 70–76
  drug names on, 70
  for generic drugs, 74–76
  for injectable medications, 162–165
  interpreting, 74–75
  for reconstitution, 182–183, 183*f*, 190
  types of print on, 72
Medication measurements, 101–136
  critical thinking exercises, 132–133
Medication orders, 76–77, 76*f*
  identifying incomplete, 77
  IV calculations for, 284–287
Medication reconciliation, 86
  calculations for, 87
  medication administration, 87
Medications
  dissolving, in vials, 190
  high-alert, 381. *see also* Anticoagulants
    ISMP list, 288*t*, 477
  injectable, 147
    dose calculation for, 165–166
    intradermal, 160, 160*f*, 161*f*
    intramuscular, 153, 161, 161*f*
      for babies, 428, 429*f*
      for children, 428, 429*f*
    label interpretation for, 162–165
    parenteral, 160

Medications (*continued*)
subcutaneous (subcut), 160, 160*f*
for children, 430–432, 430*f*
sites for, 161*f*
unit-dose, 147
vocabulary for, 147–148
liquid
calculating dosage for, 121–123
household and metric measurements for, 117
measuring, 119–123, 119*f*, 120*f*
rounding of, 118
reconstituted, 182
Clinical Alert for, 183
cost effectiveness of, 182
critical thinking exercises for, 208–209
measuring liquid medications for, 183–190, 183*f*, 184*f*
medication labels for, 182–183, 183*f*
for parenteral use, 190–191
from powders and crystals, 181–214
with prefilled vials and syringes, 193–204, 193*f*, 194*f*
shelf life of, 182
two-vial reconstitution method for, 191–192, 192*f*
types of diluents with, 191
vocabulary for, 181–182
units of, with milligrams, Clinical Alert for, 199
Medicine cups, 183, 184*f*
measuring with, 119, 119*f*
for pediatric dosages, 425*f*
Mediport, central line with, 360*f*
Meniscus, 67, 183, 183*f*
Meter (m), 101
abbreviation for, 102
English system equivalent for, 102
MethylPREDNISolone, 72
Metric measurements, 102
additional practice for, 126–129
base units of, 101, 102
calculation setup for, 104–107
clinical relevance of, 107
definition of, 102
dose calculation, 112–116
equivalent chart, 102
household measurements *vs.*, 117–118
moving decimals for, 107–112, 107*f*
notation review for, 106
prefixes and values in, 103–104, 103*t*
using ratio and proportion to find, 104–106
for volume, 110
for weight, 110
Metric Units Number Line, 103, 107*f*
Metric calibrated equipment, 66
Mg per kg calculation method, 418
Micrograms
medications in, 108–110
potential confusion with, 112
Micrograms per kilogram, 417
Milliequivalent, 124–130
Milliequivalent per liter, 124
Milliequivalent per milliliter, 124
Milligrams
confusion with, 112, 199
medications in, 108–110
Milligrams per kilogram, 417
Milliliters, 109–110
Millimeter and centimeter scale, 111, 111*f*
Milliunits, 124
Minimal effective analgesic concentration (MEAC), 256
Mixed numbers, 7
addition of, 10–11
changing improper fractions, 7
changing to improper fractions, 7–8
Mixed numbers (*continued*)
division of, 14
multiplication of, 13–14
subtraction of, 12–13
Mix-o-vial directions, 193, 193*f*
Multidose containers
Clinical Alert for, 96
vs. unit-dose containers, 73
Multiple-strength decisions, reconstituting parenteral dosages with, 190–191, 195–199, 200–204
Multiplication
of decimal, 20
of fractions and mixed numbers, 13–14

N

Nasogastric (NG) administration, 68
National drug code (NDC) number, 71
National Formulary (NF), 71
National Patient Safety Goals (NPSG), 86, 256
Needleless equipment, 155, 155*f*
Needleless infusion system, 242, 250*f*, 278*f*
Needles
disposing of, 154, 154*f*
filter, 159, 159*f*
insertion of, 161*f*
length and gauge for, 152, 152*f*
parts of, 152*f*
recapping of, 154, 154*f*
selection of, 152–160
sizes for, 152, 152*f*
Needlestick injuries
avoiding, 154
blood-borne illnesses and, 154
Clinical Alerts for, 154, 155
Neonates. *see* Infants
Nomograms, 417, 418, 422, 423
Nonparenteral (noninjectables) administration, 68
Novolog, 310*t*, 315*f*
NPSG. *see* National Patient Safety Goals (NPSG)
Numerators, 6
Nurse-activated piggyback systems, 252–253, 252*f*, 253*f*
Nurses, caregivers and, verbal communication from, 483–484
Nutrition, parenteral, 355–375
central, 357, 360, 360*f*
critical thinking exercises, 373–374
peripheral, 357
total, 356–358, 356*f*, 357*f*, 358*f*
amino acids, dextrose, and lipids in, 364
Clinical Alert for, 365
contents of, 357
kilocalories (kcal) per bag, 365
label for, validation of, 362, 362*f*, 363*f*
medication administration record, 367*f*
mL per hour to set the pump, 364
percentage of additives, 364
protocol for, 365
provider's order form for, 366*f*, 369*f*
total grams per bag, 364
vocabulary for, 355–356

O

Obstetrics, IV calculations for, 293–294
Omnicell Savvy Mobile Medication System, 84*f*
Oral diabetes medications, 333
Oral medications
administration of, 68
for children, 427
reconstitution of, 182
rounding doses for, 118
and swallowing ability, 120

Oral syringes, 120, 120*f*, 152, 152*f*, 183, 184*f*
measuring with, 119, 119*f*, 120*f*
prefilled, 118
tubing with, 120
using, 129, 129*f*
Ordering and dispensing system, computer-controlled, 83*f*
Osmolarity, 232, 237, 237*t*
Overhydration, in pediatric patients, 425
Over-the-counter (OTC) medications, 86, 391
Oxacillin sodium, diluting, 191, 192*f*

P

Pain rating scale, Wong-Baker FACES, 430
Paradigm Link blood glucose monitor, 335*f*
Parenteral administration, 68
Parenteral drugs, with vials, 191
Parenteral nutrition, 355–375
central, 357, 360, 360*f*
critical thinking exercises, 373–374
peripheral, 357
total, 356–358, 356*f*, 357*f*, 358*f*
amino acids, dextrose, and lipids in, 364
Clinical Alert for, 365
contents of, 357
kilocalories (kcal) per bag, 365
label for, validation of, 362, 362*f*, 363*f*
medication administration record, 367*f*
mL per hour to set the pump, 364
percentage of additives, 364
protocol for, 365
provider's order form for, 366*f*, 369*f*
total grams per bag, 364
vocabulary for, 355–356
Parenteral reconstituted medication, 182, 190
with multiple-strength decisions, 195–199, 200–204
Parenteral route, 148
Partial thromboplastin time (PTT), 384, 391
Patent, 58, 71
Patient
identifiers, for medication administration, 84*f*, 87
rights of, 58–60
Patient-controlled analgesia (PCA), 232
protocol for, 256, 256*f*
PCA. *see* Patient-controlled analgesia (PCA)
Peak and trough levels, 276
Pediatric dosages, 417–443
based on body weight and surface area, 418
Clinical Alerts for, 423, 424, 425, 427, 428, 429
contrasted with adult, 426, 426*t*
for IV medications, 432–436, 432*f*
for oral medications, 427
vocabulary for, 417–418
weight-based, 418–421
Pediatric patients, 417. *see also* Children; Pediatric dosages
IM injections for, 428, 429*f*
medication administration for, 419
Percentages
changing to fraction, 24
converting to decimal, 24–25
definition of, 24
finding of, 25
to make solutions, 25–26
Peripheral lines, 358
Peripheral parenteral nutrition, 357
Peripherally inserted central catheter (PICC), 358, 359*f*
Petechiae, 382
PICC line. *see* Peripherally inserted central catheter
Piggyback infusions, 257–258. *see also* Intravenous piggyback (IVPB) infusions
gravity, 250–251, 251*f*
nurse-activated, 252–253, 252*f*, 253*f*
premixed, 251–252, 251*f*
Pill splitter, 66*f*
Platelet Count, 382
Polypharmacy, and anticoagulant, 391
Postprandial, 308
Potassium chloride (KCL), Clinical Alert for, 258
Powders, 64, 65*f*, 181–214
diluents in, 191
Prefilled syringes, 150
auto-injector, 150, 151*f*, 152
oral, 66*f*
reconstituting with, 193–204, 193*f*, 194*f*
Prefilled vials, reconstituting with, 193–204, 193*f*, 194*f*
Prefixes, metric, 103–104, 103*t*
Premixed frozen IVPBs, 252
Preprandial, 308
Prescription abuse, 129
Pressure-flow infusion device, 257, 257*f*
PRN orders, MAR for, 81*f*
Proofs, compared with estimates, 46
Proportion, 41–50
definition of, 42
equivalent measurements using, 104–107
practice, 47
proving correct, 41
setting up, 46–47
solving problems of, 41
steps to, 42
Protamine sulfate, 382, 391, 392, 394
Prothrombin time (PT or Pro Time), 382, 397
Pulmonary embolus (PE), 382
Pumps
infusion syringe, 281*f*
insulin, 335
Pupil gauge, 111*f*

Q

Quality and Safety Education for Nurses (QSEN), 5
Quick-set infusion sets, 335*f*

R

Ratio, 41–50
definition of, 41–42
equivalent measurements using, 104–107
expressing in lowest terms, 42
as fraction, 41
practice, 47
setting up, 46–47
Recombinant DNA technology, 314
Reconstituted medications, 181–214, 182
Clinical Alert for, 183
cost effectiveness of, 182
critical thinking exercises for, 208–209
measuring liquid medications for, 183–190, 183*f*, 184*f*
medication labels for, 182–183, 183*f*
of parenteral dosages, with multiple-strength decisions, 195–199, 200–204
for parenteral use, 190–191
with prefilled vials and syringes, 193–204, 193*f*, 194*f*
shelf life of, 182
two-vial, 191–192, 192*f*
types of diluents with, 191
vocabulary for, 181–182
Reconstitution, 182
Red flag, 129
Refuse, right to, 59–60
Registration symbol®, 71

Respiratory administration, 68
Ringer's lactate solution, 234*f*, 235*f*
Rounding
of decimal, 16–18
of liquid medications, drop factor calculations for, 244–249, 245*f*, 247*f*
for oral medication doses, 118
Rubber latex stoppers, 159–160

S

Safe dose range (SDR), 87, 418
calculating, 418, 421
for children, 419, 424
Safe medication practices, 86–91
Clinical Alert for, 86
critical thinking exercises, 90–91
failure to perform, 86
interpretation of, 86
for medication administration. *see* Clinical Alerts
preparation for, 86–87
Saline, 233*f*
dextrose in, 235*f*, 236*f*
Saline, administer, saline, heparin (SASH), 276
Saline, administer, saline (SAS), 276
Saline flush, 249–250
Saline lock, 249–250, 250*f*
Saline lock adapter, 277*f*
Scheduled medications
measuring, 129, 130*f*
potential for use of, 129–130
Scored-medication orders, 118
Sensor glucose (SG) readings, 335
Sentinel event, 58
Sepsis, 276
Sharps container, 154, 154*f*
"Shelf life," 182
Sigma Spectrum Infusion Smart Pump, 287*f*
Silent Knight® Tablet Crushing System, 66*f*
Single injection, maximum, Clinical Alert for, 196
Single-unit-dose package, 66*f*
Sliding-scale, insulin and, 341
"Smart pumps," 287, 287*f*
Soft alert, 287, 287*f*
Solid medications
oral administration of, 64–65, 65*f*
rounding calculations for, 118
Solutes, 182
g/mL and gtt/min calculations, 260
intravenous, calculations of, 238–241
percentage of, in intravenous solutions, 236–237
tonicity of, 237*t*
Solutions, 182
hypertonic, 232, 237*t*
hypotonic, 232, 237*t*
intravenous, 232
abbreviations for, 232–236, 233*f*, 234*f*, 235*f*, 236*f*
osmolarity of, 237, 237*t*
percentage of solutes in, 236–237
isotonic, 232, 237*t*
preparing, 25–26
using fractions to change percentage to make, 25–26
Solvent, 181
Square Meter (m^2), 418
Subcutaneous (subcut) injections, 68, 160, 160*f*
for children, 430–432, 430*f*
sites for, 161*f*
Sublingual (SL) administration, 68
Subtraction
of decimal, 19–20
of fractions and mixed numbers, 12–13
Swallowing ability, checking, 120
Symbols, error-prone, 60, 62*f*-63*f*, 479–480
Syringe pump, 278*f*
Syringes
calibrations on, 149, 149*f*
checking for blood return with, 149
Clinical Alerts for, 148–149, 152
comparison of, 148*f*
for direct IV, 277
disposing of, 154, 154*f*
5-mL, 150, 150*f*
for flushing peripheral IV lines, 360
holders for, 151*f*
insulin, 311–313, 312*f*, 313*f*, 314*f*
with Luer-Lok tips, 155, 155*f*
needleless, 155*f*
oral, 120, 120*f*, 152, 152*f*, 183, 184*f*
measuring with, 119, 119*f*, 120*f*
for pediatric dosages, 425*f*
prefilled, 118
tubing with, 120
using, 129, 129*f*
parts of, 149*f*
for pediatric dosages, 425*f*
prefilled, 150
auto-injector, 150, 151*f*, 152
reconstituting with, 193–204, 193*f*, 194*f*
reading and measuring with, 149, 156
safety, 155*f*
selection of, 148–152, 148*f*, 150*f*, 151*f*, 152*f*
tuberculin, 150, 150*f*, 312
U-100 insulin, 312, 312*f*
volume practice, 157–160

T

Tablets
enteric-coated, 64, 65*f*
extended-release, 64, 65*f*
forms of, 64, 65
scored, 64, 65*f*, 66*f*, 75
Target-specific oral anticoagulants (TSOACs), new class of, 398, 399*t*
Terminology, medical, 57
Thrombocytopenia
defined, 382
heparin-induced, 385
Thrombolytic agent, 382
Times, medication, abbreviations for, 69
Titration, 276
TJC. *see* The Joint Commission (TJC)
Tonicity, 232, 237, 237*t*
Topical administration, 68
Topical prescription ointments, measurements for, 111, 111*f*
Total parenteral nutrition, 356–358, 356*f*, 357*f*, 358*f*
amino acids, dextrose, and lipids in, 364
Clinical Alert for, 365
contents of, 357
kilocalories (kcal) per bag, 365
label for, validation of, 362, 362*f*, 363*f*
medication administration record, 367*f*
mL per hour to set the pump, 364
percentage of additives, 364
protocol for, 365
provider's order form for, 366*f*, 369*f*
total grams per bag, 364
Transdermal (skin) administration, 68
Transparent measuring device, in measuring liquid medication, 183
Tuberculin syringes, 150, 150*f*, 312
Tubex syringe holder, 151*f*
Tunneled catheter, 361, 361*f*
24-hour clock, 77–79, 78*f*
Two-vial reconstitution method, 191–192, 192*f*

U

U-100 insulins, 310–311
intermediate- and rapid-acting mixtures, 318, 318*f*
intermediate-acting, 317
labels, 316–318
long-acting, 318, 318*f*
rapid-acting, 317
short-acting, 316
Unfractionated heparin (UFH), 382
Unit-dose containers, *vs.* multidose containers, 73
United States Pharmacopeia (USP), 71, 386
Units, 148
Clinical Alert for, 199
in medication dosages, 124–130
Usual dose, defined, 58

V

Values, metric, 103–104, 103*t*
Vascular access device (VAD), 276, 277
Vastus lateralis site, 161*f*
Ventrogluteal site, 161*f*
Verbal communication, from nurses to caregivers, 483–484
Verification, 101
Vials, 159, 159*f*
dissolving medications in, 190
insulin, 316, 316*f*
parenteral drugs with, 191
prefilled, reconstituting with, 193–204, 193*f*, 194*f*
Victoza pen, 314
Viscosity
defined, 148
and syringe selection, 149
Vitamin K, 382, 397, 398*f*
Volume
equivalent measures for, 110
household *vs.* metric measurements for, 109–110
Volume-control device, 278*f*

W

Warfarin (Coumadin), 397
antidote for, 397
blood-testing regimen for, 398
Clinical Alert for, 399
compared with target-specific oral anticoagulants (TSOACs), 399
discharging patient on, 398
dosing for, 397, 397*f*
drugs affecting efficacy of, 398
indications for, 384
labels for, 397*f*
missed doses of, 399
Water, dextrose in, 234*f*
Weight
equivalent measures for, 108, 110
household *vs.* metric measurements for, 108
solving mg per kg problems, 418
Weight reporting, kilogram used for, 109
West nomogram, 422, 422*f*, 423
Whole numbers, 5
changing improper fractions to, 7
Wong-Baker FACES pain rating scale, for children, 430, 430*f*

Y

Young adults, diabetes in, 308

Z

Zofran (ondansetron), 73

Metric Equivalents

Weight	Length
1000 mcg (microgram) = 1 mg (milligram)	10 mm (millimeter) = 1 cm (centimeter)
1000 mg = 1 g (gram)	100 cm = 1 m (meter)
1000 g = 1 kg (kilogram)	1000 mm = 1 m (meter)
Pound to Kilogram Conversion	1000 m = 1 km (kilometer)
2.2 lb = 1 kg (kilogram)	**Volume**
Household to Metric Length Equivalent	1000 mL (milliliter) = 1 L (liter)
1 inch = 2.54 cm (centimeter)	**Miscellaneous**
39.37 inches = 1 m (meter)	1000 milliunits = 1 Unit (U)

Approximate Equivalents of Metric and Household Measures*

Metric	Household	
5 mL	1 teaspoon (tsp)	
15 mL	1 tablespoon (Tbs),† 3 teaspoons (tsp)	½ ounce
30 mL	2 tablespoons (Tbs)	1 ounce
240 mL	1 measuring cup	8 ounces
500 mL	1 pint	1 pint or 16 ounces
1000 mL (1 liter)	1 quart	1 quart or 32 ounces
4 liters	1 gallon (gal) or 4 quarts	1 gallon (gal) or 4 quarts

*Household equipment and apothecary measurements are not a substitute for metric measurements. The volume capacity of household equipment varies greatly. The apothecary measurements are imprecise and not equal to the metric measurements. **Use Metric**. Clarify unfamiliar abbreviations with the prescriber.

†Capitalizing T for Tablespoons abbreviation helps avoid confusion with tsp (teaspoon).

Body Surface Area (BSA) Formulas

A. Formula using only metric system

$$BSA = \sqrt{\frac{\text{weight (kg)} \times \text{height (cm)}}{3600}}$$

B. Formula using only pounds and inches

$$BSA = \sqrt{\frac{\text{weight (lb)} \times \text{height (in)}}{3131}}$$